Hacker and Moore's
ESSENTIALS OF
OBSTETRICS AND
GYNECOLOGY

Hacker and Moore's
ESSENTIALS OF OBSTETRICS AND GYNECOLOGY

5th Edition

Neville F. Hacker, MD
Professor of Gynaecologic Oncology
Conjoint, University of New South Wales
Director, Gynaecological Cancer Centre
Royal Hospital for Women
Sydney, Australia

Joseph C. Gambone, DO, MPH, Executive Editor
Professor Emeritus of Obstetrics and Gynecology
David Geffen School of Medicine at UCLA
Attending Physician, Ronald Reagan UCLA Medical Center
Clinical Professor of Obstetrics and Gynecology
Western University of Health Sciences
College of Osteopathic Medicine of the Pacific
Residency Education Consultant
Arrowhead Regional Medical Center
San Bernardino, California

Calvin J. Hobel, MD
Miriam Jacobs Chair in Maternal-Fetal Medicine
Cedars-Sinai Medical Center
Professor of Obstetrics and Gynecology
Professor of Pediatrics
David Geffen School of Medicine at UCLA
Los Angeles, California

SAUNDERS
ELSEVIER

SAUNDERS
ELSEVIER

1600 John F. Kennedy Blvd.
Ste 1800
Philadelphia, PA 19103-2899

HACKER AND MOORE'S ESSENTIALS OF OBSTETRICS AND GYNECOLOGY

ISBN: 978-1-4160-5940-0
International Edition ISBN: 978-0-8089-2416-6

Notice

Knowledge and best practice in this field are constantly changing. As new research and experience broaden our knowledge, changes in practice, treatment and drug therapy may become necessary or appropriate. Readers are advised to check the most current information provided (i) on procedures featured or (ii) by the manufacturer of each product to be administered, to verify the recommended dose or formula, the method and duration of administration, and contraindications. It is the responsibility of the practitioner, relying on their own experience and knowledge of the patient, to make diagnoses, to determine dosages and the best treatment for each individual patient, and to take all appropriate safety precautions. To the fullest extent of the law, neither the Publisher nor the Editors assume any liability for any injury and/or damage to persons or property arising out of or related to any use of the material contained in this book.

Library of Congress Cataloging-in-Publication Data
Hacker, Neville F.
Hacker and Moore's essentials of obstetrics and gynecology/Neville F. Hacker, Joseph C. Gambone, Calvin J. Hobel. — 5th ed.   p. ; cm.
   Rev. ed. of: Essentials of obstetrics and gynecology / [edited by] Neville F. Hacker, J. George Moore, Joseph C. Gambone. 4th ed. c2004.
   Includes bibliographical references and index.
   ISBN 978–1–4160–5940–0
1. Gynecology. 2. Obstetrics. I. Gambone, Joseph C. II. Hobel, Calvin J. III. Essentials of obstetrics and gynecology. IV. Title. V. Title: Essentials of obstetrics and gynecology.
   [DNLM: 1. Obstetrics. 2. Genital Diseases, Female. 3. Pregnancy Complications. WQ 100 H118h 2010]

RG101.E87 2010
618—dc22

2008025860

Acquisitions Editor: James Merritt
Developmental Editor: Christine Abshire
Publishing Services Manager: Linda Van Pelt
Design Direction: Gene Harris

Printed in China

Last digit is the print number: 9 8 7 6 5 4 3 2

Dedication

This edition is dedicated to our wives, Estelle Hacker, Marge (Morris) Gambone, and Marsha Lynn Hobel.

Their understanding and support for the time and effort required to complete this project was *essential*.

Contributors

Carolyn J. Alexander, MD
Assistant Clinical Professor
David Geffen School of Medicine at UCLA
University of California at Los Angeles
Associate Director
Obstetrics and Gynecology Residency Program
Attending Physician
Division of Reproductive Endocrinology and Infertility
Department of Obstetrics and Gynecology
Cedars-Sinai Medical Center
Los Angeles, California
Puberty and Disorders of Pubertal Development;
Amenorrhea, Oligomenorrhea, and Hyperandrogenic
Disorders

Ricardo Azziz, MD, MPH, MBA
Professor and Vice-Chair
Department of Obstetrics and Gynecology
Professor
Department of Medicine
David Geffen School of Medicine at UCLA
University of California at Los Angeles
Chair
Department of Obstetrics and Gynecology
Director
Center for Androgen-Related Disorders
Cedars-Sinai Medical Center
Los Angeles, California
Puberty and Disorders of Pubertal Development;
Amenorrhea, Oligomenorrhea, and Hyperandrogenic
Disorders

Richard A. Bashore, MD
Professor Emeritus
Department of Obstetrics and Gynecology
David Geffen School of Medicine at UCLA
University of California at Los Angeles
Los Angeles, California
Fetal Surveillance During Labor;
Uterine Contractility and Dystocia

Jonathan S. Berek, MD, MMS
Professor and Chair
Department of Obstetrics and Gynecology
Stanford University School of Medicine
Stanford, California
Ovarian Cancer; Gestational Trophoblastic
Neoplasia

Narender N. Bhatia, MD
Professor
Department of Obstetrics and Gynecology
David Geffen School of Medicine at UCLA
University of California at Los Angeles
Los Angeles, California
Chief of Urogynecology
Director of Fellowship in Female Pelvic Medicine and
    Reconstructive Surgery
Harbor-UCLA Medical Center
Torrance, California
Genitourinary Dysfunction: Pelvic Organ Prolapse,
Urinary Incontinence, and Infections

Richard P. Buyalos, Jr., MD
Attending Physician
Ronald Reagan UCLA Medical Center
University of California at Los Angeles
Los Angeles, California
Attending Physician
Community Memorial Hospital
Ventura, California
Attending Physician
Los Robles Hospital
Thousand Oaks, California
Puberty and Disorders of Pubertal Development

Lony C. Castro, MD
Professor and Chair
Department of Obstetrics and Gynecology
Western University of Health Sciences
College of Osteopathic Medicine of the Pacific
Pomona, California
Maternal Fetal Medicine Specialist
Obstetrics and Gynecology
Arrowhead Regional Medical Center
San Bernardino, California
Maternal Fetal Medicine Specialist
Obstetrics and Gynecology
Riverside County Regional Medical Center
Riverside, California
  *Hypertensive Disorders of Pregnancy; Rhesus
  Isoimmunization; Common Medical and Surgical
  Conditions Complicating Pregnancy*

Ozlem Equils, MD
Associate Professor
Pediatrics
David Geffen School of Medicine at UCLA
University of California at Los Angeles
Attending Physician
Pediatric Infectious Diseases
Cedars-Sinai Medical Center
Los Angeles, California
  *Maternal Physiologic and Immunologic Adaptation
  to Pregnancy*

Bruce B. Ettinger, MD, MPH
Health Facilities Licensing and Certification Division
Los Angeles County Department of Public Health
Los Angeles, California
  *Family and Intimate Partner Violence, and Sexual
  Assault*

Michael L. Friedlander, MBChB, PhD
Conjoint Professor of Medicine
University of New South Wales
Director
Department of Medical Oncology
Prince of Wales Hospital
Consultant Medical Oncologist
Gynecological Cancer Centre
Royal Hospital for Women
Sydney, Australia
  Breast Disease: A Gynecologic Perspective

Robert H. Hayashi, MD
J. Robert Willson Professor of Obstetrics, Emeritus
Department of Obstetrics and Gynecology
University of Michigan
Ann Arbor, Michigan
  *Obstetric Hemorrhage and Puerperal Sepsis;
  Uterine Contractility and Dystocia*

Daniel A. Kahn, MD, PhD
Clinical Instructor
Department of Obstetrics and Gynecology
David Geffen School of Medicine at UCLA
University of California at Los Angeles
Los Angeles, California
  *Maternal Physiologic and Immunologic Adaptation
  to Pregnancy*

Matthew Kim, MD
Assistant Professor
Department of Obstetrics and Gynecology
David Geffen School of Medicine at UCLA
University of California at Los Angeles
Chief of Inpatient Obstetrics
Division of Maternal Fetal Medicine
Department of Obstetrics and Gynecology
Cedars-Sinai Medical Center
Los Angeles, California
  Obstetric Hemorrhage and Puerperal Sepsis

Brian J. Koos, MD, DPhil
Professor
Department of Obstetrics and Gynecology
David Geffen School of Medicine at UCLA
University of California at Los Angeles
Los Angeles, California
  *Maternal Physiologic and Immunologic Adaptation
  to Pregnancy; Fetal Surveillance During Labor*

Larry R. Laufer, CAPT, MC, USN
Voluntary Associate Professor
Obstetrics and Gynecology
University of California at San Diego
Staff Physician
Obstetrics and Gynecology
Naval Medical Center
San Diego, California
  *Amenorrhea, Oligomenorrhea, and
  Hyperandrogenic Disorders; Climacteric:
  Menopause, Peri- and Postmenopause;
  Menstrual Cycle–Influenced Disorders*

Joel B. Lench, MD
Consultant
Nurse Midwife Service
Department of Obstetrics and Gynecology
Naval Medical Center
San Diego, California
  *Vulvovaginitis, Sexually Transmitted Infections,
  and Pelvic Inflammatory Disease*

Michael C. Lu, MD, MPH
Associate Professor
Obstetrics and Gynecology, and Community Health
    Sciences
UCLA Schools of Medicine and Public Health
Ronald Reagan UCLA Medical Center
University of California at Los Angeles
Los Angeles, California
    *A Life-Course Perspective for Women's Health
    Care: Safe, Ethical and Effective Practice;
    Endocrinology of Pregnancy and Parturition;
    Antepartum Care: Preconception and Prenatal
    Care, Genetic Evaluation and Teratology, and
    Antenatal Fetal Assessment*

Ruchi Mathur, MD
Assistant Clinical Professor
Obstetrics and Gynecology
University of California at Los Angeles
Associate Director of Clinical Research,
    Recruitment and Phenotyping
Associate Director of Education
Center for Androgen-Related Disorders
Department of Obstetrics and Gynecology
Cedars-Sinai Medical Center
Los Angeles, California
    *Amenorrhea, Oligomenorrhea, and
    Hyperandrogenic Disorders*

James A. McGregor, MD, CM
Professor
Obstetrics and Gynecology
Keck School of Medicine
University of Southern California
Attending Physician
Obstetrics and Gynecology
Women's and Children's Hospital
LAC+USC Medical Center
Los Angeles, California
    *Vulvovaginitis, Sexually Transmitted Infections,
    and Pelvic Inflammatory Disease*

David R. Meldrum, MD
Clinical Professor
Department of Obstetrics and Gynecology
David Geffen School of Medicine at UCLA
University of California at Los Angeles
Los Angeles, California
Clinical Professor
Department of Reproductive Medicine
University of California at San Diego
San Diego, California
Scientific Director
Reproductive Partners Medical Group
Redondo Beach, California
    Infertility and Assisted Reproductive Technologies

Thomas R. Moore, MD
Professor and Chair
Department of Reproductive Medicine
University of California at San Diego
Professor and Chair
Reproductive Medicine
UCSD Medical Center
San Diego, California
    *Multifetal Gestation and Malpresentation;
    Obstetric Procedures*

Anita L. Nelson, MD
Professor
Department of Obstetrics and Gynecology
David Geffen School of Medicine at UCLA
University of California at Los Angeles
Los Angeles, California
Chief
Women's Health Care Programs
Obstetrics and Gynecology
Harbor-UCLA Medical Center
Torrance, California
Medical Director
Research
California Family Health Council
Los Angeles, California
    *Congenital Anomalies and Benign Conditions
    of the Vulva and Vagina; Congenital Anomalies
    and Benign Conditions of the Uterine Corpus
    and Cervix; Congenital Anomalies and Benign
    Conditions of the Ovaries and Fallopian Tubes;
    Ectopic Pregnancy; Family Planning: Reversible
    Contraception, Sterilization, and Abortion*

Dotun Ogunyemi, MD, FACOG
Associate Clinical Professor
Department of Obstetrics and Gynecology
David Geffen School of Medicine at UCLA
University of California at Los Angeles
Residency Program Director
Cedars-Sinai Medical Center
Department of Obstetrics and Gynecology
Los Angeles, California
    *Uterine Contractility and Dystocia; Common
    Medical and Surgical Conditions Complicating
    Pregnancy*

Margareta D. Pisarska, MD
Assistant Professor
Department of Obstetrics and Gynecology
University of California at Los Angeles
Director
Division of Reproductive Endocrinology and Infertility
Department of Obstetrics and Gynecology
Cedars-Sinai Medical Center
Los Angeles, California
Puberty and Disorders of Pubertal Development

Gladys A. Ramos, MD
Maternal Fetal Medicine Fellow
Department of Reproductive Medicine
University of California at San Diego
San Diego, California
Obstetric Procedures

Andrea J. Rapkin, MD
Professor and Vice-Chair
Department of Obstetrics and Gynecology
David Geffen School of Medicine at UCLA
University of California at Los Angeles
Attending Physician
Obstetrics and Gynecology
Ronald Reagan UCLA Medical Center
Los Angeles, California
Pelvic Pain

Mousa Shamonki, MD
Assistant Clinical Professor of Obstetrics
    and Gynecology
Director
In Vitro Fertilization Program
David Geffen School of Medicine at UCLA
Los Angeles, California
Ectopic Pregnancy

Christopher M. Tarnay, MD
Associate Clinical Professor
Director
Division of Female Pelvic Medicine
    and Reconstructive Surgery
Department of Obstetrics and Gynecology
David Geffen School of Medicine at UCLA
University of California at Los Angeles
Los Angeles, California
*Genitourinary Dysfunction: Pelvic Organ Prolapse,
Urinary Incontinence, and Infections*

Maryam Tarsa, MD, MAS
Assistant Professor
Department of Reproductive Medicine
University of California at San Diego
Faculty
UCSD Medical Center
San Diego, California
Multifetal Gestation and Malpresentation

John Williams III, MD
Clinical Professor
Department of Obstetrics and Gynecology
David Geffen School of Medicine at UCLA
University of California at Los Angeles
Director of Reproductive Genetics
Obstetrics and Gynecology
Cedars-Sinai Medical Center
Los Angeles, California
*Antepartum Care: Preconception and Prenatal
Care, Genetic Evaluation and Teratology, and
Antenatal Fetal Assessment*

Mark Zakowski, MD
Adjunct Associate Professor of Anesthesiology
Charles R. Drew University of Medicine and Science
Chief
Obstetric Anesthesiology
Cedars-Sinai Medical Center
Los Angeles, California
*Normal Labor, Delivery, and Postpartum Care:
Anatomic Considerations, Obstetric Analgesia
and Anesthesia, and Resuscitation of the
Newborn*

Preface to the Fifth Edition

We first would like to mention and welcome a new editor for this edition of Hacker and Moore's *Essentials of Obstetrics and Gynecology*. Calvin J. Hobel, MD, has replaced J. George (Jerry) Moore, who passed away just prior to the publication of the last edition. Dr. Hobel brings a wealth of experience as a high-risk obstetrician, with tested knowledge, wisdom, and insight.

The writing and revision of the fifth edition of *Essentials* has occurred at a time when the value of textbooks and the need for periodic revision of them is questioned by some in medical education, as well as in other fields. As the high cost of producing an accurate and authoritative text increases, along with the price that a student or resident physician must pay, these trainees and their educators are asking if the expense is an unnecessary burden. Current journal articles and the Internet are frequently mentioned as less expensive alternatives for course work. Why not get the latest information in the field?

Certainly textbooks have the disadvantage of not always containing the latest information on a topic and of having limited "shelf life." But just as newspapers and periodicals (printed or electronic) provide a "first draft" of human history, requiring frequent correction over time, medical texts should contain and document the time-tested facts of a discipline, along with newer information viewed through the prism of long-standing and safe practice. It is our belief that textbooks will continue to provide the *reliable essentials* of clinical practice. We have endeavored to revise this text only when a sufficient body of new material makes the use of the previous edition suboptimal for medical education.

Several new chapters have been added, along with extensive revision of about one third of the text. Another one third of chapters contain significant changes and new material. All of the 42 chapters in this edition have been updated. As was the case in previous editions of this text, we have included only the "essentials" of obstetrics and gynecology, making difficult choices about the breadth and depth of the material presented. Every attempt has been made to include material consistent with the learning objectives and goals proposed by the Association of Professors in Gynecology and Obstetrics (APGO), available on their website at *www.apgo.org*.

In addition to the authors and editors of this current edition, we wish to acknowledge and thank all those who have contributed to previous editions.* Their knowledge contained in their words form the foundation of this work and continue to enlighten students of obstetrics and gynecology.

We have appreciated greatly and wish to acknowledge the support and professionalism of James Merritt and his excellent production staff, particularly Christine Abshire and Linda Van Pelt, at Elsevier/Saunders.

JOSEPH C. GAMBONE (Executive Editor)
NEVILLE F. HACKER
CALVIN J. HOBEL

Contributors from previous editions
Juan J. Arce, Carol L. Archie, Martha J. Baird, A. David Barnes, Michael J. Bennett, Jennifer Blake, Clifford Bochner, J. Robert Bragonier, Charles R. Brinkman III, Michael S. Broder, Philip G. Brooks, John E. Buster, Maria Bustillo, Mary E. Carsten, Anita Bachus Chang, R. Jeffrey Chang, George Chapman, Ramen H. Chmait, Gautam Chaudhuri, Kenneth A. Conklin, Irvin M. Cushner (deceased), Alan H. DeCherney, Catherine Marin DeUgarte, William J. Dignam (deceased),

John A. Eden, Robin Farias-Eisner, Larry C. Ford (deceased), Michelle Fox, Janice I. French, Ann Garber, Anne D.M. Graham, Paul A. Gluck, William A. Growdon, John Gunning (deceased), Lewis A. Hamilton, Hunter A. Hammill, George S. Harris, James M. Heaps, Howard L. Judd (deceased), Samir Khalife, Ali Khraibi, Oscar A. Kletzky (deceased), Grace Elizabeth Kong, Thomas B. Lebherz (deceased), Ronald S. Leuchter, John K.H. Lu, Donald E. Marsden, John Marshall, Arnold L. Medearis, Robert Monoson, J. George Moore (deceased), John Morris, Suha H.N. Murad, Sathima Natarajan, Lauren Nathan, John Newnham, Tuan Nguyen, Bahij S. Nuwayhid, Gary Oakes, Aldo Palmieri, Groesbeck P. Parham, Ketan S. Patel, Anthony E. Reading, Robert C. Reiter, Jean M. Ricci (Goodman), Michael G. Ross, Edward W. Savage, William D. Schlaff, James R. Shields, Klaus J. Staisch (deceased), Eric Surrey, Khalil Tabsh, Nancy Theroux, Paul J. Toot, Maclyn E. Wade, Nathan Wasserstrum, Barry G. Wren and Linda Yielding.

Preface to the First Edition

A generation ago most schools of medicine in the United States presented courses in theoretical obstetrics and gynecology extending over a period of 18 months, supplemented by practical clerkships of 8 to 16 weeks in the third and fourth years. Most students procured as source textbooks a fairly complete compendium of obstetrics and another in gynecology. These texts not only served the students in medical school but were of great value during their housestaff training and were added to their reference library as they entered practice.

During the decade of the 1960s, theoretical obstetrics and gynecology in many institutions were condensed into a general course known as "An Introduction to Clinical Medicine" or "The Pathophysiology of Disease." Practical work in the clinics and wards was condensed into core clerkships, and in obstetrics and gynecology the "core" was generally restricted to 6 or 8 weeks, with electives available in subspecialty areas (high-risk obstetrics, gynecology oncology, reproductive endocrinology, acting internships, and outpatient gynecology). This condensation of experience into the "core" of obstetrics and gynecology during the clinical years left students with a difficult choice in selecting a textbook that would not overwhelm them with information yet would still stimulate their interest in the subject. Understandably it became increasingly difficult to hold the student responsible for a critical body of knowledge.

Textbooks prescribed for the core clerkships often do not have sufficient depth and sometimes do not possess key references or practical information. On the other hand, the classic texts of obstetrics and gynecology or gynecologic surgery are generally considered by students to be too expensive or too comprehensive for them to absorb during the clerkship. This book is a response to their dilemma. The chapters have all been written by members of the Obstetrics and Gynecology Faculty at the University of California, Los Angeles (UCLA) Medical Center and its affiliated hospitals—Harbor (LA County) General Hospital; Cedars-Sinai Medical Center; Martin Luther King, Jr., General Hospital; and Kern County Medical Center. Some authors have changed their institutional affiliations prior to the publication of the book. It is hoped that the book will serve the needs of the student, be useful during housestaff training, and be a helpful text in the medical practitioner's library. Fundamental principles and practice of obstetrics and gynecology are presented succinctly, but we have endeavored to cover all important aspects of the subject in sufficient detail to allow a reasonable understanding of the pathophysiology and a safe approach to clinical management.

The text is divided into five sections: an introductory section, obstetrics, reproductive endocrinology, gynecology, and gynecologic oncology. Special emphasis is given to family planning and important aspects of women's health. The basic operations of obstetrics and gynecology are included to allow a reasonable understanding of the technical procedures. Neville F. Hacker and J. George Moore have been responsible for the overall organization of the book. The most difficult tasks have been to maintain uniformity of style and to keep the text within 550 pages without sacrificing essential information. Calvin Hobel, John Marshall, J. George Moore, and Jonathan Berek have organized their particular sections. Neville F. Hacker has been largely responsible for the final editing of all sections.

This book would not have been possible without the special help of the following individuals, to whom we are most grateful: Gwynne Gloege, the very talented principal medical illustrator at UCLA, who was responsible for the overall uniformity and high quality of the illustrations; Yao-shi Fu, MD, and Robert Nieberg, MD, from the Department of Pathology, who provided illustrations and advice regarding gynecologic pathology; Normal Chang, who was responsible for the photography; and Linda Olt, who provided invaluable editorial assistance and also prepared the index. At WB Saunders, we are particularly grateful to Dana Dreibelbis, the Executive Editor who provided the initial inspiration and subsequent guidance for this project. Finally, this project would never have been completed without the untiring efforts, skill, and ever-cheerful countenance of Cheri Buonaguidi, the Obstetrics and Gynecology student coordinator at UCLA. She carefully read and accurately typed each version of the manuscript and worked with each of the contributors until all chapters were completed.

J. GEORGE MOORE
NEVILLE F. HACKER

Contents

PART 1 INTRODUCTION

1 A Life-Course Perspective for Women's Health Care: Safe, Ethical, and Effective Practice, 3
CALVIN J. HOBEL • MICHAEL C. LU • JOSEPH C. GAMBONE

2 Clinical Approach to the Patient, 12
JOSEPH C. GAMBONE

3 Female Reproductive Anatomy and Embryology, 22
JOSEPH C. GAMBONE

4 Female Reproductive Physiology, 34
JOSEPH C. GAMBONE

PART 2 OBSTETRICS

5 Endocrinology of Pregnancy and Parturition, 49
MICHAEL C. LU • CALVIN J. HOBEL

6 Maternal Physiologic and Immunologic Adaptation to Pregnancy, 56
BRIAN J. KOOS • DANIEL A. KAHN • OZLEM EQUILS

7 Antepartum Care: Preconception and Prenatal Care, Genetic Evaluation and Teratology, and Antenatal Fetal Assessment, 71
MICHAEL C. LU • JOHN WILLIAMS III • CALVIN J. HOBEL

8 Normal Labor, Delivery, and Postpartum Care: Anatomic Considerations, Obstetric Analgesia and Anesthesia, and Resuscitation of the Newborn, 91
CALVIN J. HOBEL • MARK ZAKOWSKI

9 Fetal Surveillance during Labor, 119
RICHARD A. BASHORE • BRIAN J. KOOS

10 Obstetric Hemorrhage and Puerperal Sepsis, 128
MATTHEW KIM • ROBERT H. HAYASHI • JOSEPH C. GAMBONE

11 Uterine Contractility and Dystocia, 139
RICHARD A. BASHORE • DOTUN OGUNYEMI • ROBERT H. HAYASHI

12 Obstetric Complications: Preterm Labor, PROM, IUGR, Postterm Pregnancy, and IUFD, 146
CALVIN J. HOBEL

13 Multifetal Gestation and Malpresentation, 160
MARYAM TARSA • THOMAS R. MOORE

14 Hypertensive Disorders of Pregnancy, 173
LONY C. CASTRO

15 Rhesus Isoimmunization, 183
LONY C. CASTRO

16 Common Medical and Surgical Conditions Complicating Pregnancy, 191
LONY C. CASTRO • DOTUN OGUNYEMI

17 Obstetric Procedures, 219
GLADYS A. RAMOS • THOMAS R. MOORE

PART 3 GYNECOLOGY

18 Congenital Anomalies and Benign Conditions of the Vulva and Vagina, 231
ANITA L. NELSON • JOSEPH C. GAMBONE

19   **Congenital Anomalies and Benign Conditions of the Uterine Corpus and Cervix, 240**
ANITA L. NELSON • JOSEPH C. GAMBONE

20   **Congenital Anomalies and Benign Conditions of the Ovaries and Fallopian Tubes, 248**
ANITA L. NELSON • JOSEPH C. GAMBONE

21   **Pelvic Pain, 256**
ANDREA J. RAPKIN • JOSEPH C. GAMBONE

22   **Vulvovaginitis, Sexually Transmitted Infections, and Pelvic Inflammatory Disease, 265**
JAMES A. MCGREGOR • JOEL B. LENCH

23   **Genitourinary Dysfunction: Pelvic Organ Prolapse, Urinary Incontinence, and Infections, 276**
CHRISTOPHER M. TARNAY • NARENDER N. BHATIA

24   **Ectopic Pregnancy, 290**
MOUSA SHAMONKI • ANITA L. NELSON • JOSEPH C. GAMBONE

25   **Endometriosis and Adenomyosis, 298**
JOSEPH C. GAMBONE

26   **Family Planning: Reversible Contraception, Sterilization, and Abortion, 305**
ANITA L. NELSON

27   **Sexuality and Female Sexual Dysfunction, 315**
JOSEPH C. GAMBONE

28   **Family and Intimate Partner Violence, and Sexual Assault, 322**
BRUCE B. ETTINGER • JOSEPH C. GAMBONE

29   **Breast Disease: A Gynecologic Perspective, 326**
NEVILLE F. HACKER • MICHAEL L. FRIEDLANDER

30   **Gynecologic Procedures, 332**
JOSEPH C. GAMBONE

PART 4 REPRODUCTIVE ENDOCRINOLOGY AND INFERTILITY

31   **Puberty and Disorders of Pubertal Development, 345**
MARGARETA D. PISARSKA • CAROLYN J. ALEXANDER • RICARDO AZZIZ • RICHARD P. BUYALOS, JR.

32   **Amenorrhea, Oligomenorrhea, and Hyperandrogenic Disorders, 355**
CAROLYN J. ALEXANDER • RUCHI MATHUR • LARRY R. LAUFER • RICARDO AZZIZ

33   **Dysfunctional Uterine Bleeding, 368**
JOSEPH C. GAMBONE

34   **Infertility and Assisted Reproductive Technologies, 371**
DAVID R. MELDRUM

35   **Climacteric: Menopause and Peri- and Postmenopause, 379**
LARRY R. LAUFER • JOSEPH C. GAMBONE

36   **Menstrual Cycle–Influenced Disorders, 386**
LARRY R. LAUFER • JOSEPH C. GAMBONE

PART 5 GYNECOLOGIC ONCOLOGY

37   **Principles of Cancer Therapy, 393**
NEVILLE F. HACKER

38   **Cervical Dysplasia and Cancer, 402**
NEVILLE F. HACKER

39   **Ovarian Cancer, 412**
JONATHAN S. BEREK

40   **Vulvar and Vaginal Cancer, 420**
NEVILLE F. HACKER

41   **Uterine Corpus Cancer, 428**
NEVILLE F. HACKER

42   **Gestational Trophoblastic Neoplasia, 435**
JONATHAN S. BEREK

Index, 443

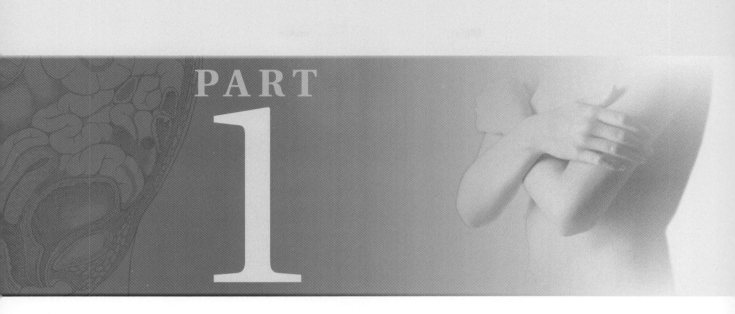

INTRODUCTION

Chapter 1

A Life-Course Perspective for Women's Health Care
SAFE, ETHICAL, AND EFFECTIVE PRACTICE

CALVIN J. HOBEL • MICHAEL C. LU • JOSEPH C. GAMBONE

Obstetrics and gynecology is an exciting and challenging area of health care. It provides students and young physicians in training with the knowledge and skills necessary to improve the health and health care of women and their children very early in their lives. The United States spends far more on health care than any other nation in the world. Despite this economic effort, it ranks poorly on most measures of overall health status. For example, for the year 2004, the United States ranked only 46th worldwide for average life expectancy and much higher than is acceptable at 42nd in infant mortality. In the year 2000, the World Health Organization ranked the U.S. health-care system only 37th out of the 191 nations whose systems were evaluated for performance. Certainly we need to improve our standing on these and other measures of performance as our health-care delivery system is refined in the coming years. In this chapter, we provide some basic principles and guidelines for improving health care and suggest several important factors that influence the health of women and their children.

Principles of Practice Management

There are four basic principles for practicing and improving health care that we would like to mention now and expand on later. First, the safety of our patients must always be paramount. In the past few years, we have made major improvements in patient safety, in large part by emphasizing teamwork and implementing practices proved effective in the airline industry. Second, we must always be true to our personal pledge made when taking the Hippocratic Oath—to adhere to ethical practices. Third, because medicine has become very complex, we must be open to a multidisciplinary approach to both diagnostic and therapeutic practice.

Quality improvement efforts, practice management skills, and effective communication are all necessary to efficiently optimize clinical outcomes. Finally and perhaps most important, we must focus on the prevention and early mitigation of disease, in addition to our continued focus on its treatment. For this reason, we emphasize an approach called a *life-course perspective for clinical practice,* beginning with preconception health, continuing throughout pregnancy, and then giving children and their mothers a **health perspective** for adopting and maintaining healthy living. Before delving more deeply into these principles of practice, some newer concepts about the origins of disease are important to mention.

LIFE-COURSE PERSPECTIVE

Where does the rubber meet the road and lead to pathology and disease during the course of life?

First, **although genetics is beginning to provide a much better understanding of the etiologic factors in poor health, it probably accounts for only about one third of the direct causes.** For example, person X with gene A has a disease, but person Y with the same gene does not. Clearly there is more to human development and disease risk than one's genetic makeup. It is thought that factors such as poverty or abnormal health behaviors and environmental conditions can influence the expression of gene A. This may occur directly, or these factors may activate another gene, A-2, downstream, which may then affect gene A. The process whereby human cells can have the same genomic makeup but different characteristics is referred to as **epigenetics. It is now thought that the effect of harmful behaviors and our environment on the expression of our genes may account for up to 40% of all premature deaths in the United States.** Two of the top behavioral factors related

3

to this premature death rate are obesity (and physical inactivity) and smoking. Environmental exposures to metals, solvents, pesticides, endocrine disruptors, and other reproductive toxicants are also major concerns.

Second, in human biology, a phenomenon called *adaptive developmental plasticity* plays a very important role in helping to adjust behavior to meet any environmental challenges. To understand human development over time (*a life-course perspective*), one must first understand what is normal and what adverse circumstances may challenge and then change normal development in the fetus. These protective modifications of growth and development may become permanent—programmed in utero to prevent fetal death. The price the fetus may pay in the long run, however, for short-term survival is a vulnerability to conditions such as obesity, hypertension, insulin resistance, atherosclerosis, and even a chronic disease such as diabetes.

In relation to individual X and individual Y with the same genomic makeup but different in utero environmental influences, metabolic changes that may be initiated in utero in response to inadequate nutritional supplies (Figure 1-1) can lead to insulin resistance and eventually the development of type 2 diabetes. These adaptive changes can even result in a reduced number of nephrons in the kidneys as a stressed fetus conserves limited nutritional resources for more important in utero organ systems. This can then lead to a greater risk for hypertension later in life. **This series of initially protective but eventually harmful developmental changes was first described in humans by David Barker, a British epidemiologist, who carefully assessed birth records of individuals and linked low birth weight to the development of hypertension, diabetes, atherosclerosis, and stroke later in life.** The association among poor fetal growth during intrauterine life, insulin resistance, and cardiovascular disease is known as the *Barker hypothesis*. The process whereby a stimulus or insult, at a sensitive or critical period of fetal development, induces permanent alterations in the structure and functions of the baby's vital organs, with lasting or lifelong consequences for health and disease, is now commonly referred to as *developmental programming*.

Third, another important concept in the life-course perspective is allostasis, which describes the body's ability to maintain stability during physiologic change. A good example of allostasis is found in the body's stress response. When the body is under stress (biological or psychological), it activates a stress response. **The sympathetic system kicks in, and adrenalin flows to make the heart pump faster and harder** (with the end result of delivering more blood and oxygen to vital organs, including the brain). **The hypothalamic-pituitary-adrenal (HPA) axis is also activated** to produce more cortisol, which has many actions to prepare the body for fight or flight.

But as soon as the fight or flight is over, the stress response is turned off. **The body's sympathetic response is counteracted by a parasympathetic response, which fires a signal through the vagal nerve to slow down the heart, and the HPA axis is shut off by cortisol through negative feedback mechanisms.** Negative feedback mechanisms are common to many biological systems and work very much like a thermostat. When the room temperature falls below a preset point, the thermostat turns on the heat. Once the preset temperature is reached, the heat turns off the thermostat. Stress turns on the HPA axis to produce cortisol. Cortisol, in turn, turns off the HPA axis to keep the stress response in check. The body has these exquisite built-in mechanisms for checks and balance to help maintain allostasis, or stability through change.

This stress response works well for acute stress; it tends to break down under chronic stress. It works well for stress one can fight off or run from, but it doesn't work as well for stress from which there is no escape. In the face of chronic and repeated stress, the body's stress response is always turned on, and over time will wear out. The body goes from being "stressed" to being "stressed out"—from a state of allostasis to **allostatic overload**. This describes the cumulative wear and tear on the body's adaptive systems from chronic stress.

The life-course perspective synthesizes both the developmental programming mechanisms of early life events and allostatic overload mechanisms of chronic life stress into a longitudinal model of health

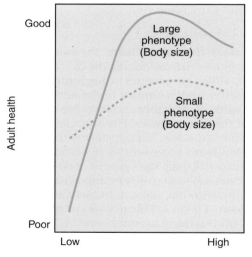

FIGURE 1-1 The potential effects of life-course nutritional determinants (intrauterine and lifelong) on subsequent adult health. *(From Bateson P, Barker D, Clutton-Brock T, et al: Developmental plasticity and human health. Nature 430:419-421, 2004. Adapted by permission from Macmillan Publishers Ltd.)*

development. It is a way of looking at life not as disconnected stages but as an integrated continuum. Thus, to promote healthy pregnancy, preconception health must first be promoted. To promote preconception health, adolescent health must be promoted, and so forth. Rather than episodic care that many women receive, as a specialty we must strive toward disease prevention and health promotion over the continuum of a woman's life course.

IMPACT ON PUBLIC HEALTH

The public health implications of the Barker hypothesis and other life-course events leading to health or the development of disease are significant. This is the beginning of an exciting era in medicine during which young physicians can begin to take charge of these events and change our health-care delivery system in a very positive way. A large part of this will occur by encouraging patients to take responsibility for improving their own health, particularly by practicing healthy behaviors early in life. They should also be encouraged to improve and maintain a healthy "green" environment. Currently, there are only a few environmental and behavioral factors that have been clearly identified as part of the Barker hypothesis. Many others are yet to be discovered.

Adaptive developmental plasticity will take place secondary to changes in genes as a result of environmental and behavioral practices. Even the controversial concept of climate change may play a role in this phenomenon. New knowledge over the next 10 to 20 years should help us to accelerate the development of focused interventions at all levels to mitigate and prevent disease and improve the health of women and their children.

Biological processes are powerful and frequently unpredictable. Physicians must decide what role they will play in a safe, ethical, and effective practice. Learning is fun and exciting, and patients who wish to be informed about their health and health care will be grateful for the wellness and good health provided to them.

The four basic principles and guidelines mentioned earlier—**patient safety, ethical practice, quality improvement,** and the need for a **focus on prevention**—are covered next.

■ *Patient Safety*

Safety in health care is not a new concept. Facilities have had safety programs in place since the early 1900s, but these programs have traditionally focused on emergency preparedness, environmental safety, security, and infection control. The term *patient safety,* meaning avoidance of medical error, was first coined by the American Society of Anesthesiologists in 1984 when they inaugurated the Anesthesia Patient Safety Foundation to give assurance that the effects of anesthesia would not harm patients.

Medical errors now rank as the fifth leading cause of death in the United States. The Institute of Medicine (IOM) published an alarming report in 1999 called *To Err Is Human: Building a Safer Health System*. This report estimated that between 44,000 and 98,000 Americans die each year as a result of medical errors. **Error is defined as failure of a planned action to be completed as intended (e.g., failing to operate when obvious signs of appendicitis are present) or the use of a wrong plan to achieve an aim (e.g., wrong diagnosis, wrong medication administered).** Medication errors alone, occurring either in or out of the hospital, are estimated to account for more than 7000 deaths annually. According to the National Council on Patient Information and Education, "more than 2/3 of all physician visits end with a prescription." An estimated 39% to 49% of all medication errors occur at the stage of drug ordering. **Patient noncompliance also contributes to medical errors.**

The United States Pharmacopoeia (USP) MED-MARK error tracking service estimates that as many as 100,000 medication errors occur annually. Because reporting is voluntary and does not include all medical facilities in the United States, the scope of the problem is likely to be much larger. A preventable adverse drug event (ADE) is one type of medication error. Administering the incorrect drug, an incorrect dose, wrong frequency, or incorrect route may cause an ADE.

A drug that cures one patient's condition may be the one that causes another patient's injury or death owing to an adverse drug reaction (ADR). The latter may account for 1 out of 5 injuries or deaths for hospitalized patients. ADRs commonly occur from an overdose, a side effect, or an interaction among several concomitantly administered drugs. **To minimize ADRs, health-care providers should avoid the following actions:**
1. **Prescribing unnecessary medications**
2. **Treating mild side effects of one drug with a second, more toxic drug**
3. **Misinterpreting a drug's side effect for a new medical problem** and prescribing another medication
4. **Prescribing a medication when there is any uncertainty about dosing**

In the absence of automated systems, health-care professionals should strive to write legibly and use only approved abbreviations and dose expressions. Most health-care facilities publish and circulate an acceptable list of appropriate abbreviations as a means of reducing medication errors.

MEDICAL ERROR REPORTING

According to the U.S. Agency for Healthcare Research and Quality (AHRQ), "Reporting is an important component of systems to improve patient safety." Incident reporting is an important and inexpensive method to detect medical error and prevent future adverse events. Unfortunately, this method may fail to affect clinical outcomes because most hospital reporting systems do not capture most errors. **Reporting should be considered a quality improvement process (focused on system failures) rather than a performance evaluation method (blaming individual providers).**

As a founding member of the National Patient Safety Foundation and the National Patient Safety Partnership, the Joint Commission on the Accreditation of Healthcare Organizations (JCAHO), now more commonly known as The Joint Commission (TJC), has formed a coalition with the USP, the American Medical Association (AMA), and the American Hospital Association (AHA) to create patient safety reporting principles. Recognizing that fear of liability discourages error reporting, TJC has advised the U.S. Congress that federal statutory protection must be afforded to those who report medical error. **An anonymous nonpunitive environment will encourage reporting.** Many states have implemented mandatory reporting systems for selected medical errors to improve patient safety and reduce errors. Others consider incident reporting and analysis as peer review activities immune from liability. **The Institute of Medicine (IOM) recommends that health-care providers be required to report errors that result in serious harm. Information collected should be made available to the public.** AHRQ publishes case summaries of reported medical errors and near misses on their website.

DISCLOSURE OF MEDICAL ERROR

The National Patient Safety Foundation (NPSF) was one of the first organizations to address the issue of disclosure. Their position, finalized in November 2000, states that **when a health-care injury occurs, the patient and family or representative is entitled to a prompt explanation of how the injury occurred and its short-term and long-term effects.** When an error contributed to the injury, the patient and family or representative should receive a truthful and compassionate explanation about the error and the remedies available to the patient. They should be informed that the factors involved in the injury will be investigated so that steps can be taken to reduce the likelihood of similar injury to other patients.

TJC now requires hospitals to disclose any serious harm caused by medical errors to the harmed parties. Disclosing error can be very difficult for physicians because they may struggle with intense feelings of incompetence, betrayal of the patient, and fear of litigation. **Studies suggest that physicians with good relationship skills are less likely to be sued. Furthermore, suits settle rapidly and for less money when errors are disclosed early. Simple rules for disclosing errors include admitting the mistake, acknowledging the listener's** **anger, speaking slowly, and stopping frequently to allow the listener to talk.** Tell the person that an error has occurred and apologize. Usually, the attending physician is the one who should disclose. Medical students should not disclose because they may not be prepared to offer advice on necessary follow-up.

▇ *Ethical Practice of Obstetrics and Gynecology*

Obstetrics and gynecology encompasses many high-profile areas of ethical concern such as in vitro fertilization (IVF) and other assisted reproductive technologies (ARTs), abortion, the use of aborted tissue for research or treatment, surrogacy, contraception for minors, and sterilization of persons with a mental illness. Nevertheless, most ethical problems in the practice of medicine arise in cases in which the medical condition or desired procedure itself presents no moral problem. **In the past, the main areas of ethical concern have related to the competence and beneficence of the physician. Current areas of ethical concern should include the goals, values, and individual and appropriate cultural preferences of the patient as well as those of the community at large.** Consideration of such issues enriches the study of obstetrics and gynecology by emphasizing that scientific knowledge and technical skills are most meaningful in a social and moral context.

ETHICAL PRINCIPLES

During the day-to-day consideration of ethical dilemmas in health care, a number of principles or ideals and the concepts derived from them are commonly accepted and taken into account. Four such principles or ideals are **nonmaleficence, beneficence, autonomy, and justice;** these are generally accepted as the major ethical concepts that apply to health care.

Nonmaleficence

The principle of *primum non nocere,* or "first, do no harm," originated from the Hippocratic school, and although few would dispute the basic concept, in day-to-day medical practice, physicians and their patients may need to accept some harm from treatment (such as necessary surgical trauma) in order to achieve a desired outcome. However, there is an ethical obligation to be certain that recommended medical treatment, surgery, or diagnostic testing is not likely to cause *more harm* than benefit.

Beneficence

The duty of beneficence, or the promotion of the welfare of patients, is an important part of the Hippocratic Oath. Most would see its strict application as an ideal rather than a duty, however. One could save many suffering people in a Third World country by practicing there or by giving a large portion of one's income in aid, but few would consider it a moral duty to do so. On the other hand, **when the concept of beneficence involves a specific patient encounter, the duty applies.** A physician prevented by conscience from participating in the performance of an abortion, for example, would generally be expected to provide lifesaving care for a woman suffering complications after such a procedure—putting her welfare first.

Autonomy

The right of self-determination is a basic concept of biomedical ethics. **To exercise autonomy, an individual must be capable of effective deliberation and be neither coerced into a particular course of action nor limited in her or his choices by external constraints.** Being capable of effective deliberation implies a level of intellectual capacity and the ability to exercise that capacity. In a number of situations, it may be reasonable to limit autonomy for the following reasons: (1) to prevent harm to others, (2) to prevent self-harm, (3) to prevent immoral acts, and (4) to benefit many others.

The concept of **informed consent** may be derived directly from the principle of autonomy and from a desire to protect patients and research subjects from harm. **There is general agreement that consent must be genuinely voluntary and made after adequate disclosure of information.** As a minimum, when a patient consents to a procedure in health care, the patient should be informed about the expectation of benefit as well as the other reasonable alternatives and possible risks that are known. Table 1-1 provides a useful checklist (PREPARED) that expands on the minimum information required.

The exercise of autonomy may cause considerable stress and conflict for those providing health care, as in the case of a woman with a ruptured ectopic pregnancy who refuses a lifesaving blood transfusion for religious reasons and dies despite the best efforts of the medical team. More complex questions may be raised by court-ordered cesarean births for the benefit of the fetus.

Justice

Justice relates to the way in which the benefits and burdens of society are distributed. The general principle that equals should be treated equally was espoused by Aristotle and is widely accepted today, but it does require that one be able to define the relevant differences between individuals and groups. Some believe all rational persons to have equal rights; others emphasize need, effort, contribution, and merit; still others seek criteria that maximize both individual and social utility. **In most Western societies, race, sex, and religion are not considered morally legitimate criteria for the distribution of benefits, although they too may be taken into account to right what are perceived to be historical wrongs, in programs of affirmative action.** When resources are scarce, issues of justice become even more acute because there are often competing claims from parties who appear equal by all relevant criteria, and the selection criteria themselves become a moral issue. Most modern societies find the *rational* rationing of health-care resources to be appropriate and acceptable (Figure 1-2).

OTHER DUTIES OF ETHICAL PRACTICE

Confidentiality is a cornerstone of the relationship between physician and patient. This duty arises from considerations of autonomy but also helps promote beneficence, as is the case with honesty. In obstetrics and gynecology, conflicts can arise, as in the case of a woman with a sexually transmitted disease who refuses to have a sexual partner informed, or a school-aged child seeking contraceptive advice or an abortion.

There are many other situations in which conflicting responsibilities make confidentiality a difficult issue. The U.S. Health Insurance Portability and Accountability Act (HIPAA) mandates strict rules that physician practices and health-care facilities must adhere to

TABLE 1-1		
THE PREPARED SYSTEM: A CHECKLIST TO ASSIST THE PATIENT AND PROVIDER IN THE PROCESS OF INFORMED CONSENT		
P	lan	The course of action being considered
R	eason	The indication or rationale
E	xpectation	The chances of benefit and failure
P	references	Cultural and patient-centered priorities (utilities) affecting choice
A	lternatives	Other reasonable options/plans
R	isks	The potential harm from plans
E	xpenses	All direct and indirect costs
D	ecision	Fully informed collaborative choice

Modified from Reiter RC, Lench JB, Gambone JC: Consumer advocacy, elective surgery, and the "Golden Era of Medicine." Obstet Gynecol 74:815, 1989.

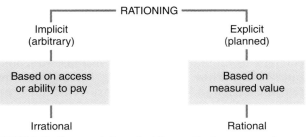

FIGURE 1-2   Representation of arbitrary rationing commonly based on access or ability to pay vs. planned clinical resource management based on measured value. *Explicit* rationing is objectionable to many despite the fact that *implicit* rationing still occurs.

regarding the confidentiality and security of patient health-care records. Some are concerned that these regulations could restrict the flow of information about patient care and may hinder efforts to improve overall performance.

Caring for a pregnant woman creates a unique **maternal-fetal relationship** because the management of the mother inevitably affects her baby. Until recently, the only way by which an obstetrician could produce a healthy baby was by maintaining optimal maternal health, but as the fetus becomes more accessible to diagnostic and therapeutic interventions, new problems emerge. **Procedures performed on behalf of the fetus may violate the personal integrity and autonomy of the mother.** The obstetrician with a dual responsibility to mother and fetus faces a potential conflict of interest. **Most conflicts will be resolved as a result of the willingness of most women to undergo considerable self-sacrifice to benefit their fetus.** When a woman refuses consent for a procedure that presents her with significant risk, her autonomy will generally be respected. However, there may be cases in which an intervention that is likely to be efficacious carries little risk to the mother and can reasonably be expected to prevent substantial harm to the fetus. These have occasionally ended in a court-ordered intervention.

Health care is a multidisciplinary activity, and respectful and collegial relationships with other health professionals are very important. Although the physician has traditionally been the only decision-maker, this situation has often caused concern among other health-care professionals. **There is increasing recognition that other clinicians involved in health care have a right to participate in any decision-making.** Physicians have not been as aware of the sensitivities of the nursing profession and other allied health professionals as they should have been. For example, the decision, no matter how it is made, to either operate or not on a newborn with severe spina bifida inevitably leaves nurses with responsibilities to the infant, the parents, and the doctor that may be in direct conflict with their personal values. They may rightly request to be party to the decision-making process, and although the exact models whereby such a goal may be achieved are debatable, physicians must be aware of the legitimate moral concerns of nurses and others involved.

And finally, health-care delivery takes place in a complex environment, and **relationships with other interested parties are becoming increasingly important.** Hospitals, health insurance companies, and governments all claim an interest in what services are made available or paid for, and this may prevent individual patients from receiving what their physician may consider optimal care. This poses moral problems not only for physicians on a case-by-case basis but also for insurance companies and society as a whole.

The interface of medicine and the law raises major ethical issues because legality and morality are not always synonymous. Professional liability insurance premiums for obstetricians are testimony to the relevance of legal issues to obstetric practice. Professional liability is affecting every major decision that is made by the practicing obstetrician and gynecologist, and under these conditions, the "tunnel vision" that ensues may obscure the ability to see clear answers to ethical questions.

◼ *Health-Care Quality Improvement*

PRACTICING MORE EFFECTIVELY

The mandate from payers (government and employers) and the public to measure and improve the effectiveness of health-care services is clear. Unfortunately, change based on adoption of national standards derived from evidence-based practice and randomized controlled trials (RCTs) alone may be too expensive and slow to meet this mandate. Furthermore, the results from RCTs may not always establish how diagnostic and therapeutic procedures actually work in clinical practice. **For these reasons, health-care organizations and physician groups must develop the tools to identify and adopt best practices and improve clinical outcomes locally.**

Paralleling the evolving science of outcomes assessment is the evolving science of outcomes improvement. Health-care organizations have adapted successful models of continuous quality improvement from industry as well as newer research or "evidence-based" models of care. Adoption of "best practice" models of care must be based on continuous reassessment of evolving practice, research, and innovation. **Methods such as the FOCUS-PDCA cycle** (Figure 1-3), **originally developed at Bell Laboratories to test small incremental changes, have been applied to health-care processes and used successfully for continuous quality improvement programs.** Use of such a standardized method has been shown to improve the effectiveness of clinical improvement efforts and accelerate the pace of needed change. Several other key clinical improvement tools are highlighted below.

CLINICAL GUIDELINES

Unintended variation in health-care processes generally connotes, and frequently results in, lower quality of care. **Clinical guidelines**, also referred to as protocols, practice parameters, algorithms, and **clinical pathways**, are tools that have been developed to reduce wasteful variation in the performance of medical and surgical procedures and to improve outcomes of care.

A guideline is a summary of optimal care processes for a medical condition stated in general terms so as to allow sufficient variation for patient differences

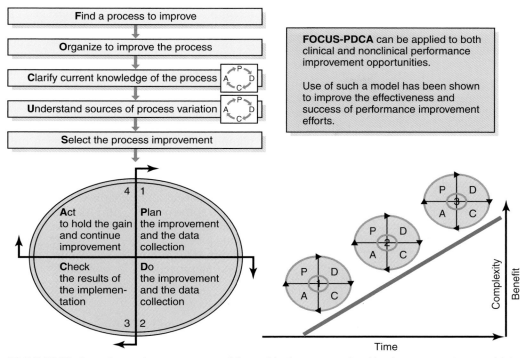

FIGURE 1-3   FOCUS-PDCA. A continuous improvement model to guide the process of making improvements now widely used in health care. *(From Langley DJ, et al: The Improvement Guide. San Francisco, Jossey-Bass, 1996.)*

and preferences. Previously, guidelines were derived largely by consensus and the opinion of experts. **More recently, these authority-based guidelines have been replaced by so-called evidence-based guidelines, which are based on objective evaluation of outcomes and the available medical literature.** Adoption of evidence-based guidelines, such as those produced by the AHRQ, the U.S. Preventive Services Task Force, and the international Cochrane Collaborative, has been shown to improve health-care outcomes and reduce costs. However, their acceptance has not been widespread in the United States, in part because of the financial consequences of their adoption.

Clinical pathways (also known as critical paths or care maps) are broad, detailed multidisciplinary guidelines that organize, sequence, and time the best or ideal management strategy, usually for a specific condition or procedure. For example, a pathway for patients undergoing hysterectomy details diagnostic and therapeutic milestones that are expected on each day of the patient's hospital stay. About 80% to 90% of patients are expected to stay on the pathway during treatment.

Disease management protocols are comprehensive approaches to patient care for an entire episode of illness (inpatient and outpatient). A disease management model provides guidelines for the continuous tracking and modification of the care plan, facilitation of care across clinical services, confirmation of service delivery, and evaluation of variances in practice and outcomes.

Focus on Prevention

The prevention and mitigation of existing disease has become an extremely important and sometimes overlooked area of effective practice. The famous American humorist, Will Rogers, said many years ago that people should only pay their doctors when they are well and not sick. This suggests a frustration that he was reflecting publicly that medical practice has neglected the promotion of wellness. As health-care treatment becomes more expensive and complex, there is a greater incentive for government, private industry, and individuals to invest in preventive services. The wise students of medical practice, including obstetrics and gynecology, will benefit from more education and training in prevention—and so will their patients. Box 1-1 contains a life-course perspective of early, effective prevention opportunities.

One recent example of a preventive intervention that is available in gynecologic practice is the vaccination against human papillomavirus (HPV) infection to prevent cervical cancer (see Chapters 22 and 38). This new technology illustrates both the promise of prevention and the controversy that can surround the use of some preventive measures.

IMMUNIZATIONS AND PREVENTIVE HEALTH SCREENING

Because public health recommendations for immunizations may change, it is best to check a reliable source periodically (e.g., www.cdc.gov) for the latest information before counseling patients. General recommendations include the following for women aged 19 to 49 years: measles, mumps, and rubella (MMR), hepatitis B, and varicella for women who are nonimmune. Additionally, vaccination against HPV is currently

---

BOX 1-1 *A Life-Course Perspective of Early Prevention Opportunities*

- Preconception counseling (Chapter 7)
- Antepartum care and nutrition counseling (Chapter 7)
- Intrapartum care and surveillance (Chapters 9 and 10)
- Newborn screening (Chapter 8 and pediatric care textbooks*)
- Well-baby visits, breastfeeding and nutrition counseling (pediatric care textbooks*)
- Childhood and adolescent screening and immunizations (pediatric care textbooks*)
- Adult preventive health screening (Table 1-2)

*For example, Kliegman R, Behrman R, Jenson H, Stanton B: Nelson's Textbooks of Pediatrics, 18th ed. Philadelphia, Elsevier Saunders, 2007.

---

recommended for girls and women aged 11 to 26 years, and a single dose of tetanus-diphtheria-pertussis (Tdap) for adults 19 to 64 years of age is now recommended to replace the next booster dose of tetanus and diphtheria toxoids (Td) vaccine. **Influenza vaccine** is recommended annually for all women older than age 50 years and for women aged 19 to 49 years who are healthcare workers, who have chronic illnesses such as heart disease or diabetes mellitus, or who are pregnant or planning to become pregnant during the flu season. **Pneumococcal vaccine** is recommended for all women aged 65 years and older, for those with chronic illness or alcoholism, and for those who are immunosuppressed. Meningococcal and hepatitis A vaccines may be indicated in some women with risk factors. Remember that MMR, varicella, and HPV vaccines are contraindicated during pregnancy.

Table 1-2 contains recommended preventive health screening procedures for women.

■ *Conclusions*

Safe, ethical, and effective practice in obstetrics and gynecology is facilitated by viewing wellness and sickness in the context of a *life-course perspective*. Effective care of the mother and fetus must begin early, even before conception, so that adverse in utero effects can be prevented or at least mitigated. The concepts of adaptive developmental plasticity and the Barker hypothesis and their potential impact on the development of disease in obstetrics and gynecology are significant.

TABLE 1-2

RECOMMENDED PREVENTIVE HEALTH SCREENING FOR WOMEN

Intervention/Procedure	Risk
Pap smear annually from age 21 yr or sexual activity; after three consecutive normal smears, every 2 to 3 yr in low-risk women from age 30 until 70 yr	Cervical dysplasia/cancer
Mammography every other year from age 40 yr and then annually from age 50 to 70 yr	Breast cancer
Smoking cessation counseling, warning second-hand smoke exposure	Lung cancer, heart disease, other health risks associated with smoking
Height and weight measurement	Overweight and obesity
Regular blood pressure screening (every 2 yr)	Hypertension and stroke
Cholesterol/lipid profile every 5 yr until age 65 yr	Heart disease
Total skin inspection and selective biopsies	Skin cancer (sun exposure)
Diet and exercise counseling	Osteoporosis, fracture, and deformity
Blood sugar study with family history, obesity, or history of gestational diabetes	Diabetes mellitus; other comorbidities associated with obesity
Sigmoidoscopy or colonoscopy every 3 to 5 yr after age 50 yr	Colorectal cancer
Cervical sampling for *Chlamydia*, *Neisseria gonorrhoeae*, syphilis, and HIV based on history	Sexually transmitted infections
PPD of tuberculin for high-risk women	Tuberculosis

HIV, human immunodeficiency virus; Pap, Papanicolaou test; PPD, purified protein derivative.

All branches of medicine, and especially obstetrics and gynecology, will face an increasing number of ethical problems in the future. It is essential that practicing obstetricians and gynecologists prepare themselves to deal with these problems, partly because managing practices in an ethical manner transforms them from mere dispensers of health care to caring, responsive, and trustworthy physicians. Also, if health-care providers do not respond to this challenge, other potentially less-qualified elements of society (e.g., legislators and special interest groups) will respond for them, to the possible detriment of both patients and physicians.

Regulatory, economic, and public pressures make the assessment and improvement of safety and quality essential in the delivery of women's health care. Optimal health outcomes can only be achieved when principles from continuous quality assessment are combined with the systematic approach of safety science and with guidelines from evidence-based medicine. Along with advances in medical science, changes in the delivery of health care, new technology, and better understanding of the causes of medical errors, the quality process must be dynamic, continuous, and patient centered.

The promising area of preventive services in obstetrics and gynecology, as well as all health care, is transforming the practice of medicine in a positive way.

SUGGESTED READING

American College of Obstetricians and Gynecologists: Ethical decision making in obstetrics and gynecology. *In* Ethics in Obstetrics and Gynecology, 2nd ed. Washington, DC, ACOG, 2004.

Bateson P, Barker D, Clutton-Brock T, et al: Developmental plasticity and human health. Nature 430:419-421, 2004.

Gambone JC, Reiter RC: Elements of a successful quality improvement and patient safety program in obstetrics and gynecology. Obstet Gynecol Clin North Am 35:129-145, 2008.

Institute of Medicine: To err is human: Building a safer health system. Washington, DC, Institute of Medicine of National Academy of Sciences, 1999.

President's Advisory Commission on Consumer Protection and Quality in the Health Care Industry. Quality first: Better health care for all Americans. Retrieved January 1, 2008, from http://www.hcqualitycommission.gov/final.

Chapter 2

Clinical Approach to the Patient

JOSEPH C. GAMBONE

As is the case in most areas of medicine, a careful history and physical examination should form the basis for patient evaluation and clinical management in obstetrics and gynecology. This chapter outlines the essential details of the clinical approach to, and evaluation of, the obstetric and gynecologic patient. Pediatric and adolescent patients, the geriatric patient, and women with disabilities all have unique gynecologic and reproductive needs, and this chapter concludes with information about their evaluation and management.

Obstetric and Gynecologic Evaluation

In few areas of medicine is it necessary to be more sensitive to the emotional and psychological needs of the patient than in obstetrics and gynecology. By their very nature, the history and physical examination may cause embarrassment to some patients. The members of the medical care team are individually and collectively responsible for ensuring that each patient's privacy and modesty are respected while providing the highest level of medical care. Box 2-1 lists the appropriate steps for the clinical approach to the patient.

Although a casual and familiar approach may be acceptable to many younger patients, it may offend others and be quite inappropriate for many older patients. Different circumstances with the same patient may dictate different levels of formality. Entrance to the patient's room should be announced by a knock and spoken identification. A personal introduction with the stated reason for the visit should occur before any questions are asked or an examination is begun. The placement of the examination table should always be in a position that maximizes privacy for the patient as other health-care professionals enter the room. Finally, any appropriate cultural beliefs and preferences for care and treatment should be recognized and respected.

Obstetric History

A complete history must be recorded at the time of the prepregnancy evaluation or at the initial antenatal visit. Several detailed standardized forms are available, but this should not negate the need for a detailed chronologic history taken personally by the physician who will be caring for the patient throughout her pregnancy. While taking the history, major opportunities will usually arise to provide counseling and explanations that serve to establish rapport and a supportive patient–physician encounter.

PREVIOUS PREGNANCIES

Each prior pregnancy should be reviewed in chronologic order and the following information recorded:

BOX 2-1 *Approach to the Patient*

The doctor should always:
- Knock before entering the patient's room.
- Identify himself or herself.
- Meet the patient initially when she is fully dressed, if possible.
- Address the patient courteously and respectfully.
- Respect the patient's privacy and modesty during the interview and examination.
- Ensure cleanliness, good grooming, and good manners in all patient encounters.
- Beware that a casual and familiar approach is not acceptable to all patients; it is generally best to avoid addressing an adult patient by her first name.
- Maintain the privacy of the patient's medical information and records.
- Be mindful and respectful of any cultural preferences.

1. **Date of delivery** (or pregnancy termination)
2. **Location of delivery** (or pregnancy termination)
3. **Duration of gestation** (recorded in weeks). When correlated with birth weight, this information allows an assessment of fetal growth patterns. The gestational age of any spontaneous abortion is of importance in any subsequent pregnancy.
4. **Type of delivery** (or method of terminating pregnancy). This information is important for planning the method of delivery in the present pregnancy. A difficult forceps delivery or a cesarean section may require a personal review of the labor and delivery records.
5. **Duration of labor** (recorded in hours). This may alert the physician to the possibility of an unusually long or short labor.
6. **Type of anesthesia.** Any complications of anesthesia should be noted.
7. **Maternal complications.** Urinary tract infections, vaginal bleeding, hypertension, and postpartum complications may be repetitive; such knowledge is helpful in anticipating and preventing problems with the present pregnancy.
8. **Newborn weight** (in grams or pounds and ounces). This information may give indications of gestational diabetes, fetal growth problems, shoulder dystocia, or cephalopelvic disproportion.
9. **Newborn gender.** This may provide insight into patient and family expectations and may indicate certain genetic risk factors.
10. **Fetal and neonatal complications.** Certain questions should be asked to elicit any problems and to determine the need to obtain further information. Inquiry should be made as to whether the baby had any problems after it was born, whether the baby breathed and cried right away, and whether the baby left the hospital with the mother.

MENSTRUAL HISTORY

A good menstrual history is essential because it is the determinant for establishing the expected date of confinement (EDC). A modification of **Nägele's rule** for establishing the EDC is to add 9 months and 7 days to the first day of the last normal menstrual period (LMP). For example:

LMP: July 20, 2008
EDC: April 27, 2009

This calculation assumes a normal 28-day cycle, and adjustments must be made for longer or shorter cycles. Any bleeding or spotting since the last normal menstrual period should be reviewed in detail and taken into account when calculating an EDC.

CONTRACEPTIVE HISTORY

This information is important for risk assessment. Oral contraceptives taken during early pregnancy have been associated with birth defects, and retained intrauterine devices (IUDs) can cause early pregnancy loss, infection, and premature delivery.

MEDICAL HISTORY

The importance of a good medical history cannot be overemphasized. In addition to common disorders, such as diabetes mellitus, hypertension, and renal disease, which are known to affect pregnancy outcome, all serious medical conditions should be recorded.

SURGICAL HISTORY

Each surgical procedure should be recorded chronologically, including date, hospital, surgeon, and complications. Trauma must also be listed (e.g., a fractured pelvis may result in diminished pelvic capacity).

SOCIAL HISTORY

Habits such as smoking, alcohol use, and other substance abuse are important factors that must be recorded and managed appropriately. The patient's contact or exposure to domesticated animals, particularly cats (which carry a risk for toxoplasmosis), is important.

The patient's type of work and lifestyle may affect the pregnancy. Exposure to solvents (carbon tetrachloride) or insulators (polychlorobromine compounds) in the workplace may lead to teratogenesis or hepatic toxicity.

◼ *Obstetric Physical Examination*

GENERAL PHYSICAL EXAMINATION

This procedure must be systematic and thorough and performed as early as possible in the prenatal period. A complete physical examination provides an opportunity to detect previously unrecognized abnormalities. Normal baseline levels must also be established, particularly those of weight, blood pressure, funduscopic (retina) appearance, and cardiac status.

PELVIC EXAMINATION

The initial pelvic examination should be done early in the prenatal period and should include the following: (1) inspection of the external genitalia, vagina, and cervix; (2) collection of cytologic specimens from the ectocervix and superficial endocervical canal; and (3) palpation of the cervix, uterus, and adnexa. The initial estimate of gestational age by uterine size becomes less accurate as pregnancy progresses. Rectal and rectovaginal examinations are also important aspects of this initial pelvic evaluation.

CLINICAL PELVIMETRY

This assessment is carried out following the bimanual pelvic examination and before the rectal examination. It is important that clinical pelvimetry be carried out systematically. The details of clinical pelvimetry are described in Chapter 8.

■ Diagnosis of Pregnancy

The diagnosis of pregnancy and its location, based on physical signs and examination alone, may be quite challenging during the early weeks of amenorrhea. Urine pregnancy tests done in the office are reliable a few days after the first missed period, and office ultrasonography is used increasingly as a routine.

SYMPTOMS OF PREGNANCY

The most common symptoms in the early months of pregnancy are amenorrhea, urinary frequency, breast engorgement, nausea, tiredness, and easy fatigability. Amenorrhea in a previously normally menstruating, sexually active woman should be considered to be caused by pregnancy until proved otherwise. Urinary frequency is most likely caused by the pressure of the enlarged uterus on the bladder.

SIGNS OF PREGNANCY

The signs of pregnancy may be divided into presumptive, probable, and positive.

Presumptive Signs

The presumptive signs are primarily those associated with skin and mucous membrane changes. Discoloration and cyanosis of the vulva, vagina, and cervix are related to the generalized engorgement of the pelvic organs and are, therefore, nonspecific. The dark discoloration of the vulva and vaginal walls is known as **Chadwick's sign.** Pigmentation of the skin and abdominal striae are nonspecific and unreliable signs. The most common sites for pigmentation are the midline of the lower abdomen (linea nigra), over the bridge of the nose, and under the eyes. The latter is called chloasma or the mask of pregnancy. Chloasma is also an occasional side effect of oral contraceptives.

Probable Signs

The probable signs of pregnancy are those mainly related to the detectable physical changes in the uterus. During early pregnancy, the uterus changes in size, shape, and consistency. Early uterine enlargement tends to be in the anteroposterior diameter so that the uterus becomes globular. In addition, because of asymmetric implantation of the ovum, one cornua of the uterus may enlarge slightly (**Piskacek's sign**). Uterine consistency becomes softer, and it may be possible to palpate or to compress the connection between the cervix and fundus. This change is referred to as **Hegar's sign.** The cervix also begins to soften early in pregnancy.

Positive Signs

The positive signs of pregnancy include the detection of a fetal heartbeat and the recognition of fetal movements. Modern Doppler techniques for detecting the fetal heartbeat may be successful as early as 9 weeks of gestation and are nearly always positive by 12 weeks. Fetal heart tones can usually be detected with a stethoscope between 16 and 20 weeks. The multiparous woman generally recognizes fetal movements between 15 and 17 weeks, whereas the primigravida usually does not recognize fetal movements until 18 to 20 weeks.

LABORATORY TESTS FOR PREGNANCY

Pregnancy Tests

Tests to detect pregnancy have revolutionized early diagnosis. Although they are considered a probable sign of pregnancy, the accuracy of these tests is very good. All commonly used methods depend on the detection of human chorionic gonadotropin (hCG) or its β subunit in urine or serum. Depending on the specific sensitivity of the test, pregnancy may be suspected even before a missed menstrual period.

Diagnostic Ultrasonography

The imaging technique of ultrasonography has made a significant contribution to the diagnosis and evaluation of pregnancy. Using real-time ultrasonography, an intrauterine gestational sac can be identified at 5 menstrual weeks (21st postovulatory day), and a fetal image can be detected by 6 to 7 weeks. A beating heart is noted at 8 weeks or even sooner with the latest equipment. Radiographic imaging, usually avoided in early pregnancy, depends on detection of the fetal skeleton, which is usually not seen until 16 weeks.

■ Gynecologic History

A full history is equally as important in evaluating the gynecologic patient as in evaluating a patient in general medicine or surgery. The history-taking must be systematic to avoid omissions, and it should be conducted with sensitivity and without haste.

PRESENT ILLNESS

The patient is asked to state her main complaint and to relate her present illness, sequentially, in her own words. Pertinent negative information should be recorded, and as much as possible, questions should be reserved until after the patient has described the course of her illness. Generally, the history provides substantial clues to the diagnosis, so it is important to evaluate fully the more common symptoms encountered in gynecologic patients.

Abnormal Vaginal Bleeding

Vaginal bleeding before the age of 9 years and after the age of 52 years is cause for concern and requires investigation. These are the limits of normal menstruation, and although the occasional woman may menstruate regularly and normally up to the age of 57 or 58 years, it is important to ensure that she is not bleeding from uterine cancer or from exogenous estrogens. Prolongation of menses beyond 7 days or bleeding between menses, except for a brief *kleine regnen* at ovulation, may connote abnormal ovarian function, uterine myomas, or endometriosis.

Abdominal Pain

Many gynecologic problems are associated with abdominal pain. The common gynecologic causes of acute lower abdominal pain are salpingo-oophoritis with peritoneal inflammation, torsion and infarction of an ovarian cyst, endometriosis, or rupture of an ectopic pregnancy. Patterns of pain radiation should be recorded and may provide an important diagnostic clue. Chronic lower abdominal pain is generally associated with endometriosis, chronic pelvic inflammatory disease, or large pelvic tumors. It may also be the first symptom of ovarian cancer.

Amenorrhea

The most common causes of amenorrhea are pregnancy and the normal menopause. It is abnormal for a young woman to reach the age of 16 years without menstruating (primary amenorrhea). Pregnancy should be suspected in a woman between 15 and 45 years of age who fails to menstruate within 35 days from the first day of her last menstruation. In a patient with amenorrhea who is not pregnant, inquiry should be made about menopausal or climacteric symptoms such as hot flashes, vaginal dryness, or mild depression.

Other Symptoms

Other pertinent symptoms of concern include dysmenorrhea, premenstrual tension, fluid retention, leukorrhea, constipation, dyschezia, dyspareunia, and abdominal distention. Lower back and sacral pain may indicate uterine prolapse, enterocele, or rectocele.

MENSTRUAL HISTORY

The menstrual history should include the age at menarche (average is 12 to 13 years), interval between periods (21 to 35 days with a median of 28 days), duration of menses (average is 5 days), and character of the flow (scant, normal, heavy, usually without clots). Any intermenstrual bleeding (metrorrhagia) should be noted. The date of onset of the LMP and the date of the previous menstrual period should be recorded. Inquiry should be made regarding menstrual cramps (dysmenorrhea); if present, the age at onset, severity, and character of the cramps should be recorded, together with an estimate of the disability incurred. Midcycle pain (*mittelschmerz*) and a midcycle increase in vaginal secretions are indicative of ovulatory cycles.

CONTRACEPTIVE HISTORY

The type and duration of each contraceptive method must be recorded, along with any attendant complications. These may include amenorrhea or thromboembolic disease with oral contraceptives; dysmenorrhea, heavy bleeding (menorrhagia), or pelvic infection with the intrauterine device; or contraceptive failure with the diaphragm, contraceptive sponge, or contraceptive cream.

OBSTETRIC HISTORY

Each pregnancy and delivery and any associated complications should be listed sequentially with relevant details and dates.

SEXUAL HISTORY

The health of, and current relationship with, the husband or partner(s) may provide insight into the present complaints. Inquiry should be made regarding any pain (dyspareunia), bleeding, or dysuria associated with sexual intercourse. Sexual satisfaction should be discussed tactfully.

PAST HISTORY

As in the obstetric history, any significant past medical or surgical history should be recorded, as should the patient's family history. A list of current medications is important.

SYSTEMIC REVIEW

A review of all other organ systems should be undertaken. Habits (tobacco, alcohol, other substance abuse), medications, usual weight with recent changes, and loss of height (osteoporosis) are important parts of the systemic review.

■ *Gynecologic Physical Examination*

GENERAL PHYSICAL EXAMINATION

A complete physical examination should be performed on each new patient and repeated at least annually. The initial examination should include the patient's height, weight, and arm span (in adolescent patients or those with endocrine problems) and should be carried out with the patient completely disrobed but suitably draped. The examination should be systematic and should include the following points.

Vital Signs

Temperature, pulse rate, respiratory rate, and blood pressure should be recorded.

General Appearance

The patient's body build, posture, state of nutrition, demeanor, and state of well-being should be recorded.

Head and Neck

Evidence of supraclavicular lymphadenopathy, oral lesions, webbing of the neck, or goiter may be pertinent to the gynecologic assessment.

Breasts

The breast examination is particularly important in gynecologic patients (see Chapters 29 and 31).

Heart and Lungs

Examination of the heart and lungs is of importance, particularly in a patient who requires surgery. The presence of a pleural effusion may be indicative of a disseminated malignancy, particularly ovarian cancer.

Abdomen

Examination of the abdomen is critical in the evaluation of the gynecologic patient. The contour, whether flat, scaphoid, or protuberant, should be noted. The latter appearance may suggest ascites. The presence and distribution of hair, especially in the area of the escutcheon, should be recorded, as should the presence of striae or operative scars.

Abdominal tenderness must be determined by placing one hand flat against the abdomen in the nonpainful areas initially, then gently and gradually exerting pressure with the fingers of the other hand (Figure 2-1). Rebound tenderness (a sign of peritoneal irritation), muscle guarding, and abdominal rigidity should be gently elicited, again first in the nontender areas. A "doughy" abdomen, in which the guarding increases gradually as the pressure of palpation is increased, is often seen with a hemoperitoneum.

It is important to palpate any abdominal mass. The size should be specifically noted. Other characteristics may be even more important, however, in suggesting the diagnosis, such as whether the mass is cystic or solid, smooth or nodular, and fixed or mobile, and whether it is associated with ascites. In determining the reason for abdominal distention (tumor, ascites, or distended bowel), it is important to percuss carefully the areas of tympany (gaseous distention) and dullness. A large tumor is generally dull on top with loops of bowel displaced to the flanks. Dullness that shifts as the patient turns onto her side (shifting dullness) is suggestive of ascites.

Back

Abnormal curvature of the vertebral column (dorsal kyphosis or scoliosis) is an important observation in evaluating osteoporosis in a postmenopausal woman. Costovertebral angle tenderness suggests pyelonephritis, whereas psoas muscle spasm may occur with gynecologic infections or acute appendicitis.

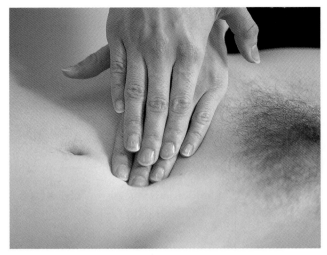

FIGURE 2-1   The abdomen is palpated by placing the left palm flat against the abdominal wall and then gently exerting pressure with the fingers of the right hand.

Extremities

The presence or absence of varicosities, edema, pedal pulsations, and cutaneous lesions may suggest pathologic conditions within the pelvis. The height of pitting edema should be noted (e.g., ankle, shin, to the knee or above).

PELVIC EXAMINATION

The pelvic examination must be conducted systematically and with careful sensitivity. The procedure should be performed with smooth and gentle movements and accompanied by reasonable explanations.

Vulva

The character and distribution of hair, the degree of development or atrophy of the labia, and the character of the hymen (imperforate or cribriform) and introitus (virginal, nulliparous, or multiparous) should be noted. Any clitorimegaly should be noted, as should the presence of cysts, tumors, or inflammation of **Bartholin's gland**. The urethra and **Skene's glands** should be inspected for any purulent exudates. The labia should be inspected for any inflammatory, dystrophic, or neoplastic lesions. Perineal relaxation and scarring should be noted because they may cause dyspareunia and defects in rectal sphincter tone. The urethra should be "milked" for any inflammatory exudates, which if found should be cultured for pathologic organisms.

Speculum Examination

The vagina and cervix should be inspected with an appropriately sized bivalve speculum (Figure 2-2), which should be warmed and lubricated with warm water only, so as not to interfere with the examination

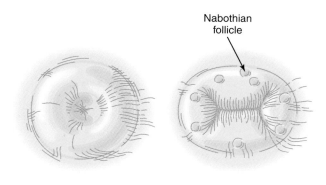

A   NULLIPAROUS   B   MULTIPAROUS

FIGURE 2-3   Cervix of a nulliparous patient (**A**) and a multiparous patient (**B**). Note the circular os in the nulliparous cervix and the transverse os, owing to lacerations at childbirth, in the multiparous cervix.

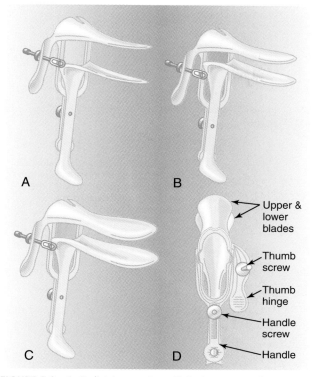

A   B

C   D

FIGURE 2-2   **A:** Pediatric speculum. **B:** Pederson speculum. **C:** Graves speculum. The Pederson speculum has narrower blades and is more appropriate for examining a nulliparous patient. **D:** Parts of a speculum.

of cervical cytology or any vaginal exudate. After gently spreading the labia to expose the introitus, the speculum should be inserted with the blades entering the introitus transversely, then directed posteriorly in the axis of the vagina with pressure exerted against the relatively insensitive perineum to avoid contacting the sensitive urethra. As the anterior blade reaches the cervix, the speculum is opened to bring the cervix into view. As the vaginal epithelium is inspected, it is important to rotate the speculum through 90 degrees, so that lesions on the anterior or posterior walls of the vagina ordinarily covered by the blades of the speculum are not overlooked. Vaginal wall relaxation should be evaluated using either a Sims' speculum or the posterior blade of a bivalve speculum. The patient is asked to bear down (Valsalva's maneuver) or to cough to demonstrate any stress incontinence. If the patient's complaint involves urinary stress or urgency, this portion of the examination should be carried out before the bladder is emptied.

The cervix should be inspected to determine its size, shape, and color. The nulliparous patient generally has a conical, unscarred cervix with a circular, centrally placed os; the multiparous cervix is generally bulbous, and the os has a transverse configuration (Figure 2-3). Any purulent cervical discharge should be cultured. Plugged, distended cervical glands (nabothian follicles) may be seen on the ectocervix. In premenopausal women, the squamocolumnar junction of the cervix is usually visible around the cervical os, particularly in patients of low parity. Postmenopausally, the junction is invariably retracted within the endocervical canal. A cervical cytologic smear (Papanicolaou, or Pap, smear) should be taken before the speculum is withdrawn. The exocervix is gently scraped with a wooden spatula, and the endocervical tissue is gently sampled with a Cytobrush.

Bimanual Examination

The bimanual pelvic examination provides information about the uterus and adnexa (fallopian tubes and ovaries). During this portion of the examination, the urinary bladder should be empty; if it is not, the internal genitalia will be difficult to delineate, and the procedure is more apt to be uncomfortable for the patient. The labia are separated, and the gloved, lubricated index finger is inserted into the vagina, avoiding the sensitive urethral meatus. Pressure is exerted posteriorly against the perineum and puborectalis muscle, which causes the introitus to gape somewhat, thereby usually allowing the middle finger to be inserted as well. Intromission of the two fingers into the depth of the vagina may be facilitated by having the patient bear down slightly.

The cervix is palpated for consistency, contour, size, and tenderness to motion. **If the vaginal fornices are absent, as may occur in postmenopausal women, it is not possible to appreciate the size of the cervix on bimanual examination.** This can be determined only on rectovaginal or rectal examination.

The uterus is evaluated by placing the abdominal hand flat on the abdomen with the fingers pressing

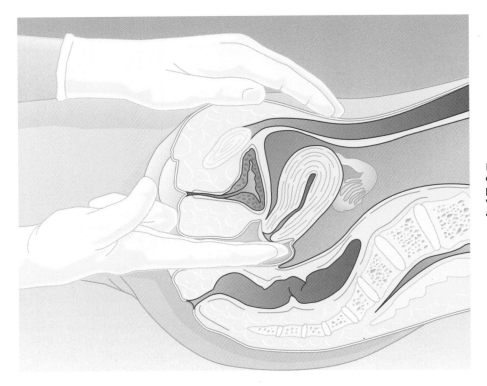

FIGURE 2-4   Bimanual evaluation of the uterus by exerting gentle pressure on the uterus with the vaginal fingers against the abdominal hand.

gently just above the symphysis pubis. With the vaginal fingers supinated in either the anterior or the posterior vaginal fornix, the uterine corpus is pressed gently against the abdominal hand (Figure 2-4). As the uterus is felt between the examining fingers of both hands, the size, configuration, consistency, and mobility of the organ are appreciated. If the muscles of the abdominal wall are not compliant or if the uterus is retroverted, the outline, consistency, and mobility must be determined by ballottement with the vaginal fingers in the fornices; in these circumstances, however, it is impossible to discern uterine size accurately.

By shifting the abdominal hand to either side of the midline and gently elevating the lateral fornix up to the abdominal hand, it may be possible to outline a right adnexal mass (Figure 2-5). The left adnexa are best appreciated with the fingers of the left hand in the vagina (Figure 2-6). The examiner should stand sideways, facing the patient's left, with the left hip maintaining pressure against the left elbow, thereby providing better tactile sensation because of the relaxed musculature in the forearm and examining hand. The **pouch of Douglas** is also carefully assessed for nodularity or tenderness, as may occur with endometriosis, pelvic inflammatory disease, or metastatic carcinoma.

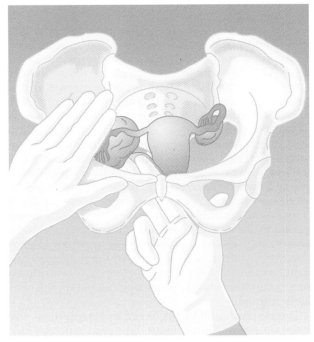

FIGURE 2-5   Bimanual examination of the right adnexa. Note that fingers of the right hand are in the vagina.

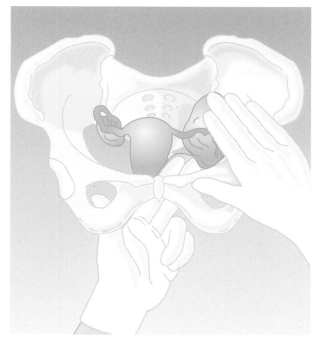

FIGURE 2-6   Bimanual examination of the left adnexa. Note that fingers of the left hand are in the vagina.

It is usually impossible to feel the normal tube, and conditions must be optimal to appreciate the normal ovary. The normal ovary has the size and consistency of a shelled oyster and may be felt with the vaginal fingers as they are passed across the undersurface of the abdominal hand. The ovaries are very tender to compression, and the patient is uncomfortably aware of any ovarian compression or movement during the examination.

It may be impossible to differentiate between an ovarian and tubal mass, and even a lateral uterine mass. Generally, left adnexal masses are more difficult to evaluate than those on the right because of the position of the sigmoid colon on the left side of the pelvis. An ultrasonic examination should be helpful for delineating these features.

RECTAL EXAMINATION

The anus should be inspected for lesions, hemorrhoids, or inflammation. Rectal sphincter tone should be recorded and any mucosal lesions noted. A guaiac test should be performed to determine the presence of occult blood.

A rectovaginal examination is helpful in evaluating masses in the cul-de-sac, the rectovaginal septum, or adnexa. It is essential in evaluating the parametrium in patients with cervical cancer. Rectal examination may also be essential in differentiating between a rectocele and an enterocele (Figure 2-7).

LABORATORY EVALUATION

Appropriate laboratory tests normally include a urinalysis, complete blood count, erythrocyte sedimentation rate, and blood chemistry analyses. Special tests, such as tumor marker and hormone assays, are performed when indicated.

ASSESSMENT

A reasonable differential diagnosis should be possible with the information gleaned from the history, physical examination, and laboratory tests. The plan of management should aim toward a chemical or histologic confirmation of the presumptive diagnosis, and the appropriate therapeutic options, along with the rationale for each option, should be recorded.

◾ Patients with Special Needs

THE PEDIATRIC AND ADOLESCENT PATIENT

Girls experience fewer gynecologic problems than do adult women, but their concerns need to be met effectively and skillfully in a way that will allay anxiety and create a positive attitude toward their gynecologic health. Unique complaints fall generally into a handful of categories: congenital anomalies, genital injuries, inflammation of the nonestrogenized genital tract, pubertal problems, and psychosexual concerns. Genital ambiguity, trauma, and vaginal bleeding in the prepubertal child are covered briefly in this chapter.

GENITAL AMBIGUITY

Dealing with genital ambiguity in the newborn requires a coordinated and timely response. **The family's psychological well-being must be addressed because they must feel confident in the gender identity of their child.** Ambiguity can result from masculinization of a female child due to exogenous hormone ingestion or maternal or fetal overproduction of androgen. It may also result from incomplete virilization of a male infant, hormonal insensitivity, gonadal dysgenesis, or chromosomal anomalies (see Chapters 31 and 32). **When assessing an infant with ambiguous genitals, fluid and electrolyte balance should be monitored and blood drawn for 17-hydroxyprogesterone and cortisol to rule out 21-hydroxylase deficiency.** Life-threatening illness may be missed in children with the salt-losing form of congenital adrenal hyperplasia (see Chapter 32).

TRAUMA

Straddle injuries are the most common cause of trauma to the genitalia of a young girl, and the injuries have a seasonal peak when bicycles come out in the spring. Most of these injuries are to the labia. Penetrating vaginal injuries can cause major intraabdominal damage with minimal external findings. **Sexual assault**

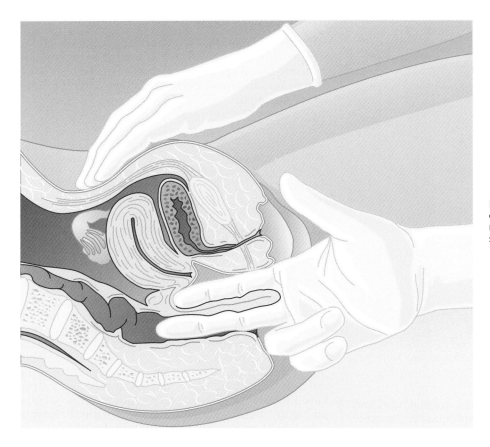

FIGURE 2-7 Rectovaginal bimanual examination. During Valsalva's maneuver, an enterocele will separate the two fingers.

must always be considered. After a life-threatening condition is ruled out, an ice pack, chilled bag of intravenous solution, or cool compress may be applied to the injured area and the child allowed to rest quietly for 20 minutes before being assessed further. Extensive injuries usually require examination under anesthesia and surgical repair.

In any case of trauma, concurrent damage to the rectum or urinary tract should be considered. **If there is any reason to suspect sexual or physical abuse, the child protection authorities must be notified, and the examination should include the collection of medicolegal evidence.**

VAGINAL BLEEDING IN THE PREPUBERTAL CHILD

Vaginal bleeding is a frequent and distressing complaint in childhood. Although it will most often be of benign cause, more serious pathologic processes must always be ruled out. Vaginal bleeding in the newborn is most often physiologic as a result of maternal estrogen withdrawal. In such cases, there should be supportive evidence of a hormonal effect, such as the presence of breast tissue and pale, engorged vaginal epithelium.

Bleeding disorders are uncommon in this age group but should be considered. Vitamin K is routinely given to the newborn, but some patients may refuse the medication.

Precocious puberty (see Chapter 31) may present with vaginal bleeding, although most commonly other evidence of maturation will have preceded the bleeding and will be evident on examination. At the very least, a pale, estrogenized vaginal epithelium will be seen, and cytologic analysis of the vagina will confirm the hormonal effect. Transient precocious puberty may occur in response to a **functional ovarian cyst,** and vaginal bleeding may be triggered by the spontaneous resolution of the cyst. **Exogenous hormonal exposure** should be considered because children have been known to ingest birth control pills. **Ovarian tumors** resulting in pseudoprecocious puberty should be ruled out.

Vulvovaginitis is common but is a diagnosis of exclusion. When bleeding is present, it is necessary to assess the vagina and to rule out a foreign body or vaginal tumor.

Vaginal tumors are the most serious possibility to be considered. **Sarcoma botryoides** classically presents with vaginal bleeding and grape-like vesicles. Fortunately, this is a rare tumor.

The Geriatric Patient

The gynecologic assessment of the elderly woman may present a special challenge. Many older patients tend to underreport their symptoms, possibly because of a belief that any new physical problems are due to the normal aging process. Also, a fear of loss of their independence may contribute to this denial, and this may lead to a delay of diagnosis and perhaps a worse prognosis. In addition to the routine gynecologic history and physical examination, these patients should be evaluated for any sensory impairment (such as visual or hearing loss), any impaired mobility, malnutrition, urinary incontinence, or confusion, which may be due to polypharmacy. Appropriate referral, when improvement can be reasonably expected, should be considered for these problems once identified.

Gynecologic conditions such as atrophic vaginitis, uterine and vaginal prolapse, and genital tract malignancies are among the more common problems encountered in the geriatric patient.

Patients with Disabilities

Women with developmental or acquired disabilities should receive the same high-quality obstetric and gynecologic care as anyone else, with a goal of sustaining their best level of functioning. Assisting families of mentally or physically disabled individuals with obstetric or gynecologic problems or attending to them in special institutions can be quite challenging. The woman with a disability is a person with special and unique needs, and communicating to her a sense of caring and respect is paramount.

SUGGESTED READING

American College of Obstetricians and Gynecologists: The initial reproductive health visit. ACOG Committee Opinion No. 335. Obstet Gynecol 100:1413-1416, 2006.

Cope Z: The Early Diagnosis of the Acute Abdomen. London, Oxford Medical Publications, 2001.

Lewis MA, Mickman JL: Approach to the patient with developmental disabilities. *In* Pregler JP, DeCherney AH (eds): Women's Health: Principles and Clinical Practice. Hamilton, Ontario, BC Decker, 2002.

Pham T: Approach to the geriatric patient. *In* Pregler JP, DeCherney AH (eds): Women's Health: Principles and Clinical Practice. Hamilton, Ontario, BC Decker, 2002.

Wilkes MS, Anderson M: Approach to the adolescent patent. *In* Pregler JP, DeCherney AH (eds): Women's Health: Principles and Clinical Practice. Hamilton, Ontario, BC Decker, 2002.

Chapter 3

Female Reproductive Anatomy and Embryology

JOSEPH C. GAMBONE

The scope of obstetrics and gynecology assumes a reasonable background in reproductive anatomy, embryology, physiology (see Chapter 4), and endocrinology (see Chapter 5 and Part 4). A physician cannot effectively practice obstetrics and gynecology without understanding the physiologic processes that transpire in a woman's life as she passes through infancy, adolescence, reproductive maturity, and the climacteric. As the various clinical problems are addressed, it is important to consider those anatomic, developmental, and physiologic changes that normally take place at key points in a woman's life cycle.

Most of this chapter deals with the disruptive deviations from normal female anatomy and physiology, whether congenital, functional, traumatic, inflammatory, neoplastic, or even iatrogenic. As the etiology and pathogenesis of clinical problems are considered, each should be studied in the context of normal anatomy, development, and physiology.

◼ Development of the External Genitalia

Before the 7th week of development, the appearance of the external genital area is the same in males and females. Elongation of the genital tubercle into a phallus with a clearly defined terminal glans portion is noted in the 7th week, and gross inspection at this time may lead to faulty sexual identification. Ventrally and caudally, the urogenital membrane, made up of both endodermal and ectodermal cells, further differentiates into the genital folds laterally and the urogenital folds medially. **The lateral genital folds develop into the labia majora, whereas the urogenital folds develop subsequently into the labia minora and prepuce of the clitoris.**

The external genitalia of the fetus are readily distinguishable as female at about 12 weeks (Figure 3-1). In the male, the urethral ostium is located conspicuously on the elongated phallus by this time and is smaller, owing to urogenital fold fusion dorsally, which produces a prominent raphe from the anus to the urethral ostium. In the female, the hymen is usually perforated by the time delivery occurs.

◼ Anatomy of the External Genitalia

The perineum represents the inferior boundary of the pelvis. It is bounded superiorly by the levator ani muscles and inferiorly by the skin between the thighs (Figure 3-2). Anteriorly, the perineum extends to the symphysis pubis and the inferior borders of the pubic bones. Posteriorly, it is limited by the ischial tuberosities, the sacrotuberous ligaments, and the coccyx. **The superficial and deep transverse perineal muscles cross the pelvic outlet between the two ischial tuberosities and come together at the perineal body. They divide the space into the urogenital triangle anteriorly and the anal triangle posteriorly.**

The urogenital diaphragm is a fibromuscular sheet that stretches across the pubic arch. It is pierced by the vagina, the urethra, the artery of the bulb, the internal pudendal vessels, and the dorsal nerve of the clitoris. Its inferior surface is covered by the crura of the clitoris, the vestibular bulbs, the greater vestibular (Bartholin's) glands, and the superficial perineal muscles. Bartholin's glands are situated just posterior to the vestibular bulbs, and their ducts empty into the introitus just below the labia minora. They are often the site of gonococcal infections and painful abscesses.

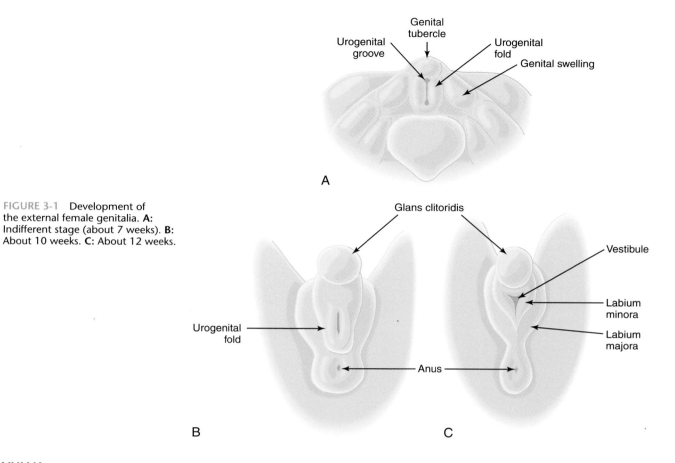

FIGURE 3-1   Development of the external female genitalia. **A:** Indifferent stage (about 7 weeks). **B:** About 10 weeks. **C:** About 12 weeks.

VULVA

The external genitalia are referred to collectively as the vulva. As shown in Figure 3-3, **the vulva includes the mons veneris, labia majora, labia minora, clitoris, vulvovaginal (Bartholin's) glands, fourchette, and perineum.** The most prominent features of the vulva, the labia majora, are large, hair-covered folds of skin that contain sebaceous glands and subcutaneous fat and lie on either side of the introitus. The labia minora lie medially and contain no hair but have a rich supply of venous sinuses, sebaceous glands, and nerves. The labia minora may vary from scarcely noticeable structures to leaf-like flaps measuring up to 3 cm in length. Anteriorly, each splits into two folds. The posterior two folds attach to the inferior surface of the clitoris, at which point they unite to form the frenulum of the clitoris. The anterior folds are united in a hood-like configuration over the clitoris, forming the prepuce. Posteriorly, the labia minora may extend almost to the fourchette.

The clitoris lies just in front of the urethra and consists of the glans, the body, and the crura. Only the glans clitoris is visible externally. The body, composed of a pair of corpora cavernosa, extends superiorly for a distance of several centimeters and divides into two crura, which are attached to the undersurface of either pubic ramus. Each crus is covered by the corresponding ischiocavernosus muscle. Each vestibular bulb (equivalent to the corpus spongiosum of the penis) extends posteriorly from the glans on either side of the lower vagina. Each bulb is attached to the inferior surface of the perineal membrane and covered by the bulbocavernosus muscle. These muscles aid in constricting the venous supply to the erectile vestibular bulbs and also act as the sphincter vaginae.

As the labia minora are spread, the vaginal introitus, guarded by the hymenal ring, is seen. Usually, the hymen is represented only by a circle of carunculae myrtiformes around the vaginal introitus. The hymen may take many forms, however, such as a cribriform plate with many small openings or a completely imperforate diaphragm.

The vestibule of the vagina is that portion of the introitus extending inferiorly from the hymenal ring between the labia minora. The fourchette represents the posterior portion of the vestibule just above the perineal body. **Most of the vulva is innervated by the branches of the pudendal nerve. Anterior to the urethra, the vulva is innervated by the ilioinguinal and**

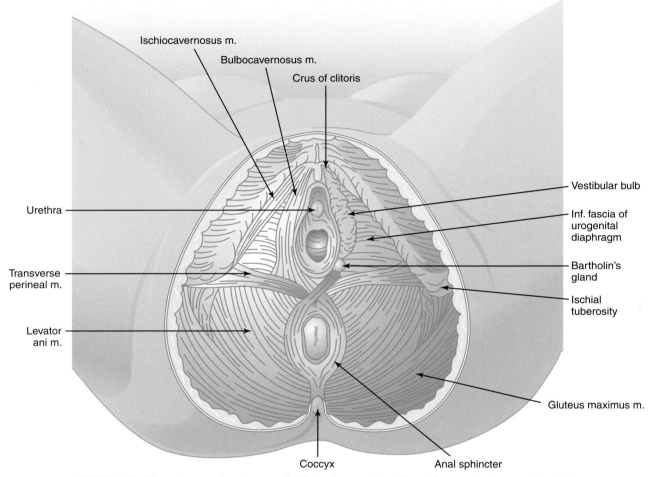

Ischiocavernosus m.

Bulbocavernosus m.

Crus of clitoris

Vestibular bulb

Urethra

Inf. fascia of urogenital diaphragm

Bartholin's gland

Transverse perineal m.

Ischial tuberosity

Levator ani m.

Gluteus maximus m.

Coccyx   Anal sphincter

FIGURE 3-2   The perineum, showing superficial structures on the left and deeper structures on the right.

genitofemoral nerves. This area is not anesthetized adequately by a pudendal block, and repair of paraurethral tears should be supplemented by additional subcutaneous anesthesia.

■ *Internal Genital Development*

The upper vagina, cervix, uterus, and fallopian tubes are formed from the paramesonephric (müllerian) ducts. Although human embryos, whether male or female, possess both paired paramesonephric and mesonephric (wolffian) ducts, **the absence of Y chromosomal influence leads to the development of the paramesonephric system with virtual total regression of the mesonephric system.** With a Y chromosome present, a testis is formed and müllerian-inhibiting substance is produced, creating the reverse situation.

Mesonephric duct development occurs in each urogenital ridge between weeks 2 and 4 and is thought to influence the growth and development of the paramesonephric ducts. **The mesonephric ducts terminate caudally by opening into the urogenital sinus.** First evidence of each paramesonephric duct is seen at 6 weeks' gestation as a groove in the coelomic epithelium of the paired urogenital ridges, lateral to the cranial pole of the mesonephric duct. **Each paramesonephric duct opens into the coelomic cavity cranially** at a point destined to become a tubal ostium. Coursing caudally at first, parallel to the developing mesonephric duct, the blind distal end of each paramesonephric duct eventually crosses dorsal to the mesonephric duct, and the two ducts approximate in the midline. **The two paramesonephric ducts fuse terminally at the urogenital septum, forming the uterovaginal primordium.** The distal point of fusion is known as the **müllerian tubercle (Müller's tubercle)** and can be seen protruding into the urogenital sinus dorsally in embryos at 9 to 10 weeks' gestation (Figure 3-4). **Later**

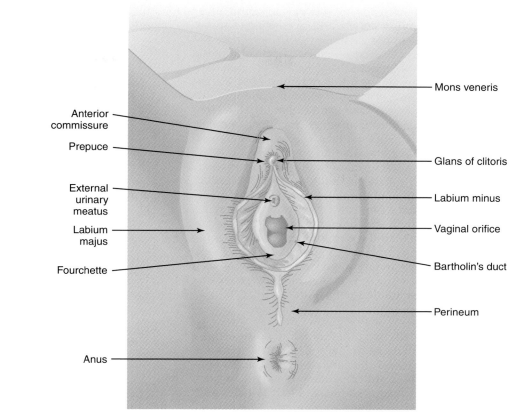

Anterior commissure

Prepuce

External urinary meatus

Labium majus

Fourchette

Anus

Mons veneris

Glans of clitoris

Labium minus

Vaginal orifice

Bartholin's duct

Perineum

FIGURE 3-3 Female external genitalia.

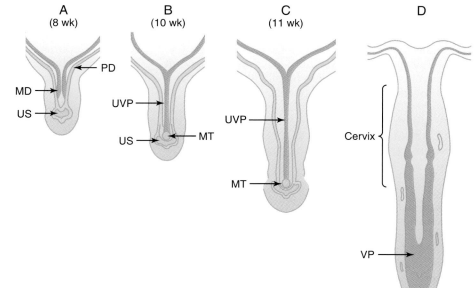

A (8 wk)

B (10 wk)

C (11 wk)

D

PD

MD

US

UVP

US

MT

UVP

MT

Cervix

VP

US

FIGURE 3-4 Early embryologic development of the genital tract (**A** to **C**) and vaginal plate (**D**). MD, mesonephric duct; MT, müllerian tubercle; PD, paramesonephric duct; UVP, uterovaginal primordium; US, urogenital sinus; VP, vaginal plate. *(Redrawn from Didusch JF, Koff AK: Contrib Embryol Carnegie Inst 24:61, 1933.)*

dissolution of the septum between the fused para-mesonephric ducts leads to the development of a single uterine fundus, cervix, and, according to some investigators, the upper vagina.

Degeneration of the mesonephric ducts is progressive from 10 to 16 weeks in the female fetus, although vestigial remnants of the latter may be noted in the adult (Gartner's duct cyst, paroöphoron, epoöphoron) (Figure 3-5). The myometrium and endometrial stroma are derived from adjacent mesenchyme; the glandular epithelium of the fallopian tubes, uterus, and cervix is derived from the paramesonephric duct.

Solid vaginal plate formation and lengthening occur from the 12th through the 20th weeks, followed by caudad to cephalad canalization, which is usually completed in utero. Controversy surrounds the relative contribution of the urogenital sinus and paramesonephric ducts to the development of the vagina, and it is uncertain whether the whole of the vaginal plate is formed secondary to growth of the endoderm of the urogenital sinus or whether the upper vagina is formed from the paramesonephric ducts.

VAGINA

The vagina is a flattened tube extending posterosuperiorly from the hymenal ring at the introitus up to the fornices that surround the cervix (Figure 3-6). **Its epithelium, which is stratified squamous in type, is normally devoid of mucous glands and hair follicles and is nonkeratinized.** Gestational exposure to diethylstilbestrol (taken by the mother) may result in columnar glands interspersed with the squamous epithelium of the upper two thirds of the vagina (vaginal adenosis). Deep to the vaginal epithelium are the muscular coats of the vagina, which consist of an inner circular and an outer longitudinal smooth muscle layer. Remnants of the mesonephric ducts may sometimes be demonstrated along the vaginal wall in the subepithelial layers and may give rise to **Gartner's duct cysts.** The adult vagina averages about 8 cm in length, although its size varies considerably with age, parity, and the status of ovarian function. An important anatomic feature is the immediate proximity of the posterior fornix of the vagina to the pouch of Douglas, which allows easy access to the peritoneal cavity from the vagina, by either culdocentesis or colpotomy.

UTERUS

The uterus consists of the cervix and the uterine corpus, which are joined by the isthmus. The uterine isthmus represents a transitional area wherein the endocervical epithelium gradually changes into the endometrial lining. In late pregnancy, this area elongates and is referred to as the lower uterine segment.

The cervix is generally 2 to 3 cm in length. In infants and children, the cervix is proportionately longer

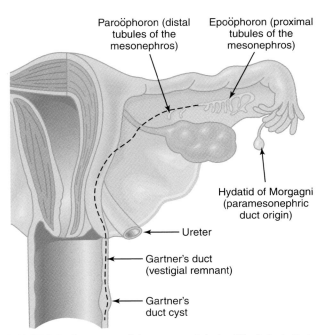

FIGURE 3-5   Remnants of the mesonephric (wolffian) ducts that may persist in the anterolateral vagina or adjacent to the uterus within the broad ligament or mesosalpinx.

than the uterine corpus (Figure 3-7). The portion that protrudes into the vagina and is surrounded by the fornices is covered with a nonkeratinizing squamous epithelium. **At about the external cervical os, the squamous epithelium covering the ectocervix changes to simple columnar epithelium, the site of transition being referred to as the squamocolumnar junction.** The cervical canal is lined by irregular, arborized, simple columnar epithelium, which extends into the stroma as cervical "glands" or crypts.

The uterine corpus is a thick, pear-shaped organ, somewhat flattened anteroposteriorly, that consists of largely interlacing smooth muscle fibers. The endometrial lining of the uterine corpus may vary from 2 to 10 mm in thickness (which may be measured by ultrasonic imaging), depending on the stage of the menstrual cycle. Most of the surface of the uterus is covered by the peritoneal mesothelium.

Four paired sets of ligaments are attached to the uterus (Figure 3-8). Each round ligament inserts on the anterior surface of the uterus just in front of the fallopian tube, passes to the pelvic side wall in a fold of the broad ligament, traverses the inguinal canal, and ends in the labium majus. **The round ligaments are of little supportive value in preventing uterine prolapse** but help to keep the uterus anteverted. **The uterosacral ligaments** are condensations of the endopelvic fascia that arise

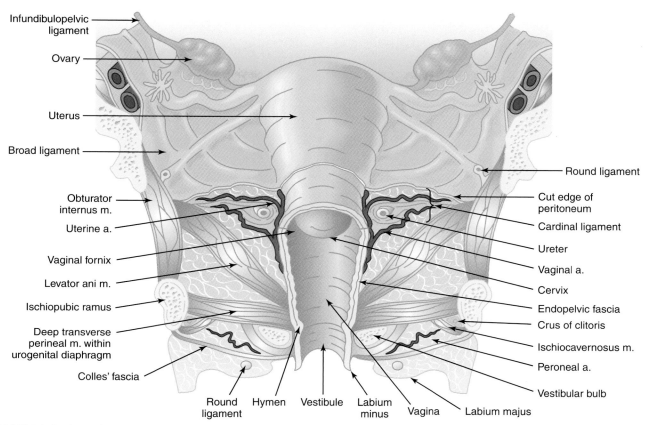

Infundibulopelvic ligament

Ovary

Uterus

Broad ligament

Obturator internus m.

Uterine a.

Vaginal fornix

Levator ani m.

Ischiopubic ramus

Deep transverse perineal m. within urogenital diaphragm

Colles' fascia

Round ligament

Cut edge of peritoneum

Cardinal ligament

Ureter

Vaginal a.

Cervix

Endopelvic fascia

Crus of clitoris

Ischiocavernosus m.

Peroneal a.

Vestibular bulb

Round ligament   Hymen   Vestibule   Labium minus   Vagina   Labium majus

FIGURE 3-6   Coronal section of the pelvis at the level of the uterine isthmus and ischial spines, showing the ligaments supporting the uterus.

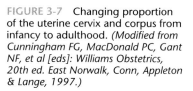
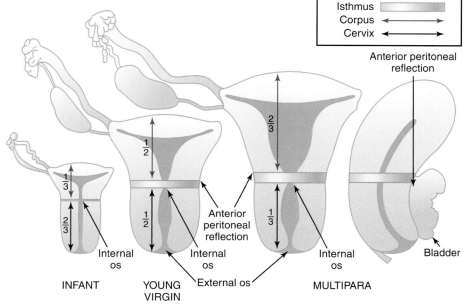

FIGURE 3-7   Changing proportion of the uterine cervix and corpus from infancy to adulthood. *(Modified from Cunningham FG, MacDonald PC, Gant NF, et al [eds]: Williams Obstetrics, 20th ed. East Norwalk, Conn, Appleton & Lange, 1997.)*

Isthmus
Corpus
Cervix

Anterior peritoneal reflection

$\frac{2}{3}$

$\frac{1}{2}$

$\frac{1}{3}$

$\frac{2}{3}$

$\frac{1}{2}$

$\frac{1}{3}$

Internal os

Internal os

Internal os

Bladder

Anterior peritoneal reflection

External os

INFANT

YOUNG VIRGIN

MULTIPARA

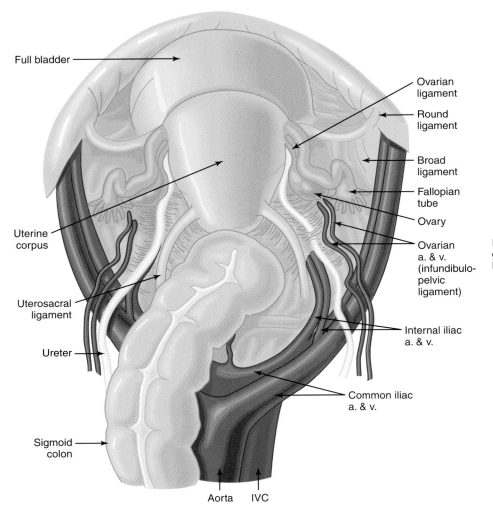

Full bladder

Ovarian ligament

Round ligament

Broad ligament

Fallopian tube

Ovary

Uterine corpus

Ovarian a. & v. (infundibulo-pelvic ligament)

Uterosacral ligament

Internal iliac a. & v.

Ureter

Common iliac a. & v.

Sigmoid colon

Aorta   IVC

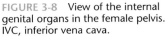

FIGURE 3-8   View of the internal genital organs in the female pelvis. IVC, inferior vena cava.

from the sacral fascia and insert into the posteroinferior portion of the uterus at about the level of the isthmus. These ligaments contain sympathetic and parasympathetic nerve fibers that supply the uterus. They provide important support for the uterus and are also significant in precluding the development of an enterocele. **The cardinal ligaments (Mackenrodt's)** are the other important supporting structures of the uterus that prevent prolapse. They extend from the pelvic fascia on the lateral pelvic walls and insert into the lateral portion of the cervix and vagina, reaching superiorly to the level of the isthmus. **The pubocervical ligaments** pass anteriorly around the bladder to the posterior surface of the pubic symphysis.

In addition, there are four peritoneal folds. Anteriorly, **the vesicouterine fold** is reflected from the level of the uterine isthmus onto the bladder. Posteriorly, **the rectouterine fold** passes from the posterior

wall of the uterus, to the upper fourth of the vagina, and thence onto the rectum. The pouch between the cervix and vagina anteriorly and rectum posteriorly forms a cul-de-sac, called the pouch of Douglas. Laterally, the **two broad ligaments** each pass from the side of the uterus to the lateral wall of the pelvis. Between the two leaves of each broad ligament are contained the fallopian tube, the round ligament, and the ovarian ligament, in addition to nerves, blood vessels, and lymphatics. **The fold of broad ligament containing the fallopian tube is called the mesosalpinx.** Between the end of the tube and ovary and the pelvic side wall, where the ureter passes over the common iliac vessels, is the infundibulopelvic ligament, which contains the vessels and nerves for the ovary. The ureter may be injured when this ligament is ligated during a salpingo-oophorectomy procedure.

FALLOPIAN TUBES

The oviducts are bilateral muscular tubes (about 10 cm in length) with lumina that connect the uterine cavity with the peritoneal cavity. They are enclosed in the medial four fifths of the superior aspect of the broad ligament. The tubes are lined by a ciliated, columnar epithelium that is thrown into branching folds. That segment of the tube within the wall of the uterus is referred to as the **interstitial portion.** The medial portion of each tube is superior to the round ligament, anterior to the ovarian ligament, and relatively fixed in position. This nonmobile portion of the tube has a fairly narrow lumen and is referred to as the **isthmus.** As the tube proceeds laterally, it is located anterior to the ovary; it then passes around the lateral portion of the ovary and down toward the cul-de-sac. The **ampullary and fimbriated portions** of the tube are suspended from the broad ligament by the mesosalpinx and are quite mobile. The mobility of the fimbriated end of the tube plays an important role in fertility. The ampullary portion of the tube is the most common site of ectopic pregnancies.

◼ Normal Embryologic Development of the Ovary

The earliest anatomic event in gonadogenesis is noted at about 4 weeks' gestational age (i.e., 4 weeks from conception), when a thickening of the peritoneal, or coelomic, epithelium on the ventromedial surface of the urogenital ridge occurs. A bulging **genital ridge** is subsequently produced by rapid proliferation of the coelomic epithelium in an area that is medial, but parallel, to the mesonephric ridge. Before 5 weeks, this indifferent gonad consists of germinal epithelium surrounding the internal blastema, a primordial mesenchymal cellular mass designated to become the ovarian medulla. After 5 weeks, projections from the germinal epithelium extend like spokes into the mesenchymal blastema to form **primary sex cords.** Soon thereafter at 7 weeks, a testis can be identified histologically if the embryo has a Y chromosome. In the absence of a Y chromosome, definitive ovarian characteristics do not appear until somewhere between 12 and 16 weeks.

As early as 3 weeks' gestation, relatively large primordial germ cells appear intermixed with other cells in the endoderm of the yolk sac wall of the primitive hindgut. These germ cell precursors migrate along the hindgut dorsal mesentery (Figure 3-9) and are all contained in the mesenchyme of the undifferentiated urogenital ridge by 8 weeks' gestation. Subsequent replication of these cells by mitotic division occurs, with maximal mitotic activity noted up to 20 weeks and cessation noted by term. These oogonia, the end result of this germ cell proliferation, are incorporated into the cortical sex cords of the genital ridge.

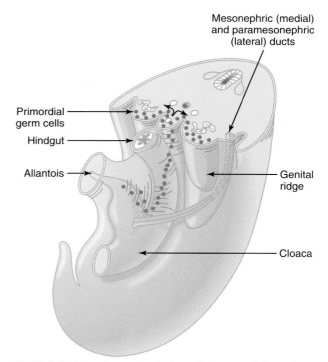

FIGURE 3-9   Migratory path of primordial germ cells from the yolk sac, along the hindgut mesentery, to the urogenital ridge at about 5 weeks.

Histologically, the first evidence of follicles is seen at about 20 weeks, with germ cells surrounded by flattened cells derived from the cortical sex cords. These flattened cells are recognizable as granulosa cells of coelomic epithelial origin and theca cells of mesenchymal origin. The oogonia enter the prophase of the first meiotic division and are then called **primary oocytes** (see Chapter 4). It has been estimated that more than 2 million primary oocytes, or their precursors, are present at 20 weeks' gestation, but only about 300,000 to 500,000 primordial follicles are present by 7 years of age.

Regression of the primary sex cords in the medulla produces the **rete ovarii,** which are found histologically in the hilus of the ovary along with another testicular analogue called **Leydig's cells,** which are thought to be derived from mesenchyme. Vestiges of the rete ovarii and of the degenerating mesonephros may also be noted at times in the mesovarium or mesosalpinx. Structural homologues in males and females are shown in Table 3-1.

ANATOMY OF THE OVARIES

The ovaries are oval, flattened, compressible organs, about 3 × 2 × 2 cm in size. They are situated on the superior surface of the broad ligament and are

TABLE 3-1

STRUCTURAL HOMOLOGUES IN MALES AND FEMALES

Primordia	Female	Male	Major Determining Factors
GONADAL			
Germ cells	Oogonia	Spermatogonia	Sex chromosomes
Coelomic epithelium	Granulosa cells	Sertoli cells	
Mesenchyme	Theca cells	Leydig cells	
Mesonephros	Rete ovarii	Rete testis	
DUCTAL			
Paramesonephric (müllerian) duct	Fallopian tubes Uterus Superior 2/3 of vagina	Hydatid testis	Absence of Y chromosome
Mesonephric (wolffian) duct	Gartner's duct	Vas deferens Seminal vesicles	Testosterone Müllerian inhibiting factor
Mesonephric tubules	Epoöphoron	Epididymis	
	Paroöphoron	Efferent ducts	
EXTERNAL GENITALIA			
Urogenital sinus	Vaginal contribution Skene's glands Bartholin's glands	Prostate Prostatic utricle Cowper's glands	Presence or absence of testosterone, dihydrotestosterone (DHT), and 5α-reductase enzyme
Genital tubercle	Clitoris	Penis	
Urogenital folds	Labia minora	Corpora spongiosa	
Genital folds	Labia majora	Scrotum	

suspended between the ovarian ligament medially and the suspensory ligament of the ovary or infundibulopelvic ligament laterally and superiorly. Each occupies a position in the ovarian fossa (of Waldeyer), which is a shallow depression on the lateral pelvic wall just posterior to the external iliac vessels and anterior to the ureter and hypogastric vessels. In endometriosis and salpingo-oophoritis, the ovaries may be densely adherent to the ureter. Generally, the serosal covering and the tunica albuginea of the ovary are quite thin, and developing follicles and corpora lutea are readily visible.

The blood supply to the ovaries is provided by the long ovarian arteries, which arise from the abdominal aorta immediately below the renal arteries. These vessels course downward and cross laterally over the ureter at the level of the pelvic brim, passing branches to the ureter and the fallopian tube. The ovary also receives substantial blood supply from the uterine artery through the uterine-ovarian arterial anastomosis. **The venous drainage from the right ovary is directly into the inferior vena cava, whereas that from the left ovary is into the left renal vein** (Figure 3-10).

ANATOMY OF THE URETERS

The ureters extend 25 to 30 cm from the renal pelves to their insertion into the bladder at the trigone. Each descends immediately under the peritoneum, crossing the pelvic brim beneath the ovarian vessels just anterior to the bifurcation of the common iliac artery. In the true pelvis, the ureter initially courses inferiorly, just anterior to the hypogastric vessels, and stays closely attached to the peritoneum. It then passes forward along the side of the cervix and beneath the uterine artery toward the trigone of the bladder.

LYMPHATIC DRAINAGE

The lymphatic drainage of the vulva and lower vagina is principally to the inguinofemoral lymph nodes and then to the external iliac chains (see Figure 3-10). The lymphatic drainage of the cervix takes place through the parametria (cardinal ligaments) to the pelvic nodes (the hypogastric, obturator, and external iliac groups) and then to the common iliac and para-aortic chains. The lymphatic drainage from the endometrium is through the broad ligament and infundibulopelvic ligament to the pelvic and para-aortic chains. The

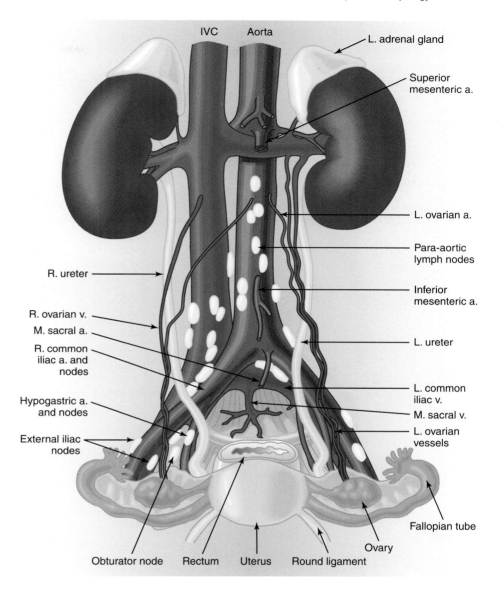

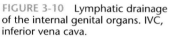

FIGURE 3-10   Lymphatic drainage of the internal genital organs. IVC, inferior vena cava.

ANATOMY OF THE LOWER ABDOMINAL WALL

lymphatics of the ovaries pass via the infundibulopelvic ligaments to the pelvic and para-aortic nodes (see Figure 3-10).

Because most intraabdominal gynecologic operations are performed through lower abdominal incisions, it is important to review the anatomy of the lower abdominal wall with special reference to the muscles and fasciae. After transecting the skin, subcutaneous fat, superficial fascia (Camper's), and deep fascia (Scarpa's), the anterior rectus sheath is encountered (Figure 3-11). **The rectus sheath is a strong fibrous compartment formed by the aponeuroses of the three lateral abdominal wall muscles.** The aponeuroses meet in the midline to form the linea alba and partially encase the two rectus abdominis muscles. The composition of the rectus sheath differs in its upper and lower portions. Above the midpoint between the umbilicus and the symphysis pubis, the rectus muscle is encased anteriorly by the aponeurosis of the external oblique and the anterior lamina of the internal oblique aponeurosis and posteriorly by the aponeurosis of the transversus abdominis and the posterior lamina of the internal oblique aponeurosis. **In the lower fourth of the abdomen, the posterior aponeurotic layer of the sheath terminates in a free crescentic margin, the semilunar fold of Douglas.**

Each rectus abdominis muscle, encased in the rectus sheath on either side of the midline, extends from the

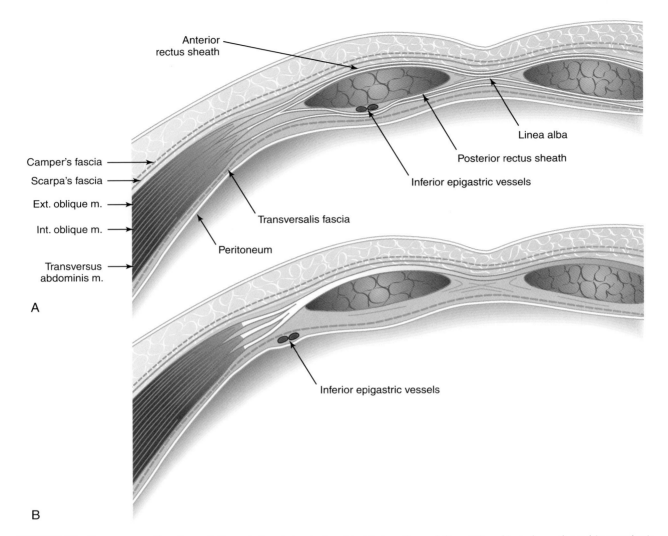

Anterior rectus sheath

Camper's fascia

Scarpa's fascia

Ext. oblique m.

Int. oblique m.

Transversus abdominis m.

Linea alba

Posterior rectus sheath

Inferior epigastric vessels

Transversalis fascia

Peritoneum

A

Inferior epigastric vessels

B

FIGURE 3-11   Transverse section through the anterior abdominal wall just below the umbilicus (**A**) and just above the pubic symphysis (**B**). Note the absence of the posterior rectus sheath in **B**.

superior aspect of the symphysis pubis to the anterior surface of the fifth, sixth, and seventh costal cartilages. A variable number of tendinous intersections (three to five) crosses each muscle at irregular intervals, and any transverse rectus surgical incision forms a new fibrous intersection during healing. The muscle is not attached to the posterior sheath and, following separation from the anterior sheath, can be retracted laterally, as in the Pfannenstiel incision. **Each rectus muscle has a firm aponeurosis at its attachment to the symphysis pubis, and this tendinous aponeurosis can be transected if necessary to improve exposure, as in the Cherney incision,** and resutured securely during closure of the abdominal wall.

The inferior epigastric arteries arise from the external iliac arteries and proceed superiorly just lateral to the rectus muscles between the transversalis fascia and the peritoneum. They enter the rectus sheaths at the level of the semilunar line and continue their course superiorly just posterior to the rectus muscles. In a transverse rectus muscle–cutting incision, the epigastric arteries can be retracted laterally or ligated to allow a wide peritoneal incision.

ABDOMINAL WALL INCISIONS

The most commonly used lower abdominal incision in gynecologic surgery is the Pfannenstiel incision (Figure 3-12). Although it does not always give

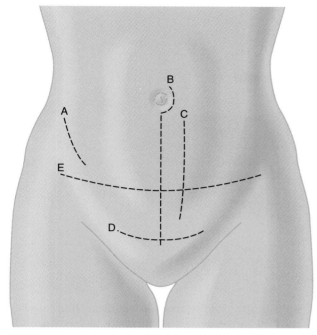

FIGURE 3-12 Abdominal wall incisions: McBurney (**A**), lower midline (**B**), left lower paramedian (**C**), Pfannenstiel or Cherney (**D**), and transverse, Maylard, or Bardenheuer (**E**).

sufficient exposure for extensive operations, it has cosmetic advantages in that it is generally only 2 cm above the symphysis pubis, and the scar is later covered by the pubic hair. Because the rectus abdominis muscles are not cut, eviscerations and wound hernias are extremely uncommon. **For extensive pelvic procedures (e.g., radical hysterectomy and pelvic lymphadenectomy), a transverse muscle–cutting incision (Bardenheuer or Maylard) at a slightly higher level in the lower abdomen gives sufficient exposure.** In addition, the skin incision falls within the lines of Langer, so a good cosmetic result can be expected. When it is anticipated that upper abdominal exploration will be necessary, such as in a patient with suspected ovarian cancer, a midline incision through the linea alba or a paramedian vertical incision is indicated.

SUGGESTED READING

Agur AMR (ed): Grant's Atlas of Anatomy, 9th ed. Baltimore, Williams & Wilkins, 1991.

Clemente CD: Anatomy: An Atlas of the Human Body, 4th ed. Baltimore, Williams & Wilkins, 1997.

Cunningham EG, MacDonald PC, Gant NF, et al (eds): Williams Obstetrics, 20th ed., Norwalk, Conn, Appleton & Lange, 1997.

Chapter 4

Female Reproductive Physiology

JOSEPH C. GAMBONE

◼ *The Menstrual Cycle*

Each menstrual cycle represents a complex interaction among the hypothalamus, pituitary gland, ovaries, and endometrium. Cyclic changes in gonadotropins (peptide hormones) and steroid hormones induce functional as well as morphologic changes in the ovary, resulting in follicular maturation, ovulation, and corpus luteum formation. Similar changes at the level of the endometrium allow for successful implantation of the developing embryo or a physiologic shedding of the menstrual endometrium when an early pregnancy does not occur.

The reproductive cycle can be viewed from the perspective of each of the aforementioned organ systems. The cyclic changes within the hypothalamic-pituitary axis, ovary, and endometrium are approached separately in this chapter, but these endocrinologic events occur in concert in a uniquely integrated fashion. In addition, fertilization, implantation, and placentation are discussed.

◼ *Hypothalamic-Pituitary Axis*

PITUITARY GLAND

The pituitary gland lies below the hypothalamus at the base of the brain within a bony cavity (sella turcica) and is separated from the cranial cavity by a condensation of dura mater overlying the sella turcica (diaphragma sellae). The pituitary gland is divided into two major portions (Figure 4-1). **The neurohypophysis, which consists of the posterior lobe (pars nervosa), the neural stalk (infundibulum), and the median eminence, is derived from neural tissue and is in direct continuity with the hypothalamus and central nervous system. The adenohypophysis, which consists of the pars** distalis (anterior lobe), pars intermedia (intermediate lobe), and pars tuberalis—which surrounds the neural stalk—is derived from ectoderm.

The arterial blood supply to the median eminence and the neural stalk (pituitary portal system) represents a major avenue of transport for hypothalamic secretions to the anterior pituitary.

The neurohypophysis serves primarily to transport oxytocin and vasopressin (antidiuretic hormone) along neuronal projections from the supraoptic and paraventricular nuclei of the hypothalamus to their release into the circulation.

The anterior pituitary contains different cell types that produce six protein hormones: follicle-stimulating hormone (FSH), luteinizing hormone (LH), thyroid-stimulating hormone (TSH), prolactin, growth hormone (GH), and adrenocorticotropic hormone (ACTH).

The gonadotropins, FSH and LH, are synthesized and stored in cells called **gonadotrophs,** whereas TSH is produced by **thyrotrophs.** FSH, LH, and TSH are glycoproteins, consisting of α and β subunits. The α subunits of FSH, LH, and TSH are identical. The same α subunit is also present in human chorionic gonadotropin (hCG). The β subunits are individual for each hormone. The half-life for circulating LH is about 30 minutes, whereas that of FSH is several hours. The difference in half-lives may account, at least in part, for the differential secretion patterns of these two gonadotropins.

Prolactin is secreted by **lactotrophs.** Unlike the case with other peptide hormones produced by the adenohypophysis, **pituitary release of prolactin is under tonic inhibition by the hypothalamus.** The half-life for circulating prolactin is about 20 to 30 minutes. In addition to its lactogenic effect, prolactin may directly

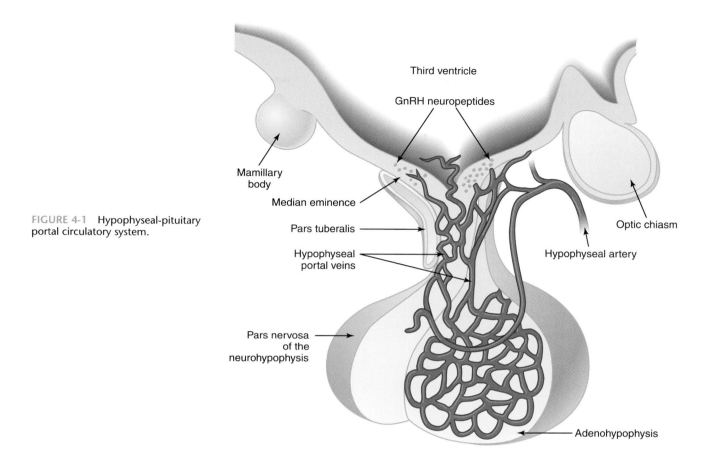

Third ventricle

GnRH neuropeptides

Mamillary body

Median eminence

Pars tuberalis

Hypophyseal portal veins

Optic chiasm

Hypophyseal artery

Pars nervosa of the neurohypophysis

Adenohypophysis

FIGURE 4-1   Hypophyseal-pituitary portal circulatory system.

or indirectly influence hypothalamic, pituitary, and ovarian functions in relation to the ovulatory cycle, particularly in the pathologic state of chronic hyperprolactinemia (see Chapter 32).

GONADOTROPIN SECRETORY PATTERNS

A normal ovulatory cycle can be divided into a follicular and a luteal phase (Figure 4-2). The follicular phase begins with the onset of menses and culminates in the preovulatory surge of LH. The luteal phase begins with the onset of the preovulatory LH surge and ends with the first day of menses.

Decreasing levels of estradiol and progesterone from the regressing corpus luteum of the preceding cycle initiate an increase in FSH by a negative feedback mechanism, which stimulates follicular growth and estradiol secretion. A major characteristic of follicular growth and estradiol secretion is explained by the two-gonadotropin (LH and FSH), two-cell (theca cell and granulosa cell) theory of ovarian follicular development. According to this theory, there are separate

cellular functions in the ovarian follicle wherein LH stimulates the theca cells to produce androgens (androstenedione and testosterone) and FSH then stimulates the granulosa cells to convert these androgens into estrogens (androstenedione to estrone and testosterone to estradiol), as depicted in Figure 4-3. Initially, at lower levels of estradiol, there is a negative feedback effect on the ready-release form of LH from the pool of gonadotropins in the pituitary gonadotrophs. As estradiol levels rise later in the follicular phase, there is a positive feedback on the release of storage gonadotropins, resulting in the LH surge and ovulation. The latter occurs 36 to 44 hours after the onset of this midcycle LH surge. With pharmacologic doses of progestins contained in contraceptive pills, there is a profound negative feedback effect on gonadotropin-releasing hormone (GnRH) so that none of the gonadotropin pool (ready-release or storage) is released. Hence, ovulation is (generally) blocked (see Chapter 26).

During the luteal phase, both LH and FSH are significantly suppressed through the negative feedback

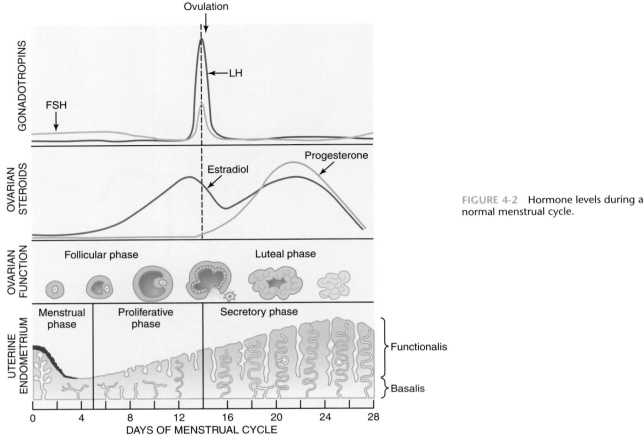

FIGURE 4-2 Hormone levels during a normal menstrual cycle.

effect of elevated circulating estradiol and progesterone. This inhibition persists until progesterone and estradiol levels decline near the end of the luteal phase as a result of corpus luteal regression, should pregnancy fail to occur. The net effect is a slight rise in serum FSH, which initiates new follicular growth for the next cycle. The duration of the corpus luteum's functional regression is such that menstruation generally occurs 14 days after the LH surge in the absence of pregnancy.

HYPOTHALAMUS

Five different small peptides or biogenic amines that affect the reproductive cycle have been isolated from the hypothalamus. All exert specific effects on the hormonal secretion of the anterior pituitary gland. They are **GnRH, thyrotropin-releasing hormone (TRH), somatotropin release-inhibiting factor (SRIF) or somatostatin, corticotropin-releasing factor (CRF), and prolactin release-inhibiting factor (PIF).** Only GnRH and PIF are discussed in this chapter.

GnRH is a decapeptide that is synthesized primarily in the arcuate nucleus. It is responsible for the synthesis and release of both LH and FSH. Because it usually

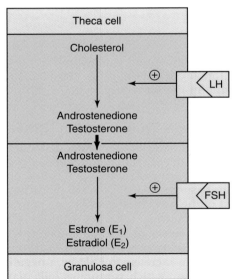

FIGURE 4-3 The two-gonadotropin (LH and FSH), two-cell (theca cell on top and granulosa cell below) theory of follicular development. Each cell is theorized to perform separate functions; LH stimulates the production of androgens (androstenedione and testosterone) in the theca cell, and FSH stimulates the aromatization of these androgens to estrogens, estrone, and estradiol in the granulosa cell.

causes the release of more LH than FSH, it is less commonly called LH-releasing hormone (LH-RH) or LH-releasing factor (LRF). **Both FSH and LH appear to be present in two different forms within the pituitary gonadotrophs. One is a releasable form and the other a storage form.** GnRH reaches the anterior pituitary through the hypophyseal portal vessels and stimulates the synthesis of both FSH and LH, which are stored within gonadotrophs. Subsequently, GnRH activates and transforms these molecules into releasable forms. GnRH can also induce immediate release of both LH and FSH into the circulation. Some recent research that found receptors for GnRH in other tissues including the ovary suggests that GnRH may have a direct effect on ovarian function as well.

GnRH is secreted in a pulsatile fashion throughout the menstrual cycle as depicted in Figure 4-4. The frequency of GnRH release, as assessed indirectly by measurement of LH pulses, varies from about every 90 minutes in the early follicular phase to every 60 to 70 minutes in the immediate preovulatory period. During the luteal phase, pulse frequency decreases while pulse amplitude increases. A considerable variation among individuals has been identified.

Intravenous and subcutaneous administration of exogenous pulsatile GnRH has been used to induce ovulation in selected women who are not ovulating as a result of hypothalamic dysfunction. **A continuous (nonpulsatile) infusion of GnRH results in a reversible inhibition of gonadotropin secretion through a process of "downregulation" or desensitization of pituitary gonadotrophs.** This represents the basic mechanism of action for the GnRH agonists (nonapeptides, containing only nine amino acids) that have been successfully used in the therapy of such ovarian hormone–dependent disorders as endometriosis, leiomyomas, hirsutism, and precocious puberty.

Several mechanisms control the secretion of GnRH. **Estradiol appears to enhance hypothalamic release of GnRH and may help induce the midcycle LH surge by increasing GnRH release or by enhancing pituitary responsiveness to the decapeptide.** Gonadotropins have an inhibitory effect on GnRH release. Catecholamines may play a major regulatory role as well. Dopamine is synthesized in the arcuate and periventricular nuclei and may have a direct inhibitory effect on GnRH secretion through the tuberoinfundibular tract that projects onto the median eminence. Serotonin also appears to inhibit GnRH pulsatile release, whereas norepinephrine stimulates it. Endogenous opioids suppress release of GnRH from the hypothalamus in a manner that may be partially regulated by ovarian steroids.

The hypothalamus produces PIF, which exerts chronic inhibition of prolactin release from the lactotrophs. A number of pharmacologic agents (e.g., chlorpromazine) that affect dopaminergic mechanisms

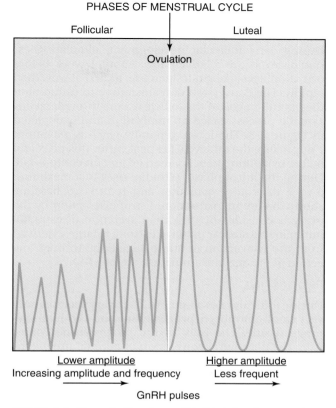

PHASES OF MENSTRUAL CYCLE

FIGURE 4-4 The pulsatile release of GnRH during the normal menstrual cycle.

influence prolactin release. Dopamine itself is secreted by hypothalamic neurons into the hypophyseal portal vessels and inhibits prolactin release directly within the adenohypophysis. Based on these observations, it has been proposed that hypothalamic dopamine may be the major PIF. In addition to the regulation of prolactin release by PIF, the hypothalamus may also produce prolactin-releasing factors (PRFs) that can elicit large and rapid increases in prolactin release under certain conditions, such as breast stimulation during nursing. All PIFs and PRFs have not been clearly characterized biochemically as of 2008. TRH serves to stimulate prolactin release as well. This phenomenon may explain the association between primary hypothyroidism (with secondary TRH elevation) and hyperprolactinemia. **The precursor protein for GnRH, called GnRH-associated peptide (GAP), has been identified to be both a potent inhibitor of prolactin secretion and an enhancer of gonadotropin release. These findings suggest that this GnRH-associated peptide may also be a physiologic PIF** and could explain the inverse relationship between gonadotropin and prolactin secretions seen in many reproductive states.

Ovarian Cycle

ESTROGENS

During early follicular development, circulating estradiol levels are relatively low. About 1 week before ovulation, levels begin to increase, at first slowly, then rapidly. The conversion of testosterone to estradiol in the granulosa cell of the follicle occurs through an enzymatic process called aromatization and is depicted in Figure 4-3. The levels generally reach a maximum 1 day before the midcycle LH peak. After this peak and before ovulation, there is a marked and precipitous fall. During the luteal phase, estradiol rises to a maximum 5 to 7 days after ovulation and returns to baseline shortly before menstruation. Estrone secretion by the ovary is considerably less than secretion of estradiol but follows a similar pattern. Estrone is largely derived from the conversion of androstenedione through the action of the enzyme aromatase (Figure 4-5).

PROGESTINS

During follicular development, the ovary secretes only very small amounts of progesterone and 17α-hydroxyprogesterone. The bulk of the progesterone comes from the peripheral conversion of adrenal pregnenolone and pregnenolone sulfate. Just before ovulation, the unruptured but luteinizing graafian follicle begins to produce increasing amounts of progesterone. At about this time, a marked increase also occurs in serum 17α-hydroxyprogesterone. The elevation of basal body temperature is temporally related to the central effect of progesterone. As with estradiol, secretion of progestins by the corpus luteum reaches a maximum 5 to 7 days after ovulation and returns to baseline shortly before menstruation. Should pregnancy occur, progesterone levels and therefore basal body temperature remain elevated.

ANDROGENS

Both the ovary and the adrenal glands secrete small amounts of testosterone, but most of the testosterone is derived from the metabolism of androstenedione, which is also secreted by both the ovary and the adrenal gland. Near midcycle, an increase occurs in plasma androstenedione, which reflects enhanced secretion from the follicle. During the luteal phase, a second rise occurs in androstenedione, which reflects enhanced secretion by the corpus luteum. The adrenal gland also secretes androstenedione in a diurnal pattern similar to that of cortisol. The ovary secretes small amounts of the very potent dihydrotestosterone (DHT), but the bulk of DHT is derived from the conversion of androstenedione and testosterone. The majority of dehydroepiandrosterone (DHEA) and virtually all DHEA sulfate (DHEA-S), which are weak androgens, are secreted by the adrenal glands, although small amounts of DHEA are secreted by the ovary.

SERUM-BINDING PROTEINS

Circulating estrogens and androgens are mostly bound to specific sex hormone–binding globulins (SHBG) or to serum albumin. The remaining fraction

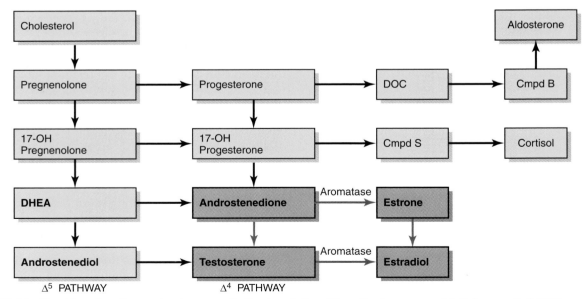

FIGURE 4-5　Steroidogenic pathways showing aromatization in red. Cmpd B, corticosterone; cmpd S, II-deoxycortisol; DOC, desoxycorticosterone; OH, hydroxylase.

of sex hormones is unbound (free), and this is the biologically active fraction. It is unclear whether steroids bound to serum proteins (e.g., albumin) are accessible for tissue uptake and utilization. The synthesis of SHBG in the liver is increased by estrogens and thyroid hormones but decreased by testosterone.

PROLACTIN

Serum prolactin levels do not change strikingly during the normal menstrual cycle. Both the serum level of prolactin and prolactin release in response to TRH are somewhat more elevated during the luteal phase than during the mid-follicular phase of the cycle. This suggests that high amounts of circulating estradiol and progesterone may enhance prolactin release. **Prolactin release varies throughout the day, with the highest levels occurring during sleep.**

Prolactin may participate in the control of ovarian steroidogenesis. Prolactin concentrations in follicular fluid change markedly during follicular growth. The highest prolactin concentrations are seen in small follicles during the early follicular phase. Prolactin concentrations in the follicular fluid may be inversely related to the production of progesterone. In addition, hyperprolactinemia may alter gonadotropin secretion. Despite these observations, the physiologic role of prolactin during the normal menstrual cycle has not been clearly established.

FOLLICULAR DEVELOPMENT

Primordial follicles undergo sequential development, differentiation, and maturation until a mature graafian follicle is produced. The follicle then ruptures, releasing the ovum. Subsequent luteinization of the ruptured follicle produces the corpus luteum.

At about 8 to 10 weeks of fetal development, oocytes become progressively surrounded by precursor granulosa cells, which then separate themselves from the underlying stroma by a basal lamina. This oocyte–granulosa cell complex is called a **primordial follicle.** In response to gonadotropin and ovarian steroids, the follicular cells become cuboidal, and the stromal cells around the follicle become prominent. This process, which takes place in utero (i.e., in the fetal ovary) at between 20 and 24 weeks' gestation, results in a primary follicle. As granulosa cells proliferate, a clear gelatinous material surrounds the ovum, forming the **zona pellucida.** This larger unit is called a **secondary follicle**.

In the adult ovary, **a graafian follicle** forms as the innermost three or four layers of rapidly multiplying granulosa cells become cuboidal and adherent to the ovum (**cumulus oophorus**). In addition, a fluid-filled antrum forms among the granulosa cells.

As the liquor continues to accumulate, the antrum enlarges, and the centrally located primary oocyte migrates eccentrically to the wall of the follicle. The innermost layer of granulosa cells of the cumulus, which are in close contact with the zona pellucida, become elongated and form the **corona radiata.** The corona radiata is released with the oocyte at ovulation. Covering the granulosa cells is a thin basement membrane, outside of which connective tissue cells organize themselves into two coats: the **theca interna** and **theca externa**.

During each cycle, a cohort of follicles is recruited for development. Among the many developing follicles, only one usually continues differentiation and maturation into a follicle that ovulates. The remaining follicles undergo atresia. On the basis of in vitro measurement of local steroid levels, growing follicles can be classified as either estrogen predominant or androgen predominant. **Follicles greater than 10 mm in diameter are usually estrogen predominant, whereas smaller follicles are usually androgen predominant.** Mature preovulatory follicles reach mean diameters of about 18 to 25 mm. Furthermore, in estrogen-predominant follicles, antral FSH concentrations continue to rise while serum FSH levels decline beginning at the mid-follicular phase. In smaller, androgen-predominant follicles, antral fluid FSH values decrease while serum FSH levels decline; thus, the intrafollicular steroid milieu appears to play an important role in determining whether a follicle undergoes maturation or atresia. Additional follicles may be "rescued" from atresia by administration of exogenous gonadotropins.

Follicular maturation is dependent on the local development of receptors for FSH and LH. FSH receptors are present on granulosa cells. Under FSH stimulation, granulosa cells proliferate, and the number of FSH receptors per follicle increases proportionately. Thus, the growing primary follicle is increasingly more sensitive to stimulation by FSH; as a result, estradiol levels increase. Estrogens, particularly estradiol, enhance the induction of FSH receptors and act synergistically with FSH to increase LH receptors.

During early stages of folliculogenesis, LH receptors are present only on the theca interna layer. LH stimulation induces steroidogenesis and increases the synthesis of androgens by thecal cells. In nondominant follicles, high local androgen levels may enhance follicular atresia. However, in the follicle destined to reach ovulation, FSH induces aromatase enzyme and its receptor formation within the granulosa cells. As a result, androgens produced in the theca interna of the dominant follicle diffuse into the granulosa cells and are aromatized into estrogens. **FSH also enhances the induction of LH receptors on the granulosa cells of the follicle that is destined to ovulate.** These are essential for the appropriate response to the LH surge, leading to the final stages of maturation, ovulation, and the luteal phase production of progesterone. Thus, **the presence of greater numbers of FSH receptors and granulosa cells and increased induction of aromatase enzyme and its receptors may differentiate between the follicle of the initial cohort that will develop normally and those that will undergo atresia.**

Growth factors such as insulin, insulin-like growth factor (IGF), fibroblast growth factor (FGF), and epidermal growth factor (EGF) may also play significant mitogenic roles in folliculogenesis, including enhanced responsiveness to FSH.

OVULATION

The preovulatory LH surge initiates a sequence of structural and biochemical changes that culminate in ovulation. **Before ovulation, a general dissolution of the entire follicular wall occurs, particularly the portion that is on the surface of the ovary. Presumably this occurs as a result of the action of proteolytic enzymes.** With degeneration of the cells on the surface, a stigma forms, and the follicular basement membrane finally bulges through the stigma. When this ruptures, the oocyte, together with the corona radiata and some cumulus oophora cells, is expelled into the peritoneal cavity, and ovulation takes place.

Ovulation is now known from ultrasonic studies to be a gradual phenomenon, with the collapse of the follicle taking from several minutes to as long as an hour or more. The oocyte adheres to the surface of the ovary, allowing an extended period during which the muscular contractions of the fallopian tube may bring it in contact with the tubal epithelium. Probably both muscular contractions and tubal ciliary movement contribute to the entry of the oocyte into, and the transportation along, the fallopian tube. Ciliary activity may not be essential because some women with immotile cilia also become pregnant.

At birth, primary oocytes are in the prophase of the first meiotic division. They continue in this phase until the next maturation division occurs in conjunction with the midcycle LH surge. **A few hours preceding ovulation, the chromatin is resolved into distinct chromosomes, and meiotic division takes place with unequal distribution of the cytoplasm to form a secondary oocyte and the first polar body. Each element contains 23 chromosomes, each in the form of two monads.** The second maturation spindle forms immediately, and the oocyte remains at the surface of the ovary. No further development takes place until after ovulation and fertilization have occurred. At that time, and before the union of the male and female pronuclei, another division occurs to reduce the chromosomal component of the egg pronucleus to 23 single chromosomes (22 plus X or Y), each composed of the one monad. The ovum and a second polar body are thus formed. The first polar body may also divide.

LUTEINIZATION AND CORPUS LUTEUM FUNCTION

After ovulation and under the influence of LH, the granulosa cells of the ruptured follicle undergo luteinization. These luteinized granulosa cells, plus the surrounding theca cells, capillaries, and connective tissue, form the corpus luteum, which produces copious amounts of progesterone and some estradiol. **The normal functional life span of the corpus luteum is about 9 to 10 days.** After this time it regresses, and unless pregnancy occurs, menstruation ensues, and the corpus luteum is gradually replaced by an avascular scar called a *corpus albicans*. The events occurring in the ovary during a complete cycle are shown in Figure 4-6.

■ *Histophysiology of the Endometrium*

The endometrium is uniquely responsive to the circulating progestins, androgens, and estrogens. It is this responsiveness that gives rise to menstruation and makes implantation and pregnancy possible.

Functionally, the endometrium is divided into two zones: (1) the **outer portion,** or **functionalis,** that undergoes cyclic changes in morphology and function during the menstrual cycle and is sloughed off at menstruation; and (2) the **inner portion,** or **basalis,** that remains relatively unchanged during each menstrual cycle and, after menstruation, provides stem cells for the renewal of the functionalis. **Basal arteries** are regular blood vessels found in the basalis, whereas **spiral arteries** are specially coiled blood vessels seen in the functionalis.

The cyclic changes in histophysiology of the endometrium can be divided into three stages: the menstrual phase, the proliferative or estrogenic phase, and the secretory or progestational phase.

MENSTRUAL PHASE

Because it is the only portion of the cycle that is visible externally, the first day of menstruation is taken as day 1 of the menstrual cycle. The first 4 to 5 days of the cycle are defined as the menstrual phase. **During this phase, there is disruption and disintegration of the endometrial glands and stroma, leukocyte infiltration, and red blood cell extravasation.** In addition to this sloughing of the functionalis, there is a compression of the basalis due to the loss of ground substances. Despite these degenerative changes, early evidence of renewed tissue growth is usually present at this time within the basalis of the endometrium.

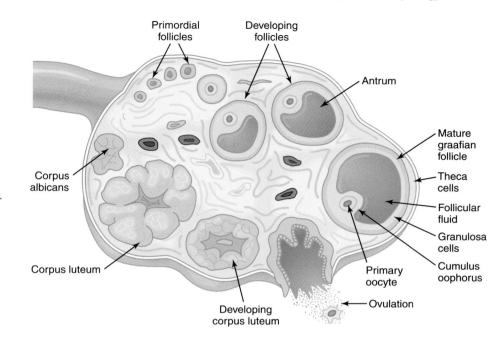

FIGURE 4-6 Schematic representation of the sequence of events occurring in the ovary during a complete follicular cycle. *(Adapted from Yen SC, Jaffe R [eds]: Reproductive Endocrinology. Philadelphia, WB Saunders, 1978.)*

Labels on figure: Primordial follicles; Developing follicles; Antrum; Mature graafian follicle; Theca cells; Follicular fluid; Granulosa cells; Cumulus oophorus; Primary oocyte; Ovulation; Developing corpus luteum; Corpus luteum; Corpus albicans

PROLIFERATIVE PHASE

The proliferative phase is characterized by endometrial proliferation or growth secondary to estrogenic stimulation. Because the bases of the endometrial glands lie deep within the basalis, these epithelial cells are not destroyed during menstruation.

During this phase of the cycle, the large increase in estrogen secretion causes marked cellular proliferation of the epithelial lining, the endometrial glands, and the connective tissue of the stroma (Figure 4-7). Numerous mitoses are present in these tissues, and there is an increase in the length of the spiral arteries, which traverse almost the entire thickness of the endometrium. By the end of the proliferative phase, cellular proliferation and endometrial growth have reached a maximum, the spiral arteries are elongated and convoluted, and the endometrial glands are straight, with narrow lumens containing some glycogen.

SECRETORY PHASE

Following ovulation, progesterone secretion by the corpus luteum stimulates the glandular cells to secrete glycogen, mucus, and other substances. The glands become tortuous and the lumens are dilated and filled with these substances. The stroma becomes edematous. Mitoses are rare. The spiral arteries continue to extend into the superficial layer of the endometrium and become convoluted (Figure 4-8).

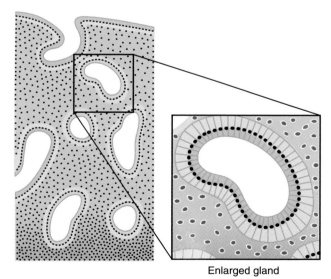

Enlarged gland

FIGURE 4-7 Early proliferative phase endometrium. Note the regular, tubular glands lined by pseudostratified columnar cells.

The marked changes that occur in endometrial histology during the secretory phase permit relatively precise timing (dating) of secretory endometrium.

If pregnancy does not occur by day 23, the corpus luteum begins to regress, secretion of progesterone and estradiol declines, and the endometrium undergoes

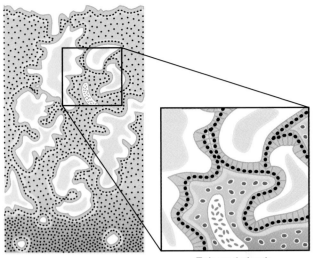

Enlarged glands

FIGURE 4-8   Late secretory phase endometrium. Note the tortuous, saw-toothed appearance of the endometrial glands with secretions in the lumens. The stroma is edematous and necrotic during this stage, leading to sloughing of the endometrium at the time of menstruation.

involution. About 1 day before the onset of menstruation, marked constriction of the spiral arterioles takes place, causing ischemia of the endometrium followed by leukocyte infiltration and red blood cell extravasation. It is thought that these events occur secondary to prostaglandin production by the endometrium. The resulting necrosis causes menstruation or sloughing of the endometrium. Thus, menstruation, which clinically marks the beginning of the menstrual cycle, is actually the terminal event of a physiologic process that enables the uterus to be prepared to receive another conceptus.

Spermatogenesis, Sperm Capacitation, and Fertilization

Fertilization, or conception, is the union of male and female pronuclear elements. Conception normally takes place in the fallopian tube, after which the fertilized ovum continues to the uterus, where implantation occurs and development of the conceptus continues.

Spermatogenesis requires about 74 days. Together with transportation, a total of about 3 months elapses before sperm are ejaculated. The sperm achieve motility during their passage through the epididymis, but sperm capacitation, which renders them capable of fertilization in vivo, does not occur until they are removed from the seminal plasma after ejaculation. Interestingly, sperm aspirated from the epididymis and

testis can be used to achieve fertilization in vitro employing intracytoplasmic injection techniques directly into the ooplasm.

Estrogen levels are high at the time of ovulation, resulting in an increased quantity, decreased viscosity, and favorable electrolyte content of the cervical mucus. These are the ideal characteristics for sperm penetration. **The average ejaculate contains 2 to 5 mL of semen; 40 to 300 million sperm may be deposited in the vagina, 50% to 90% of which are morphologically normal.** Fewer than 200 sperm achieve proximity to the egg. Only one sperm fertilizes a single egg released at ovulation.

The major loss of sperm occurs in the vagina following coitus, with expulsion of the semen from the introitus playing an important role. In addition, digestion of sperm by vaginal enzymes, destruction by vaginal acidity, phagocytosis of sperm along the reproductive tract, and further loss from passage through the fallopian tube into the peritoneal cavity all diminish the number of sperm capable of achieving fertilization.

Those sperm that do migrate from the alkaline environment of the semen to the alkaline environment of the cervical mucus exuding from the cervical os are directed along channels of lower-viscosity mucus into the cervical crypts where they are stored for later ascent. Two waves of passage to the tubes may occur. **Uterine contractions, probably facilitated by prostaglandin in the seminal plasma, propel sperm to the tubes within 5 minutes.** Some evidence indicates that these sperm may not be as capable of fertilization as those that arrive later largely under their own power. Sperm may be found within the peritoneal cavity for long periods, but it is not known whether they are capable of fertilization. **Ova are usually fertilized within 12 hours of ovulation.**

Capacitation is the physiologic change that sperm must undergo in the female reproductive tract before fertilization. Human sperm can also undergo capacitation after a short incubation in defined culture media without residence in the female reproductive tract, which allows for in vitro fertilization (see Chapter 34).

The acrosome reaction is one of the principal components of capacitation. The acrosome, a modified lysosome, lies over the sperm head as a kind of "chemical drill-bit" designed to enable the sperm to burrow its way into the oocyte (Figure 4-9). The overlying plasma membrane becomes unstable and eventually breaks down, releasing **hyaluronidase**, a neuraminidase, and **corona-dispersing enzyme. Acrosin**, bound to the remaining inner acrosomal membrane, may play a role in the final penetration of the zona pellucida. The latter contains species-specific receptors for the plasma membrane. After traversing the zona, the postacrosomal region of the sperm head fuses with the oocyte membrane, and the sperm nucleus is incorporated

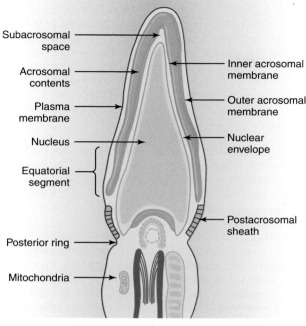

Subacrosomal space

Acrosomal contents

Plasma membrane

Nucleus

Equatorial segment

Posterior ring

Mitochondria

Inner acrosomal membrane

Outer acrosomal membrane

Nuclear envelope

Postacrosomal sheath

FIGURE 4-9   The sperm head.

into the ooplasm. This process triggers release of the contents of the cortical granules that lie at the periphery of the oocyte. This cortical reaction results in changes in the oocyte membrane and zona pellucida that prevent the entrance of further sperm into the oocyte. **The process of capacitation may be inhibited by a factor in the semen, thus preserving maximal release of enzyme to allow effective penetration of the corona and zona pellucida surrounding the oocyte.** The cellular investments of the oocyte may further activate the sperm, thus facilitating penetration to the oocyte membrane. The corona is not required for normal fertilization to occur because its removal has no effect on the rate or quality of fertilization in vitro. The major function of these surrounding granulosa cells and their intercellular matrix may be to serve as a sticky mass that causes adherence to the ovarian surface and to the mucosa of the tubal epithelium.

Following penetration of the oocyte, the sperm nucleus decondenses to form the male pronucleus, which approaches and finally fuses with the female pronucleus at syngamy to form the zygote. **Fertilization restores the diploid number of chromosomes and determines the sex of the zygote.** In couples with infertility resulting from severe sperm abnormalities, fertilization and subsequent pregnancy can be successfully achieved after the injection of a single sperm, with or without its tail, into the cytoplasm of the oocyte (see Chapter 34).

■ Cleavage, Morula, Blastocyst

Following fertilization, cleavage occurs. This consists of a rapid succession of mitotic divisions that produce a mulberry-like mass known as a morula. **Fluid is secreted by the outer cells of the morula, and a single fluid-filled cavity develops, known as the blastocyst cavity.** An inner-cell mass can be defined, attached eccentrically to the outer layer of flattened cells; the latter becomes the trophoblast. The embryo at this stage of development is called a **blastocyst,** and the zona pellucida disappears at about this time. A blastocyst cell can be removed and tested for genetic imperfections without harming further development of the conceptus.

■ Implantation

The fertilized ovum reaches the endometrial cavity about 3 days after ovulation.

Hormones influence egg transport. Estrogen causes "locking" of the egg in the tube, and progesterone reverses this action. Prostaglandins have diverse effects. Prostaglandin E relaxes the tubal isthmus, whereas prostaglandin F stimulates tubal motility. It is unknown whether abnormalities of egg transportation play a role in infertility, but in animal studies, acceleration of ovum transportation causes a failure of implantation. Additional cytokines may be released by the tubal epithelium and embryo to enhance embryo transportation and development and to signal the impending implantation to the endometrium.

Initial embryonic development primarily occurs in the ampullary portion of the fallopian tube with subsequent rapid transit through the isthmus. This process takes about 3 days. **On reaching the uterine cavity, the embryo undergoes further development for 2 to 3 days before implanting.** The zona is shed, and the blastocyst adheres to the endometrium, a process that is probably dependent on the changes in the surface characteristics of the embryo, such as electrical charge and glycoprotein content. A variety of proteolytic enzymes may play a role in separating the endometrial cells and digesting the intercellular matrix.

Initially, the wall of the blastocyst facing the uterine lumen consists of a single layer of flattened cells. The thicker opposite wall has two zones: the **trophoblast** and the **inner cell mass (embryonic disk).** The latter differentiates at 7.5 days into a thick plate of **primitive "dorsal" ectoderm** and an underlying layer of **"ventral" endoderm. A group of small cells appears between the embryonic disk and trophoblast. A space develops within them, which becomes the amniotic cavity.**

Under the influence of progesterone, decidual changes occur in the endometrium of the pregnant uterus. The endometrial stromal cells enlarge and form

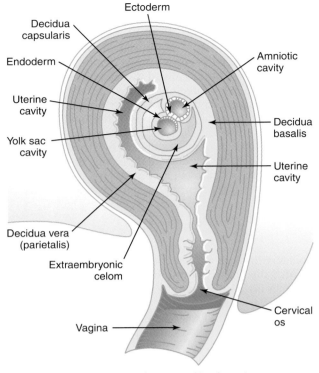

Ectoderm

Decidua
capsularis

Endoderm

Uterine
cavity

Yolk sac
cavity

Decidua vera
(parietalis)

Extraembryonic
celom

Vagina

Amniotic
cavity

Decidua
basalis

Uterine
cavity

Cervical
os

FIGURE 4-10   Early stage of implantation.

polygonal or round decidual cells. The nuclei become round and vesicular, and the cytoplasm becomes clear, slightly basophilic, and surrounded by a translucent membrane. During pregnancy, the decidua thickens to a depth of 5 to 10 mm. The **decidua basalis** is the decidual layer directly beneath the site of implantation. **Integrins**, a class of proteins involved in cell-to-cell adherence, peak within the endometrium at the time of implantation and may play a significant role. Additional growth factors act in a synergistic fashion to enhance the implantation process. The **decidua capsularis** is the layer overlying the developing ovum and separating it from the rest of the uterine cavity. The **decidua vera** (parietalis) is the remaining lining of the uterine cavity (Figure 4-10). The space between the decidua capsularis and decidua vera is obliterated by the 4th month with fusion of the capsularis and vera.

The decidua basalis enters into the formation of the basal plate of the placenta. The spongy zone of the decidua basalis consists mainly of arteries and dilated veins. **The decidua basalis is invaded extensively by trophoblastic giant cells, which first appear as early as the time of implantation.** Minute levels of hCG appear in the maternal serum at this time. **Nitabuch's layer** is a zone of fibrinoid degeneration where the trophoblast meets the decidua. When the decidua is defective, as in placenta accreta, Nitabuch's layer is absent.

When the free blastocyst contacts the endometrium after 4 to 6 days, the syncytiotrophoblast, a syncytium of cells, differentiates from the cytotrophoblast. **At about 9 days, lacunae, irregular fluid-filled spaces, appear within the thickened trophoblastic syncytium.** This is soon followed by the appearance of maternal blood within the lacunae as maternal tissue is destroyed and the walls of the mother's capillaries are eroded.

▇ *Placenta*

As the blastocyst burrows deeper into the endometrium, the trophoblastic strands branch to form the solid, primitive villi traversing the lacunae. The villi, which are first distinguished about the 12th day after fertilization, are the essential structures of the definitive placenta. Located originally over the entire surface of the ovum, the villi later disappear except over the most deeply implanted portion, the future placental site.

Embryonic mesenchyme first appears as isolated cells within the cavity of the blastocyst. When the cavity is completely lined with mesoderm, it is termed the **extraembryonic celom.** Its membrane, the **chorion,** is composed of trophoblast and mesenchyme. When the solid trophoblast is invaded by a mesenchymal core, presumably derived from cytotrophoblast, secondary villi are formed.

Maternal venous sinuses are tapped about 15 days after fertilization. By the 17th day, both fetal and maternal blood vessels are functional, and a placental circulation is established. The fetal circulation is completed when the blood vessels of the embryo are connected with chorionic blood vessels that are formed from cytotrophoblast. Proliferation of cellular trophoblasts at the tips of the villi produces cytotrophoblastic columns that progressively extend through the peripheral syncytium. Cytotrophoblastic extensions from columns of adjacent villi join together to form the cytotrophoblastic shell, which attaches the villi to the decidua. By the 19th day of development, the cytotrophoblastic shell is thick. Villi contain a central core of chorionic mesoderm, where blood vessels are developing, and an external covering of syncytiotrophoblasts or syncytium.

By 3 weeks, the relationship of the chorion to the decidua is evident. The greater part of the chorion, denuded of villi, is designated the **chorion laeve** (smooth chorion). Until near the end of the 3rd month, the chorion laeve remains separated from the amnion by the **extraembryonic celomic cavity.** Thereafter, amnion and chorion are in intimate contact. The villi adjacent to the decidua basalis enlarge and branch (**chorion frondosum**) and progressively assume the form of the fully developed human placenta (Figure 4-11). **By 16 to 20 weeks, the chorion laeve contacts and fuses with the decidua vera, thus obliterating most of the uterine cavity.**

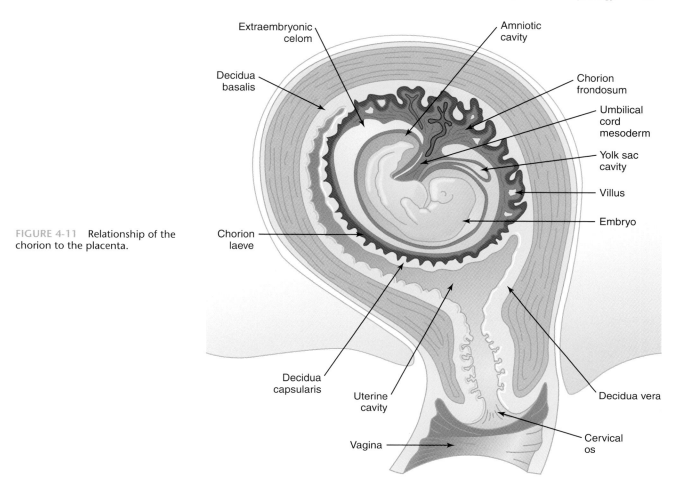

FIGURE 4-11 Relationship of the chorion to the placenta.

Labels (clockwise from top left): Extraembryonic celom · Amniotic cavity · Decidua basalis · Chorion frondosum · Umbilical cord mesoderm · Yolk sac cavity · Villus · Embryo · Chorion laeve · Decidua capsularis · Uterine cavity · Decidua vera · Vagina · Cervical os

▥ *Amniotic Fluid*

Throughout normal pregnancy, the amniotic fluid compartment allows the fetus room for growth, movement, and development. Without amniotic fluid, the uterus would contract and compress the fetus. **In cases of leakage of amniotic fluid early in the first trimester, the fetus may develop structural abnormalities including facial distortion, limb reduction, and abdominal wall defects secondary to uterine compression.**

Toward mid-pregnancy (20 weeks), the amniotic fluid becomes increasingly important for fetal pulmonary development. The latter requires a fluid-filled respiratory tract and the ability of the fetus to "breathe" in utero, moving amniotic fluid into and out of the lungs. **The absence of adequate amniotic fluid during mid-pregnancy is associated with pulmonary hypoplasia at birth, which is often incompatible with life.**

The amniotic fluid also has a protective role for the fetus. It contains antibacterial activity and acts to inhibit the growth of potentially pathogenic bacteria.

During labor and delivery, the amniotic fluid continues to serve as a protective medium for the fetus, aiding dilation of the cervix. The premature infant, with its fragile head, may benefit most from delivery with the amniotic membranes intact (en caul). In addition, the amniotic fluid may serve as a means of communication for the fetus. Fetal maturity and readiness for delivery may be signaled to the maternal uterus through fetal urinary hormones excreted into the amniotic fluid.

SUGGESTED READING

Adashi E: The ovarian cycle. *In* Yen SSC, Jaffe RB, (eds): Reproductive Endocrinology, 4th ed. Philadelphia, WB Saunders, 1997.

Olive DL, Palter SF: Reproductive physiology. *In* Berek and Novak's Gynecology, 14th ed. Philadelphia, Lippincott Williams & Wilkins, 2007.

Speroff L, Glass RH, Kase NG: Clinical Gynecologic Endocrinology and Fertility, 6th ed. Baltimore, Williams & Wilkins, 1999.

Strauss J, Gurpide E: The endometrium: Regulation and dysfunction. *In* Yen SSC, Jaffe RB, (eds): Reproductive Endocrinology, 4th ed. Philadelphia, WB Saunders, 1997.

Yen SSC: The human menstrual cycle: Neuroendocrine regulation. *In* Yen SSC, Jaffe RB, (eds): Reproductive Endocrinology, 4th ed. Philadelphia, WB Saunders, 1997.

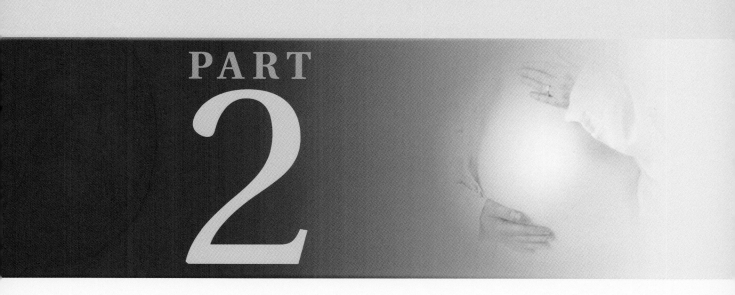

PART 2

OBSTETRICS

Chapter 5

Endocrinology of Pregnancy and Parturition

MICHAEL C. LU • CALVIN J. HOBEL

Women undergo major endocrinologic and metabolic changes that establish, maintain, and terminate pregnancy. The aim of these changes is the safe delivery of an infant who can survive outside of the uterus. The maturation of the fetus and the adaptation of the mother are regulated by a variety of hormones. This chapter deals with the properties, functions, and interactions of the most important of these hormones as they relate to pregnancy and parturition.

Fetoplacental Unit

The concept of the fetoplacental unit is based on observations of the interactions of hormones of fetal and maternal origin. **The fetoplacental unit largely controls the endocrine events of the pregnancy.** Although the fetus, the placenta, and the mother all provide input, the fetus appears to play the most active and controlling role of the three in its growth and maturation, and probably also in the events that lead to parturition.

FETUS

The adrenal gland is the major endocrine component of the fetus. In mid-pregnancy, it is larger than the fetal kidney. The fetal adrenal cortex consists of an outer definitive, or adult, zone and an inner, fetal, zone. The definitive zone later develops into the three components of the adult adrenal cortex: the zona fasciculata, the zona glomerulosa, and the zona reticularis. During fetal life, the definitive zone secretes primarily glucocorticoids and mineralocorticoids. **The fetal zone, at term, constitutes 80% of the fetal gland and primarily secretes androgens during fetal life.** It involutes following delivery and completely disappears by the end of the first year of life. The fetal adrenal medulla synthesizes and stores catecholamines, which play an important role in maintaining fetal homeostasis.

The role of the fetal adrenal during fetal growth and maturation is not completely understood.

PLACENTA

The placenta produces both steroid and peptide hormones in amounts that vary with gestational age. Precursors for progesterone synthesis come from the maternal circulation. **Because of the lack of the enzyme 17α-hydroxylase, the human placenta cannot directly convert progesterone to estrogen** but must use androgens, largely from the fetal adrenal gland, as its source of precursor for estrogen production.

MOTHER

The mother adapts to pregnancy through major endocrinologic and metabolic changes. **The ovaries produce progesterone in early pregnancy** until its production shifts to the placenta. **The maternal hypothalamus and posterior pituitary produce and release oxytocin,** which causes uterine contractions and milk letdown. **The anterior pituitary produces prolactin,** which stimulates milk production. Several important changes in maternal metabolism are described later in the chapter.

Hormones

The fetoplacental unit produces a variety of hormones to support the maturation of the fetus and the adaptation of the mother.

PEPTIDE HORMONES

Human Chorionic Gonadotropin

Human chorionic gonadotropin (hCG) is secreted by trophoblastic cells of the placenta and maintains pregnancy. This hormone is a glycoprotein with a molecular weight of 40,000 to 45,000 and **consists of two subunits: alpha (α) and beta (β).** The α subunit is shared with luteinizing hormone (LH) and thyroid-stimulating hormone (TSH). **The specificity of hCG is related to its β subunit (β-hCG),** and a radioimmunoassay that is specific for the β subunit allows positive identification of hCG. The presence of hCG at times other than pregnancy signals the presence of an hCG-producing tumor, usually a hydatidiform mole, choriocarcinoma, or embryonal carcinoma (a germ cell tumor).

During pregnancy, hCG begins to rise 8 days after ovulation (9 days after the midcycle LH peak). This provides the basis for virtually all immunologic or chemical pregnancy tests. With continuing pregnancy, hCG values peak at 60 to 90 days and then decline to a moderate, more constant level. **For the first 6 to 8 weeks of pregnancy, hCG maintains the corpus luteum and thereby ensures continued progesterone output until progesterone production shifts to the placenta.** Titers of hCG are usually abnormally low in patients with an ectopic pregnancy or threatened abortion and abnormally high in those with trophoblastic disease (e.g., moles or choriocarcinoma). This hormone may also regulate steroid biosynthesis in the placenta and the fetal adrenal gland and stimulate testosterone production in the fetal testicle. Although immune suppression has been ascribed to hCG, this effect has not been verified.

Human Placental Lactogen

Human placental lactogen (hPL) originates in the placenta. It is a single-chain polypeptide with a molecular weight of 22,300, and it resembles pituitary growth hormone and human prolactin in structure. Maternal serum concentrations parallel placental weight, rising throughout gestation to maximum levels in the last 4 weeks. At term, hPL accounts for 10% of all placental protein production. Low values are found with threatened abortion and intrauterine fetal growth restriction. **Human placental lactogen antagonizes the cellular action of insulin and decreases maternal glucose utilization, which increases glucose availability to the fetus.** This may play a role in the pathogenesis of gestational diabetes.

Corticotropin-Releasing Hormone

During pregnancy the major source of corticotropin-releasing hormone (CRH) is the placenta, and it can be measured as early as 12 weeks of gestation when it passes into the fetal circulation. This 41–amino acid peptide stimulates fetal adrenocorticotropic hormone (ACTH) secretion, which in turn stimulates the fetal adrenal to secrete dehydroepiandrosterone sulfate (DHEA-S), an important precursor of estrogen production by the placenta. The fetal adrenal gland early in pregnancy does not have the enzymes to produce cortisol, but as gestational age increases, it becomes more responsive. **Fetal cortisol stimulates placental CRH release, which then stimulates fetal ACTH secretion, completing a positive feedback loop that plays an important role in the activation and amplification of labor, both preterm and term.** Elevated levels of CRH in mid-gestation have been found to be associated with an increased risk for subsequent preterm labor.

Prolactin

Prolactin is a peptide from the anterior pituitary with a molecular weight of about 20,000. Normal nonpregnant levels are about 10 ng/mL. **During pregnancy, maternal prolactin levels rise in response to increasing maternal estrogen output that stimulates the anterior pituitary lactotrophs. The main effect of prolactin is stimulation of postpartum milk production.** In the second half of pregnancy, prolactin secreted by the fetal pituitary may be an important stimulus of fetal adrenal growth. Prolactin may also play a role in fluid and electrolyte shifts across the fetal membranes.

STEROID HORMONES

Progesterone

Progesterone is the most important human progestogen. **In the luteal phase, it induces secretory changes in the endometrium, and in pregnancy, higher levels induce decidual changes.** Up to the 6th or 7th week of pregnancy, the major source of progesterone (in the form of 17-OH progesterone) is the ovary. Thereafter, the placenta begins to play the major role. **If the corpus luteum of pregnancy is removed before 7 weeks and continuation of the pregnancy is desired, progesterone should be given to prevent spontaneous abortion.** Circulating progesterone is mostly bound to carrier proteins, and less than 10% is free and physiologically active.

The myometrium receives progesterone directly from the venous blood draining the placenta. Progesterone prevents uterine contractions and may also be involved in establishing an immune tolerance for the products of conception. Progesterone also suppresses gap junction formation, placental CRH expression, and the actions of estrogen, cytokines, and prostaglandin. This steroid hormone therefore **plays a central role in maintaining uterine quiescence** throughout most of pregnancy.

The fetus inactivates progesterone by transformation to corticosteroids or by hydroxylation or conjugation to inert excretory products. However, the placenta can convert these inert materials back to progesterone. Steroid biochemical pathways are shown in Figure 5-1.

Estrogens

Both fetus and placenta are involved in the biosynthesis of estrone, estradiol, and estriol. Cholesterol is converted to pregnenolone and pregnenolone

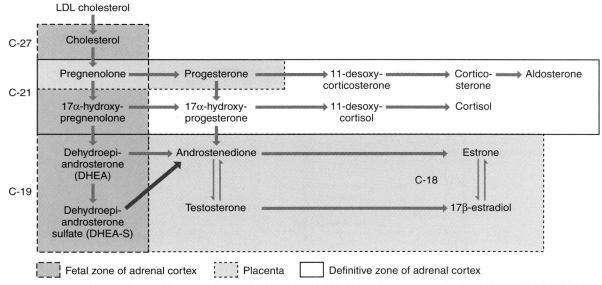

FIGURE 5-1   Main pathways of steroid hormone biosynthesis. Adrenal DHEA is largely transported as its sulfate, DHEA-S, which can also be formed from steroid sulfates starting with cholesterol sulfate. LDL, low-density lipoprotein.

sulfate in the placenta. These precursors are converted to DHEA-S largely in the fetal, and to a lesser extent the maternal, adrenals. The DHEA-S is further metabolized by the placenta to estrone (E1) and, through testosterone, to estradiol (E2). **Estriol (E3), the most abundant estrogen in human pregnancy, is synthesized in the placenta from 16α-hydroxy-DHEA-S, which is produced in the fetal liver from adrenal DHEA-S.** Placental sulfatase is required to deconjugate 16α-hydroxy-DHEA-S before conversion to E3 (Figure 5-2). Steroid sulfatase activity in the placenta is high except in rare cases of sulfatase deficiency.

A sudden decline of estriol in the maternal circulation may indicate fetal compromise in neurologically intact fetuses. Anencephalic fetuses lack a hypothalamus and have hypoplastic anterior pituitary and adrenal glands; thus, estriol production is only about 10% of normal.

Androgens

During pregnancy, androgens originate mainly in the fetal zone of the fetal adrenal cortex. Androgen secretion is stimulated by ACTH and hCG, the latter being effective primarily in the first half of pregnancy, when it is present in high concentration. The fetal adrenal favors production of DHEA over testosterone and androstenedione. **Fetal androgens enter the umbilical and placental circulation and serve as precursors for estradiol and estriol** (see Figure 5-1).

The fetal testis also secretes androgens, particularly testosterone, which is converted within target cells to **dihydrotestosterone** (DHT), which is required for the

development of male external genitalia. The main trophic stimulus appears to be hCG.

Glucocorticoids

Cortisol is derived from circulating cholesterol (see Figure 5-1). Maternal plasma cortisol concentrations rise throughout pregnancy, and the diurnal rhythm of cortisol secretion persists. The plasma level of transcortin rises in pregnancy, probably stimulated by estrogen, and the plasma-free cortisol concentration doubles.

Both the fetal adrenal and the placenta participate in cortisol metabolism. The fetal adrenal is stimulated by ACTH, originating from the fetal pituitary, to produce both cortisol and DHEA-S. In contrast to DHEA-S, which is produced in the fetal zone, cortisol originates in the definitive zone (see Figure 5-1). Toward the end of pregnancy **cortisol promotes differentiation of type II alveolar cells and the biosynthesis and release of surfactant into the alveoli.** Surfactant decreases the force required to inflate the lungs. Insufficiency of surfactant leads to respiratory distress in the premature infant, which can cause death. **Cortisol also plays an important role in the activation of labor,** increasing the release of placental CRH and prostaglandins.

OTHER HORMONES AND TRANSMITTERS

Oxytocin

The oxytocic prohormone, which originates in the supraoptic and paraventricular nuclei of the maternal hypothalamus, migrates down the nerve fibers, and oxytocin accumulates at the nerve endings in the posterior pituitary. Oxytocin is a nonapeptide, which

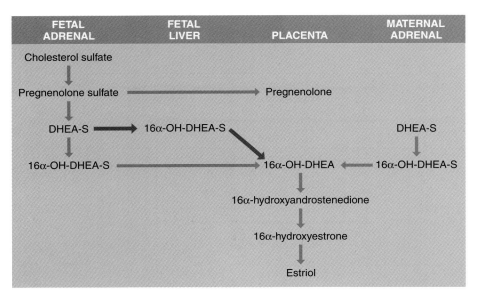

FIGURE 5-2 Formation of estriol in the fetal-placental unit.

is released from the posterior pituitary by various stimuli, such as distention of the birth canal and mammary stimulation. **Oxytocin causes uterine contractions, but impairment of oxytocin production, as in diabetes insipidus, does not interfere with normal labor.** Fluctuations in circulating oxytocin levels before the onset of labor do not correspond to changes in uterine activity. Maternal serum oxytocin levels rise only during the first stage of labor. Oxytocin can be administered to induce labor, especially in term pregnancies, or to increase the frequency and strength of contractions during spontaneous labor.

Relaxin

Relaxin is a peptide hormone that originates mostly from the ovary. In the human, it reaches its peak concentration in the maternal circulation at the 10th week of pregnancy and then declines. Relaxin is associated with the softening of the cervix, which is one of the anatomic signs of pregnancy. **Its primary function appears to be in promoting implantation of the embryo by facilitating angiogenesis.** During hyperstimulation of the ovaries of women undergoing in vitro fertilization (IVF), the ovaries produce excessive levels of relaxin. This excess of relaxin has been shown to be associated with shortening of the cervix and an increased risk for preterm labor.

Prostaglandins and Leukotrienes

Prostaglandins are a family of ubiquitous, biologically active lipids that are involved in a broad range of physiologic and pathophysiologic responses. **They are not true hormones** in that they are not synthesized in one gland and transported through the circulating blood to a target organ. Rather, they are synthesized at or near

their site of action. **Prostaglandin E_2 (PGE_2) and prostaglandin $F_{2\alpha}$ ($PGF_{2\alpha}$), prostacyclin, and thromboxane A_2 are synthesized in the endometrium, myometrium, the fetal membranes, decidua, and placenta. PGE_2 and $PGF_{2\alpha}$ cause contraction of the uterus.** Their receptors in the myometrium are downregulated during pregnancy. Prostaglandins can also cause contraction of other smooth muscles, such as those of the intestinal tract. Hence, when used pharmacologically, prostaglandins may give rise to undesirable side effects such as nausea, vomiting, and diarrhea. The amniotic fluid concentrations of PGE_2 and $PGF_{2\alpha}$ rise throughout pregnancy and increase further during spontaneous labor. Levels are lower in women who require oxytocin for induction of labor than in women going into spontaneous labor. Administration of PGE_2 or $PGF_{2\alpha}$ by various routes induces labor or abortion at any stage of gestation. **Various synthetic prostaglandin derivatives are currently in use to terminate pregnancy at any stage and to induce labor at term.**

Prostaglandins are thought to play a major role in the initiation and control of labor. **Prostaglandin synthesis begins with the formation of arachidonic acid, an obligatory precursor of the prostaglandins of the "2" series (i.e., PGE_2, $PGF_{2\alpha}$).** Arachidonic acid is stored in esterified form as glycerophospholipid in the trophoblastic membranes. The initial step is the hydrolysis of glycerophospholipids, which is catalyzed by phospholipase A_2 or C. **Phospholipase A_2 preferentially acts on chorionic phosphatidyl ethanolamine to release arachidonic acid** (Figure 5-3). Free arachidonic acid does not accumulate. Labor appears to be accompanied by a cascade of events in the chorion, amnion, and decidua that releases arachidonic acid from its stored form and converts it to active prostaglandins. 17β-Estradiol

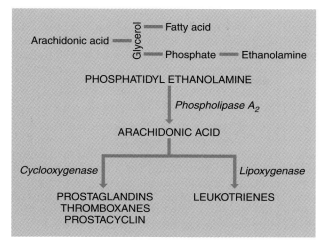

FIGURE 5-3 Diagram of prostaglandin and leukotriene biosynthesis.

stimulates several enzymes active in the synthesis of prostaglandins from arachidonic acid.

There are two cyclooxygenase isoenzymes referred to as COX-1, or PGHS-1, and COX-2, or PGHS-2. These isoenzymes originate from separate genes. COX-1 is expressed in quiescent cells, whereas COX-2 is inducible and is expressed at sites of inflammation upon cell activation and potentiates the inflammatory process. COX-1 mRNA expression is low in fetal membranes and does not change with gestational age, whereas COX 2 mRNA expression in the amnion increases with gestational age.

Increased phospholipase A_2 activity may lead to premature labor. Endocervical, intrauterine, or urinary tract infections are often associated with premature labor. Many of the organisms producing these infections have phospholipase A_2 activity, which could produce free arachidonic acid, followed by prostaglandin synthesis, which could trigger labor.

Prostaglandin synthetase inhibitors can prolong gestation. Nonsteroidal antiinflammatory drugs (NSAIDs) inhibit phospholipase A_2, whereas aspirin-like drugs inhibit cyclooxygenase. Because PGE_2 keeps the ductus arteriosus open, premature closure of the ductus may occur after ingestion of NSAIDs or aspirin in large amounts or for a prolonged period of time, resulting in fetal pulmonary hypertension and death.

An additional pathway for arachidonic acid metabolism is the conversion of arachidonic acid to leukotrienes (see Figure 5-3). Both prostaglandins and leukotrienes induce decidualization, which means that they initiate changes in the endometrium to facilitate implantation of the fertilized ovum.

Although $PGF_{2\alpha}$ is more potent in producing uterine contractile activity, PGE_2 is the most potent prostaglandin for ripening the cervix by inducing changes in the connective tissue. Hence, PGE_2 and its synthetic derivatives are clinically useful for cervical ripening before the induction of labor or abortion.

Changes in Maternal Metabolism

Maternal metabolism adapts to pregnancy through endocrinologic regulation, as described subsequently.

ANGIOTENSIN-ALDOSTERONE

Aldosterone is a mineralocorticoid synthesized in the zona glomerulosa of the adrenal cortex. The main source in pregnancy is the maternal adrenal. The fetal adrenal and the placenta do not participate significantly in aldosterone production, although the fetal adrenal is capable of synthesizing it. Aldosterone secretion is regulated by the renin-angiotensin system. Increased renin formed in the kidney converts angiotensinogen (renin-substrate) to angiotensin I, which is further metabolized to angiotensin II, which in turn stimulates aldosterone secretion. Aldosterone stimulates the absorption of sodium and the secretion of potassium in the distal tubule of the kidney, thereby maintaining sodium and potassium balance. Renin-substrate (a plasma protein) concentration rises in pregnancy. It is thought that the high concentrations of progesterone and estrogen present during pregnancy stimulate renin and renin-substrate formation, thus giving rise to increased levels of angiotensin II and greater aldosterone production. Aldosterone secretion rates decline in pregnancy-induced hypertension and, in some cases, may fall below nonpregnant levels.

CALCIUM METABOLISM

Although calcium absorption is increased in pregnancy, total maternal serum calcium declines. The fall in total calcium parallels that of serum albumin because about half of the total calcium is bound to albumin. Ionic calcium, the physiologically important calcium fraction, remains essentially constant throughout pregnancy because of increased maternal production of parathyroid hormone. In late pregnancy, coinciding with maximal calcification of the fetal skeleton, increased serum parathyroid hormone enhances both maternal intestinal absorption of calcium and bone resorption. The latter counteracts the inhibition of bone resorption caused by increased circulating estrogen. Urinary calcium excretion is decreased.

Calcium ions are actively transported across the placenta, and fetal serum levels of total as well as ionized calcium are higher than maternal levels in late pregnancy. High fetal ionic calcium suppresses fetal parathyroid hormone production, and parathyroid hormone does not cross the placenta. Furthermore, calcitonin production is stimulated, thus providing the fetus with ample calcium for calcification of the skeleton. In the first 24 to 48 hours postpartum, the total serum calcium concentration in the neonate usually falls, while the phosphorus concentration rises. Both adjust to adult levels within 1 week.

■ *Parturition*

Parturition means childbirth, and labor is the physiologic process by which a fetus is expelled from the uterus to the outside world.

BIOCHEMICAL BASIS OF CONTRACTION

Muscle contraction is brought about by the sliding of actin and myosin filaments fueled by adenosine triphosphate (ATP) and calcium. **Although skeletal muscle requires innervation, contraction of smooth muscles such as the myometrium is triggered primarily by hormonal stimuli.** Hormonal receptors have been found in the myometrial cell membrane.

The binding of oxytocin and prostaglandins to their respective receptors activates phospholipase C, which hydrolyzes phosphatidylinositol bisphosphate, a lipid present in the cell membrane, to inositol trisphosphate and diacylglycerol (Figure 5-4). Inositol trisphosphate induces release of calcium from the sarcoplasmic reticulum, an intracellular calcium storage area. The resulting high intracellular free calcium concentration enables the myofibrils of the myometrium to contract. Subsequently, the calcium is pumped back into the sarcoplasmic reticulum with the help of ATP, and more calcium may enter from the extracellular fluid through both voltage-operated and receptor-operated channels that open briefly.

Unlike the heart, in which the bundle of His is present, no anatomic structures for synchronization of contractions have been found in the uterus. Instead, contraction spreads as current flows from cell to cell through areas of low resistance. Such areas are associated with gap junctions, which become especially prominent at parturition. **Estradiol and prostaglandins promote the appearance of gap junctions,** whereas progesterone opposes this action of estradiol.

HORMONAL CONTROL OF GESTATIONAL LENGTH AND INITIATION OF LABOR

Gestational length is under the hormonal control of the fetus in most species. Each species, however, has not only a unique gestational length, but also unique mechanisms for controlling the length of gestation. Thus, although animal models provide important insight, they do not provide specific information concerning the control of the human gestational length or the mechanisms controlling initiation of labor.

Animal Models

Most studies have been conducted in the sheep, where the fetus appears to control the onset of labor. The fetal hypothalamus stimulates the fetal pituitary to secrete ACTH, which brings about a surge of cortisol from the fetal adrenal. The cortisol surge induces the placental enzyme 17α-hydroxylase and formation of androgens, which are estrogen precursors (see Figure 5-1), simultaneously decreasing progesterone formation. The rise in the estrogen-to-progesterone ratio leads to (1) greater secretion of prostaglandins; (2) formation of myometrial gap junctions, which provide areas of low resistance to current flow and increase coordinated uterine contractions; (3) cervical ripening; and (4) the onset of labor. Administered ACTH, glucocorticoids, or dexamethasone can also initiate parturition. Removal of the fetal pituitary or adrenal, both of which are required for the cortisol surge, results in prolonged pregnancy.

In a breed of Guernsey cows with a genetic defect resulting in fetal pituitary and adrenal dysfunction, pregnancy is prolonged, and normal vaginal delivery does not occur. **In the rabbit, parturition directly follows a decline in progesterone production secondary to a decline in corpus luteum function.** Abortion can be prevented by administration of progesterone.

The Human

The process of normal spontaneous human parturition can be divided into four phases.

PHASE 0: QUIESCENCE. Throughout the majority of pregnancy, the uterus remains relatively quiescent. Myometrial activity is inhibited during pregnancy by various substances, but **progesterone appears to play a central role in maintaining uterine quiescence.** Rare uterine contractions that occur during the quiescent phase are of low frequency and amplitude and are poorly coordinated; these are commonly referred to as **Braxton-Hicks contractions** in women. The poor coordination

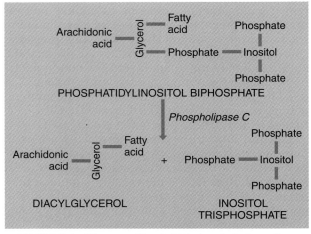

FIGURE 5-4   Diagram of inositol trisphosphate formation.

of these contractions is primarily due to an absence of gap junctions in the pregnant myometrium.

PHASE 1: ACTIVATION. **Normally, the signals for myometrial activation can come from uterine stretch as a result of fetal growth, or from activation of the fetal hypothalamic-pituitary-adrenal (HPA) axis as a result of fetal maturation, or both.** Uterine stretch has been shown in animal models to increase gap junctions and contraction-associated proteins in the myometrium. It is currently thought that once fetal maturity has been reached (as determined by as yet unknown mechanisms), the fetal hypothalamus increases CRH secretion, which in turn stimulates ACTH expression by the fetal pituitary and cortisol and androgen production by the fetal adrenals. Recent data from pregnant mice suggest that the fetus signals the initiation of labor by secreting a major lung surfactant protein, SP-A, into the amniotic fluid.

These data support a critical role for the fetal HPA axis in the initiation of parturition because surfactant protein synthesis is stimulated by glucocorticoids. **The concept of a role for the fetal lung in the initiation of parturition is particularly attractive because the fetal lung is the last major organ to mature.**

PHASE 2: STIMULATION. Phase 2 involves a progressive cascade of events leading to a common pathway of parturition, and involving uterine contractility, cervical ripening, and decidual/fetal membrane activation. **This cascade probably begins with placental production of CRH.** Placental CRH synthesis is stimulated by glucocorticoids, in contrast to the inhibitory effect of glucocorticoids on maternal hypothalamic CRH synthesis. Placental CRH enters into the fetal circulation and, in turn, promotes fetal cortisol and DHEA-S production. This positive feedback loop is progressively amplified, thereby driving the process forward from fetal HPA activation to parturition and the placental production of estrogens.

For most of pregnancy, uterine quiescence is maintained by the action of progesterone. At the end of pregnancy in most mammals, maternal progesterone levels fall, and estrogen levels rise. In human and nonhuman primate pregnancies, progesterone and estrogen concentrations continue to rise throughout pregnancy until delivery of the placenta. A functional progesterone withdrawal may occur in women and nonhuman primates by alterations in progesterone receptor (PR) expression. **There are two progesterone receptors (PRA and PRB) in the human myometrium.** In contrast to PRB, which increases progesterone action, **PRA inhibits progesterone action.** The ratio of PRA to PRB in the myometrium in labor is increased, which in effect results in a progesterone withdrawal.

Functional progesterone withdrawal results in functional estrogen predominance, in part as a result **of the increase in placental estrogen production.** The expression of estrogen receptor (ER) isoform, ERα, is normally suppressed by progesterone, but as the expression of PRA increases relative to that of PRB, so does the expression of ERα in the laboring myometrium. The rising expression of ERα facilitates increased estrogen action. Increasing estrogen levels also enhance expression of many estrogen-dependent contraction associated proteins (CAPs), including connexin 43 (gap junctions), oxytocin receptor, prostaglandin receptors, COX-2 (which results in prostaglandin production), and myosin light-chain kinase (MLCK), which stimulate myometrial contractility and labor.

The progressive cascade of biological processes leads to a common pathway of parturition, involving cervical ripening, uterine contractility, and decidual/fetal membrane activation. **Cervical ripening** is largely mediated by the actions of prostaglandins, **uterine contractility** by the actions of gap junctions and MLCK, and **decidual/fetal membrane activation** by the actions of enzymes such as metalloproteinases, which ultimately lead to rupture of the membranes.

PHASE 3: INVOLUTION. During expulsion of the fetus, there is a dramatic increase in the release of maternal oxytocin, which facilitates the initiation of the final phase of labor. **Phase 3 involves placental separation and continued uterine contractions.** Placental separation occurs by cleavage along the plane of the decidua basalis. Uterine contraction is essential to prevent bleeding from large venous sinuses that are exposed after delivery of the placenta and is primarily affected by oxytocin. This is further supported by oxytocin letdown during early breastfeeding.

To summarize, labor is a release from the state of functional quiescence maintained during pregnancy due, in large part, to the lack of myometrial gap junctions and the actions of progesterone. It is hoped that future research in this important area will further our knowledge and improve our ability to prevent premature labor and delivery, currently the leading cause of perinatal mortality.

SUGGESTED READING

Behrman RE, Butler AS (eds): Preterm birth: Causes, consequences, and prevention. Institute of Medicine: Committee on Understanding Premature Birth and Assuring Healthy Outcomes, Board on Health Sciences Policy. Washington, DC, National Academies Press, 2007.

Challis JRG: Mechanism of parturition and preterm labor. Obstet Gynecol Surv 55:650-660, 2000.

Jeyabalan A, Shroff SG, Novak J, Conrad KP: The vascular actions of relaxin. Adv Exp Med Biol 612:65-87, 2007.

Norwitz ER, Robinson JN, Challis JRG: The control of labor. N Engl J Med 341:660-666, 1999.

Vidaeff AC, Ramin SM: Potential biochemical events associated with initiation of labor. Curr Med Chem 15:614-619, 2008.

Chapter 6

Maternal Physiologic and Immunologic Adaptation to Pregnancy

BRIAN J. KOOS • DANIEL A. KAHN • OZLEM EQUILS

Maternal physiologic adjustments to pregnancy are designed to support the requirements of fetal homeostasis and growth without unduly jeopardizing maternal well-being. This is accomplished by remodeling maternal systems to deliver energy and growth substrates to the fetus and to remove inappropriate heat and waste products. There appears to be a privileged immunologic sanctuary for the fetus and placenta during pregnancy.

Normal Values in Pregnancy

The normal values for several hematologic, biochemical, and physiologic indices during pregnancy differ markedly from those in the nonpregnant range and may also vary according to the duration of pregnancy. These alterations are shown in Table 6-1.

Cardiovascular System

CARDIAC OUTPUT

The hemodynamic changes associated with pregnancy are summarized in Table 6-2. Retention of sodium and water during pregnancy accounts for a total body water increase of 6 to 8 L, two thirds of which is located in the extravascular space. The total sodium accumulation averages 500 to 900 mEq by the time of delivery. **The total blood volume increases by about 40% above nonpregnant levels, with wide individual variations.** The plasma volume rises as early as the 6th week of pregnancy and reaches a plateau by about 32 to 34 weeks' gestation, after which little further change occurs. The increase averages 50% in singleton pregnancies and approaches 70% with a twin gestation. The red blood cell mass begins to increase at the start of the second trimester and continues to rise throughout pregnancy.

By the time of delivery, it is 20% to 35% above nonpregnant levels. **The disproportionate increase in plasma volume compared with the red cell volume results in hemodilution with a decreased hematocrit reading, sometimes referred to as physiologic anemia of pregnancy.** If iron stores are adequate, the hematocrit tends to rise from the second to the third trimester.

Cardiac output rises by the 10th week of gestation; it reaches about 40% above nonpregnant levels by 20 to 24 weeks, after which there is little change. The rise in cardiac output, which peaks while blood volume is still rising, reflects increases mainly in stroke volume and, to a lesser extent, in heart rate. With twin and triplet pregnancies, the changes in cardiac output are greater than those seen with singleton pregnancies.

The cardiovascular responses to exercise are altered during pregnancy. **For any given level of exercise, oxygen consumption is higher in pregnant than in nonpregnant women.** Similarly, the cardiac output for any level of exercise is also increased during pregnancy compared with that seen in a nonpregnant state, and the maximum cardiac output is reached at lower levels of exercise. It is not clear that any of the changes in hemodynamic responses to exercise are detrimental to mother and fetus, but it suggests that maternal cardiac reserves are lowered during pregnancy and that shunting of blood away from the uterus might occur during or after exercise.

INTRAVASCULAR PRESSURES

Systolic pressure falls only slightly during pregnancy, whereas diastolic pressure decreases more markedly; this reduction begins in the first trimester, reaches its nadir in mid-pregnancy, and returns toward nonpregnant levels by term. These changes reflect the elevated cardiac output and reduced peripheral resistance

TABLE 6-1

COMMON LABORATORY VALUES IN PREGNANCY

Test	Normal Range (Nonpregnant)	Change in Pregnancy	Timing
SERUM CHEMISTRIES			
Albumin	3.5-4.8 g/dL	↓ 1 g/dL	Most by 20 wk, then gradual
Calcium (total)	9-10.3 mg/dL	↓ 10%	Gradual fall
Chloride	95-105 mEq/L	No significant change	Gradual rise
Creatinine (female)	0.6-1.1 mg/dL	↓ 0.3 mg/dL	Most by 20 wk
Fibrinogen	1.5-3.6 g/L	↑ 1-2 g/L	Progressive
Glucose, fasting (plasma)	65-105 mg/dL	↓ 10%	Gradual fall
Potassium (plasma)	3.5-4.5 mEq/L	↓ 0.2-0.3 mEq/L	By 20 wk
Protein (total)	6.5-8.5 g/dL	↓ 1 g/dL	By 20 wk, then stable
Sodium	135-145 mEq/L	↓ 2-4 mEq/L	By 20 wk, then stable
Urea nitrogen	12-30 mg/dL	↓ 50%	1st trimester
Uric acid	3.5-8 mg/dL	↓ 33%	1st trimester, rise at term
URINE CHEMISTRIES			
Creatinine	15-25 mg/kg/day (1-1.4 g/day)	No significant change	
Protein	Up to 150 mg/day	Up to 250-300 mg/day	By 20 wk
Creatinine clearance	90-130 mL/min/ 1.73 m^2	↓ 40%-50%	By 16 wk
SERUM ENZYMATIC ACTIVITIES			
Amylase	23-84 IU/L	↑ 50%-100%	
Transaminase			
Glutamic pyruvic (SGPT)	5-35 mU/mL	No significant change	
Glutamic oxaloacetic (SGOT)	5-40 mU/mL	No significant change	
Hematocrit (female)	36%-46%	↓ 4%-7%	Bottoms at 30-34 wk
Hemoglobin (female)	12-16 g/dL	↓ 1.5-2 g/dL	Bottoms at 30-34 wk
Leukocyte count	4.8-10.8 × 10^3/mm^3	↑ 3.5 × 10^3/mm^3	Gradual
Platelet count	150-400 × 10^3/mm^3	Slight decrease	
SERUM HORMONE VALUES			
Cortisol (plasma)	8-21 g/dL	↑ 20 g/dL	
Prolactin (female)	25 ng/mL	↑ 50-400 ng/mL	Gradual, peaks at term
Thyroxine (T$_4$), total	5-11 g/dL	↑ 5 g/dL	Early sustained
Triiodothyronine (T$_3$), total	125-245 ng/dL	↑ 50%	Early sustained

Data from Main DM, Main EK: Obstetrics and Gynecology: A Pocket Reference. Chicago, Year Book, 1984, p 7.

TABLE 6-2

CARDIOVASCULAR CHANGES IN PREGNANCY

Parameter	Amount of Change	Timing
Arterial blood pressures		
Systolic	↓ 4-6 mm Hg	All bottom at 20-24 wk, then rise gradually to prepregnancy
Diastolic	↓ 8-15 mm Hg	values at term
Mean	↓ 6-10 mm Hg	
Heart rate	↑ 12-18 beats/min	1st, 2nd, 3rd trimesters
Stroke volume	↑ 10%-30%	1st and 2nd trimesters, then stable until term
Cardiac output	↑ 33%-45%	Peaks in early 2nd trimester, then stable until term

Data from Main DM, Main EK: Obstetrics and Gynecology: A Pocket Reference. Chicago, Year Book, 1984, p 18.

that characterize pregnancy. Toward the end of pregnancy, vasoconstrictor tone, and with it blood pressure, normally increases. The normal, modest rise of arterial pressure as term approaches should be distinguished from the development of pregnancy-induced hypertension or preeclampsia. Pregnancy does not alter central venous pressures.

Blood pressure, as measured with a sphygmomanometer cuff around the brachial artery, varies with posture. In late pregnancy, arterial pressure is higher when the gravid woman is sitting compared with lying supine. When elevations in blood pressure are clinically detected during pregnancy, it is customary to repeat the measurement with the patient lying on her side. This practice usually introduces a systematic error. In the lateral position, the blood pressure cuff around the brachial artery is raised about 10 cm above the heart. This leads to a hydrostatic fall in measured pressure, yielding a reading about 7 mm Hg lower than if the cuff were at heart level, as occurs during sitting or supine measurements.

MECHANICAL CIRCULATORY EFFECTS OF THE GRAVID UTERUS

As pregnancy progresses, the enlarging uterus displaces and compresses various abdominal structures, including the iliac veins and inferior vena cava (and probably also the aorta), with marked effects. The supine position accentuates this venous compression, producing a fall in venous return and hence cardiac output. In most gravid women, a compensatory rise in peripheral resistance minimizes the fall in blood pressure. In up to 10% of gravid women, however, a significant fall occurs in blood pressure accompanied by symptoms of nausea, dizziness, and even syncope. This **supine hypotensive syndrome** is relieved by changing position to the side. The expected baroreflexive tachycardia, which normally occurs in response to other maneuvers that reduce cardiac output and blood pressure, does not accompany caval compression. In fact, bradycardia is often associated with the syndrome.

The venous compression by the gravid uterus elevates pressure in veins that drain the legs and pelvic organs, thereby exacerbating varicose veins in the legs and vulva and causing hemorrhoids. The rise in venous pressure is the major cause of the lower extremity edema that characterizes pregnancy. The hypoalbuminemia associated with pregnancy also shifts the balance of the other major factor in the Starling equation (colloid osmotic pressure) in favor of fluid transfer from the intravascular to the extracellular space. Because of venous compression, the rate of blood flow in the lower veins is also markedly reduced, causing a predisposition to thrombosis. The various effects of caval compression are somewhat mitigated by the development of a paravertebral collateral circulation that permits blood from the lower body to bypass the occluded inferior vena cava.

During late pregnancy, the uterus can also partially compress the aorta and its branches. This is thought to account for the observation in some patients of lower pressure in the femoral artery compared with that in the brachial artery. This aortic compression can be accentuated during uterine contractions and may be a cause of fetal distress when a patient is in the supine position. This phenomenon has been referred to as the Posiero effect. Clinically, it can be suspected when the femoral pulse is not palpable.

REGIONAL BLOOD FLOW

Blood flow to most regions of the body increases and reaches a plateau relatively early in pregnancy. Notable exceptions occur in the uterus, kidney, breasts, and skin, in each of which blood flow increases with gestational age. **Two of the major increases (those to the kidney and to the skin) serve purposes of elimination: the kidney of waste material and the skin of heat.** Both processes require plasma rather than whole blood, which gives point to the disproportionate increase of plasma over red blood cells in the blood expansion.

Early in pregnancy, renal blood flow increases to levels about 30% above nonpregnant levels and remains unchanged as pregnancy advances. This change accounts for the increased creatinine clearance and lower serum creatine level. Engorgement of the breasts begins early in gestation, with mammary blood flow increasing 2 to 3 times in later pregnancy. The skin blood flow increases slightly during the third trimester, reaching 12% of cardiac output.

There is little information on the distribution of blood flow to other organ systems during pregnancy. The uterine blood flow increases from about 100 mL/min in the nonpregnant state (2% of cardiac output) to about 1200 mL/min (17% of cardiac output) at term. Uterine blood flow and thus gas and nutrient transfer to the fetus are vulnerable. **When maternal cardiac output falls, blood flow to the brain, kidneys, and heart is supported by a redistribution of cardiac output, which shunts blood away from the uteroplacental circulation.** Similarly, changes in perfusion pressure can lead to decreases in uterine blood flow. Because the uterine vessels are maximally dilated during pregnancy, little autoregulation can occur to improve uterine blood flow.

CONTROL OF CARDIOVASCULAR CHANGES

The precise mechanisms accounting for the cardiovascular changes in pregnancy have not been fully elucidated. The rise in cardiac output and fall in peripheral resistance during pregnancy may be explained in terms of the circulatory response to an arteriovenous shunt, represented by the uteroplacental circulation. The elevations in cardiac output and uterine blood flow follow different time courses in pregnancy, however, with the former reaching its maximum in the second trimester and the latter increasing to term.

A unifying hypothesis suggests that the elevations in circulating steroid hormones, in combination with increases in production of aldosterone and vasodilators such as prostaglandins, atrial natriuretic peptide, nitric oxide, and probably others, reduce arterial tone

TABLE 6-3

LUNG VOLUMES AND CAPACITIES IN PREGNANCY

Test	Definition	Change in Pregnancy
Respiratory rate	Breaths/minute	No significant change
Tidal volume	The volume of air inspired and expired at each breath	Progressive rise throughout pregnancy of 0.1-0.2 L
Expiratory reserve volume	The maximum volume of air that can be additionally expired after a normal expiration	Lowered by about 15% (0.55 L in late pregnancy compared with 0.65 L postpartum)
Residual volume	The volume of air remaining in the lungs after a maximum expiration	Falls considerably (0.77 L in late pregnancy compared with 0.96 L postpartum)
Vital capacity	The maximum volume of air that can be forcibly inspired after a maximum expiration	Unchanged, except for possibly a small terminal diminution
Inspiratory capacity	The maximum volume of air that can be inspired from resting expiratory level	Increased by about 5%
Functional residual capacity	The volume of air in lungs at resting expiratory level	Lowered by about 18%
Minute ventilation	The volume of air inspired or expired in 1 min	Increased by about 40% as a result of the increased tidal volume and unchanged respiratory rate

Data from Main DM, Main EK: Obstetrics and Gynecology: A Pocket Reference. Chicago, Year Book, 1984, p 14.

and increase venous capacitance. **These changes, along with the development of arteriovenous shunts, appear responsible for the increase in blood volume and the hyperdynamic (high-flow, low-resistance) circulation of pregnancy.** The same hormonal changes cause relaxation in the cytoskeleton of the maternal heart, which allows the end-diastolic volume (and stroke volume) to increase.

OXYGEN-CARRYING CAPACITY OF BLOOD

Plasma volume expands proportionately more than red blood cell volume, leading to a fall in hematocrit. Optimal pregnancy outcomes are generally achieved with a maternal hematocrit of 33% to 35%. Hematocrit readings below about 27% or above about 39% are associated with less favorable outcomes. **Despite the relatively low "optimal" hematocrit, the arteriovenous oxygen difference in pregnancy is below nonpregnant levels.** This supports the concept that the hemoglobin concentration in pregnancy is more than sufficient to meet oxygen-carrying requirements.

Pregnancy requires about 1 g of elemental iron: 0.7 g for mother and 0.3 g for the placenta and fetus. A high proportion of women in the reproductive age group enter pregnancy without sufficient stores of iron to meet the increased needs of pregnancy.

▆ Respiratory System

The major respiratory changes in pregnancy involve three factors: the mechanical effects of the enlarging uterus, the increased total body oxygen consumption, and the respiratory stimulant effects of progesterone.

RESPIRATORY MECHANICS IN PREGNANCY

The changes in lung volume and capacities associated with pregnancy are detailed in Table 6-3. Assessment of mechanical changes during pregnancy reveals that the diaphragm at rest rises to a level of 4 cm above its usual resting position. The chest enlarges in transverse diameter by about 2.1 cm. Simultaneously, the subcostal angle increases from an average of 68.5 degrees to 103.5 degrees during the latter part of gestation. The increase in uterine size cannot completely explain the changes in chest configuration because these mechanical changes occur early in gestation.

As pregnancy progresses, the enlarging uterus elevates the resting position of the diaphragm. This results in less negative intrathoracic pressure and a decreased resting lung volume; that is, a decrease in functional residual capacity (FRC). The enlarging uterus produces no impairment in diaphragmatic or thoracic muscle motion. Hence, the vital capacity (VC) remains unchanged. **These characteristics—reduced FRC with unimpaired VC—are analogous to those seen in a pneumoperitoneum** and contrast with those seen in severe obesity or abdominal binding, where the elevation of the diaphragm is accompanied by decreased excursion of the respiratory muscles. Reductions in both the expiratory reserve volume and the residual volume contribute to the reduced FRC.

OXYGEN CONSUMPTION AND VENTILATION

Total body oxygen consumption increases about 15% to 20% in pregnancy. About half of this increase is accounted for by the uterus and its contents. The remainder is accounted for mainly by increased maternal renal and cardiac work. Smaller increments are due to greater breast tissue mass and to increased work of the respiratory muscles.

In general, a rise in oxygen consumption is accompanied by cardiorespiratory responses that facilitate oxygen delivery (i.e., by increases in cardiac output and alveolar ventilation). To the extent that elevations in cardiac output and alveolar ventilation keep pace with the rise in oxygen consumption, the arteriovenous oxygen difference and the arterial partial pressure of carbon dioxide (PCO_2), respectively, remain unchanged. **In pregnancy, the elevations in both cardiac output and alveolar ventilation are greater than those required to meet the increased oxygen consumption.** Hence, despite the rise in total body oxygen consumption, the arteriovenous oxygen difference and arterial PCO_2 both fall. The fall in PCO_2 (to 27-32 mm Hg), by definition, indicates hyperventilation.

The rise in minute ventilation reflects an approximate 40% increase in tidal volume at term; the respiratory rate does not change during pregnancy. During exercise, pregnant subjects show a 38% increase in minute ventilation and a 15% increase in oxygen consumption above comparable levels for postpartum subjects.

When injected into normal nonpregnant subjects, progesterone increases ventilation. The central chemoreceptors become more sensitive to CO_2 (i.e., the curve describing the ventilatory response to increasing CO_2 has a steeper slope). **Such increased respiratory sensitivity to CO_2 is characteristic of pregnancy and probably accounts for the hyperventilation of pregnancy.**

In summary, both at rest and with exercise, minute ventilation and, to a lesser extent, oxygen consumption are increased during pregnancy over the nonpregnant control values. The respiratory stimulating effect of progesterone is probably responsible for the disproportionate increase in minute ventilation over oxygen consumption.

ALVEOLAR-ARTERIAL GRADIENT AND ARTERIAL BLOOD GAS MEASUREMENTS

The hyperventilation of pregnancy results in a respiratory alkalosis. Renal compensatory bicarbonate excretion leads to a final maternal blood pH between 7.40 and 7.45. During labor (without conduction anesthesia), the hyperventilation associated with each contraction produces a further transient fall in PCO_2. By the end of the first stage of labor, when cervical dilation is complete, a decrease in arterial PCO_2 persists, even between contractions.

In general, when alveolar PCO_2 falls during hyperventilation, alveolar partial pressure of oxygen (PO_2) shows a corresponding rise, leading to a rise in arterial PO_2. In the first trimester, the mean arterial PO_2 may be 106 to 108 mm Hg. There is a slight downward trend in arterial PO_2 as pregnancy proceeds. This reflects, at least in part, an increased alveolar-arterial gradient, possibly resulting from the decrease in FRC discussed previously, which leads to a ventilation-perfusion mismatch.

DYSPNEA OF PREGNANCY

In general, airway resistance is unchanged or even decreased in pregnancy. **Despite the absence of obstructive or restrictive effects, dyspnea is a common symptom in pregnancy. Some studies have suggested that dyspnea may be experienced at some time during pregnancy by as many as 60% to 70% of women.** Although the mechanism has not been established, the dyspnea of pregnancy may involve the increased sensitivity and lowered threshold to PCO_2.

◾ *Renal Physiology*

ANATOMIC CHANGES IN THE URINARY TRACT

The urinary collecting system, including the calyces, renal pelves, and ureters, undergoes marked dilation in pregnancy, as is readily seen on intravenous urograms. It begins in the first trimester, is present in 90% of women at term, and may persist until the 12th to 16th postpartum week. Progesterone appears to produce smooth muscle relaxation in various organs, including the ureter. **As the uterus enlarges, partial obstruction of the ureter occurs at the pelvic brim in both the supine and the upright positions.** Because of the relatively greater effect on the right side, some have ascribed a role to the dilated ovarian venous plexus. Ovarian venous drainage is asymmetric, with the right vein emptying into the inferior vena cava and the left into the left renal vein.

RENAL BLOOD FLOW AND GLOMERULAR FILTRATION RATE

Renal plasma flow and the glomerular filtration rate (GFR) increase early in pregnancy, with maximum plateau elevations of at least 40% to 50% above nonpregnant levels by mid-gestation, and then remain unchanged to term. As was true for cardiac output, renal blood flow and GFR (clinically measured as the creatinine clearance) reach their peak relatively early in pregnancy, before the greatest expansion in intravascular and extracellular volume occurs. **The elevated GFR is reflected in lower serum levels of creatinine and urea nitrogen,** as noted in Table 6-1.

Pregnancy is associated with large reductions in resistance in the afferent and efferent arterioles of the renal arteries, which appears to involve **vasorelaxation induced by relaxin, endothelin, and nitric oxide.** The resulting rise in renal plasma flow accounts for the hyperfiltration.

RENAL TUBULAR FUNCTION

Although 500 to 900 mEq of sodium is retained during pregnancy, sodium balance is maintained with exquisite precision. Despite the large amounts of sodium consumed daily (100 to 300 mEq), only 20 to 30 mEq of sodium is retained every week. Pregnant women given high or low sodium diets are able to demonstrate decreases or increases in sodium tubular reabsorption, respectively, which maintain sodium and fluid balance.

Pregnant women also maintain fluid balance with no change in the concentrating or diluting ability of the kidney. Plasma osmolarity is reduced by about 10 mOsm/kg of water. Potassium metabolism during pregnancy is unchanged, although about 350 mEq of potassium is retained during pregnancy for fetoplacental development and expansion of maternal red cell mass.

The hyperventilation (low $PaCO_2$) of pregnancy results in respiratory alkalosis, which is compensated by renal excretion of bicarbonate. As a result, maternal renal buffering capacity is reduced.

FLUID VOLUMES

The maternal extracellular volume, which consists of intravascular and interstitial components, increases throughout pregnancy, leading to a state of physiologic extracellular hypervolemia. The intravascular volume, which consists of plasma and red cell components, increases about 50% during pregnancy. Maternal interstitial volume shows its greatest increase in the last trimester.

The magnitude of the rise in maternal plasma volume correlates with the size of the fetus; it is particularly marked in cases of multiple gestation. Multiparous women with poor reproductive histories show smaller increments in plasma volume and GFR when compared with those with a history of normal pregnancies and normal-sized babies.

RENIN-ANGIOTENSIN SYSTEM IN PREGNANCY

Plasma concentrations of renin, renin substrate, and angiotensin I and II are increased during pregnancy. **Renin levels remain elevated throughout pregnancy,** with at least a portion of the renin circulating in a high-molecular-weight form.

The uterus, like the kidney, can produce renin, and extremely high concentrations of renin occur in the amniotic fluid. The physiologic role of uterine renin has not been established.

▓ *Homeostasis of Maternal Energy Substrates*

The metabolic regulation of energy substrates, including glucose, amino acids, fatty acids, and ketone bodies, is complex and interrelated.

INSULIN EFFECTS AND GLUCOSE METABOLISM

In pregnancy, the insulin response to glucose stimulation is augmented. By the 10th week of normal pregnancy and continuing to term, fasting concentrations of insulin are elevated and those of glucose reduced. Until mid-gestation, these changes are accompanied by enhanced intravenous glucose tolerance (although oral glucose tolerance remains unchanged). **Glycogen synthesis and storage by the liver increases, and gluconeogenesis is inhibited.** Thus, during the first half of pregnancy, the anabolic actions of insulin are potentiated.

After early pregnancy, insulin resistance emerges, so glucose tolerance is impaired. The fall in serum glucose for a given dose of insulin is reduced compared with the response in earlier pregnancy. Elevation of circulating glucose is prolonged after meals, although fasting glucose remains reduced, as in early pregnancy.

A variety of humoral factors derived from the placenta have been suggested to account for the anti-insulin environment of the latter part of pregnancy. Perhaps the most important are cytokines and human placental lactogen (hPL), which antagonize the peripheral effects of insulin. An increase in levels of free cortisol and other hormones may also be involved in the insulin resistance of pregnancy.

LIPID METABOLISM

The potentiated anabolic effects of insulin that characterize early pregnancy lead to the inhibition of lipolysis. **During the second half of pregnancy, however, probably as a result of rising hPL levels, lipolysis is augmented, and fasting plasma concentrations of free fatty acids are elevated.** Teleologically, the free fatty acids act as substrates for maternal energy metabolism, whereas glucose and amino acids cross the placenta to the fetus. In the humoral milieu of the second half of the pregnancy, the increased free fatty acids lead to ketone body (β-hydroxybutyrate and acetoacetate) formation. Pregnancy is thus associated with an increased risk for ketoacidosis, especially after prolonged fasting.

In the context of maternal lipid metabolism, the most dramatic lipid change in pregnancy is the rise in fasting triglyceride concentration.

▓ *Placental Transfer of Nutrients*

The transfer of substances across the placenta occurs by several mechanisms, including simple diffusion, facilitated diffusion, and active transport. **Low molecular size and lipid solubility promote simple diffusion.** Substances with molecular weights greater than

TABLE 6-4

MATERNAL-FETAL TRANSFER DURING PREGNANCY

Function	Substance	Placental Transfer
Glucose homeostasis	Glucose	Excellent—"facilitated diffusion"
	Amino acids	Excellent—active transport
	Free fatty acids (FFA)	Very limited—essential FFA only
	Ketones	Excellent—diffusion
	Insulin	No transfer
	Glucagon	No transfer
Thyroid function	Thyroxine (T_4)	Very poor—diffusion
	Triiodothyronine (T_3)	Poor—diffusion
	Thyrotropin-releasing hormone (TRH)	Good
	Thyroid-stimulating immunoglobulin (TSI)	Good
	Thyroid-stimulating hormone (TSH)	Negligible transfer
	Propylthiouracil	Excellent
Adrenal hormones	Cortisol	Excellent transfer and active placental conversion of cortisol to cortisone beginning at mid-pregnancy[*]
	ACTH	No transfer
Parathyroid function	Calcium	Active transfer against gradient
	Magnesium	Active transfer against gradient
	Phosphorus	Active transfer against gradient
	Parathyroid hormone	Not transferred
Immunoglobulins	IgA	Minimal passive transfer
	IgG	Good—both passive and active transport from 7 wk gestation
	IgM	No transfer

[*]At mid-gestation, placental 11-β hydroxysteroid dehydrogenase converts cortisol to cortisone.

Data from Main DM, Main EK: Obstetrics and Gynecology: A Pocket Reference. Chicago, Year Book, 1984, p 37.

1000 Daltons, such as polypeptides and proteins, cross the placenta slowly, if at all.

Amino acids are actively transported across the placenta, making fetal levels higher than maternal levels. Glucose is transported by facilitated diffusion, leading to rapid equilibrium with only a small maternal-fetal gradient. **Glucose is the main energy substrate of the fetus** although amino acids and lactate may contribute up to 25% of fetal oxygen consumption. The degree and mechanism of placental transfer of these and other substances are summarized in Table 6-4.

■ *Other Endocrine Changes*

THYROID

The thyroid gland undergoes moderate enlargement during pregnancy. This is not due to elevation of thyroid-stimulating hormone (TSH), which remains unchanged. Placenta-derived human chorionic gonadotropin (hCG) has a TSH effect on the thyroid gland, which can result in abnormally low levels of TSH in the first trimester, when hCG concentrations are highest.

Circulating thyroid hormone exists in two primary active forms: thyroxine (T_4) and triiodothyronine (T_3). The former circulates in higher concentrations, is more highly protein bound, and is less metabolically potent than T_3, for which it may serve as a prohormone. Circulating T_4 is bound to carrier proteins, about 85% to thyroxine-binding globulin (TBG) and most of the remainder to another protein, thyroxine-binding prealbumin. It is believed that only the unbound fraction of the circulating hormone is biologically active. **TBG is increased during pregnancy because the high estrogen levels induce increased hepatic synthesis.** The body responds by raising total circulating levels of T_4 and T_3, and the net effect is that the free, biologically active concentration of each hormone is unchanged. Therefore, clinically, the free T_4 index, which corrects

TABLE 6-5

ANALYSIS OF WEIGHT GAIN IN PREGNANCY

Tissues and Fluids	Increase in Weight (Grams) Up to:			
	10 wk	20 wk	30 wk	40 wk
Fetus	5	300	1500	3400
Placenta	20	170	430	650
Amniotic fluid	30	350	750	800
Uterus	140	320	600	970
Mammary gland	45	180	360	405
Blood	100	600	1300	1250
Interstitial fluid (no edema or leg edema)	0	30	80	1680
Maternal stores	310	2050	3480	3345
Total weight gained	650	4000	8500	12,500

Data from Hytten F, Chamberlain G (eds): Clinical Physiology in Obstetrics. Oxford, Blackwell Scientific, 1980, p 221.

the total circulating T_4 for the amount of binding protein, is an appropriate measure of thyroid function, with the same normal range as in the nonpregnant state. **Only minimal amounts of thyroid hormone cross the placenta.**

ADRENAL

Adrenocorticotropic hormone (ACTH) and plasma cortisol levels are both elevated from 3 months' gestation to delivery. Although less so than thyroid hormones, circulating cortisol is also primarily bound to a specific plasma protein, corticosteroid-binding globulin (CBG), or transcortin. **Unlike the level of thyroid hormones, the mean unbound level of cortisol is elevated in pregnancy;** there is also some loss of the diurnal variation that characterizes its concentration in nonpregnant women.

Weight Gain in Pregnancy

The average weight gain in pregnancy uncomplicated by generalized edema is 12.5 kg (28 lb). The components of this weight gain are indicated in Table 6-5. The products of conception constitute only about 40% of the total maternal weight gain.

Placental Transfer of Oxygen and Carbon Dioxide

FETAL OXYGENATION

The placenta receives 60% of the combined ventricular output, whereas the postnatal lung receives a greater proportion of the cardiac output. Unlike the lung, which consumes little of the oxygen it transfers, **a significant percentage of the oxygen derived from maternal blood at term is consumed by placental tissue.** The degree of functional shunting of placental blood past exchange sites is about 10-fold greater than in the lung. A major cause of this functional shunting is probably a mismatch between maternal and fetal blood flow at the exchange sites, analogous to the ventilation-perfusion inequalities that occur in the lung.

The uteroplacental circulation subserves fetal gas exchange. Oxygen, carbon dioxide, and inert gases cross the placenta by simple diffusion. The rate of transfer is proportional to the difference in gas tension across the placenta and the surface area of the placenta; and the transfer rate is inversely proportional to diffusion distance between maternal and fetal blood. The placenta normally does not pose a significant barrier to respiratory gas exchange, unless it becomes separated (abruption placenta) or edematous (severe hydrops fetalis).

Figure 6-1 depicts the anatomic distribution of uterine and umbilical blood flow and O_2 transfer across the placenta. A **maternal shunt,** which describes the fraction of blood shunted to the myoendometrium and is estimated to constitute 20% of uterine blood flow, is depicted. Similarly, a **fetal shunt,** which supplies blood to the placenta and fetal membranes and accounts for 19% of umbilical blood flow, is shown. The **maternal-to-fetal** PO_2 and PCO_2 gradients are calculated from measurements of gas tensions in the uterine and umbilical arteries and veins. **The umbilical vein of the fetus, like the pulmonary vein of the adult, carries the circulation's most highly oxygenated blood.** The umbilical venous PO_2 of about 28 mm Hg is relatively low by adult standards. This relatively low fetal tension is essential for survival in utero because a high PO_2 initiates physiologic adjustments (e.g., closure of the ductus arteriosus and vasodilation of the pulmonary

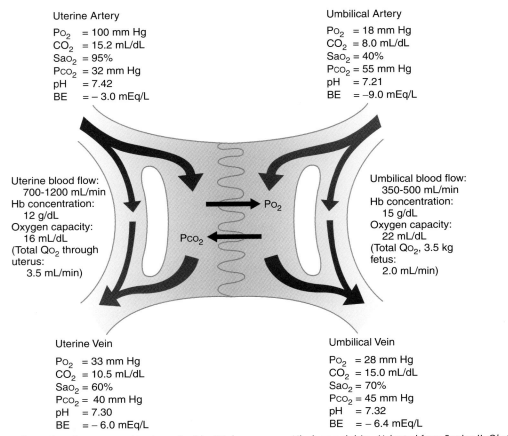

Uterine Artery

P_{O_2} = 100 mm Hg
CO_2 = 15.2 mL/dL
Sa_{O_2} = 95%
P_{CO_2} = 32 mm Hg
pH = 7.42
BE = −3.0 mEq/L

Umbilical Artery

P_{O_2} = 18 mm Hg
CO_2 = 8.0 mL/dL
Sa_{O_2} = 40%
P_{CO_2} = 55 mm Hg
pH = 7.21
BE = −9.0 mEq/L

Uterine blood flow:
700-1200 mL/min
Hb concentration:
12 g/dL
Oxygen capacity:
16 mL/dL
(Total Q_{O_2} through uterus:
3.5 mL/min)

Umbilical blood flow:
350-500 mL/min
Hb concentration:
15 g/dL
Oxygen capacity:
22 mL/dL
(Total Q_{O_2}, 3.5 kg fetus:
2.0 mL/min)

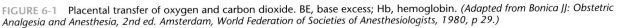

Uterine Vein

P_{O_2} = 33 mm Hg
CO_2 = 10.5 mL/dL
Sa_{O_2} = 60%
P_{CO_2} = 40 mm Hg
pH = 7.30
BE = −6.0 mEq/L

Umbilical Vein

P_{O_2} = 28 mm Hg
CO_2 = 15.0 mL/dL
Sa_{O_2} = 70%
P_{CO_2} = 45 mm Hg
pH = 7.32
BE = −6.4 mEq/L

FIGURE 6-1 Placental transfer of oxygen and carbon dioxide. BE, base excess; Hb, hemoglobin. *(Adapted from Bonica JJ: Obstetric Analgesia and Anesthesia, 2nd ed. Amsterdam, World Federation of Societies of Anesthesiologists, 1980, p 29.)*

vessels) that normally occur in the neonate but would be harmful in utero.

Although not involved in respiratory gas exchange, fetal breathing movements are critically involved in lung development and in the development of respiratory regulation. Fetal breathing differs from that in the adult in that it is episodic, sensitive to fetal glucose concentrations, and inhibited by hypoxia. Because of its sensitivity to acute O_2 deprivation, fetal breathing is used clinically as indicator of the adequacy of fetal oxygenation.

FETAL AND MATERNAL HEMOGLOBIN DISSOCIATION CURVES

Most of the oxygen in blood is carried by hemoglobin in red blood cells. The maximum amount of oxygen carried per gram of hemoglobin, that is, the amount carried at 100% saturation, is fixed at 1.37 mL. The hemoglobin flow rates depend on blood flow rates and hemoglobin concentration. The uterine blood flow at term has been estimated at 700 to 1200 mL/min, with about 75% to 88% of this entering the intervillous space.

The umbilical blood flow has been estimated at 350 to 500 mL/min, with more than 50% going to the placenta (see Figure 6-1).

The hemoglobin concentration of the blood determines its oxygen-carrying capacity, which is expressed in milliliters of oxygen per 100 mL of blood. In the fetus at or near term, the hemoglobin concentration is about 18 g/dL, and oxygen-carrying capacity is 20 to 22 mL/dL. Maternal oxygen-carrying capacity of blood, which is generally proportional to hemoglobin concentration, is lower than that of the fetus.

The affinity of hemoglobin for oxygen, which is reflected as the percent saturation at a given oxygen tension, depends on chemical conditions. As is illustrated in Figure 6-2, **when compared with that in nonpregnant adults, the binding of oxygen by hemoglobin is much greater in the fetus under standard conditions of P_{CO_2}, pH, and temperature.** In contrast, maternal affinity is lower under these conditions, with 50% of hemoglobin saturated with O_2 at a P_{O_2} of 26.5 mm Hg (P_{50}) for mother compared with 20 mm Hg for the fetus.

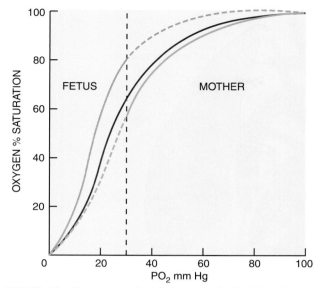

FIGURE 6-2   The oxygen dissociation curve for fetal blood compared with maternal blood. The central continuous curve (in red) is for normal adult blood under standard conditions. A vertical line at an oxygen partial pressure of 30 mm Hg divides the curves. The fetal curve normally operates below that level (to the left) and the maternal curve above it (to the right). *(Adapted from Hytten F, Chamberlain G [eds]: Clinical Physiology in Obstetrics, 2nd ed. Oxford, Blackwell, 1991, p 418.)*

In vivo, the greater fetal temperature and lower pH shift the O_2-dissociation curve to the right, while the lower maternal temperature and higher pH shift the maternal curve to the left. As a result, the O_2-dissociation curves for the fetal and maternal blood are not too dissimilar at the site of placental transfer. Maternal venous blood probably has an O_2 saturation of about 73% and a PO_2 of about 36 mm Hg, and the corresponding values for blood in the umbilical vein are about 63% and 28 mm Hg. As the only source of O_2 for the fetus, blood in the umbilical vein has a higher O_2 saturation and PO_2 than blood in the fetal circulation (Figure 6-3). In the presence of a low fetal arterial PO_2, fetal oxygenation is maintained by a high rate of blood flow to fetal tissues, which is supported by a very high cardiac output. This feature, along with the lower P_{50} of fetal blood, results in normal O_2 delivery to fetal organs.

The decrease in the affinity of hemoglobin for oxygen produced by a fall in pH is referred to as the Bohr effect. Because of the unique situation in the placenta, a double Bohr effect facilitates oxygen transfer from mother to fetus. When CO_2 and fixed acids are transferred from fetus to mother, the associated rise in fetal pH increases the fetal red blood cell's affinity for oxygen uptake. The concomitant reduction in maternal blood pH decreases oxygen affinity and promotes its unloading of oxygen from maternal red cells.

▪ *Fetal Circulation*

Several anatomic and physiologic factors must be noted in considering the fetal circulation (Table 6-6; see Figure 6-3).

The normal adult circulation is a series circuit with blood flowing through the right heart, the lungs, the left heart, the systemic circulation, and finally the right heart. In the fetus, the circulation is a parallel system with the cardiac outputs from the right and left ventricles directed primarily to different vascular beds. For example, the right ventricle, which contributes about 65% of the combined output, pumps blood primarily through the pulmonary artery, ductus arteriosus, and descending aorta. Only a small fraction of right ventricular output flows through the pulmonary circulation. The left ventricle supplies blood mainly to the tissues supplied by the aortic arch, such as the brain. **The fetal circulation is a parallel circuit characterized by channels (ductus venosus, foramen ovale, and ductus arteriosus) and preferential streaming, which function to maximize the delivery of more highly oxygenated blood to the upper body and brain, less highly oxygenated blood to the lower body, and very low blood flow to the nonfunctional lungs.**

The umbilical vein, carrying oxygenated (80% saturated) blood from the placenta to the fetal body, enters the portal system. A portion of this umbilical-portal blood passes through the hepatic microcirculation, where oxygen is extracted, and thence through the hepatic veins into the inferior vena cava. **Most of the blood bypasses the liver through the ductus venosus, which directly enters the inferior vena cava, which also receives the unsaturated (25% saturated) venous return from the lower body.** Blood reaching the heart through the inferior vena cava has an oxygen saturation of about 70%, which represents the most highly oxygenated blood in the heart. About one third of blood returning to the heart from the inferior vena cava preferentially streams across the right atrium, mixing with blood from the superior vena cava to the foramen ovale into the left atrium, where it mixes with the relatively meager pulmonary venous return. Blood flows from the left atrium into the left ventricle, and then to the ascending aorta.

The proximal aorta, carrying the most highly saturated blood leaving the heart (65%), gives off branches to supply the brain and upper body. Most of the blood returning through the inferior vena cava enters the right atrium, where it mixes with the unsaturated blood returning through the superior vena cava (25% saturated). Right ventricular outflow (O_2 saturation of 55%) enters the aorta through the ductus arteriosus, and the descending aorta supplies the lower body with blood having less O_2 saturation (about 60%) than that flowing to the brain and the upper body.

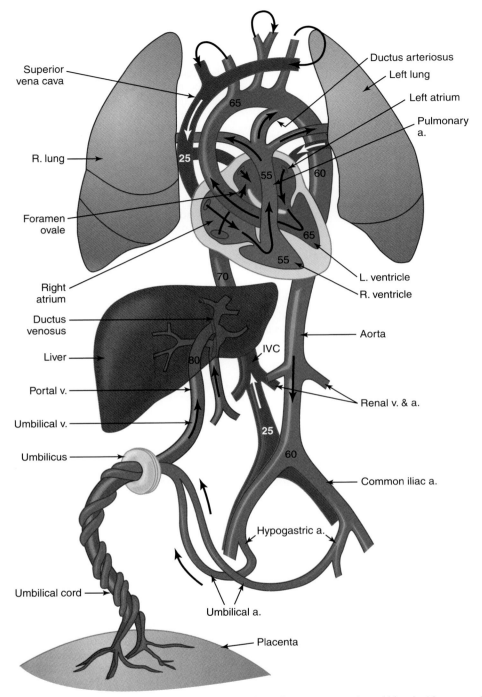

FIGURE 6-3 The fetal circulation. Numbers represent approximate values of percent saturation of blood with oxygen in utero. *(Adapted from Parer JJ: Fetal circulation. In Sciarra JJ [ed]: Obstetrics and Gynecology, Vol 3: Maternal and Fetal Medicine. Hagerstown, MD, Harper & Row, 1984, p 2.)*

TABLE 6-6

COMPONENTS OF THE FETAL CIRCULATION

Fetal Structure	From/To	Adult Remnant
Umbilical vein	Umbilicus/ductus venosus	Ligamentum teres hepatis
Ductus venosus	Umbilical vein/inferior vena cava (bypasses liver)	Ligamentum venosum
Foramen ovale	Right atrium/left atrium	Closed atrial wall
Ductus arteriosus	Pulmonary artery/descending aorta	Ligamentum arteriosum
Umbilical artery	Common iliac artery/umbilicus	Superior vesical arteries; lateral vesicoumbilical ligaments

Data from Main DM, Main EK: Obstetrics and Gynecology: A Pocket Reference. Chicago, Year Book, 1984, p 34.

The role of the ductus arteriosus must be emphasized. **Right ventricular output enters the pulmonary trunk, from which its major portion, owing to the high vascular resistance of the pulmonary circulation, bypasses the lungs by flowing through the ductus arteriosus to the descending aorta.** Although the descending aorta supplies branches to the lower fetal body, the major portion of descending aortic flow goes to the umbilical arteries, which carry deoxygenated blood to the placenta.

CHANGES IN THE ANATOMY OF THE CARDIOVASCULAR SYSTEM AFTER BIRTH

The following changes occur after birth (see Table 6-6):
1. **Elimination of the placental circulation, with interruption and eventual obliteration of the umbilical vessels**
2. **Closure of the ductus venosus**
3. **Closure of the foramen ovale**
4. **Gradual constriction and eventual obliteration of the ductus arteriosus**
5. **Dilation of the pulmonary vessels and establishment of the pulmonary circulation**

The elimination of the umbilical circulation, closure of the vascular shunts, and establishment of the pulmonary circulation will change the vascular circuitry of the neonate from an "in parallel" system to an "in series" system.

Immunology of Pregnancy

Nearly 60 years ago, Peter Medawar recognized the apparent paradox of the immunologic evasion of the semiallogenic fetus to maternal response. He proposed three hypotheses to explain this paradox: (1) anatomic separation of mother and fetus; (2) antigenic immaturity of the fetus; or (3) immunologic "inertness" (tolerance) of the mother. In the intervening years, **it has become apparent that both the mother and her fetus are immunologically aware of one another and yet tolerance exists for the most part.** Furthermore, while the maternal immune response during pregnancy is qualitatively different, pregnancy does *not* result in an overall maternal immunosuppression.

It is clear that the growth and development of a semiallogeneic conceptus within an immunologically competent mother depends on the manner in which pregnancy alters the immune regulatory mechanisms. Historically, attention in addressing the "Medawar paradox" has focused exclusively on the mother, but it is now known that mammalian fetuses are capable of mounting immune responses in utero. The interplay between the fetal and maternal immune systems is complex and is a current active area on investigation.

INNATE AND ADAPTIVE IMMUNITY

Mammalian (including human) immune systems have two fundamental responses: an early "innate" and a later more specific and robust adaptive response.

The innate immune system response is the first line of defense and includes surface barriers (mucosal immunity), saliva, tears, nasal secretions, perspiration, blood and tissue monocyte-macrophages, natural killer (NK) cells, endothelial cells, polymorphonuclear neutrophils, the complement system, dendritic cells, and the normal microbial flora. **The adaptive immune system is composed of cell-mediated (T lymphocytes) and humoral (B lymphocytes-antibodies) responses.** Activation of T and consequently B lymphocytes is critical for the development of lifelong memory immune responses.

Innate immune cells have evolutionary acquired mechanisms that recognize the foreign nature of the inciting antigen and mount a transient protection within hours. There is no need for major histocompatibility complex (MHC) molecules. **The epithelial cell interaction with the antigens induces the release of cytokines and chemokines, which attract the macrophages, dendritic cells, and NK cells.** Macrophages and neutrophils then engulf and lyse the pathogens and produce cytokines. NK cells play the key role in destroying the virally infected cells. Damaged epithelial cells lead to the activation of complements. Complements can directly kill the microbes by punching holes in their membrane and indirectly by opsonizing them, which facilitates their phagocytosis. Complements also promote the inflammatory cell recruitment. **The cytokines released from the immune cells activate the vascular endothelial cells, increasing permeability, allowing immune effector cells to penetrate into the tissues**.

The critical link between the innate immune response and the adaptive immune response is antigen presentation. Foreign proteins that are phagocytosed are processed intracellularly, and then expressed on the cell surface complexed with MHC II. Additionally, the presenting cells provide critical secondary signals (through cell surface molecules) that are permissive for appropriate T-cell activation. **Among the most efficient antigen-presenting cells are dendritic cells.**

Dendritic cells play a key role in alerting the adaptive immune responses. Immature dendritic cells engulf the pathogens, carry them to the lymph nodes, and present them to CD4$^+$ T lymphocytes. Activated T cells develop surface receptors for specific foreign antigens and undergo clonal proliferation. Cytotoxic (activated) T cells can directly kill target cells expressing viral antigens together with MHC I. In contrast to antigens presented in the context of MHC II, **a portion of all cellular proteins are expressed on the cell surface of all normal cells in the context of MHC I.** By this mechanism, the immune system can determine whether a cell is producing self proteins or if the cell has been altered (e.g., by virus) to produce foreign proteins.

Once CD4$^+$ T cells are activated, they can direct an immune response by secreting proteins (cytokines) that activate surrounding cells. By secreting interferon-γ and interleukin-2 (IL-2), a CD4$^+$ T cell induces a cellular immune response through CD8$^+$ "killer" T cells. By secreting IL-4 and IL-5, CD4$^+$ T cells promote B cells to proliferate and differentiate for immunoglobulin (antibody) production. B cells exposed to antigen for the first time produce immunoglobulin M (IgM). As the affinity of the immunoglobulin (antibody) increases, the B cell undergoes a genetic rearrangement and may produce a variety of different antibodies. The most specific are usually of the IgG subtype. IgG crosses the placenta and will accumulate into the fetus.

DEVELOPMENT OF FETAL IMMUNITY

The innate immune effector cells first arise from hematopoietic progenitors noted in the blood islands of the yolk sac. By 8 embryonic weeks, the fetal liver becomes the source of these cells, and by 20 weeks, the fetal bone marrow takes over.

Macrophage-like cells arise from the yolk sac around 4 weeks; by 16 weeks, a fetus has the same number of circulating macrophages as adults, but they are less functional. The fetus has fewer tissue macrophages. Immature granulocytes can be found in the fetal spleen and liver by 8 weeks. NK cells are detected in the liver by 8 to 13 weeks and complements 2 and 4 by 8 weeks. C1, 3, 5, 7, 9 are found in the serum by 18 weeks. Maternal complements do not cross placenta into the fetus. The complement system continues to mature after parturition, and adult levels are reached by 1 year of age. Skin, one of the main innate barriers, completes its development 2 to 3 weeks after birth.

The cellular component of the adaptive immunity, T cells, are also derived from hematopoietic progenitors that are first seen in the blood islands of the yolk sac by 8 weeks. To differentiate into activated T cells, they must first migrate to the thymus gland, a relatively large organ in the fetus, the sole function of which appears to be to nurture and develop T cells. After maturation, T cells develop into either CD4 or CD8 types according to the surface receptor expressed. By 16 weeks, the thymus contains T cells in proportion to those found in the adult. **In the newborn, the proportion of CD4 helper T cells and CD8 T cells is similar to that in the adult. However interferon-γ production is less efficient in fetal CD4 helper T cells.**

Fetal B cells are first detected in the liver by 8 weeks, and around the second trimester, B-cell production is mostly from the bone marrow. Fetal B cells secrete IgG or IgA during the second trimester, but IgM antibodies are not secreted until the third trimester. Cord IgM levels greater than 20 mg/dL suggest an intrauterine infection. **Maternal IgG crosses the placenta as early as the late first trimester, but the efficiency of the transport is poor until 30 weeks.** Significant passive immunity can be transferred to the fetus in this manner, and **for this reason, premature infants are not as well protected by maternal antibodies. IgM, because of its larger molecular size, is unable to cross the placenta.** The other immunoglobulins (IgA, IgD, and IgE) are also confined to the maternal compartment, but the fetus can make its own IgA and IgM.

Physiologically, newborns have higher neutrophil and lymphocyte counts. The neutrophil counts decrease by 1 week of age, whereas lymphocyte counts continue to rise. **The proportion of lymphocytes and absolute lymphocyte counts are higher in neonates compared with adults.**

IMMUNOBIOLOGY OF THE MATERNAL-FETAL INTERACTION

Pregnancy poses a special immunologic problem. The embryo must implant and cause a portion (placenta) to invade the uterine lining in order to gain access to the maternal circulation for nutrition and gas exchange. The maintenance of the antigenically dissimilar fetus in the uterus of the mother is of primary importance in obstetrics. The total picture of immune regulation at the maternal-fetal interface is yet to be elucidated, but the following is a synopsis of the current level of understanding.

The primary sites of modulation of the maternal response are the uterus, regional lymphatics, and placenta. **In the uterus, NK-cell–mediated inflammation is necessary for the appropriate attachment and penetration of the fertilized egg into the uterine wall and for early placental development,** whereas increased suppressive T cells, the presence of molecules that inactivate the previously activated maternal lymphocytes (CTLA4), and the absence of B cells provide the needed immune quiescence to allow for successful pregnancy. The placenta and the membranes provide the key barrier in protecting the growing fetus from microbial pathogens and toxins circulating in the mother's blood. **Syncytiotrophoblast, which makes up the cell barrier between the fetal and maternal blood in the placenta, does not express classic self and nonself MHC I and II molecules.** Deeper trophoblastic cells do not express MHC II, but some express MHC I and are not stimulatory. This allows protection from invading microbes but at the same time prevents the destruction of the fetus.

HLA-G suppresses the adaptive and innate immune responses in the placenta and promotes the release of antiinflammatory cytokines such as IL-10. The soluble forms of HLA-G are found in the blood of pregnant women. HLA-G is thought to act by suppressing the activity of uterine NK cells, which normally destroy cells that *lack* the expression of MHC I.

The understanding of mechanisms of immune regulation is largely derived from the study of autoimmune diseases. Many disease-free individuals possess potentially autoreactive T cells. A variety of mechanisms regulate the response of CD4+ T cells so that they don't react against self antigens. Naïve T helper cells have the potential to become a variety of specialized T cells. There are now four well-recognized possibilities, each with a unique role and ability to cross-regulate. T_H1 cells drive cell-mediated immunity by secreting IL-2 and interferon-γ. T_H2 cells drive humoral reactions (antibody and B cell) by secreting IL-4. Regulatory T cells are a subtype that suppresses ongoing cellular immune reactions through cell contact. Lastly, there is a newly described proinflammatory population of T cells (T_H17) that secrete IL-17. These T_H17 cells under normal circumstances are important for the clearance of parasites, bacteria, and fungi, but under pathologic conditions, they appear to play a crucial role in the development of autoimmune disease. One of the hallmarks of T-cell regulation is the ability of these specialized T-cell populations to cross-regulate.

IMMUNOLOGIC RESPONSE DURING NORMAL PREGNANCY

The mother's immunologic defense system remains intact during pregnancy. While allowing the fetus to grow, the mother must still be able to protect herself and her fetus from infection and antigenically foreign substances. **The nonspecific (innate) mechanisms of the immunologic system (including phagocytosis and the inflammatory response) are not affected by pregnancy. The specific (adaptive) mechanisms of the immune response (humoral and cellular) are also not significantly affected.** In fact, women with renal transplants do not experience any reduction in serious episodes of acute rejection during pregnancy. No significant change occurs in the leukocyte count. The percentage of B or T lymphocytes is not appreciably altered, nor is there any consistent alteration in their performance during pregnancy. Immunoglobulin levels do not change in pregnancy, and vaccine responses are preserved.

However, **pregnant women are at higher risk for severe infection and death from certain pathogens** such as viruses (hepatitis, influenza, varicella, cytomegalovirus, polio), bacteria (*Listeria*, streptococcus, gonorrhea, salmonella, leprosy), and parasites (malaria, coccidioidomycosis) compared with nonpregnant women. The underlying mechanism for this selective immune suppression is not clearly understood.

ROLE OF IMMUNOLOGY IN PREGNANCY-ASSOCIATED CONDITIONS

The major pregnancy-associated immunologic disease process is hemolytic disease of the newborn. Rh factor incompatibility, which is the most important of these conditions, is discussed in Chapter 15.

Hemolytic disease secondary to non-Rh sensitization and the destruction of lymphocytes or platelets secondary to sensitization against specific surface antigens have the same pathogenesis. Fetal cellular antigens leak into the maternal circulation, primarily at birth, and initiate an immune response. The reaction to these foreign antigens (primarily Rh) leads to a humoral response. Initially, only a weak IgM response can be measured. In a subsequent pregnancy, the maternal immune system undergoes a memory response, and highly specific IgG molecules are secreted by memory plasma cells. These antibodies cross the placenta and attach to the fetal Rh-bearing RBCs. The consequence is the sequestration and destruction of fetal RBCs in the fetal spleen, leading occasionally to profound fetal anemia and hydrops.

Although the Rhesus antigen (Rh) is the most common cause of fetal alloimmunization-induced fetal anemia, other antigens are also implicated. The Kell antigen has the additional problem that the maternal IgG against Kell also suppresses erythropoiesis in the fetal bone marrow. **ABO incompatibility does not lead to a significant maternal immune response to fetal antigens.** Thus, the nature of the antigen is important, but the reason certain antigens are potentially pathogenic is poorly understood.

SUGGESTED READING

Fineman JR, Clyman R, Heymann MA: Fetal cardiovascular physiology. *In* Creasy RK, Resnick R, Iams JD (eds): Maternal-Fetal Medicine. Principles and Practice, 5th ed. Philadelphia, WB Saunders, 2004, pp 169-180.

Kahn DA, Koos BJ: Maternal physiology during pregnancy. *In* Decherney AH, Nathan L, Goodwin TM, Laufer N (eds): Current Diagnosis and Treatment. Obstetrics & Gynecology, 10th ed. New York, McGraw-Hill, 2007, pp 149-158.

Koos BJ: Breathing and sleep states in the fetus and at birth. *In* Marcus CL, Carroll JL, Donnelly DF, Loughlin GM (eds): Sleep and Breathing in Children, 2nd ed. New York, Informa Healthcare, 2008, pp 1-17.

Terness P, Kallikourdis M, Betz A, et al: Tolerance signaling molecules and pregnancy: IDO, galectins, and the renaissance of regulatory T cells. Am J Reprod Immunol 58:238, 2007.

Chapter 7

Antepartum Care
PRECONCEPTION AND PRENATAL CARE, GENETIC EVALUATION AND TERATOLOGY, AND ANTENATAL FETAL ASSESSMENT

MICHAEL C. LU • JOHN WILLIAMS III • CALVIN J. HOBEL

▒ Preconception Care

Ideally, prenatal care should begin before pregnancy. Organogenesis begins early in pregnancy, and placental development starts with implantation at 7 days postconception. Poor placental development has been linked to such pregnancy complications as preeclampsia, preterm birth, and intrauterine growth restriction and may play a role in fetal programming of chronic diseases in later life. By the time most pregnant women have their first prenatal visit, it is often too late to prevent some birth defects or defective placental development.

More importantly, **early prenatal care is often too late to restore allostasis**. Allostasis refers to the body's ability to maintain stability through change. Examples include feedback inhibition on the hypothalamic-pituitary-adrenal (HPA) axis to keep the body's stress response in check, or modulation of the body's inflammatory response by the HPA axis. In the face of chronic and repeated stress (psychological or biologic), however, these systems can wear out. If a woman enters pregnancy with worn-out allostatic systems (e.g., dysregulated stress or inflammatory response), she may be more vulnerable to a number of pregnancy complications, including preterm birth.

The growing recognition of the limits of prenatal care and the importance of women's health before pregnancy has drawn increasing attention to preconception care. As defined by the U.S. Centers for Disease Control and Prevention, preconception care is a set of interventions that aim to identify and modify biomedical, behavioral, and social risks to a woman's health or pregnancy outcome through prevention and management. The American College of Obstetricians and Gynecologists (ACOG) recommends that a routine visit by any woman who may, at some time, become pregnant presents an opportunity to promote preconception health, whether or not she is planning on getting pregnant. Men should also get preconception care, though the content of preconception care for men is less well defined.

Several models of preconception care have been developed. **Major components of preconception care include risk assessment, health promotion, and medical and psychosocial interventions and follow-up**, as summarized in Table 7-1. There is currently no consensus on the timing of preconception care, probably because there are different ideas about what preconception care should be or do. For some, preconception care means a single prepregnancy checkup a few months before couples attempt to conceive. A single visit, however, may be too little too late to address some problems (e.g., promoting smoking cessation or healthy weight) and will miss those pregnancies that are unintended at the time of conception (about half of all pregnancies in the United States). For others, preconception care means all well-woman care, from prepubescence to menopause. In practice, however, asking providers to squeeze more into an already hurried routine visit may not be feasible, and some components (e.g., genetic screening or laboratory testing) may not be indicated for every woman at every visit.

Preconception care is probably more than a single prepregnancy visit and less than all well-woman care. A good place to start is to ask every woman at every visit about her reproductive life plan. A **reproductive life plan** is a set of personal goals about having or not having children based on personal values and resources, and a plan to achieve those goals. The provider should ask the woman if she plans to have any (more) children, and how long she plans to wait until she (next) becomes pregnant. If it is within the next 1 or 2 years,

TABLE 7-1

ELEMENTS OF PRECONCEPTION COUNSELING AND CARE

Major Components of Preconception Care	Risk Assessment
Reproductive life plan	Ask your patient if she plans to have any (more) children and how long she plans to wait until she (next) becomes pregnant. Help her develop a plan to achieve those goals.
Past reproductive history	Review prior adverse pregnancy outcomes, such as fetal loss, birth defects, low birth weight, and preterm birth, and assess ongoing biobehavioral risks that could lead to recurrence in a subsequent pregnancy.
Past medical history	Ask about past medical history such as rheumatic heart disease, thromboembolism, or autoimmune diseases that could affect future pregnancy. Screen for ongoing chronic conditions such as hypertension and diabetes.
Medications	Review current medication use. Avoid category X drugs and most category D drugs unless potential maternal benefits outweigh fetal risks (see Box 7-1). Review use of over-the-counter medications, herbs, and supplements.
Infections and immunizations	Screen for periodontal, urogenital, and sexually transmitted infections as indicated. Discuss TORCH (toxoplasmosis, other, rubella, cytomegalovirus, and herpes) infections and update immunization for hepatitis B, rubella, varicella, Tdap (combined tetanus, diphtheria, and pertussis), human papillomavirus, and influenza vaccines as needed.
Genetic screening and family history	Assess risk for chromosomal or genetic disorders based on family history, ethnic background, and age. Offer cystic fibrosis screening. Discuss management of known genetic disorders (e.g., phenylketonuria, thrombophilia) before and during pregnancy.
Nutritional assessment	Assess anthropometric (body mass index), biochemical (e.g., anemia), clinical, and dietary risks.
Substance abuse	Ask about smoking, alcohol, drug use. Use T-ACE (tolerance, annoyed, cut down, eye opener) or CAGE (cut-down, annoyed, guilty, eye-opener) questions to screen for alcohol and substance abuse.
Toxins and teratogens	Review exposures at home, neighborhood, and work. Review Material Safety Data Sheet and consult local Teratogen Information Service as needed.
Psychosocial concerns	Screen for depression, anxiety, intimate-partner violence, and major psychosocial stressors.
Physical examination	Focus on periodontal, thyroid, heart, breasts, and pelvic examination.
Laboratory tests	Check complete blood count, urinalysis, type and screen, rubella, syphilis, hepatitis B, HIV, cervical cytology; screen for gonorrhea, chlamydia, and diabetes in selected populations. Consider thyroid-stimulating hormone.
Major Components of Preconception Care	**Health promotion**
Family planning	Promote family planning based on a woman's reproductive life plan. For women who are not planning on getting pregnant, promote effective contraceptive use and discuss emergency contraception.
Healthy weight and nutrition	Promote healthy prepregnancy weight through exercise and nutrition. Discuss macronutrients and micronutrients, including 5-a-day and daily intake of multivitamin containing folic acid.
Health behaviors	Promote such health behaviors as nutrition, exercise, safe sex, effective use of contraception, dental flossing, and use of preventive health services. Discourage risk behaviors such as douching, nonuse of seat belt, smoking, and alcohol and substance abuse.
Stress resilience	Promote healthy nutrition, exercise, sleep, and relaxation techniques; address ongoing stressors such as intimate partner violence; identify resources to help patient develop problem-solving and conflict resolution skills, positive mental health, and relational resilience.
Healthy environments	Discuss household, neighborhood, and occupational exposures to metals, organic solvents, pesticides, endocrine disruptors, and allergens. Give practical tips such as how to reduce exposures during commuting or picking up dry cleaning.

BOX 7-1 *FDA* Fetal Drug Risk Classification (approximate percent of drugs in each category)*

Category A (<5%)	Controlled studies in women fail to demonstrate a risk to the fetus in the first trimester.
Category B (50%)	Animal-reproduction studies have not demonstrated a fetal risk, but there are no controlled studies in pregnant women.
Category C (40%)	Studies in animals have revealed adverse effects on the fetus (teratogenic or embryocidal or other), and there are no controlled studies in women.
Category D (<5%)	There is positive evidence of human fetal risk, but the benefits from use in pregnant women may be acceptable despite the risk.
Category X (<5%)	Studies in animals or human beings have demonstrated fetal abnormalities, and the risk of the use of the drug in pregnant women clearly outweighs any possible benefit. The drug is contraindicated in women who are or may become pregnant.

*Food and Drug Administration.

In 2008 the U.S. FDA proposed an overhaul of how pregnancy and breastfeeding information should be included on provider labeling for prescription drugs. The proposed new labeling would eliminate the current lettering system (above), which is not required to be updated as new information becomes available and, according to experts, can be misleading. The proposed new system would provide brief bulleted information instead of a letter designation on the potential benefits and risks for the mother and the fetus and how these risks may change the course of pregnancy. The proposed new system would require drug labels to be updated as new data emerge. The U.S. FDA website *(www.fda.gov)* should be consulted for the latest information on the new system and on drug risk during pregnancy and breastfeeding.

the provider should bring her and her partner back for a full assessment and counseling. The schedule of follow-up visits should be individualized according to identified risks. If she does not plan on becoming pregnant in the next 1 to 2 years or ever, the provider should continue to provide well-woman care but make sure she has effective contraception if needed and update her reproductive life plan at every routine visit. **Because about half of all pregnancies in the United States are unplanned, preconception counseling is recommended for every woman of reproductive age.**

One example of how preconception care can improve obstetric outcomes is the **opportunity to counsel and appropriately change dietary behavior.** Women in the reproductive age group should be instructed to take multivitamins containing folic acid and in addition omega-3 fatty acids. Women who are underweight (body mass index [BMI] <19) have a greater risk for having a low-birth-weight or premature infant, and women who are obese (BMI >29) are at significantly greater risk for obstetric complications, including pregnancy-induced hypertension, diabetes mellitus, and fetal macrosomia. It is important that nutrition be balanced for at least 3 months before conception. Attempts at weight loss too soon before conception may have deleterious effects on fetal development.

Prenatal Care

The three basic components of prenatal care are (1) early and continuing risk assessment, (2) health promotion, and (3) medical and psychosocial interventions and follow-up. Risk assessment includes a complete history, a physical examination, laboratory tests, and assessment of fetal growth and well-being. Health promotion consists of providing information on proposed care, enhancing general knowledge of pregnancy and parenting, and promoting and supporting healthful behaviors. Interventions include treatment of any existing illness, provision of social and financial resources, and referral to and consultation with other specialized providers.

THE FIRST PRENATAL VISIT

The first prenatal visit provides an opportunity to assess or review medical, reproductive, family, genetic, nutritional, and psychosocial histories. Women whose health may be seriously jeopardized by the pregnancy, such as those with Eisenmenger's syndrome or a history of peripartum cardiomyopathy, should be counseled about the option of terminating the pregnancy. Such reproductive histories as preterm birth, low birth weight, preeclampsia, stillbirth, congenital anomalies, and gestational diabetes are important to obtain because of the substantial risk for recurrence. Women with prior cesarean delivery should be asked about the circumstances of the delivery, and discussion about options for the mode of delivery for the current pregnancy should be initiated. Additionally, **the importance of screening women for domestic violence cannot be overemphasized.** As many as 20% of women are physically abused during pregnancy (most studies report a prevalence that clusters around 4% to 8%), making abuse more common than preeclampsia, diabetes, and other conditions that are routinely screened for during prenatal care.

Standardized forms have been developed to facilitate overall prenatal risk assessment. One such system is the Problem Oriented Prenatal Risk Assessment System, or POPRAS (www.POPRAS.com).

A complete physical examination should be performed. Clinicians should be familiar with physical findings associated with normal pregnancy, such as systolic murmurs, exaggerated splitting, and S_3 during cardiac auscultation, or spider angiomas, palmar erythema, linea nigra, and striae gravidarum on inspection of the skin. During the breast examination, clinicians should **initiate discussion about breastfeeding.** A pelvic examination should be performed and **Pap smear status documented or obtained**.

Prenatal laboratory testing should be undertaken as outlined in Table 7-1, if not done during preconception care. **Screening for and treating asymptomatic bacteriuria** significantly reduces the risk for pyelonephritis and preterm delivery.

Women who are **Rh negative** should receive $Rh_O(D)$ immune globulin (Rh_O-GAM) at 28 weeks of gestation and postpartum and at any time when sensitization may occur (e.g., threatened abortion or invasive procedures such as amniocentesis and chorionic villus sampling). **Rubella vaccination is contraindicated during pregnancy**, and pregnant women who are found to be seronegative should be vaccinated immediately postpartum. **Syphilis testing** is mandated by law in virtually all states. Early diagnosis and treatment of syphilis can reduce perinatal morbidity. Women who test negative for **hepatitis B surface antigen** and are at high risk for hepatitis B infection (e.g., health-care workers) are candidates for vaccination before and during pregnancy. Infants born to women who test positive for hepatitis B surface antigen should receive both hepatitis B immune globulin (HBIG) and hepatitis B vaccine within 12 hours of birth, followed by two more injections of hepatitis B vaccine in the first 6 months of life.

Voluntary and confidential **HIV counseling and testing** should be offered and documented in the medical record. Diagnosis and treatment significantly reduce the risk for vertical transmission. **Other tests, such as screening for sexually transmitted infections like gonorrhea and chlamydia, are generally considered routine.** All pregnant women at high risk for **tuberculosis** should be screened with a purified protein derivative (PPD) skin test when they begin prenatal care.

Additionally, the clinician should use the first prenatal visit to confirm pregnancy and determine viability, estimate gestational age and due date, diagnose and deal with early pregnancy loss, provide genetic counseling and information about teratology, and provide advice on alleviating unpleasant symptoms during pregnancy. Information about nutrition, behavioral changes to expect, and the benefits of breastfeeding should be provided as prenatal care progresses. **Clinical**

pelvimetry should be performed sometime before labor begins**.

Confirming Pregnancy and Determining Viability

Women most commonly present to the clinician after missed menses. **About 30% to 40% of all pregnant women will have some bleeding during early pregnancy (e.g., implantation bleeding),** which may be mistaken for a period. Therefore, a pregnancy test should be performed in all women of reproductive age who present with abnormal vaginal bleeding.

The pregnancy test detects human chorionic gonadotropin (hCG) in the serum or the urine. **The most widely used standard is the First International Reference Preparation (1st IRP). The hCG molecule is first detectable in serum 6 to 8 days after ovulation.** A titer of less than 5 IU/L is considered negative, and a level above 25 IU/L is a positive result. Values between 6 and 24 IU/L are considered equivocal, and the test should be repeated in 2 days. **A concentration of about 100 IU/L is reached about the date of expected menses.** Most qualitative urine pregnancy tests can detect hCG above 25 IU/L.

It is important to differentiate a normal pregnancy from a nonviable or ectopic gestation. In the first 30 days of a normal gestation, the level of hCG doubles every 2.2 days. In patients whose pregnancies are destined to abort, the level of hCG rises more slowly, plateaus, or declines.

The use of transvaginal ultrasonography has improved the accuracy of predicting viability in early pregnancies. Using transvaginal ultrasonography, the gestational sac should be seen at 5 weeks of gestation or a mean hCG level of about 1500 IU/L (1st IRP). The fetal pole should be seen at 6 weeks or a mean hCG level of about 5200 IU/L. Fetal cardiac motion should be seen at 7 weeks or a mean hCG level of about 17,500 IU/L. **The presence of a gestational sac of 8 mm (mean sac diameter) without a demonstrable yolk sac, 16 mm without a demonstrable embryo, or the absence of fetal cardiac motion in an embryo with a crown-rump length of greater than 5 mm indicates probable embryonic demise.** When there is any doubt about these measurements, it is best to repeat the evaluation in 1 week before terminating the pregnancy.

INCIDENCE OF EARLY PREGNANCY LOSS

Because the incidence of conception is unknown, the incidence of spontaneous abortion (miscarriage) cannot be determined with certainty. **Spontaneous abortion occurs in 10% to 15% of clinically recognizable pregnancies.** The term *biochemical pregnancy* refers to the presence of hCG in the blood of a woman 7 to 10 days after ovulation but in whom menstruation occurs when expected. In other words, conception has occurred, but spontaneous loss of the gestation takes place without prolongation of the menstrual cycle. When both clinical and biochemical pregnancies are considered, evidence would suggest that **more than 50% of all conceptions are lost, the majority in the 14 days following conception.**

Real-time ultrasonography has been extensively used to monitor the intrauterine events of the first trimester of pregnancy. **If a live, appropriately grown fetus is present at 8 weeks' gestation, the fetal loss rate over the next 20 weeks (up to 28 weeks) is on the order of 3%.**

TYPES OF SPONTANEOUS ABORTION

The terms and definitions in the remainder of this chapter refer only to clinically recognizable pregnancies.

Threatened Abortion

The term *threatened abortion* is used **when a pregnancy is complicated by vaginal bleeding before the 20th week.** Pain may not be a prominent feature of threatened abortion, although a lower abdominal dull ache sometimes accompanies the bleeding. Vaginal examination at this stage usually reveals a closed cervix. About one third of pregnant women have some degree of vaginal bleeding during the first trimester, **and 25% to 50% of threatened abortions eventually result in loss of the pregnancy.**

Inevitable Abortion

In a case of inevitable abortion, **a clinical pregnancy is complicated by both vaginal bleeding and cramp-like lower abdominal pain.** The cervix is frequently partially dilated, contributing to the inevitability of the process.

Incomplete Abortion

In addition to vaginal bleeding, cramp-like pain, and cervical dilation, an incomplete abortion involves **the passage of products of conception,** often described by the woman as looking like pieces of skin or liver.

Complete Abortion

In complete abortion, after **passage of all the products of conception,** the uterine contractions and bleeding abate, the cervix closes, and the uterus is smaller than the period of amenorrhea would suggest. In addition, the symptoms of pregnancy are no longer present, and the pregnancy test becomes negative.

Missed Abortion

The term *missed abortion* is used when **the fetus has died but is retained in the uterus,** usually for more than 6 weeks. Because **coagulation problems may develop,** fibrinogen levels should be checked weekly until the fetus and placenta are expelled (spontaneously) or removed surgically.

Recurrent Abortion

Three successive spontaneous abortions usually occur before a patient is considered as a recurrent aborter. Many clinicians feel that two successive first-trimester losses or a single second-trimester spontaneous abortion is justification for an evaluation of a couple for the causes of the pregnancy losses (see page 77, "Patients Who Require Genetic Counseling").

ETIOLOGY

Although many factors may result in the loss of a single pregnancy, relatively few factors are present consistently in couples who abort recurrently. Cause-and-effect relationships in individual patients are frequently difficult to determine.

General Maternal Factors

Infection with *Mycoplasma, Listeria,* or *Toxoplasma* should be specifically sought in women with recurrent abortions because despite being found infrequently, they are all treatable with antibiotics. **Maternal smoking and alcohol consumption are associated with an increased incidence of chromosomally normal abortions.** Women who smoke 20 or more cigarettes daily and consume more than seven standard alcoholic drinks per week have a fourfold increased risk for spontaneous abortion. There is a doubling of the risk for spontaneous abortion with as few as two drinks a week.

There is very little evidence that a sudden physical or emotional shock can cause pregnancy loss, but psychodynamic factors may contribute to recurrent abortion in a few cases.

Three medical disorders are commonly linked to spontaneous abortion: **(1) diabetes mellitus, (2) hypothyroidism,** and **(3) systemic lupus erythematosus (SLE).** The evidence linking diabetes mellitus with spontaneous abortion is not conclusive, and severe hypothyroidism is more often associated with disordered ovulation than spontaneous abortion. Up to 40% of clinical pregnancies are lost in women with SLE, and such patients have an increased risk for pregnancy loss before developing the clinical stigmata of the disease (see Chapter 16).

The risk for abortion increases with maternal age (Table 7-2). If a live fetus is demonstrated by ultrasonography at 8 weeks' gestational age, however, fewer than 2% will abort spontaneously when the mother is younger than 30 years of age. If she is older than 40 years, the risk exceeds 10%, and it may be as high as 50% at age 45 years. **The probable explanation is the increased incidence of chromosomally abnormal conceptus in older women.**

TABLE 7-2

NUMBER OF PREGNANCIES, SPONTANEOUS ABORTIONS, AND SPONTANEOUS ABORTION RATES BY MATERNAL AGE AT FIRST PREGNANCY

Age at LMP (yr)	Pregnancies	Spontaneous Abortions	Spontaneous Abortion Rate (%)
<30	1856	208	11.2
30-35	590	85	14.4
36-40	82	15	18.3
>40	25	14	56.0

LMP, last menstrual period.

Combined data from Alberman E: Maternal age and spontaneous abortion. *In* Bennett MJ, Edmonds DK (eds): Spontaneous and Recurrent Abortion. Oxford, Blackwell Scientific Publications, 1987.

Local Maternal Factors

No prospective study has been able to demonstrate unequivocally that a normal pregnancy can be lost as a result of abnormal hormone production by either the corpus luteum or the placenta. In addition to this, no controlled trial of exogenous hormones has been able to demonstrate any benefit, and there is some evidence that exogenous sex steroids may indeed be teratogenic.

Uterine abnormalities, including cervical incompetence, congenital abnormalities of the uterine fundus (as may result from gestational exposure to diethylstilbestrol), and acquired abnormalities of the uterine fundus are known to be associated with pregnancy loss.

Cervical incompetence occurs under a number of circumstances. The incompetence is usually the result of trauma. This occurs most frequently from mechanical dilation of the cervix at the time of termination of pregnancy, but it may also occur at the time of curettage. **The diagnosis of cervical incompetence is usually made when a mid-trimester pregnancy is lost with a clinical picture of sudden unexpected rupture of the membranes, followed by painless expulsion of the products of conception.**

There continues to be controversy surrounding cervical incompetence, with some experts suggesting that cervical incompetence is, in most instances, a variant of preterm delivery, occurring at a time when there is an associated finding of asymptomatic ascending infection.

When cervical incompetence is suspected during pregnancy (e.g., history of cervical incompetence in a previous pregnancy or of cone biopsy of the cervix), sequential ultrasonography of the cervix and lower uterine segment may identify the problem before a pregnancy loss occurs.

A **congenitally abnormal uterus** may be associated with pregnancy loss in both the first and second trimesters. Surgical correction of the abnormality, particularly with a history of second-trimester loss, is frequently successful. The diagnosis of these abnormalities is made by either hysterography or hysteroscopy. Complete evaluation of the congenitally abnormal uterus usually requires laparoscopic, hysteroscopic, and hysterographic examination before any management plan can be made.

The most commonly acquired abnormalities of the uterus with the potential to affect fecundity are **submucous fibroids.** Although these tend to occur more frequently in women in their late 30s, they should be considered when investigating pregnancy loss in all women. Removal of submucous fibroids and large (>6 cm) intramural ones is associated with improved fecundity, especially when they distort the endometrial cavity. Subserous fibroids do not appear to affect fecundity.

Intrauterine adhesions result from trauma to the basal layer of the endometrium from previous surgery or infection. When most of the uterine cavity has been obliterated (Asherman's syndrome), amenorrhea results; but much more frequently, fewer intrauterine adhesions (synechiae) are present with reasonably normal menses, and these lesions are not even suspected until a pregnancy is attempted and lost. Surgical correction of these intrauterine adhesions is recommended to improve fecundity.

Fetal Factors

The most common cause of spontaneous abortion is a significant genetic abnormality of the conceptus. In spontaneous first-trimester abortions, about two thirds of fetuses have significant chromosomal anomalies, with about half of these being autosomal trisomies and most of the remainder being triploid, tetraploid, or 45 X monosomies. Fortunately, most of these are not inherited from either mother or father and are single nonrecurring events. **When seen on ultrasonography before spontaneous abortion occurs, many such pregnancies appear to consist of an empty gestational sac.** When a fetus is present in many late first-trimester and early second-trimester abortions, it is often significantly abnormal, either genetically or morphologically. It seems that nature has a way of identifying some of its major mistakes and causing them to abort.

Chromosomal Factors

Occasionally, fetal chromosomal abnormalities occur as a result of a chromosomal rearrangement (balanced translocation, inversion) in either parent. Therefore, **karyotyping is important for evaluation** of couples suffering from recurrent abortion.

Immunologic Factors

A successful pregnancy depends on a number of immunologic factors that allow the host (mother) to retain an antigenically foreign product (fetus) without rejection taking place (see Chapter 6). The precise mechanism of this immunologic anomaly is not fully understood, but the immunologic functioning of some women, particularly those who abort recurrently, is different from that of women who carry pregnancies to term. The immunologic relationship between male and female in such a couple may be regarded as abnormal, and in some instances, treatment of this condition may result in a successful pregnancy.

MANAGEMENT
Threatened Abortion

A threatened abortion is best managed by an ultrasonic examination to determine whether the fetus is present and, if so, whether it is alive. **Of those in whom a live fetus is present, 94% will produce a live baby,** although the incidence of preterm delivery in these cases may be somewhat higher than in those who do not bleed in the first trimester. **Once a live fetus has been demonstrated to the couple on ultrasonography, management consists essentially of reassurance;** however, they should be encouraged to undergo first trimester screening for chromosome abnormalities such as trisomy 13, 18, or 21. There is no need for admission to hospital nor is there any evidence that bed rest improves the prognosis.

Incomplete Abortion

Until bleeding has stopped or is minimal, it is best to insert an intravenous line and take blood for grouping and cross-matching because shock may occur from hemorrhage or sepsis. **Once the patient's condition is stable, the remaining products of conception should be evacuated from the uterus under appropriate pain control.** These tissues should be sent for pathologic evaluation. An incomplete abortion that is infected must be managed vigorously. Delay in treatment may result in overwhelming sepsis that may lead to renal and hepatic failure, disseminated intravascular coagulation (DIC), and even death.

Missed Abortion

Suspected missed abortion should be confirmed by ultrasound. **Once the diagnosis has been made, it is appropriate to evacuate the retained products of conception surgically** to minimize the risk for sepsis and DIC and to reduce the extent of hemorrhage and the degree of pain that accompanies the spontaneous expulsive process.

General Management Considerations

When the patient is Rh negative and does not have Rh (anti-D) antibodies, **prophylactic Rh$_o$(D) immune globulin (Rh$_o$-GAM) should be administered.** All couples who have had a pregnancy loss should be seen and counseled some weeks after the event. At this time, questions that the couple may have can be answered, the findings of any pathologic studies discussed, and reassurance given about their chances of reproductive success in the future.

Recurrent Abortion

As far as the mother is concerned, it is appropriate to rule out the presence of systemic disorders such as **diabetes mellitus, SLE,** and **thyroid disease,** and it is also necessary to test for the presence of a lupus anticoagulant. **Paternal and maternal chromosomes** should be evaluated, and **hysteroscopy or hysterography** should be performed to evaluate the uterine cavity. Given the possibility of the pregnancy losses being caused by infectious agents, it is also appropriate to rule out the presence of *Mycoplasma, Listeria, Toxoplasma, Treponema,* cytomegalovirus, and *Brucella.*

More than half of couples with recurrent losses will have normal findings during an evaluation. When a specific etiologic factor is found, appropriate management often leads to reproductive success. Many of the **congenital abnormalities of the uterus** can now be diagnosed using pelvic ultrasonography and may no longer require laparotomy for repair. **Cervical incompetence** is managed by the placement of a cervical suture (cerclage) at the level of the internal os, and this suture is best placed in the first trimester, after a live fetus has been demonstrated on ultrasonography. **The effectiveness of prophylactic cervical cerclage (see Chapters 17 and 19) in preventing recurrent loss from cervical incompetence has not been conclusively established.**

Estimating Gestational Age and Date of Confinement

Gestational age should be determined during the first prenatal visit. Accurate determination of gestational age may become important later in pregnancy for the management of obstetric conditions such as preterm labor, intrauterine growth restriction, and postdate pregnancy. Clinical assessment to determine gestational age is usually appropriate for the woman with regular menstrual cycles and a known last menstrual period that was confirmed by an early examination.

Estimated date of confinement (EDC) or "due date" may be determined by adding 9 months and 7 days to the first day of the last menstrual period.

Ultrasonography may also be used to estimate gestational age. Measurement of **fetal crown-rump length between 6 and 11 weeks of gestation** can define gestational age to within 7 days. At 12 to 20 weeks, gestational age can be determined within 10 days by the average of multiple measurements (**e.g., biparietal diameter, femur length, abdominal and head circumferences**). Thereafter, measurements become less reliable with advancing gestation (±3 weeks in the third trimester).

■ Patients Who Require Genetic Counseling

Ideally, couples should receive preconception counseling before they decide to have children, so that genetic disease in the couple or their families may be identified before pregnancy. The major reason couples are referred for prenatal diagnosis is advanced maternal age. Women older than 34 years have an increased risk for having children with chromosomal abnormalities. Other indications for genetic counseling and prenatal diagnosis are listed in Box 7-2.

CONGENITAL AND HEREDITARY DISORDERS

Chromosomal Disorders

Chromosomal abnormalities occur in 0.5% of live births, but the incidence associated with spontaneous abortions is much higher and is estimated to be about 50%. The most common chromosomal abnormalities among liveborn infants are sex chromosomal aneuploidy (e.g., Turner syndrome [45 XO], Klinefelter syndrome [47 XXY]), balanced Robertsonian translocations (translocations within group D or between

groups D and G), and autosomal trisomies (e.g., Down syndrome; Figure 7-1).

Women older than 34 years are at increased risk for giving birth to children with autosomal trisomies (e.g., trisomy 21, 13, or 18) or sex chromosomal abnormalities (e.g., triple X syndrome, Klinefelter syndrome). The overall risk for Down syndrome (trisomy 21) is 1 per 800 live births. It increases to about 1 per 300 live births for women who are 35 to 39 years of age and to about 1 in 80 for those 40 to 45 years of age (Table 7-3). The incidence of Down syndrome diagnosed at the time of chorionic villus sampling (CVS) or amniocentesis is considerably higher. In women 35 to 39 years of age, the rate is about 1 in 125; in those 40 to 45, it is about 1 in 20. The discrepancy between the rate of occurrence at delivery and that at prenatal diagnosis is believed to be due in part to fetal loss in the second and third trimester.

Ninety-five percent of cases of Down syndrome are due to meiotic nondisjunctional events leading to 47 chromosomes with an extra copy of chromosome number 21, whereas 4% are due to an unbalanced translocation. Parents of a child with translocation Down syndrome have rearrangements between chromosome 21 and chromosomes 14, 15, 21, or 22. The remaining 1% of individuals with Down syndrome have the mosaic type, which consists of two populations of cells, one with 46 and one with 47 chromosomes.

A couple who has previously had a child with trisomy 21 (Down syndrome) or with a meiotic nondisjunctional type of chromosomal abnormality is believed to be at a small but definite increased risk (about 1%) of giving birth to another child with a chromosomal abnormality and should be referred for prenatal diagnosis.

BOX 7-2 *Indications for Genetic Counseling and Prenatal Diagnosis Other than Age*

1. A previous child with or a family history of birth defects, chromosomal abnormality, or known genetic disorder
2. A previous child with undiagnosed mental retardation
3. A previous baby who died in the neonatal period
4. Multiple fetal losses
5. Abnormal serum marker screening results
6. Consanguinity
7. Maternal conditions predisposing the fetus to congenital abnormalities
8. A current pregnancy history of teratogenic exposure
9. A fetus with suspected abnormal ultrasonic findings
10. A parent who is a known carrier of a genetic disorder

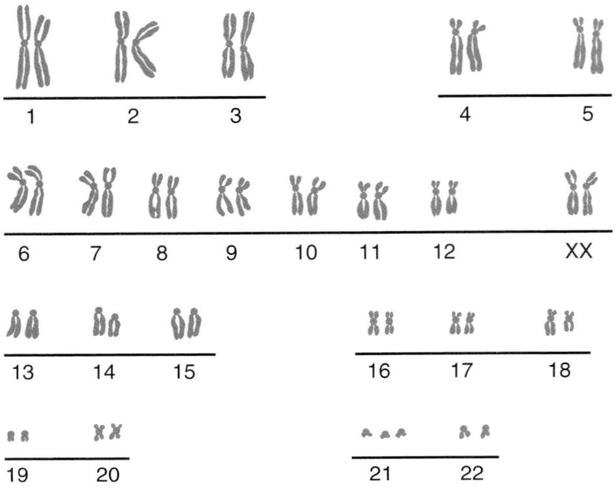

FIGURE 7-1 Karyotype of a patient with Down syndrome (47 XX + 21).

TABLE 7-3

RISK TABLE FOR CHROMOSOMAL ABNORMALITIES BY MATERNAL AGE AT TERM

Age at Term (yr)	Risk for Trisomy 21*	Risk for Any Chromosomal Abnormality†,‡
15	1:1578	1:454
16	1:1572	1:475
17	1:1565	1:499
18	1:1556	1:525
19	1:1544	1:555
20	1:1528	1:525
21	1:1507	1:525
22	1:1481	1:499
23	1:1447	1:499
24	1:1404	1:475
25	1:1351	1:475
26	1:1286	1:475
27	1:1208	1:454
28	1:1119	1:434
29	1:1018	1:416
30	1:909	1:384
31	1:796	1:384
32	1:683	1:322
33	1:574	1:285
34	1:474	1:243
35	1:384	1:178
36	1:307	1:148
37	1:242	1:122
38	1:189	1:104
39	1:146	1:80
40	1:112	1:62
41	1:85	1:48
42	1:65	1:38
43	1:49	1:30
44	1:37	1:23
45	1:28	1:18
46	1:21	1:14
47	1:15	1:10
48	1:11	1:8
49	1:8	1:6
50	1:6	Data not available

*Data from Chuckle HA, Wald NJ, Thompson SC: Estimating a woman's risk of having a pregnancy associated with Down's syndrome using her age and serum alpha-fetoprotein level. Br J Obstet Gynaecol 94:387, 1987.

†Adapted from Hook EB: Rates of chromosomal abnormalities at different maternal ages. Obstet Gynecol 58:282-285, 1981.

‡Risk for any chromosomal abnormality includes the risk for trisomy 21 and 18 in addition to trisomy 13, 47 XXY, 47 XYY, Turner syndrome genotype, and other clinically significant abnormalities. 47 XXX is not included.

Approximately 1 in 500 individuals carries a balanced structural chromosomal rearrangement such as a translocation or inversion. Blood chromosomal studies should be performed on a couple after three or more spontaneous abortions because in about 3% to 5% of such couples, one member is a carrier of a balanced rearrangement. The recurrence risk for spontaneous abortions, abnormal offspring, or both is greatly increased among translocation carriers, and it can be estimated according to the type of translocation and which parent carries the translocation. For example, if the mother carries a balanced 14;21 robertsonian translocation, the risk for a child with an unbalanced translocation resulting in Down syndrome is 10% to 15%. However, if the father carries the translocation, the risk for an affected child is 2% to 3%. **These couples should be alerted to the advisability of prenatal diagnosis because of their increased risk for having liveborn children with unbalanced translocations.**

Using **fluorescent in situ hybridization** (FISH), a labeled chromosome-specific DNA segment or probe is hybridized to metaphase, prophase, or interphase chromosomes and visualized with fluorescent microscopy. FISH analysis has led to the identification of a number of genetic syndromes that could not previously be detected because the chromosomal deletion in these syndromes is beyond the resolution of banded chromosomal analysis. Syndromes identified by FISH analysis include Prader-Willi, Angelman, DiGeorge, and Williams syndromes. Trisomies can also be identified in interphase cells with FISH probes.

Single Gene Disorders

Single gene disorders are relatively uncommon. They follow the laws of mendelian inheritance and may be passed from generation to generation, as with autosomal dominant disorders, or affect siblings without a family history of other affected family members, as in autosomal recessive disorders. Males may be affected with healthy females transmitting the abnormal gene, as in X-linked recessive disorders.

Autosomal Dominant Disorders

In autosomal dominant disorders, only one abnormal gene is necessary for disease manifestation. **The affected individual has a 50% chance of passing the gene and the disorder on to offspring.** The unaffected offspring cannot pass on the gene or the disorder. The occurrence and transmission of the genes are not influenced by gender. A spontaneous mutation of genetic material in the germ cells of clinically normal parents can also result in an affected offspring.

The hallmark of autosomal dominant disease is the variable expressivity. It is important to determine whether a child is affected by a spontaneous mutation or is the product of a parent with minimal expression of the same gene. A careful history and physical examination of family members, in addition to biochemical, radiologic, or histologic testing, may be necessary to determine the parents' genetic status.

Some of the common autosomal dominant disorders include tuberous sclerosis, neurofibromatosis, achondroplasia, craniofacial synostosis, adult-onset polycystic kidney disease, and several types of muscular dystrophy.

Autosomal Recessive Disorders

With autosomal recessive disorders, two affected genes must be present for manifestation of the disease. Usually there is no family history, but if a family history exists, siblings of either sex are equally likely to be affected. Consanguineous couples are at an increased risk for having a child who is homozygous for a deleterious recessive gene, with subsequent pregnancies being at 25% risk for producing a similarly affected child.

Many autosomal recessive disorders may be diagnosed prenatally. Biochemical genetic disorders (e.g., Tay-Sachs disease) can be diagnosed by enzymatic assay, whereas others (e.g., sickle cell disorders, β-thalassemia, and cystic fibrosis) can be diagnosed by DNA analysis from amniocytes or chorionic villi.

GENETIC SCREENING FOR AUTOSOMAL RECESSIVE DISORDERS

Carrier screening programs for autosomal recessive disorders have traditionally focused on high-risk populations, in which the frequency of heterozygotes is greater than in the general population. Screening for Tay-Sachs disease among Eastern European Jewish and French Canadian populations has proved to be particularly successful in the recognition of couples at 25% risk for having offspring affected with this fatal disease. Table 7-4 lists selected autosomal recessive disorders for which genetic screening has been initiated.

The most common gene carried by North American whites is the cystic fibrosis (CF) gene (carrier frequency, 1/25). With the use of recombinant DNA technology, the CF gene has been mapped to

chromosome 7, and a gene deletion (*AF508*) has been found in about 70% of carriers. More than 400 mutations have been identified in the CF gene. **Genetic counseling is essential in offering CF carrier detection because 15% of carriers (and maybe more depending on ethnic group) remain undetected, and the limitations of the testing must be explained.** At present, carrier detection is offered to individuals with a family history of CF, partners of identified CF carriers, parents of a fetus with ultrasonic findings of an echogenic bowel, those who donate sperm, and any parent who requests carrier testing.

Sex-Linked Disorders

Sex-linked disorders, caused by recessive genes located on the X chromosome, primarily affect males, whereas unaffected (or mildly affected) females carry the deleterious gene. There is no male-to-male transmission of X-linked disorders. Using gene mapping technology, many sex-linked disorders such as **Duchenne muscular dystrophy (DMD) or fragile X syndrome** can now be diagnosed by CVS or amniocentesis. X-linked disorders can occur because of new mutations of genetic material as a sporadic event or from the inheritance of the X-linked recessive gene from the carrier mother.

Fragile X syndrome is an X-linked disorder that is the second most common form of mental retardation after Down syndrome, and the most common form of inherited mental retardation. It has an incidence of 1 per 1500 males and 1 per 2500 females. Mental impairment is variable in heterozygous females. The fragile X syndrome is caused by triplet repeat expansion in the long arm of the X chromosome. Using molecular genetic techniques, the number of triplet repeats can be measured in affected individuals to confirm a suspected diagnosis of fragile X or fragile X carrier status. In women who have a family history of mental retardation, genetic counseling is recommended for consideration of fragile X testing in the patient or family member.

Multifactorial Disorders

Many birth defects are inherited in a multifactorial fashion, which means that both genes and the environment play a role. Common multifactorial disorders include cleft lip or palate, neural tube defects (spina bifida or anencephaly), congenital heart defects, and pyloric stenosis.

Neural tube defects occur in about 1 per 1000 births in the United States. In Northern Ireland, Wales, and Scotland, the incidence of neural tube defects is 6 to 8 per 1000 births. Both anencephaly (congenital absence of the forebrain) and spina bifida (open spine) are believed to occur before 30 days' gestation because of failure of the neural tube to close. Newborns with

TABLE 7-4

SELECTED AUTOSOMAL RECESSIVE DISEASES IN DEFINED ETHNIC GROUPS		
Disease	**Ethnic Group**	**Carrier Frequency**
Sickle cell disease	Blacks	1/10
Cystic fibrosis	Whites	1/25
Tay-Sachs disease	Jews, French Canadians	1/30
Thalassemia	Mediterraneans, Southeast Asians	1/25

anencephaly are stillborn or die within the first few days of life. Newborns with spina bifida have a variable course, depending on the site of the lesion and whether it is a **meningocele** (herniation of the meninges through an open spinal defect with cord remaining in its usual position) or a **myelocele** (herniation of the spinal cord). **Folic acid has been shown to lower the risk for neural tube defects, and women who have had an infant with a neural tube defect should take vitamins plus 4 mg of folic acid daily before conception. Because neural tube closure is complete by 28 days postconception, initiating folic acid after the first 28 days has no prophylactic value.**

With multifactorial disorders in general, and with neural tube defects in particular, a couple who has had one affected child has an increased risk of about 3% for having another similarly affected child.

Maternal Ultrasonic and Serum Marker Screening

There are multiple approaches available for maternal screening for fetal aneuploidy. Traditionally, second-trimester screening has been the standard approach. First-trimester screening was introduced in the late 1990s.

FIRST-TRIMESTER SCREENING

A combination of **maternal age, fetal nuchal translucency (NT) thickness, and maternal serum-free β-human chorionic gonadotrophin (β-hCG) and pregnancy-associated plasma protein-A (PAPP-A) are included in the first-trimester screen.** Maternal age alone has only a 30% detection rate. In the early 1990s,

an association was reported between fetal chromosomal abnormalities and the finding of an abnormally increased nuchal translucency (an echo-free area at the back of the fetal neck) between 10 and 14 weeks' gestational age (Figure 7-2). **Increased nuchal translucency has been associated with both chromosomal abnormalities and other congenital anomalies.** Elevated levels of free β-hCG and low levels of plasma protein-A are associated with an increased risk for Down syndrome. A multicenter study in the United States reported that combining first-trimester maternal serum screening markers with nuchal translucency and maternal age showed a detection rate for Down syndrome of 79% with a positive screening rate of 5%. Anatomic and radiographic studies have shown absence or hypoplasia of the nasal bones in fetuses with Down syndrome. Visualization of the nasal bone on first-trimester ultrasound has been shown to reduce the risk for Down syndrome (see Figure 7-1), whereas nonvisualization (absence) has been associated with increased risk. **The addition of nasal bone assessment to nuchal lucency measurement and serum biochemistry can increase the Down syndrome detection rate to 93% with a screen positive rate of 5%.**

SECOND-TRIMESTER SCREENING

Traditionally, a woman was offered the serum triple screening test that measures **alpha fetoprotein (AFP), hCG,** and **unconjugated estriol (UE3) at 16 to 20 weeks of gestation.** Amniotic fluid alpha-fetoprotein (AFP) levels are frequently elevated in blood samples of women carrying fetuses affected with neural tube defects. **Approximately 80% to 85% of all open neural tube defects can be detected by maternal serum AFP (MSAFP).** In addition to open neural tube defects, ventral wall defects (gastroschisis or omphalocele) can cause elevations of MSAFP.

If the MSAFP level is elevated, an ultrasound is done to rule out multiple gestation, fetal demise, or inaccurate gestational age (all of which can give false-positive results). If none of these factors are present, amniocentesis is recommended to determine the amniotic fluid AFP level and to measure acetylcholinesterase (AChE). **Acetylcholinesterase is a protein that is present only if there is an open neural tube defect.**

An association between low maternal serum AFP and Down syndrome has been noted. The combination of low MSAFP, elevated hCG, and low UE3 levels (triple screen) has a detection rate for Down syndrome of about 70%, with a positive screen result in about 5% of all pregnancies.

Low MSAFP, low hCG, and low UE3 levels can also be used to screen for trisomy 18. With the addition of inhibin A, the quadruple screen increases the Down syndrome detection rate to 81%, with a positive screen result in 5% of pregnancies.

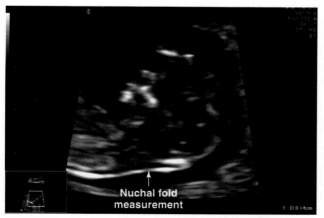

Nuchal fold measurement

FIGURE 7-2 Ultrasound image of fetal head at 12 weeks and 0 days showing a lucent area at the posterior aspect of the fetal neck that can be measured. Normal values for this measurement and the risk associated with abnormal measurements are based on gestational age as determined by crown-rump length.

COMBINED FIRST- AND SECOND-TRIMESTER SCREENING

In an attempt to improve the detection rate and minimize the screen positive rate and the number of invasive procedures, a few studies have been conducted to evaluate the concept of combining first- and second-trimester screening. **The approaches that have been proposed include integrated screening and sequential screening.**

With integrated screening, the first- and second-trimester results are combined into a single risk calculation and are not reported until after the second-trimester results are available. This approach **has been found to have the highest sensitivity and to be the most cost effective. Sequential screening** involves performance of both first- and second-trimester screening with disclosure of the first-trimester results for clinical management.

It is not uncommon for one or more of the biomarkers to be abnormal in the presence of a chromosomally normal fetus. An elevated level of β-hCG or AFP and low levels of PAPP-A or UE3 are associated with complications of pregnancy such as preterm birth, intrauterine growth restriction, and preeclampsia. Thus, these pregnancies require close follow-up.

Genetic counseling is an essential component of screening programs. It provides education and alleviates anxiety in patients with abnormal test results. Patients must be informed of the differences between screening results and diagnostic testing.

◼ *Diagnostic Procedures*

Recombinant DNA technology, coupled with first-trimester fetal tissue sampling, has enhanced the growth and development of prenatal diagnosis. Obstetric procedures, such as ultrasonography, amniocentesis, chorionic villus sampling, and cordocentesis (percutaneous umbilical blood sampling [PUBS]) are currently used during prenatal diagnosis. These procedures are described and discussed in Chapter 17.

◼ *Teratology*

A teratogen is any agent or factor that can cause abnormalities of form or function (birth defects) in an exposed fetus. Such abnormalities include fetal wastage and intrauterine fetal growth restriction, malformations due to abnormal growth and morphogenesis, fetal endocrine disruption, and abnormal central nervous system performance.

It was not until the teratogenic effects of rubella infection were demonstrated in 1941 that any notable consideration was given to environmental factors and their potentially deleterious effects on human pregnancy. In the succeeding decades, the susceptibility of the fetus to many environmental factors has been appreciated.

Probably the best known teratogen is **thalidomide,** which was shown to cause phocomelia and other malformations in the offspring of mothers who had been given the drug during pregnancy. It is the only example of a teratogen that, when introduced to the pregnant population, led to a dramatic epidemic of a specific malformation; withdrawal of the drug led to a virtual disappearance of the malformation.

Although drugs are the most obvious source for teratogenic exposure, chemical waste disposals, alcohol, tobacco, cosmetics, and occupational agents contain substances that individuals are exposed to such as fertilizers and insecticides. Some of these agents are known teratogens, whereas the fetal effects of others are not known.

EXPOSURE

Results of the Collaborative Perinatal Project indicate that more than 900 different drugs are taken by pregnant women in the United States and that **40% of women take medication during the first trimester, when organogenesis occurs.** During the first trimester alone, as many as 32% of pregnant women are exposed to analgesics (mostly aspirin), 18% to immunizing agents, 16% to antimicrobial and antiparasitic agents, and 6% to sedatives, tranquilizers, and antidepressants.

PRINCIPLES OF TERATOLOGY

Fetal Susceptibility

The efficacy of a particular teratogen is, in part, dependent on the genetic makeup of both mother and fetus, as well as on a number of factors related to the maternal-fetal environment. For instance, many congenital abnormalities, such as oral clefts, congenital heart disease, and neural tube defects, are inherited through multifactorial inheritance.

Dose

Depending on the particular teratogen, there may be (1) no apparent effect at a low dose, (2) an organ-specific malformation at an intermediate dose, or (3) a spontaneous abortion at a high dose. Additionally, smaller doses administered over several days may produce a different effect from a single large dose.

Timing

Three stages of teratogenic susceptibility may be identified on the basis of gestational age. Before implantation (1 week postovulation in humans), there is no demonstrable teratogenic insult. **The most vulnerable stage is from day 17 to day 56 postconception (or day**

31 to day 71 by gestational age), during the period of organogenesis. The timing determines which organ system or systems are affected. Unfortunately, most women do not realize they are pregnant until this critical period of development is well under way. From about the 4th month of pregnancy to the end of gestation, embryonic development consists primarily of increasing organ size. With the exception of a limited number of tissues (brain and gonads), teratogenic exposure after the 4th month usually causes decreased growth without malformation.

Nature of Teratogenic Agents

Although few agents are known to cause serious malformations in a large proportion of exposed individuals, there are probably hundreds of potentially teratogenic agents, given the right set of circumstances (susceptible fetus, embryologically vulnerable period, large teratogenic dose). Furthermore, certain drugs combined with other drugs may be capable of producing malformations, although neither agent would be teratogenic when taken alone.

TERATOGENIC AGENTS

Teratogens may be assigned to three broad categories: (1) drugs and chemical agents, (2) infectious agents, and (3) radiation. The list that follows is far from exhaustive. Pharmaceutical agents have their fetal risk classification (as of 2008; see Box 7-1) in parentheses following the drug name.

Alcohol

The adverse effects of ethanol (D) on fetal development were not fully realized until the 1970s. The frequency of the fetal alcohol syndrome runs as high as 0.2%, whereas an additional 0.4% of newborns show less severe features of the disorder (Box 7-3).

Antianxiety Agents

Antianxiety agents are currently used by a significant number of pregnant women. Data regarding their teratogenicity are conflicting, although exposure to meprobamate (D) or chlordiazepoxide (D) has been associated with a greater than fourfold increase in severe congenital anomalies. Fluoxetine (B) is now the drug of choice for anxiety and depression during pregnancy and is considered safe to continue even in women who breastfeed. The risk for recurrence of significant depression during pregnancy is too great to routinely discontinue treatment during pregnancy.

Antineoplastic Agents

Aminopterin (X) and methotrexate (D), both of which are folic acid antagonists, have been clearly established as teratogens. Exposure before 40 days' gestation is lethal to the embryo; later exposure during the first trimester produces fetal effects, including intrauterine growth restriction, craniofacial anomalies, abnormal positioning of extremities, mental retardation, early miscarriage, stillbirth, and neonatal death.

Alkylating agents, including busulfan (D), chlorambucil (D), cyclophosphamide (D), and nitrogen mustard (D), have been associated with fetal anomalies such as severe intrauterine growth restriction, fetal death, cleft palate, microphthalmia, limb reduction anomalies, and poorly developed external genitalia. During the first trimester, the teratogenic risks may be as high as 30%.

Anticoagulants

COUMARIN DERIVATIVES. Use of warfarin (Coumadin [D]) during the first trimester is associated with an increased risk for spontaneous abortion, intrauterine growth restriction, central nervous system defects (including mental retardation), stillbirth, and a characteristic syndrome of craniofacial features known as the fetal warfarin syndrome. Embryologically, the most vulnerable time appears to be between 6 and 9 weeks after conception. As many as 30% of exposed fetuses suffer serious teratogenic consequences, or loss of the pregnancy occurs. Warfarin easily crosses the placenta, causing bleeding problems in the fetus, and is excreted in breast milk.

HEPARIN. Heparin (B) has major advantages over coumarin anticoagulants during pregnancy because it does not cross the placenta. Reported risks include

BOX 7-3 *Clinical Features of Fetal Alcohol Syndrome*

Craniofacial
Eyes: Short palpebral fissures, ptosis, strabismus, epicanthic folds, myopia, microphthalmia
Ears: Poorly formed concha, posterior rotation
Nose: Short, hypoplastic philtrum
Mouth: Prominent lateral palatine ridges, micrognathia, cleft lip or palate, faulty enamel
Maxilla: Hypoplastic

Cardiac
Murmurs, atrial septal defect, ventricular septal defect, tetralogy of Fallot

Central Nervous System
Mild to moderate mental retardation, microcephaly, poor coordination, hypotonia

Growth
Prenatal-onset growth deficiency

Muscular
Hernias of diaphragm, umbilicus, or groin

Skeletal
Pectus excavatum, abnormal palmar creases, nail hypoplasia, scoliosis

prematurity and fetal demise. Because no specific malformation syndrome has been described, these abnormalities may be more closely related to the maternal disease necessitating the heparin use.

Anticonvulsants

About 1 in 200 pregnant women is epileptic. Box 7-4 lists the etiologic factors that may play a role in the congenital abnormalities associated with in utero exposure to anticonvulsants. The complexity in providing genetic counseling for pregnant epileptic women is underscored when considering the interactive effects of these factors, the effect of combined anticonvulsant treatment, and the genetic aspects of the disease itself. The goals of counseling include providing the patient with the teratogenic risks of her medication, the risk for seizures during pregnancy, the effect of pregnancy on seizures, and the risk for development of epilepsy in her offspring. **From a medication standpoint, the benefits of seizure prevention need to be weighed against the teratogenicity of the drug.**

DIPHENYLHYDANTOIN (DILANTIN [D]). A specific syndrome, known as the **fetal hydantoin syndrome,** has been described, the clinical features of which include **craniofacial abnormalities, limb reduction defects, prenatal-onset growth restriction, mental deficiency, and cardiovascular anomalies.** About 10% of exposed fetuses demonstrate fetal hydantoin syndrome, whereas an additional 30% may have isolated features of the syndrome. Hydantoins may also have a prenatal carcinogenic effect because several exposed infants with signs of fetal hydantoin syndrome have subsequently developed neuroblastomas.

ANTICONVULSANTS. Trimethadione (Tridione [D]) and paramethadione (Paradione [D]), used to treat petit mal epilepsy, have been associated with a characteristic malformation syndrome in exposed fetuses. **The clinical features include craniofacial abnormalities, prenatal-onset growth restriction, an increased frequency of mental retardation, and cardiovascular**

abnormalities. Because of this serious teratogenic potential and because petit mal epilepsy is rare during reproductive years, **oxazolidinedione anticonvulsants are contraindicated during pregnancy.**

VALPROIC ACID. Valproic acid (D) use during pregnancy is associated with a 1% to 2% risk for open spina bifida. Other findings reported to be associated with valproic acid exposure include cardiac defects, skeletal defects, and craniofacial malformations.

CARBAMAZEPINE. As with valproic acid, carbamazepine (Tegretol [C]) exposure during pregnancy is associated with an **increased risk for fetal spina bifida** and is an indication for amniotic fluid AFP analysis. Some studies have reported a specific malformation pattern that includes minor craniofacial defects, fingernail hypoplasia, and developmental delay, which are features that would be unlikely to be detected prenatally.

PHENOBARBITAL. The true teratogenicity of phenobarbital (D) is difficult to assess because other drugs are usually taken in combination with this agent, but the risk appears to be very low. **Potential complications of phenobarbital include neonatal withdrawal symptoms and neonatal hemorrhage.**

Hormones

ESTROGEN-PROGESTIN COMBINATIONS. A large number of pregnant women are exposed to progestins or estrogen-progestin combinations because they continue taking birth control pills, unaware that they are pregnant. Recent analyses have failed to confirm any teratogenicity, and the U.S. Food and Drug Administration has removed the product insert warnings. **The main abnormality associated with the use of strongly androgenic progestins during pregnancy is masculinization of the external genitalia in female fetuses, with a risk of up to 2%.**

DIETHYLSTILBESTROL. Diethylstilbestrol (DES [X]), which in the past was widely used in the treatment of "threatened abortion," has clearly been established as a fetal teratogen and carcinogen when used in human pregnancy. **DES exposure poses an increased risk for cervical abnormalities and uterine malformations** (see Figure 19-2) **as well as for vaginal clear cell adenocarcinomas in female offspring.** Exposed males may be at increased risk for testicular abnormalities, infertility, and testicular malignancy.

Miscellaneous Agents

RETINOIDS. Isotretinoin (Accutane [X]) is prescribed for cystic acne or for acne that has not responded to other forms of treatment. **Exposure during pregnancy is clearly associated with a specific malformation**

BOX 7-4 *Etiologic Factors that May Play a Role in Anticonvulsant Teratogenicity*

Antiepileptic Drugs
Dose, serum levels, metabolism, teratogenicity, metabolic interactions

Genetic Predisposition
Maternal, paternal, and fetal metabolism

Maternal Disease
Teratogenicity, underlying disease, seizures

pattern that includes central nervous system, cardiovascular, and craniofacial defects (especially ear abnormalities). The central nervous system findings include hydrocephaly, facial nerve palsies, and cortical blindness. Microcephaly with severe ear anomalies, microtia, and cleft palate are common findings. The risk for spontaneous abortion or congenital malformations is greater than 50% in patients who take isotretinoin throughout the first trimester.

Etretinate (X), used for severe psoriasis, has been similarly associated with a characteristic malformation pattern. However, unlike isotretinoin, which has a half-life of less than 1 day, etretinate has a half-life of months, leading to a longer risk period even after the agent has been discontinued.

TOBACCO SMOKING. Maternal tobacco smoking interferes with prenatal growth, including birth weight, birth length, and head circumference. The teratogenic effects are related to the extent of maternal exposure to tobacco and include an increased risk for spontaneous abortion, fetal death, neonatal death, and prematurity. Pregnant women should be strongly encouraged to avoid smoking (or secondhand smoke). They should continue to abstain after delivery because secondhand smoke exposure is associated with an increased risk for respiratory diseases in infants and children.

ILLICIT DRUGS. Prenatal cocaine exposure, particularly among chronic abusers, has been associated with **fetal malformations, particularly genitourinary tract anomalies; behavioral abnormalities have also been documented in such fetuses.**

INFECTIOUS AGENTS. The exact frequency of significant infection during pregnancy is not known, but it is probably between 15% and 25%. **Viruses, bacteria, and parasites may have serious effects on the fetus, including fetal death, growth delay, congenital malformations, and mental deficiency.** In more recent years, the AIDS epidemic has had a significant impact on pregnancy management.

RADIATION. Prenatal ionizing radiation exposure occurs frequently as a result of therapeutic or diagnostic medical and dental procedures. **The medical effects of ionizing radiation are dose dependent and include teratogenesis, mutagenesis, and carcinogenesis.** The most critical period appears to be from about 2 to 6 weeks after conception. Exposures before 2 weeks produce either a lethal effect or no effect at all. Teratogenicity is still a possibility after 5 weeks, but the risk for deleterious consequences is relatively small.

Theoretically, any dose of ionizing radiation at a critical time could cause fetal damage. In most circumstances, diagnostic levels of radiation do not produce a teratogenic risk in the developing fetus.

■ Advice during Pregnancy

One of the most important functions of prenatal care is to provide information and support to the woman for self-care. The Cochrane pregnancy and childbirth database (www.cochrane.org) has compiled systematic reviews on the effectiveness of advice and interventions during pregnancy and can be a useful source of information for prenatal care providers. The following sections examine advice given on alleviating unpleasant symptoms, nutrition, lifestyle, and breastfeeding.

ALLEVIATING UNPLEASANT SYMPTOMS DURING PREGNANCY

Nausea and vomiting complicate up to 70% of pregnancies. Eating small, frequent meals and avoiding greasy or spicy foods may help. Also, having protein snacks at night, saltine crackers at the bedside, and room-temperature sodas is a nonpharmacologic approach that may provide some relief. **When medication is deemed necessary, antihistamines appear to be the drug of choice,** although no single product has been satisfactorily tested for efficacy and safety. **Vitamin B_6 (pyridoxine) and acupressure ("sea sickness arm bands") may be effective.** Patients with dehydration and electrolyte abnormalities from vomiting (hyperemesis gravidarum) should be evaluated for possible secondary causes, and they may need hospitalization for rehydration and antiemetic therapy.

Heartburn affects about two thirds of women at some stage of pregnancy, resulting from progesterone-induced relaxation of the esophageal sphincter. Avoiding lying down immediately after meals and elevating the head of the bed may help reduce heartburn. When these simple measures fail, antacids, such as calcium carbonate, should be used.

Constipation is a troublesome problem for many women in pregnancy, secondary to decreased colonic motility. Dietary modification, including increased fiber and water intake, can help lessen this problem. Stool softeners may be used in combination with bulking agents. Irritant laxatives should be reserved for short-term use in refractory cases.

Hemorrhoids are caused by increased venous pressure in the rectum. Increased rest, with elevation of the legs, and avoidance of constipation are recommended.

Leg cramps are experienced by almost half of all pregnant women, particularly at night and in the later months of pregnancy. Massage and stretching may afford some relief during an attack. Both calcium and sodium chloride appear to help reduce leg cramps in pregnancy.

Backaches are common during pregnancy and are lessened by avoiding excessive weight gain. Additionally, exercise, sensible shoes, and specially shaped pillows can offer relief. In cases of muscle spasm or strain, analgesics (such as acetaminophen), rest, and heat may lessen the symptoms.

NUTRITIONAL COUNSELING

Although the nutritional care plan should be individualized, every woman can benefit from nutritional education that includes counseling on weight gain, dietary guidelines, physical activity, avoidance of harmful substances and unsafe foods, and breastfeeding. The appropriate weight gain during pregnancy is listed in Table 7-5. Recommended rates of weight gain per week during the second and third trimesters are 1.1 pound, 0.9 pound, and 0.66 pound for pregnant women who are underweight, normal weight, and overweight, respectively. **Inadequate weight gain has been associated with low birth weight, whereas excessive weight gain has been associated with fetal macrosomia and maternal obesity, because of the difficulty of the mother returning to her prepregnancy body weight.** Women should avoid fasting (>13 hours without food) or skipping meals. This behavior is associated with accelerated ketosis and a greater risk for preterm delivery. They should have five feedings per day (breakfast, lunch, afternoon snack, dinner, and bedtime snack). **Pregnant women should never skip breakfast.**

Weight gain is an important consideration during pregnancy, and the clinician should emphasize the right amount of nutrition over the right amount of weight gain. Normal pregnancy requires an increase in daily caloric intake of 300 kcal.

LIFESTYLE ADVICE

Women should be advised to rest when tired and should be reassured that the **fatigue usually abates by the 4th month of pregnancy.** Normal prepregnancy activity levels are usually acceptable. Advice regarding work should be individualized to the nature of the work, the health status of the woman, and the condition of the pregnancy. Work that requires prolonged standing, shift or night work, and high cumulative occupational fatigue has been associated with an increased risk for low birth weight and prematurity. When working conditions involve occupational fatigue or stress, a change in work during pregnancy should be recommended by the prenatal care provider.

Women should be advised to continue to exercise during pregnancy, unless there is pregnancy-induced hypertension, preterm labor or rupture of membranes, intrauterine growth restriction, incompetent cervix, persistent second- or third-trimester bleeding, or medical conditions that severely restrict physiologic adaptations to exercise during pregnancy. They should avoid exercise in the supine position after the first trimester and should be encouraged to modify the intensity of their exercise according to maternal symptoms. Any type of exercise involving the potential for loss of balance or even mild abdominal trauma should be avoided.

Travel is acceptable under most circumstances. Prolonged sitting increases the risk for thrombus formation and thromboembolism. Pregnant women should be encouraged to ambulate periodically when taking a long flight or car ride. Support stockings may help reduce lower limb edema and varicose veins. International travel that places the patient at a high risk for infectious disease (such as travel to areas with a high rate of transmission of malaria or typhoid fever) should be avoided, whenever possible. When such travel cannot be avoided, appropriate vaccinations should be administered. For specific recommendations go to www.cdc.gov and select "Traveler's Health." Live attenuated virus vaccinations are generally contraindicated in pregnancy, but inactivated virus vaccines may be acceptable.

Women should be reassured that increased, unchanged, and decreased levels of sexual activity can all be normal during pregnancy. Abstinence or condom use may be advisable if there is an increased risk for preterm labor or repeated pregnancy loss, or in women with a history of persistent second- or third-trimester bleeding.

BREASTFEEDING

Breastfeeding has been shown to significantly reduce morbidity and improve cognitive development during infancy and childhood. Providers should initiate discussion with the pregnant woman and her family regarding breastfeeding during the first visit, including possible barriers to breastfeeding, such as prior poor experiences, misinformation, or nonsupportive work environment. Partners, peers, and other family members or friends may also exert an important influence on a woman's decision to breastfeed. Referral to a childbirth preparation class or a lactation consultant may provide additional encouragement to breastfeeding.

FOLLOW-UP VISITS

Additional prenatal visits are routinely scheduled every 4 weeks until 28 weeks' gestation, every 2 to 3 weeks until 36 weeks' gestation, and then weekly until delivery.

TABLE 7-5		
APPROPRIATE WEIGHT GAIN IN PREGNANCY		
	BMI	Recommended Weight Gain (pounds)
Underweight	<19	28–40
Normal	19–25	25–35
Overweight	>25	15–25

The schedule of these follow-up visits, however, should be tailored to the needs of individual patients. The regularity of scheduled prenatal visits should be sufficient to allow the clinician to monitor the progression of the pregnancy, provide education and recommended screening and interventions, assess the well-being of the fetus and mother, reassure the mother, and detect and treat medical and psychosocial complications.

During each regularly scheduled visit, the clinician should evaluate blood pressure, weight, urine protein and glucose, uterine size for progressive growth, and fetal heart rate. After the woman reports quickening (first sensation of fetal movement, on average at 20 weeks' gestation) and at each subsequent visit, she should be asked about **fetal movements.** Between 24 and 34 weeks, women should be **taught warning symptoms of preterm labor** (uterine contractions, leakage of fluid, vaginal bleeding, low pelvic pressure, or low back pain). Patients at risk may require additional visits to assess signs and symptoms of preterm labor. Beginning in the late second trimester, they should also be **taught to recognize the warning symptoms of preeclampsia** (frontal headache, visual changes, hand or facial swelling, epigastric or right upper quadrant pain). **Near term, they should be instructed on the symptoms of labor.**

Beginning at 28 weeks, systematic examination of the abdomen is carried out at each prenatal visit to **identify the lie** (e.g., longitudinal, transverse, oblique), **presentation** (e.g., vertex, breech, shoulder), **and position** (e.g., flexion, extension, or rotation of the occiput) of the fetus. This can be accomplished by the **maneuvers of Leopold.** The **first maneuver** involves palpating the fundus to determine which part of the fetus occupies the fundus. The head is round and hard, whereas the breech is irregular and soft. The **second maneuver** involves palpating either side of the abdomen to determine on which side the fetal back lies. The fetal back is linear and firm, whereas the extremities have multiple parts. The **third maneuver** involves grasping the presenting part between the thumb and third finger just above the pubic symphysis to determine the presenting part. The **fourth maneuver** involves palpating for the brow and the occiput of the fetus to determine fetal head position when the fetus is in a vertex presentation. This is best accomplished with the examiner facing the patient's feet and placing both hands on either side of the lower abdomen just above the inlet. By exerting pressure in the direction of the pelvic inlet, the hand running along the back will bump into the occiput if the head is extended, whereas the hand on the same side of the small parts will bump into the brow if the head is flexed. If there is a question about the presentation of the fetus, a real-time ultrasound may be performed.

Depending on the practice setting and population, either universal or selective **screening for gestational diabetes** should be performed between 24 and 28 weeks of gestation. Risk factors for selective screening include family history of diabetes; previous birth of a macrosomic, malformed, or stillborn baby; hypertension; glycosuria; maternal age of 30 years or older; or previous gestational diabetes. Repeat measurements of **hemoglobin or hematocrit levels** early in the third trimester have been recommended. Tests **for sexually transmitted infections** (e.g., syphilis) may also be repeated at 32 to 36 weeks of gestation if the woman has specific risk factors for these diseases. The Centers for Disease Control and Prevention recommend **universal screening for maternal colonization of** group B streptococcus at 35 to 37 weeks of gestation. The value of selective ultrasound for specific indications has been clearly established; the value of routine ultrasound in low-risk pregnancies remains undetermined. Ultrasonic examination during pregnancy is not harmful, but controlled trials have failed to demonstrate that routine ultrasonic examinations for dating in early pregnancy, anatomic survey in mid-pregnancy, or assessment of fetal growth in late pregnancy improve perinatal outcome.

▓ *Assessment of Fetal Well-Being*

During the past 20 years, electronic advances have provided new technology that has made the fetus more accessible and has allowed visualization of the fetus and recording of intrauterine fetal events. A combination of the nonstress test, contraction stress test, and real-time ultrasonic assessment is used to assess fetal well-being. Figure 7-3 presents an algorithm that may be used to follow a high-risk pregnancy.

MATERNAL SELF-ASSESSMENT OF FETAL WELL-BEING

A simple technique (kick counting) may be used to assess fetal well-being. The mother assesses fetal movement (kick counts) each evening on her left side. She should recognize 10 movements in 1 hour, and if she does not, she should retest in 1 hour. If she still does not have 10 fetal movements in 1 hour, she should contact her doctor or present for fetal assessment of well-being.

NONSTRESS TEST ASSESSMENT

The first step in the assessment of fetal well-being is the nonstress test. With the mother resting in the left lateral supine position, a continuous fetal heart rate tracing is obtained using external Doppler equipment. The mother reports each fetal movement, and the effects of the fetal movements on heart rate are determined. **A normal fetus responds to fetal movement with an acceleration in fetal heart rate of 15 beats/minute or more above the baseline for at least 15 seconds** (Figure 7-4). If at least two such accelerations occur

ANTENATAL TESTING GUIDELINES

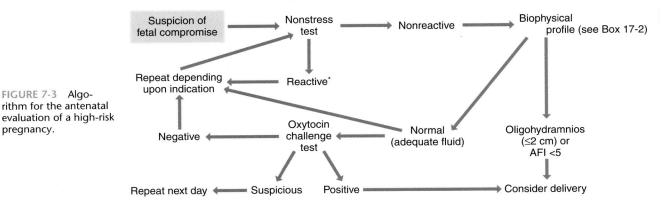

FIGURE 7-3   Algorithm for the antenatal evaluation of a high-risk pregnancy.

*All pregnancies complicated by IUGR or postdatism should have a complete biophysical profile that includes an ultrasonic evaluation.

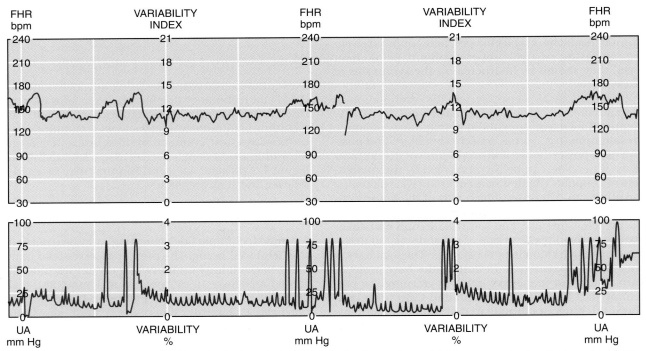

FIGURE 7-4   Reactive nonstress test. Note the fetal heart rate (FHR) accelerations with most fetal movements, denoted by spikes above 75 mm Hg in lower panel. bpm, Beats per minute.

in a 20-minute interval, the fetus is regarded as being healthy, and the test is said to be reactive. A nonreactive nonstress test is shown in Figure 7-5.

ULTRASONIC ASSESSMENT

The next step in prenatal assessment is to determine the adequacy of amniotic fluid volume by real-time ultrasonography. Reduced fluid (oligohydramnios) suggests fetal compromise. Oligohydramnios can be defined as an amniotic fluid index (AFI) of less than 5 cm. **The AFI represents the sum of the linear measurements (in centimeters) of the largest amniotic fluid pockets noted on ultrasonic inspection of each of the four quadrants of the gestational sac.** When amniotic fluid is reduced, the fetus is more likely to become compromised as a result of umbilical cord compression.

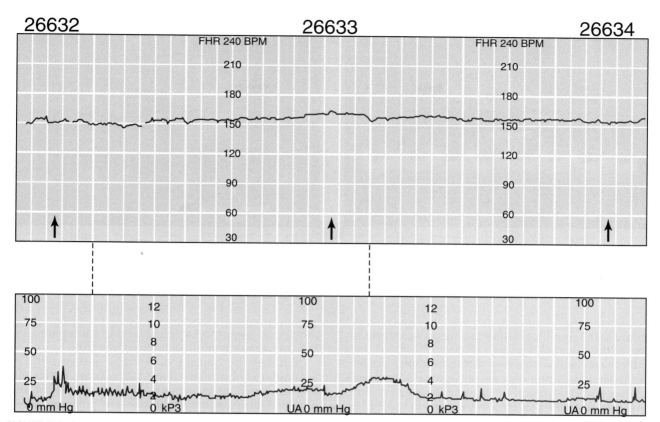

FIGURE 7-5 Nonreactive nonstress test. Note the lack of beat-to-beat variability and the lack of acceleration of the fetal heart rate (FHR) with fetal movements (*arrows*). bpm, Beats per minute.

Excessive amniotic fluid (polyhydramnios; AFI > 23 cm) can be a sign of poor control in a diabetic pregnancy or an indication that the fetus may have an anomaly. **Fetal breathing (chest wall movements) and fetal movements (stretching and rotational movements) are also used to assess the fetus.** A fetus who has at least 30 breathing movements in 10 minutes or 3 body movements in 10 minutes is considered healthy. A combination of a **reactive nonstress test, adequate amniotic fluid, adequate fetal breathing, adequate fetal movements, and adequate tone** is frequently referred to as a **normal biophysical profile.** Each parameter is given a score of 2. A normal profile equals 10. Table 7-6 lists the recommended frequency for biophysical profile testing based on the high-risk condition.

UMBILICAL ARTERY DOPPLER ASSESSMENT

During the ultrasonic assessment, it is easy to assess fetal umbilical artery vascular resistance as an index of fetal health performing pulse wave Doppler assessment. A normal systolic-to-diastolic (S/D) ratio (Figure 7-6) suggests normal flow when the S/D ratio is low, indicating low fetal-placental vascular resistance. When flow becomes abnormal, there is complete loss

TABLE 7-6

RECOMMENDED FREQUENCY FOR BIOPHYSICAL PROFILE TESTING	
High-Risk Condition	**Frequency**
IUGR	
Mild	Weekly
Moderate*	Twice weekly
DIABETES MELLITUS	
Class A	Weekly, 37 to 40 wk
	Twice weekly, beyond 40 wk
Class B and worse	Twice weekly, beginning at 34 wk
POST-TERM PREGNANCY	Twice weekly, beginning at 42 wk
Decreased fetal movements	Weekly
Other high-risk conditions	Weekly
Maternal or physician concern	Weekly

*For severe IUGR, delivery is usually indicated.
IUGR, intrauterine growth restriction.

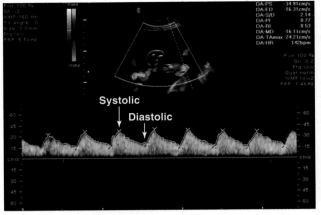

FIGURE 7-6   Fetal umbilical artery Doppler assessment at 31 weeks and 3 days showing a series of Doppler waveforms with systolic (upper) peaks marked with X (+37 cm/sec) and lower X marking diastole at (+21 cm/sec). The systolic-to-diastolic ratio is calculated as 2.14 (*upper right corner*), and normal for this gestational age is <3.2.

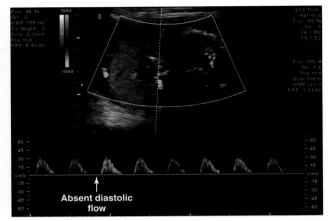

FIGURE 7-7   Fetal umbilical artery Doppler assessment at 26 weeks and 5 days in a case with reduced amniotic fluid (small lucent pocket left of midline with Doppler assessment of cord artery). The systolic-to-diastolic ratio cannot be calculated as in Figure 7-6 because of absent diastolic flow. Only systolic flow can be measured (+30 cm/sec).

of flow in the umbilical artery during diastole from the fetus to the placenta (Figure 7-7). When the fetus is very ill, there can be reversed flow during diastole, whereby the deflection during diastole is negative (downward, −cm/second) and blood in the umbilical artery flows backward from the placenta to the fetus in the umbilical artery. Under the latter condition, the fetus should be delivered expeditiously.

CONTRACTION STRESS TEST

The contraction stress test is a test for uteroplacental dysfunction, a condition that may occur in a high-risk pregnancy. **A dilute infusion of oxytocin is given to establish at least three uterine contractions in 10 minutes. If late decelerations are observed with each contraction, the test is positive (abnormal).** If only one deceleration is observed, the test is suspicious. When the test is positive, the baby should usually be delivered.

PREVENTIVE HEALTH CARE

Management before and during pregnancy presents an opportunity for patient education and the practice of preventive medicine. **Childbirth preparation classes for both the patient and her husband are very educational, particularly during the first pregnancy.** The presence and encouragement of the baby's father can be most helpful during labor and delivery. These classes provide an important opportunity for both parents to enhance bonding to the infant before birth.

Although preconception, prenatal, and obstetric information is of primary importance, other topics that may have lifelong relevance can be introduced and emphasized during antepartum care. The pregnancy itself is frequently a strong motivator for women to eliminate potentially harmful habits or dietary patterns and to become more aware of their general health. Therefore, a systematic approach to the dissemination of preventive health-care information is generally well received by the pregnant woman.

SUGGESTED READING

American Academy of Pediatrics, the American College of Obstetricians, Gynecologists: Guidelines for Perinatal Care: 4th ed, Elk Grove Village, Ill, American Academy of Pediatrics, 1997.

Invasive prenatal testing for fetal aneuploidy: ACOG Committee Opinion No. 88. Obstet Gynecol 110:1449–1457, 2007.

Liston R, Sawchuck D, Young D: Fetal health surveillance: Antepartum and intrapartum consensus guideline. Society of Obstetricians and Gynecologists of Canada. British Columbia Prenatal Health Program. [Erratum in J Obstet Gynaecol Can 29:909, 2007.]. J Obstet Gynaecol Can 29:S3-S56, 2007.

Mennuti MT: Genetic screening in reproductive health care. Clin Obstet Gynecol 51:3-33, 2008.

Rayburn WF: What you need to know about medication safety in pregnancy. OBG Management 19(11):66-82, 2007.

Chapter 8

Normal Labor, Delivery, and Postpartum Care

ANATOMIC CONSIDERATIONS, OBSTETRIC ANALGESIA AND ANESTHESIA, AND RESUSCITATION OF THE NEWBORN

CALVIN J. HOBEL • MARK ZAKOWSKI

Labor is a process that permits a series of extensive physiologic changes in the mother to allow for the delivery of her fetus through the birth canal. **It is defined as progressive cervical effacement and dilation resulting from regular uterine contractions that occur at least every 5 minutes and last 30 to 60 seconds.**

The role of the obstetrician is to anticipate and manage abnormalities that may occur to either the maternal or the fetal process. When a decision is made to intervene, it must be considered carefully because each intervention carries not only potential benefits but also potential risks. In most cases, the best management may be close observation and, when necessary, cautious intervention.

◼ Anatomic Characteristics of the Fetal Head and Maternal Pelvis

Vaginal delivery necessitates the accommodation of the fetal head to the bony pelvis.

FETAL HEAD

The head is the largest and least compressible part of the fetus. Thus, from an obstetric viewpoint, it is the most important part, whether the presentation is cephalic or breech.

The fetal skull consists of a base and a vault (cranium). The base of the skull has large, ossified, firmly united, and noncompressible bones. This serves to protect the vital structures contained within the brain stem.

The cranium consists of the occipital bone posteriorly, two parietal bones bilaterally, and two frontal and temporal bones anteriorly. The cranial bones at birth are thin, weakly ossified, easily compressible, and interconnected only by membranes. These features allow them to overlap under pressure and to change shape to conform to the maternal pelvis, a process known as "**molding.**"

Sutures

The membrane-occupied spaces between the cranial bones are known as sutures. The **sagittal suture** lies between the parietal bones and extends in an anteroposterior direction between the fontanelles, dividing the head into right and left sides (Figure 8-1). The **lambdoid suture** extends from the posterior fontanelle laterally and serves to separate the occipital from the parietal bones. The **coronal suture** extends from the anterior fontanelle laterally and serves to separate the parietal and frontal bones. The **frontal suture** lies between the frontal bones and extends from the anterior fontanelle to the glabella (the prominence between the eyebrows).

Fontanelles

The membrane-filled spaces located at the point where the sutures intersect are known as fontanelles, the most important of which are the **anterior and posterior fontanelles.** Clinically, they are even more useful in diagnosing the fetal head position than the sutures.

The **posterior fontanelle** closes at 6 to 8 weeks of life, whereas the **anterior fontanelle** does not become ossified until about 18 months. This allows the skull to accommodate the tremendous growth of the infant's brain after birth.

The anterior fontanelle (**bregma**) is found at the intersection of the sagittal, frontal, and coronal sutures. It is diamond shaped and measures about 2 × 3 cm, and it is much larger than the posterior fontanelle. The posterior fontanelle is Y- or T-shaped and is found at the junction of the sagittal and lambdoid sutures.

Landmarks

The fetal skull is characterized by a number of landmarks. Moving from front to back, they include the following (Figure 8-2):

1. **Nasion** (the root of the nose)
2. **Glabella** (the elevated area between the orbital ridges)
3. **Sinciput (brow)** (the area between the anterior fontanelle and the glabella)
4. **Anterior fontanelle (bregma)**—diamond shaped
5. **Vertex** (the area between the fontanelles and bounded laterally by the parietal eminences)
6. **Posterior fontanelle (lambda)**—Y or T shaped
7. **Occiput** (the area behind and inferior to the posterior fontanelle and lambdoid sutures)

Diameters

Several diameters of the fetal skull are important (see Figures 8-1 and 8-2). The **anteroposterior diameter** presenting to the maternal pelvis depends on the degree of flexion or extension of the head and is important because the various diameters differ in length. The following measurements are considered average for a term fetus:

1. **Suboccipitobregmatic (9.5 cm),** the presenting anteroposterior diameter when the head is well flexed, as in an occipitotransverse or occipitoanterior position; it extends from the undersurface of the occipital bone at the junction with the neck to the center of the anterior fontanelle.
2. **Occipitofrontal (11 cm),** the presenting anteroposterior diameter when the head is deflexed, as in an occipitoposterior presentation; it extends from the external occipital protuberance to the glabella.
3. **Supraoccipitomental (13.5 cm),** the presenting anteroposterior diameter in a brow presentation and the longest anteroposterior diameter of the head; it extends from the vertex to the chin.
4. **Submentobregmatic (9.5 cm),** the presenting anteroposterior diameter in face presentations; it extends from the junction of the neck and lower jaw to the center of the anterior fontanelle.

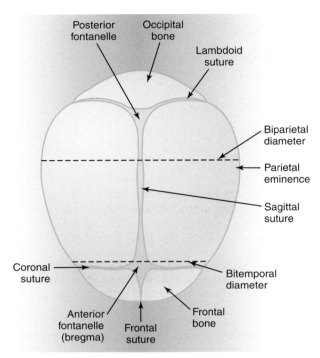

FIGURE 8-1 Superior view of the fetal skull showing the sutures, fontanelles, and transverse diameters.

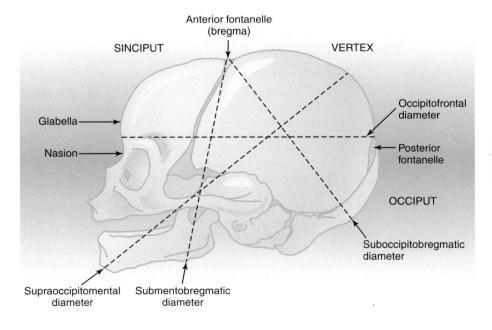

FIGURE 8-2 Lateral view of the fetal skull showing the prominent landmarks and the anteroposterior diameters.

The **transverse diameters** of the fetal skull are as follows:

1. **Biparietal (9.5 cm),** the largest transverse diameter; it extends between the parietal bones.
2. **Bitemporal (8 cm),** the shortest transverse diameter; it extends between the temporal bones.

The average circumference of the term fetal head, measured in the occipitofrontal plane, is 34.5 cm.

PELVIC ANATOMY

Bony Pelvis

The bony pelvis is made up of four bones: the sacrum, coccyx, and two innominates (composed of the ilium, ischium, and pubis). These are held together by the sacroiliac joints, the symphysis pubis, and the sacrococcygeal joint. The union of the pelvis and the vertebral column stabilizes the pelvis and allows weight to be transmitted to the lower extremities.

The **sacrum** consists of five fused vertebrae. The anterior-superior edge of the first sacral vertebra is called the **promontory,** which protrudes slightly into the cavity of the pelvis. The anterior surface of the sacrum is usually concave. It articulates with the ilium at its upper segment, with the coccyx at its lower segment, and with the sacrospinous and sacrotuberous ligaments laterally.

The **coccyx** is composed of three to five rudimentary vertebrae. It articulates with the sacrum, forming a joint, and occasionally the bones are fused.

The pelvis is divided into the false pelvis above and the true pelvis below the linea terminalis. The false pelvis is bordered by the lumbar vertebrae posteriorly, an iliac fossa bilaterally, and the abdominal wall anteriorly. Its only obstetric function is to support the pregnant uterus.

The true pelvis is a bony canal and is formed by the sacrum and coccyx posteriorly and by the ischium and pubis laterally and anteriorly. Its internal borders are solid and relatively immobile. The posterior wall is twice the length of the anterior wall. The true pelvis is the area of concern to the obstetrician because its dimensions are sometimes not adequate to permit passage of the fetus.

Pelvic Planes

The pelvis is divided into the following four planes for descriptive purposes:

1. **The pelvic inlet**
2. **The plane of greatest diameter**
3. **The plane of least diameter**
4. **The pelvic outlet**

These planes are imaginary, flat surfaces that extend across the pelvis at different levels. Except for the plane of greatest diameter, each plane is clinically significant.

The **plane of the inlet** is bordered by the pubic crest anteriorly, the iliopectineal line of the innominate bones laterally, and the promontory of the sacrum posteriorly. The fetal head enters the pelvis through this plane in the transverse position.

The **plane of greatest diameter** is the largest part of the pelvic cavity. It is bordered by the posterior midpoint of the pubis anteriorly, the upper part of the obturator foramina laterally, and the junction of the 2nd and 3rd sacral vertebrae posteriorly. The fetal head rotates to the anterior position in this plane.

The **plane of least diameter** is the most important from a clinical standpoint because most instances of arrest of descent occur at this level. It is bordered by the lower edge of the pubis anteriorly, the ischial spines and sacrospinous ligaments laterally, and the lower sacrum posteriorly. Low transverse arrests generally occur in this plane.

The **plane of the pelvic outlet** is formed by two triangular planes with a common base at the level of the ischial tuberosities. The anterior triangle is bordered by the subpubic angle at the apex, the pubic rami on the sides, and the bituberous diameter at the base. The posterior triangle is bordered by the sacrococcygeal joint at its apex, the sacrotuberous ligaments on the sides, and the bituberous diameter at the base. This plane is the site of a low pelvic arrest.

Pelvic Diameters

The diameters of the pelvic planes represent the amount of space available at each level. The key measurements for assessing the capacity of the maternal pelvis include the following:

1. **The obstetric conjugate of the inlet**
2. **The bispinous diameter**
3. **The bituberous diameter**
4. **The posterior sagittal diameter at all levels**
5. **The curve and length of the sacrum**
6. **The subpubic angle**

The average lengths of the diameters of each pelvic plane are listed in Table 8-1.

Pelvic Inlet

The pelvic inlet has five important diameters (Figure 8-3). The anteroposterior diameter is described by one of two measurements. The **true conjugate (anatomic conjugate)** is the anatomic diameter and extends from the middle of the sacral promontory to the superior surface of the pubic symphysis. The **obstetric conjugate** represents the actual space available to the fetus and extends from the middle of the sacral promontory to the closest point on the convex posterior surface of the symphysis pubis.

The **transverse diameter** is the widest distance between the iliopectineal lines. Each **oblique diameter** extends from the sacroiliac joint to the opposite ilio-pectineal eminence.

The **posterior sagittal diameter** extends from the anteroposterior and transverse intersection to the middle of the sacral promontory.

Plane of Greatest Diameter

The plane of greatest diameter has two noteworthy diameters. The **anteroposterior diameter** extends from the midpoint of the posterior surface of the pubis to the junction of the 2nd and 3rd sacral vertebrae. The **transverse diameter** is the widest distance between the lateral borders of the plane.

TABLE 8-1		
AVERAGE LENGTH OF PELVIC PLANE DIAMETERS		
Pelvic Plane	**Diameter**	**Average Length (cm)**
Inlet	True (anatomic) conjugate	11.5
	Obstetric conjugate	11
	Transverse	13.5
	Oblique	12.5
	Posterior sagittal	4.5
Greatest diameter	Diagonal conjugate	12.75
	Transverse	12.5
Midplane	Anteroposterior	12
	Bispinous	10.5
	Posterior sagittal	4.5-5
Outlet	Anatomic anteroposterior	9.5
	Obstetric anteroposterior	11.5
	Bituberous	11
	Posterior sagittal	7.5

Plane of Least Diameter (Midplane)

The plane of least diameter has three important diameters. The **anteroposterior diameter** extends from the lower border of the pubis to the junction of the fourth and fifth sacral vertebrae. The **transverse (bispinous) diameter** extends between the ischial spines. The **posterior sagittal diameter** extends from the midpoint of the bispinous diameter to the junction of the fourth and fifth sacral vertebrae.

Pelvic Outlet

The pelvic outlet has four important diameters (Figure 8-4). The **anatomic anteroposterior diameter** extends from the inferior margin of the pubis to the tip of the coccyx, whereas the **obstetric anteroposterior diameter** extends from the inferior margin of the pubis to the sacrococcygeal joint. The **transverse (bituberous) diameter** extends between the inner surfaces of the ischial tuberosities, and the **posterior sagittal diameter** extends from the middle of the transverse diameter to the sacrococcygeal joint.

PELVIC SHAPES

Based on the general bony architecture, the pelvis may be classified into four basic types (Figure 8-5).

Gynecoid

The gynecoid pelvis is the classic female type of pelvis and is found in about 50% of women. It has the following characteristics:
1. Round at the inlet, with the widest transverse diameter only slightly greater than the anteroposterior diameter
2. Side walls straight
3. Ischial spines of average prominence
4. Large sacrospinous notch

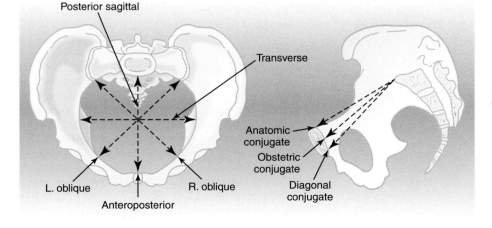

FIGURE 8-3   Pelvic inlet and its diameters.

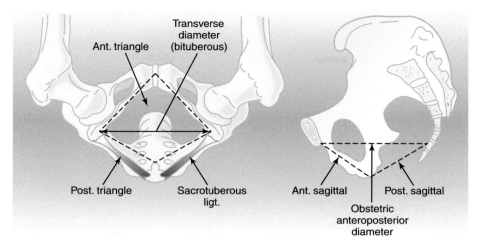

FIGURE 8-4   Pelvic outlet and its diameters.

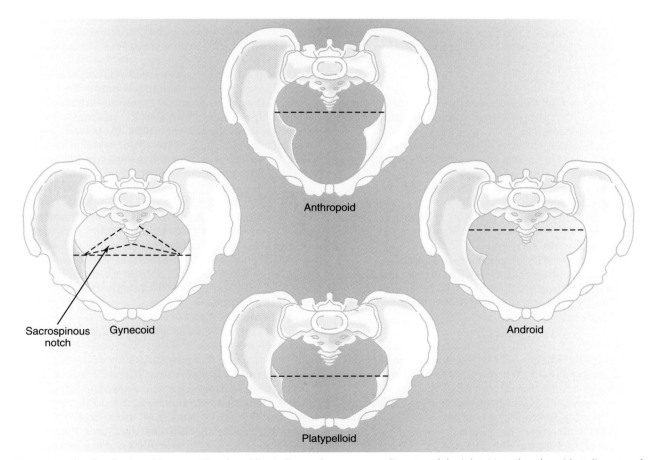

FIGURE 8-5   The four basic pelvic types. The *dotted line* indicates the transverse diameter of the inlet. Note that the widest diameter of the inlet is posteriorly situated in an android or anthropoid pelvis. The gynecoid pelvis illustrates the location of the sacrosciatic notch, present in all pelvic types.

5. Well-curved sacrum
6. Spacious subpubic arch, with an angle of about 90 degrees

These features create a cylindrical shape that is spacious throughout. The fetal head generally rotates into the occipitoanterior position in this type of pelvis.

Android

The android pelvis is the typical male type of pelvis, and it is found in less than 30% of women and has the following characteristics:
1. Triangular inlet with a flat posterior segment and the widest transverse diameter closer to the sacrum than in the gynecoid type
2. Convergent side walls with prominent spines
3. Shallow sacral curve
4. Long and narrow (small) sacrospinous notch
5. Narrow subpubic arch

This type of pelvis has limited space at the inlet and progressively less space as one moves down the pelvis, owing to the funneling effect of the side walls, sacrum, and pubic rami. Thus, the amount of space is restricted at all levels. The fetal head is forced to be in the occipitoposterior position to conform to the narrow anterior pelvis. Arrest of descent is common at the midpelvis.

Anthropoid

The anthropoid pelvis resembles that of the anthropoid ape. It is found in about 20% of women and has the following characteristics:
1. A much larger anteroposterior than transverse diameter, creating a long narrow oval at the inlet
2. Side walls that do not converge
3. Ischial spines that are not prominent but are close, owing to the overall shape
4. Variable, but usually posterior, inclination of the sacrum
5. Small sacrospinous notch
6. Narrow, outwardly shaped subpubic arch

The fetal head can engage only in the anteroposterior diameter and usually does so in the occipitoposterior position because there is more space in the posterior pelvis.

Platypelloid

The platypelloid pelvis is best described as being a flattened gynecoid pelvis. It is found in only 3% of women, and it has the following characteristics:
1. A short anteroposterior and wide transverse diameter creating an oval-shaped inlet
2. Straight or divergent side walls
3. Posterior inclination of a flat sacrum
4. A wide bispinous diameter
5. Long but small sacrospinous notch
6. A wide subpubic arch

The overall shape is that of a gentle curve throughout. The fetal head has to engage in the transverse diameter.

ENGAGEMENT

Engagement occurs when the widest diameter of the fetal presenting part has passed through the pelvic inlet. In cephalic presentations, the widest diameter is biparietal; in breech presentations, it is intertrochanteric.

The station of the presenting part in the pelvic canal is defined as its level above or below the plane of the ischial spines. The level of the ischial spines is assigned as "zero" station, and each centimeter above or below this level is given a minus or plus designation, respectively, for a total length of 10 cm.

In most women, the bony presenting part is at the level of the ischial spines when the head has become engaged. The fetal head usually engages with its sagittal suture in the transverse diameter of the pelvis. The head position is considered to be **synclitic** when the biparietal diameter is parallel to the pelvic plane and the sagittal suture is midway between the anterior and posterior planes of the pelvis. When this relationship is not present, the head is considered to be **asynclitic** (Figure 8-6).

There is a distinct advantage to having the head engage in asynclitism in certain situations. In a synclitic presentation, the biparietal diameter entering the pelvis measures 9.5 cm; but when the parietal bones enter the pelvis in an asynclitic manner, the presenting diameter measures 8.75 cm. Therefore, asynclitism permits a larger head to enter the pelvis than would be possible in a synclitic presentation.

CLINICAL PELVIMETRY

The diameters that can be clinically evaluated can be assessed at the time of the first prenatal visit to screen for obvious pelvic contractions, although some obstetricians believe that it is better to wait until later in pregnancy when the soft tissues are more distensible and the examination is less uncomfortable and possibly more accurate.

The clinical evaluation is started by assessing the pelvic inlet. The pelvic inlet can be evaluated clinically for its anteroposterior diameter. The obstetric conjugate can be estimated from the diagonal conjugate, which is obtained on clinical examination (see Figure 8-3).

The diagonal conjugate is approximated by measuring from the lower border of the pubis to the sacral promontory using the tip of the second finger and the point where the base of the index finger meets the pubis (Figure 8-7). The **obstetric conjugate** is then estimated by subtracting 1.5 to 2 cm, depending on the height and inclination of the pubis. Often the middle finger of the examining hand cannot reach the sacral

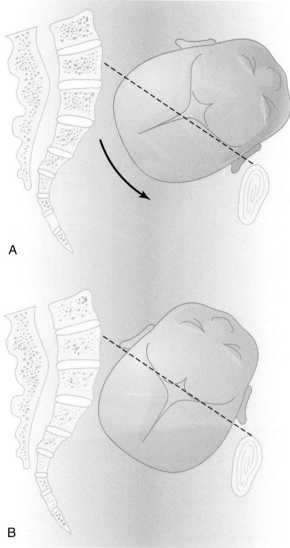

A

B

FIGURE 8-6   Anterior asynclitism entering the pelvis (**A**), and synclitism in the pelvis (**B**).

promontory; thus, the obstetric conjugate is considered adequate. If the diagonal conjugate is greater than or equal to 11.5 cm, the anteroposterior diameter of the inlet is considered to be adequate.

The anterior surface of the sacrum is then palpated to assess its curvature. The usual shape is concave. A flat or convex shape may indicate anteroposterior constriction throughout the pelvis.

The midpelvis cannot accurately be measured clinically in either the anteroposterior or transverse diameter. A reasonable estimate of the size of the midpelvis, however, can be obtained as follows. **The pelvic side walls can be assessed to determine whether they**

are convergent rather than having the normal, almost parallel, configuration. The ischial spines are palpated carefully to assess their prominence, and several passes are made between the spines to approximate the bispinous diameter. The length of the sacrospinous ligament is assessed by placing one finger on the ischial spine and one finger on the sacrum in the midline. The average length is 3 fingerbreadths. If the sacrospinous notch that is located lateral to the ligament can accommodate two-and-a-half fingertips, the posterior midpelvis is most likely of adequate dimensions. A short ligament suggests a forward inclination of the sacrum and a narrowed sacrospinous notch (see Figure 8–5, pg 95).

Finally, the pelvic outlet is assessed. This is done by first placing a fist between the ischial tuberosities. An 8.5-cm distance is considered an adequate transverse diameter. The posterior sagittal measurement should also be greater than 8 cm. The infrapubic angle is assessed by placing a thumb next to each inferior pubic ramus and then estimating the angle at which they meet. An angle of less than 90 degrees is associated with a contracted transverse diameter in the midplane and outlet.

Radiologic Assessment of the Pelvis

When an accurate measurement of the pelvis is indicated, nuclear magnetic resonance imaging (MRI) may be used. The advantage of MRI over x-ray or computed tomography (CT) for pelvic assessment is the lack of ionizing radiation exposure.

Indications

1. **Clinical evidence or obstetric history suggestive of pelvic abnormalities.**
2. **A history of pelvic trauma.**

It should always be questioned whether the results obtained by radiologic assessment will have sufficient influence on the patient's management to make the investigation worthwhile.

PREPARATION FOR LABOR

Before actual labor begins, a number of physiologic preparatory events usually occur.

Lightening

Two or more weeks before labor, the fetal head in most primigravid women settles into the brim of the pelvis. In multigravida, this often does not occur until early in labor. **Lightening** may be noted by the mother as a flattening of the upper abdomen and an increased prominence of the lower abdomen.

False Labor

During the last 4 to 8 weeks of pregnancy, the uterus undergoes irregular contractions that normally are painless. Such contractions appear unpredictably and

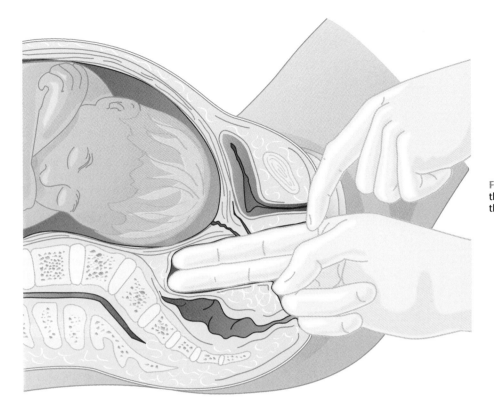

FIGURE 8-7 Clinical estimation of the diagonal conjugate diameter of the pelvis.

sporadically and can be rhythmic and of mild intensity. In the last month of pregnancy, these contractions may occur more frequently, sometimes every 10 to 20 minutes, and with greater intensity. **These Braxton Hicks contractions are considered false labor in that they are not associated with progressive cervical dilation or effacement.** They may serve a physiologic role in preparing the uterus and cervix for true labor.

Cervical Effacement

Before the onset of parturition, the cervix is frequently noted to soften as a result of increased water content and collagen lysis. Simultaneous effacement, or thinning of the cervix, occurs as it is taken up into the lower uterine segment (Figure 8-8B). Consequently, patients often present in early labor with a cervix that is already partially effaced. As a result of cervical effacement, the mucous plug within the cervical canal may be released. The onset of labor may thus be heralded by the passage of a small amount of blood-tinged mucus from the vagina (**"bloody show"**).

STAGES OF LABOR

There are four stages of labor, each of which is considered separately. These stages in actuality are definitions of progress during labor, delivery, and the puerperium.

The first stage is from the onset of true labor to complete dilation of the cervix. The second stage is from complete dilation of the cervix to the birth of the baby. The third stage is from the birth of the baby to delivery of the placenta. The fourth stage is from delivery of the placenta to stabilization of the patient's condition, usually at about 6 hours postpartum.

First Stage of Labor

PHASES. The first stage of labor consists of two phases: a latent phase, during which cervical effacement and early dilation occur, and an active phase, during which more rapid cervical dilation occurs (Figure 8-9). Although cervical softening and early effacement may occur before labor, during the first stage of labor, the entire cervical length is retracted into the lower uterine segment.

LENGTH. The length of the first stage may vary in relation to parity; primiparous patients generally experience a longer first stage than do multiparous patients (Table 8-2). Because the latent phase may overlap considerably with the preparatory phase of labor, its duration is highly variable. It may also be influenced by other factors, such as sedation and stress. The active phase begins when the cervix is 3 to 4 cm dilated

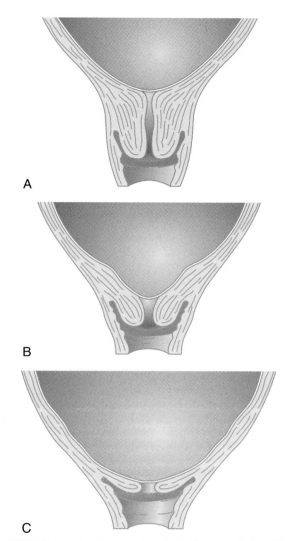

A

B

C

FIGURE 8-8 **A:** The absence of cervical effacement before labor. **B:** Cervix being progressively taken up into the lower segment of the uterus (about 50% effaced). **C:** Cervix fully taken up (i.e., cervix is completely effaced).

TABLE 8-2

CHARACTERISTICS OF NORMAL LABOR		
Characteristic	Primipara	Multipara
Duration of first stage	6-18 hr	2-10 hr
Rate of cervical dilation during active phase	1 cm/hr	1.2 cm/hr
Duration of second stage	30 min to 3 hr	5-30 min
Duration of third stage	0-30 min	0-30 min

completion of cervical dilation, the second stage commences. Thereafter, only the descent, flexion, and rotation of the presenting part are available to assess the progress of labor.

CLINICAL MANAGEMENT OF THE FIRST STAGE. Certain steps should be taken in the clinical management of the patient during the first stage of labor.

MATERNAL POSITION. The mother may ambulate provided that intermittent monitoring ensures fetal well-being and the presenting part is engaged in patients with ruptured membranes. **If she is lying in bed, the lateral recumbent position should be encouraged** to ensure perfusion of the uteroplacental unit.

ADMINISTRATION OF FLUIDS. Because of decreased gastric emptying during labor, **oral fluids are best avoided.** However, fasting results in the more rapid development of ketosis in pregnant women. Placement of a 16- to 18-gauge venous catheter is advisable during the active phase of labor. Recently, it has been shown that **giving at least 125 mL/hour of 10% dextrose (D) in normal saline (NS),** compared with 5% D/NS or just NS, **results in significantly shorter labors**. Thus, this intravenous route is used to both hydrate the patient with crystalloids and provide calories during labor, to administer oxytocin after the delivery of the placenta, and for the treatment of any unanticipated emergencies.

INVESTIGATIONS. Every woman admitted in labor should have a hematocrit or hemoglobin measurement and a blood clot held in the event that a crossmatch is needed. Blood group, Rhesus (Rh) type, and an antibody screen should be done if these are not known. It is also important to know the hepatitis B status of the mother so that a pediatrician can be notified if the mother is positive. Additionally, a voided urine specimen should be checked for the presence of protein and glucose.

MATERNAL MONITORING. Maternal pulse rate, blood pressure, respiratory rate, and temperature should be recorded every 1 to 2 hours in normal labor and more frequently if indicated. Fluid balance, particularly urine output and intake, should be monitored carefully.

ANALGESIA. Adequate analgesia is important during the first stage of labor (see later in this chapter).

in the presence of regularly occurring uterine contractions. **The minimal dilation during the active phase of the first stage is nearly the same for primiparous and multiparous women: 1 and 1.2 cm/hour, respectively.** If progress is slower than this, evaluation for uterine dysfunction, fetal malposition, or cephalopelvic disproportion should be undertaken.

MEASUREMENT OF PROGRESS. During the first stage, the progress of labor may be measured in terms of cervical effacement, cervical dilation, and descent of the fetal head. The clinical pattern of the uterine contractions alone is not an adequate indication of progress. After

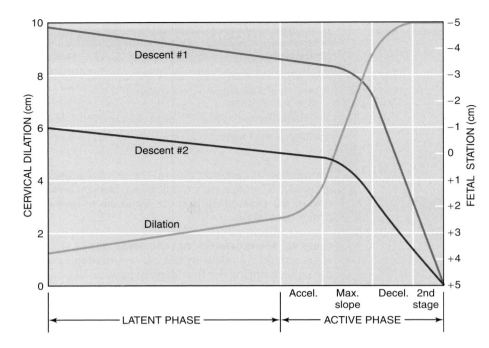

FIGURE 8-9   Cervical dilation and descent of the fetal head during labor. The first descent curve represents a fetus with a floating presenting part at the onset of labor, whereas the second represents a fetus with the presenting part fixed in the pelvis before labor. *(Modified from Friedman EA: Labor: Evaluation and Management, 2nd ed. East Norwalk, CT, Appleton-Century-Crofts, 1978, p 41.)*

FETAL MONITORING. The fetal heart rate should be evaluated either by auscultation with a De Lee stethoscope, by external monitoring with Doppler equipment, or by internal monitoring with a fetal scalp electrode. In uncomplicated pregnancies, continuous electronic fetal monitoring is not necessary, as several studies have demonstrated that intermittent auscultation of the fetal heart rate, when performed in conjunction with a 1:1 nurse-to-patient ratio, results in comparable outcomes. **In patients with no significant obstetric risk factors, the fetal heart rate should be auscultated or the electronic monitor tracing evaluated at least every 30 minutes in the active phase of the first stage of labor and at least every 15 minutes in the second stage of labor.** In patients with obstetric risk factors, the fetal heart rate should be auscultated or the electronic monitoring tracing evaluated at least every 15 minutes during the active phase of the first stage of labor (immediately following a uterine contraction), and at least every 5 minutes during the second stage.

UTERINE ACTIVITY. Uterine contractions should be monitored every 30 minutes by palpation for their frequency, duration, and intensity. **For high-risk pregnancies, uterine contractions should be monitored continuously along with the fetal heart rate.** This can be achieved electronically using either an external tocodynamometer or an internal pressure catheter in the amniotic cavity. The latter is particularly of value when a patient's labor is being augmented with oxytocin (Pitocin).

VAGINAL EXAMINATION. During the latent phase, particularly when the membranes are ruptured, vaginal examinations should be done sparingly to decrease the risk for an intrauterine infection. **In the active phase, the cervix should be assessed about every 2 hours to determine the progress of labor.** Cervical effacement and dilation, the station and position of the presenting part, and the presence of molding or caput in vertex presentations should be recorded.

AMNIOTOMY. The artificial rupture of fetal membranes may provide information on the volume of amniotic fluid and the presence or absence of meconium. In addition, rupture of the membranes may cause an increase in uterine contractility. **Amniotomy incurs risks for chorioamnionitis if labor is prolonged and for umbilical cord compression or cord prolapse if the presenting part is not engaged.**

Second Stage of Labor

At the beginning of the second stage, the mother usually has a desire to bear down with each contraction. This abdominal pressure, together with the uterine contractile force, combines to expel the fetus. During the second stage of labor, **fetal descent must be monitored carefully** to evaluate the progress of labor. Descent is measured in terms of progress of the presenting part through the birth canal.

In cephalic presentations, the shape of the fetal head may be altered during labor, making the assessment of descent more difficult. **Molding** is the alteration of the relationship of the fetal cranial bones to each other as

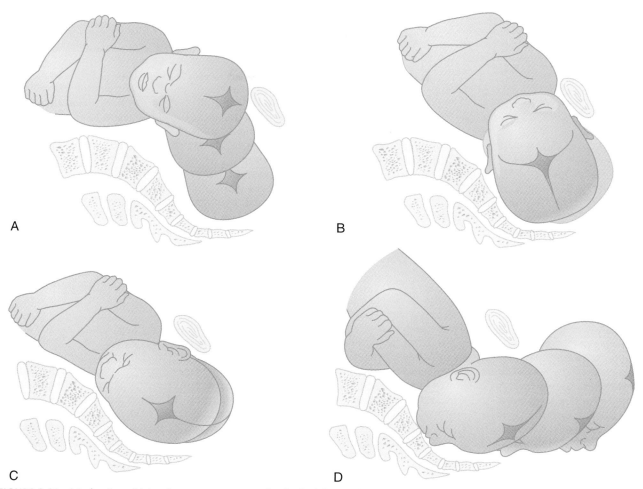

FIGURE 8-10   Mechanism of labor for a vertex presentation in the left occipitotransverse position. **A:** Flexion and descent. **B** and **C:** Continued descent and commencement of internal rotation. **D:** Completion of internal rotation to the occipitoanterior position followed by delivery of the head by extension.

a result of the compressive forces exerted by the bony maternal pelvis. Some molding is necessary for delivery under normal circumstances. If cephalopelvic disproportion is present, the amount of molding will be more pronounced. **Caput** is a localized, edematous swelling of the scalp caused by pressure of the cervix on the presenting portion of the fetal head. The development of both molding and caput can create a false impression of fetal descent.

The second stage generally takes from 30 minutes to 3 hours in primigravid women and from 5 to 30 minutes in multigravida.

MECHANISM OF LABOR. Six movements of the baby enable it to adapt to the maternal pelvis: descent, flexion, internal rotation, extension, external rotation, and expulsion (Figure 8-10). These movements are discussed here for both an occipitoanterior and occipitoposterior

position at engagement. The mechanism of labor for other presentations is discussed in Chapter 13.

DESCENT. Descent is brought about by the force of the uterine contractions, maternal bearing-down (Valsalva) efforts, and, if the patient is upright, gravity.

FLEXION. Partial flexion exists before labor as a result of the natural muscle tone of the fetus. During descent, resistance from the cervix, walls of the pelvis, and pelvic floor cause further flexion of the cervical spine, with the baby's chin approaching its chest. **In the occipitoanterior position, the effect of flexion is to change the presenting diameter from the occipitofrontal to the smaller suboccipitobregmatic** (see Figure 8-2). In the occipitoposterior position, complete flexion may not occur, resulting in a larger presenting diameter, which may contribute to a longer labor.

INTERNAL ROTATION. In the occipitoanterior positions, the fetal head, which enters the pelvis in a transverse or oblique diameter, rotates so that the occiput turns anteriorly toward the symphysis pubis. Internal rotation probably occurs as the fetal head meets the muscular sling of the pelvic floor. It is often not accomplished until the presenting part has reached the level of the ischial spines (zero station) and therefore is engaged. In the occipitoposterior positions, the fetal head may rotate posteriorly, so the occiput turns toward the hollow of the sacrum.

EXTENSION. The flexed head in an occipitoanterior position continues to descend within the pelvis. Because the vaginal outlet is directed upward and forward, extension must occur before the head can pass through it. As the head continues its descent, there is bulging of the perineum followed by crowning. **Crowning** occurs when the largest diameter of the fetal head is encircled by the vulvar ring. At this time, the vertex has reached station +5. When necessary, an incision in the perineum (**episiotomy**) may aid in reducing perineal resistance, although **current management is to allow the fetus to deliver without an episiotomy**. The head is born by rapid extension as the occiput, sinciput, nose, mouth, and chin pass over the perineum.

In the **occipitoposterior position**, the head is born by a combination of flexion and extension. At the time of crowning, the posterior bony pelvis and the muscular sling encourage further flexion. The forehead, sinciput, and occiput are born as the fetal chin approaches the chest. Subsequently, the occiput falls back as the head extends, and the nose, mouth, and chin are born.

EXTERNAL ROTATION. In both the occipitoanterior and occipitoposterior positions, the delivered head now returns to its original position at the time of engagement to align itself with the fetal back and shoulders. Further head rotation may occur as the shoulders undergo an internal rotation to align themselves anteroposteriorly within the pelvis.

EXPULSION. Following external rotation of the head, the anterior shoulder delivers under the symphysis pubis, followed by the posterior shoulder over the perineal body and the body of the child.

CLINICAL MANAGEMENT OF THE SECOND STAGE. As in the first stage, certain steps should be taken in the clinical management of the second stage of labor.

MATERNAL POSITION. With the exception of avoiding the supine position, the mother may assume any comfortable position for effective bearing down.

BEARING DOWN. With each contraction, the mother should be encouraged to hold her breath and bear down with expulsive efforts. This is particularly important for patients with regional anesthesia because their reflex sensations may be impaired.

FETAL MONITORING. During the second stage, the fetal heart rate should be monitored continuously or evaluated every 5 minutes in patients with obstetric risk factors. Fetal heart rate decelerations (head compression or cord compression) with recovery following the uterine contraction may occur normally during this stage.

VAGINAL EXAMINATION. Progress should be recorded about every 30 minutes during the second stage. Particular attention should be paid to the descent and flexion of the presenting part, the extent of internal rotation, and the development of molding or caput. During the second stage of labor, the retracted cervix is no longer palpable.

DELIVERY OF THE FETUS. When delivery is imminent, the patient is usually placed in the lithotomy position, and the skin over the lower abdomen, vulva, anus, and upper thighs is cleansed with an antiseptic solution. Uncomplicated deliveries, particularly in multiparous women, may be carried out in the **supine position** with the thighs flexed. The **left lateral position** may be used to deliver patients with hip or knee joint deformities that prevent adequate flexion, or for patients with a superficial or deep venous thrombosis in one of the lower extremities.

As the perineum becomes flattened by the crowning head, an episiotomy may be performed to prevent perineal lacerations. **The performance of episiotomies may result in a higher proportion of lacerations that involve the anal sphincter (third degree) or anal mucosa (fourth degree). Although these more extensive lacerations may be surgically repaired, there is an increasing awareness of the occasional complication of anal incontinence of gas or feces following vaginal delivery.**

To facilitate delivery of the fetal head, a **Ritgen maneuver** may be performed (Figure 8-11). The right hand, draped with a towel, exerts upward pressure through the distended perineal body, first to the supraorbital ridges and then to the chin. This upward pressure, which increases extension of the head and prevents it from slipping back between contractions, is counteracted by downward pressure on the occiput with the left hand. A recent (2008) randomized trial from Sweden found simple manual perineal support to be equally effective.

Once the head is delivered, the airway is cleared of blood and amniotic fluid using a bulb suction device. The oral cavity is cleared initially and then the nares are cleared. Suction of the nares is not performed if fetal distress or meconium-stained liquor is present because it may result in gasping and aspiration of pharyngeal contents. A second towel is used to wipe secretions from the face and head.

After the airway has been cleared, an index finger is used to check whether the umbilical cord encircles the neck. If so, the cord can usually be slipped over the infant's head. If the cord is too tight, it can be cut between two clamps.

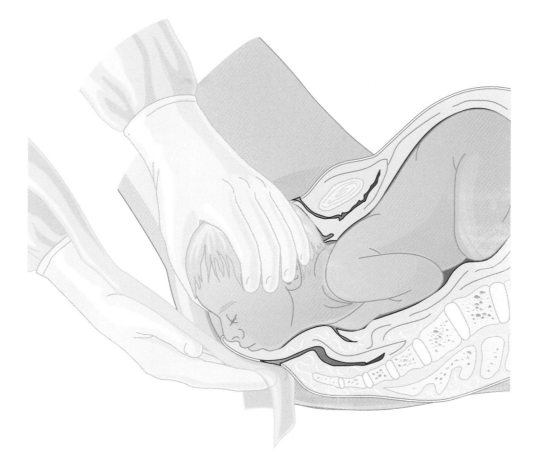

FIGURE 8-11   Ritgen's maneuver. The fingers of the right hand, pressing posterior to the rectum, are used to extend the head while counterpressure is applied to the occiput by the left hand to allow for a more controlled delivery of the fetal head. Simple manual support of the perineum using one or both hands may be equally effective.

Following delivery of the head, the shoulders descend and rotate into the anteroposterior diameter of the pelvis and are delivered (Figure 8-12). **Delivery of the anterior shoulder is aided by gentle downward traction on the externally rotated head. The brachial plexus may be injured if excessive force is used.** The posterior shoulder is delivered by elevating the head. Finally, the body is slowly extracted by traction on the shoulders.

After delivery, blood will be infused from the placenta into the newborn if the baby is held below the mother's introitus. Usually, the cord is clamped and cut within 15 to 20 seconds. Delayed cord clamping can result in neonatal hyperbilirubinemia as additional blood is transferred from the placenta to the newborn infant. The newborn is then placed under an infant warmer.

Third Stage of Labor

Immediately after the baby's delivery, the cervix and vagina should be thoroughly inspected for lacerations and surgical repair performed if necessary. The cervix, vagina, and perineum may be more readily examined before the separation of the placenta because no uterine bleeding should be present to obscure visualization.

DELIVERY OF THE PLACENTA. Separation of the placenta generally occurs within 2 to 10 minutes of the end of the second stage of labor. Squeezing of the fundus to hasten placental separation is not recommended because it may increase the likelihood of passage of fetal cells into the maternal circulation.

Signs of placental separation are as follows: (1) a fresh show of blood from the vagina, (2) the umbilical cord lengthens outside the vagina, (3) the fundus of the uterus rises up, and (4) the uterus becomes firm and globular. Only when these signs have appeared should the assistant attempt traction on the cord. With gentle traction and counterpressure between the symphysis and fundus to prevent descent of the uterus into the pelvis, the placenta is delivered.

Following delivery of the placenta, attention should be paid to any uterine bleeding that may originate

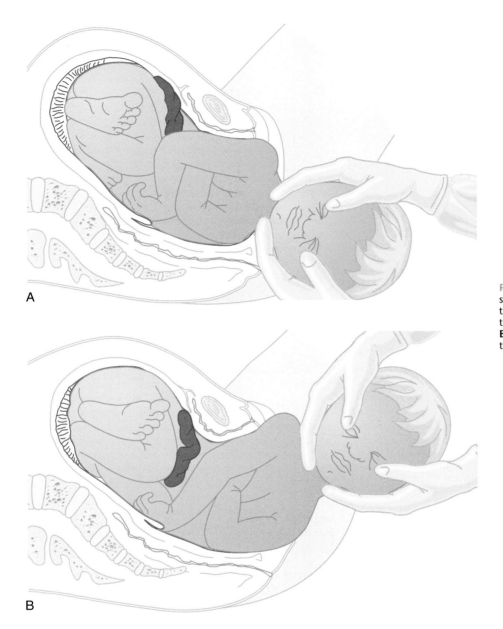

A

B

FIGURE 8-12 Delivery of the shoulders. **A:** Gentle downward traction on the head is applied to deliver the anterior shoulder. **B:** Gentle upward traction is used to deliver the posterior shoulder.

from the placental implantation site. Uterine contractions, which reduce this bleeding, may be hastened by uterine massage and the use of oxytocin. **It is routine to add 20 U of oxytocin to the intravenous infusion after the baby has been delivered.** The placenta should be examined to ensure its complete removal and to detect placental abnormalities. If the patient is at risk for postpartum hemorrhage (e.g., because of anemia, prolonged oxytocic augmentation of labor, multiple gestation, or hydramnios), manual removal of the placenta, manual exploration of the uterus, or both may be necessary.

PERINEAL LACERATIONS. Perineal lacerations, with or without episiotomy, may be classified as follows:

- **First degree:** A laceration involving the vaginal epithelium or perineal skin
- **Second degree:** A laceration extending into the subepithelial tissues of the vagina or perineum with or without involvement of the muscles of the perineal body
- **Third degree:** A laceration involving the anal sphincter
- **Fourth degree:** A laceration involving the rectal mucosa

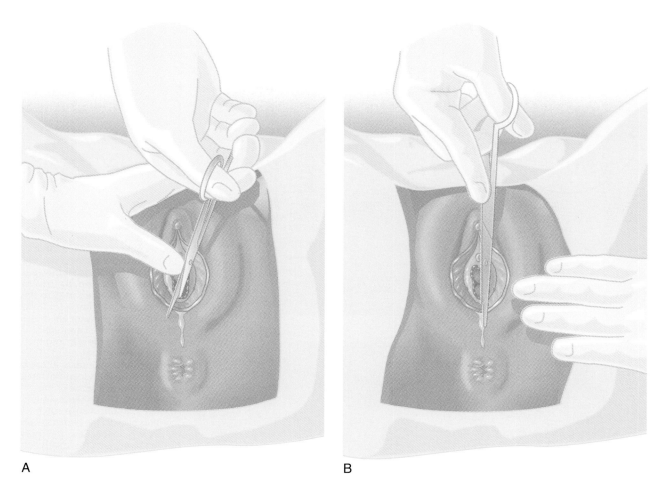

A   B

FIGURE 8-13   **A:** Mediolateral episiotomy. **B:** Midline episiotomy.

If an episiotomy has been performed (Figure 8-13), it should be repaired as illustrated in Figure 8-14. Absorbable sutures (00) should be used, and a rectal examination should ensure that the sutures have not inadvertently transected the rectal mucosa. A third-degree tear (Figure 8-15) should be repaired as shown in Figure 8-16.

Fourth Stage of Labor

The hour immediately following delivery requires close observation of the patient. Blood pressure, pulse rate, and uterine blood loss must be monitored closely. It is during this time that postpartum hemorrhage commonly occurs, usually because of uterine relaxation, retained placental fragments, or unrepaired lacerations. Occult bleeding (e.g., vaginal hematoma formation) may manifest as pelvic pain. An increase in pulse rate, often out of proportion to any decrease in blood pressure, may indicate hypovolemia.

Induction and Augmentation of Labor

Induction of labor is the process whereby labor is initiated by artificial means; **augmentation** is the artificial stimulation of labor that has begun spontaneously.

In the absence of the natural onset of labor, pharmacologic methods may be used to initiate labor. However, labor should be induced only after appropriate assessment of the mother and fetus and an explanation to the patient of the indications for induction. In the absence of a medical indication for labor induction, fetal maturity should be confirmed by either appropriate pregnancy dating, ultrasonic measurements, or amniotic fluid analysis (e.g., lecithin/sphingomyelin [L/S] ratio).

Cervical effacement and softening (ripening) occur before the onset of spontaneous labor. Cervical ripening frequently does not occur before a decision about labor induction, yet the success of induction is dependent on these necessary changes in the cervix.

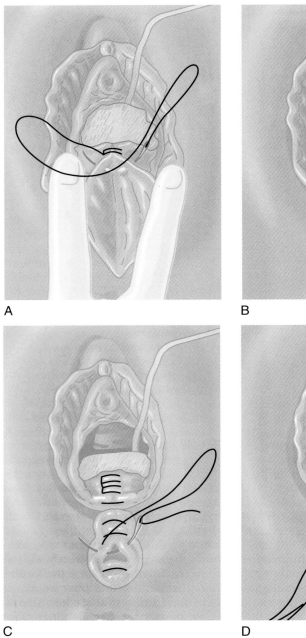

FIGURE 8-14   **A:** Repair of a midline episiotomy. A taped sponge is placed in the upper vagina, and a continuous locked 00 or 000 absorbable suture closes the vaginal epithelium from the apex to the hymeneal ring. **B:** Three interrupted sutures are used to close the deep perineal fascia (of Colles) and underlying levator ani muscles. The vaginal epithelial suture is brought below the skin into the subcutaneous tissue.
C: The same continuous suture is used to close the superficial fascia down to the anal edge of the episiotomy. **D:** The same suture is used as a subcuticular stitch coming back to the hymeneal ring, where it is doubly tied. The sponge is then removed. (This is very important.)

A

B

C

D

Several mechanical and pharmacologic approaches promote cervical ripening before the actual induction of uterine contractions. Local application of prostaglandins may be used. Currently approved pharmacologic treatments include intravaginal application of prostaglandin E_2 using a vaginal insert called **Cervidil** (on a string), which can be removed quickly if the medication causes hyperstimulation. **Cytotec**, a synthetic prostaglandin E_1 analogue, has been approved

for cervical ripening. One 25-μg tablet placed intravaginally effectively initiates cervical ripening. Although prostaglandin administration has been demonstrated to shorten the duration of labor induction, the impact on cesarean birth rates due to failed induction has been minimal.

Other methods of cervical ripening may include intrauterine placement of catheters or the use of osmotic dilators (see Figure 26-4). Manual separation of

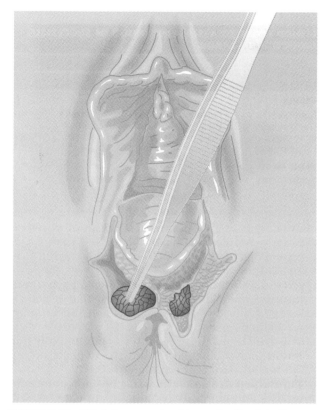

FIGURE 8-15 Third-degree perineal tear extending into the rectum and avulsing the circular rectal sphincter.

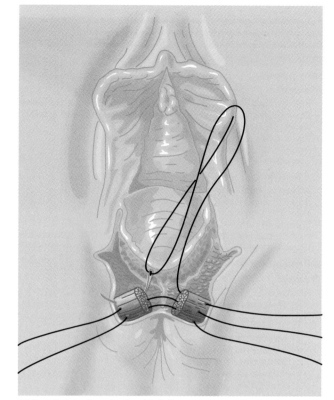

FIGURE 8-16 Repair of a third-degree tear involves approximating the fascia surrounding the rectal sphincter muscle and reapproximating the vaginal tears with locked continuous sutures. The process is then completed as with a midline episiotomy repair.

the chorioamnion from the lower uterine segment does not necessarily speed the onset of labor. Although controversial, **artificial rupture of the membranes** may be used to increase uterine activity, and perhaps to speed cervical change, when performed in conjunction with administration of oxytocin.

In addition to cervical ripening, induction of labor requires the initiation of effective uterine contractions. Oxytocin is identical to the natural pituitary peptide, and it is the only drug approved for induction and augmentation of labor. Pitocin is the synthetic preparation. The physician must be fully aware of the indications and the contraindications for the use of oxytocin (Table 8-3). **In general, induction of labor before term is indicated only when the continuation of pregnancy represents a significant risk to the fetus or mother. In some situations, induction may be indicated at term, as in the case of premature rupture of the membranes.** Induction at term for convenience is not appropriate unless the patient has a history of previous precipitous delivery (less than 3 hours) or lives an unusually long distance from the hospital.

In general, any condition that makes normal labor dangerous for the mother or fetus is a contraindication to induction or augmentation of labor. The most common contraindication has been prior uterine surgery in which there has been complete transection of the uterine wall. However, **a previous lower transverse incision is no longer considered a contraindication to a trial of labor.** This is referred to as vaginal birth after cesarean (VBAC).

Induction of labor before term for maternal or fetal indications **must not be undertaken without the assessment of fetal pulmonary maturity,** provided that a delay will not jeopardize the mother or fetus. **Fetal lung maturity can most often be accelerated within 24 to 48 hours by the use of glucocorticoids.**

TECHNIQUE FOR INDUCTION AND AUGMENTATION OF LABOR

A hospital obstetric service must establish guidelines for the proper use of oxytocin for induction and augmentation of labor. In general, an assessment and plan of management must be outlined in the patient's medical record. Indications for induction of labor should be clearly stated. It is helpful to assess the likelihood of

TABLE 8-3

INDICATIONS AND CONTRAINDICATIONS FOR INDUCTION AND AUGMENTATION OF LABOR

Induction	Augmentation
INDICATIONS	
Maternal	
Preeclampsia	Abnormal labor (in the presence
Diabetes mellitus	of inadequate uterine activity)
Heart disease	Prolonged latent phase
Prolonged pregnancy	Prolonged active phase
Intrauterine growth restriction (IUGR)	
Fetoplacental	
Abnormal fetal testing	
Rh incompatibility	
Fetal abnormality	
Premature rupture of membranes (PROM)	
Chorioamnionitis	
CONTRAINDICATIONS	
Maternal	
Absolute	Same contraindications as for
Contracted pelvis	maternal and fetoplacental
Relative	
Prior uterine surgery	
Classic cesarean birth	
Complete transection of uterus (myomectomy, reconstruction)	
Overdistended uterus	
Fetoplacental	
Preterm fetus without lung maturity	
Acute fetal distress	
Abnormal presentation	

TABLE 8-4

BISHOP SCORE TO ASSESS LIKELIHOOD OF SUCCESSFUL INDUCTION OF LABOR

Physical Findings	Rating			
	0	1	2	3
CERVIX				
Position	Posterior	Mid	Anterior	—
Consistency	Firm	Medium	Soft	—
Effacement (%)	0-30	40-50	60-70	≥80
Dilation (cm)	0	1-2	3-4	≥5
FETAL HEAD				
Station (cm)	−3	−2	−1	+1

as uterine hypertonus or fetal distress develops. Because oxytocin has a half-life of 3 to 5 minutes, its physiologic effect will diminish quickly (within 15 to 30 minutes) after discontinuation.

2. **A dilute infusion must be used and "piggybacked" into the main intravenous line** so that it can be stopped quickly if necessary, without interrupting the main intravenous route.

3. **The drug is best infused with a calibrated infusion pump** that can be easily adjusted to effect the required infusion rate accurately.

4. **The induction of labor for a specific indication generally should not exceed 72 hours.** In patients with a low Bishop score, it is not unusual for an induction to progress slowly. If the cervix effaces and dilates, it is recommended that the membranes be ruptured on the third day. If adequate progress is not made within 12 hours of rupturing the membranes, a cesarean delivery may be performed.

5. **If adequate labor is established, the infusion rate and the concentration may be reduced,** especially during the second stage of labor. This principle avoids the risks of hyperstimulation and fetal distress, which frequently occur once labor has been established.

Substantial variation exists regarding the initial dose, incremental dose, and time interval between dose increments when oxytocin is used for labor induction and augmentation. Well-performed clinical studies have supported both low-dose (1 to 30 mU/min) and high-dose (4 to 40 mU/min) protocols, as seen in Table 8-5. It is not surprising that many protocols use "moderate" doses of oxytocin. Generally, intervals between dose increments should be no less than 20 minutes to permit time for steady-state plasma levels of oxytocin to be achieved and to prevent an increased risk for uterine hyperstimulation.

COMPLICATIONS. The use of oxytocin for the induction and augmentation of labor can cause three major complications. First, an excessive infusion rate can cause

success by a careful pelvic examination to determine the **Bishop score,** which evaluates the status of the cervix and the station of the fetal head (Table 8-4). A high score (9 to 13) is associated with a high likelihood of a vaginal delivery, whereas a low score (<5) is associated with a decreased likelihood of success (65% to 80%). Before induction is begun, the patient's blood must be typed and screened for antibodies. A blood specimen should be held in the laboratory in case crossmatching becomes necessary. **Continuous electronic monitoring of the fetal heart rate and uterine activity is required during induction.** An internal uterine catheter for monitoring uterine pressure is suggested if intensity cannot be adequately assessed.

Oxytocin Infusion

Several principles should be followed when oxytocin is used to induce or augment labor:

1. **Oxytocin must be given intravenously** to allow it to be discontinued quickly if a complication such

TABLE 8-5

METHOD OF OXYTOCIN INFUSION FOR INDUCTION OR AUGMENTATION

SOLUTION

10 units of oxytocin in 1000 mL of 5% dextrose or balanced salt solution (10 mU/mL)

ADMINISTRATION

Piggyback into main IV line; administer solution by infusion pump

	Low-Dose Protocol	High-Dose Protocol
Starting dose	1 mU/min	4 mU/min
Increment	1 mU/min	4 mU/min
Interval	20 min	20 min
Limited by	5 contractions in 10 min	7 contractions in 15 min
Maximal dose	20-30 mU/min	40 mU/min

hyperstimulation and thereby cause fetal distress from ischemia. In rare situations, a tetanic contraction can occur and lead to **rupture of the uterus.** Second, because oxytocin has a similar structure to antidiuretic hormone, it has an intrinsic **antidiuretic effect** and will increase water reabsorption from the glomerular filtrate. **Severe water intoxication with convulsions and coma can occur** rarely when oxytocin is infused continuously for more than 24 hours. Third, prolonged infusion of oxytocin can result in **uterine muscle fatigue** (nonresponsiveness) and **postdelivery uterine atony** (hypotonus), which can increase the risk for postpartum hemorrhage.

◼ *Puerperium*

The puerperium consists of the period following delivery of the baby and placenta to about 6 weeks postpartum. During the puerperium, the reproductive organs and maternal physiology return toward the prepregnancy state, although menses may not return for much longer.

ANATOMIC AND PHYSIOLOGIC CHANGES

Involution of the Uterus

Through a process of tissue catabolism, the uterus rapidly decreases in weight from about 1000 g at delivery to 100 to 200 g at about 3 weeks postpartum. The cervix similarly loses its elasticity and regains its prepregnancy firmness. For the first few days after delivery, the uterine discharge (lochia) appears red (**lochia rubra**), owing to the presence of erythrocytes. After 3 to 4 days, the lochia becomes paler (**lochia serosa**), and by the 10th day, it assumes a white or yellow-white color (**lochia alba**). Foul-smelling lochia suggests endometritis.

Vagina

Although the vagina may never return to its prepregnancy state, the supportive tissues of the pelvic floor gradually regain their former tone. Women who deliver vaginally should be taught and encouraged to perform Kegel exercises (intermittent tightening of the perineal muscles) to maintain and improve the supportive tissues of the pelvic floor.

Cardiovascular System

Immediately after delivery, there is a marked increase in peripheral vascular resistance due to the removal of the low-pressure uteroplacental circulatory shunt. The cardiac output and plasma volume gradually return to normal during the first 2 weeks of the puerperium. As a result of the loss of plasma volume and the diuresis of extracellular fluid, a marked weight loss occurs in the first week.

Psychosocial Changes

It is fairly common for women to exhibit a mild degree of depression a few days after delivery. The **"postpartum blues"** are probably due to both emotional and hormonal factors. With understanding and reassurance from both family and physician, this usually resolves without consequence. **Any prolonged episodes of depression during or after pregnancy should receive urgent attention.**

Return of Menstruation and Ovulation

In women who do not nurse, menstrual flow usually returns by 6 to 8 weeks, although this is highly variable. Although ovulation may not occur for several months, particularly in nursing mothers, contraceptive counseling and use should be emphasized during the puerperium to avoid an undesired pregnancy.

◼ *Breastfeeding*

There are many advantages to breastfeeding. First, **breast milk is the ideal food for the newborn, is inexpensive, and is usually in good supply.** Second, **breastfeeding accelerates the involution of the uterus** because suckling stimulates the release of oxytocin, thereby causing increased uterine contractions. Third, and probably most important, **there are immunologic advantages for the baby from breastfeeding.** Various types of maternal antibodies are present in breast milk. The predominant immunoglobulin is secretory immunoglobulin A (IgA), which provides protection in the infant's gut by preventing attachment of harmful bacteria (e.g., *Escherichia coli*) to cells on the mucosal surface. This prevents the bacteria from penetrating the bowel wall. It is also thought that maternal lymphocytes pass through the infant's gut wall and initiate immunologic processes that are not yet well understood. **Breastfeeding** thereby **provides the newborn with passive immunity** against certain infectious diseases until its own immune mechanisms become fully functional by 3 to 4 months.

LACTATION

Various hormones, such as estrogen, progesterone, human chorionic gonadotropin, cortisol, insulin, prolactin, and placental lactogen, play an important role in preparing the breasts for lactation. **At delivery, two events are instrumental in initiating lactation. First is the drop in placental hormones, particularly estrogen.** Before delivery, these hormones interfere with the lactogenic action of prolactin. **Second, suckling stimulates the release of prolactin and oxytocin.** The latter causes contraction of the myoepithelial cells in the alveoli and milk ducts. The suckling stimulus is thought to be important for milk production, as well as for the ejection of colostrum and milk.

On about the second day after delivery, colostrum is secreted. Its content is composed mostly of protein, fat, and minerals. It is the colostrum that contains secretory IgA. **After about 3 to 6 days, the colostrum is replaced by mature milk.** The content of milk varies considerably depending on the nutritional status of the mother and the gestational age at the time of delivery. In general, the major components of breast milk are proteins, lactose, water, and fat. The major proteins synthesized in the human breast, which are unique and are not found in cows' milk, are casein, lactalbumin, and ß-lactoglobulin. Essential amino acids are delivered from the mother's blood, and some of the nonessential amino acids can be synthesized in the breast. In addition, breast milk is a source of omega-3 fatty acids, which are important for early brain development.

LACTATION SUPPRESSION

When the mother chooses not to breastfeed, lactation suppression is indicated. **The simplest, and probably safest, method to accomplish this is to use a tight-fitting bra.** If breast distention does occur, pumping only makes the situation worse. Ice packs should be applied and the discomfort managed with analgesics.

COMPLICATIONS OF BREASTFEEDING

Cracked Nipples

If the nipples of the breast become fissured, nursing may become difficult. Because fissures are also a portal of entry for bacteria, they should be managed aggressively with a nipple shield and an appropriate cream, such as lanolin or Masse breast cream. Further breastfeeding should be temporarily stopped. Milk can be expressed manually until the nipples heal, at which time breastfeeding can be resumed.

Mastitis

This is an uncommon complication of breastfeeding and usually develops after 2 to 4 weeks. The first symptoms are usually slight fever and chills. These are followed by redness of a segment of the breast, which becomes indurated and painful. **The etiologic agent is usually *Staphylococcus aureus*, which originates from the infant's oral pharynx.** Milk should be obtained from the breast for culture and sensitivity, and the mother should be started on a regimen of antibiotics immediately. **Because most staphylococcal organisms are penicillinase producing, a penicillinase-resistant antibiotic, such as dicloxacillin, should be used.** Breastfeeding may be discontinued but is not contraindicated. An appropriate antibiotic should be continued for 7 to 10 days. If a breast abscess ensues, it should be surgically drained. A breast pump can be used to maintain lactation until the infection has cleared if nursing is discontinued.

Drug Passage to the Newborn

Because an infant may ingest up to 500 mL of breast milk per day, maternally administered drugs that pass into breast milk may have a significant effect on the infant. The amount of drug found in breast milk depends on the maternal dose, the rate of maternal clearance, the physicochemical properties of the drug, and the composition of the breast milk with respect to fat and protein. The gestational age of the infant may also be a determinant of the ultimate drug effect. Table 8-6 lists selected drugs with their reported newborn effects.

Interconception Care

Women who have poor pregnancy outcomes, such as preterm births and perinatal deaths, are at greater risk for having the same problems with subsequent pregnancies. Programs are now offering comprehensive interconception care to address conditions that have been shown to cause poor outcomes with interventions that could mitigate or eliminate any recurrence. The rationale for this approach is to provide continuous obstetric care rather than episodic care triggered by another pregnancy. Studies are underway to determine the value of these programs.

Obstetric Analgesia and Anesthesia

The goal of obstetric analgesia and anesthesia is to provide effective pain relief for the mother during the course of labor and delivery that is safe for her and her baby and that has minimal or no adverse effects on the progress and outcome of labor. Anesthetic practices have evolved to include an increased reliance on highly

TABLE 8-6

EFFECTS OF MATERNAL DRUG INGESTION ON BREASTFEEDING INFANTS

Drug	Reported Infant Effects
SEDATIVE-HYPNOTICS	
Diazepam	Sedation
ANTIPSYCHOTICS	
Chlorpromazine	No adverse effects reported
Haloperidol	No adverse effects reported
NONNARCOTIC ANALGESICS	
Acetaminophen	No adverse effects reported
Salicylates	Theoretical risk for platelet dysfunction
ANTICONVULSANTS*	
Phenobarbital	Sedation
Phenytoin	Sedation, decreased sucking
NARCOTICS	
Heroin	May cause addiction
Methadone	Infant death reported
Meperidine	No adverse effects reported
ANTIBIOTICS	
Penicillin	May modify bowel flora, cause allergy, or interfere with sepsis work-up
Ampicillin	Same as for penicillin
Erythromycin	Same as for penicillin
Nitrofurantoin	Theoretical risk for hemolytic anemia in infants with glucose-6-phosphate dehydrogenase deficiency
Tetracycline	Same as for penicillin; theoretical risk for discoloration of teeth and inhibition of bone growth
DIGOXIN	No adverse effects reported
THYROID DRUGS	
Thyroxine	May interfere with screening for hypothyroidism
Propylthiouracil	Nodular goiter
ANTIHYPERTENSIVES	
Methyldopa	No adverse effects reported
Propranolol	No adverse effects reported
THEOPHYLLINE	One case of infant irritability following maternal administration of a rapidly absorbed oral preparation

*See Chapters 7 and 16.

effective and safe regional anesthetic techniques, using low-concentration combinations of narcotics and local anesthetics in order to minimize the adverse effects of each. Maternal anesthetic risk has also declined owing to the increased awareness of the safety benefits of regional over general anesthesia for cesarean birth. **Maternal mortality due to anesthesia has decreased to less than 1 in 500,000 mothers.**

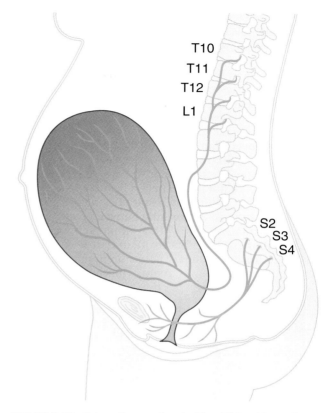

FIGURE 8-17   Pain pathways of parturition. T10 to L1 supply innervation to the uterus, L1 to S4 supply pain pathways to the vagina and deep pelvic structures, S2 to S4 supply nerve fibers to the pudendal nerve.

UTERINE BLOOD FLOW

Uterine blood flow at term accounts for 700 to 900 mL/min (about 12% of maternal cardiac output) and is not autoregulated. Regional analgesia or anesthesia may increase uterine blood flow, especially in preeclamptic patients, by relieving pain and stress and reducing circulating catecholamines. Regional analgesia or anesthesia may also decrease uterine blood flow if hypotension occurs and is not properly and promptly treated. Adequate hydration (e.g., 1000 mL of lactated Ringer's), 30 to 60 minutes before regional anesthesia, helps improve uterine blood flow and mitigates the risk for hypotension. If hypotension does occur (>15% below baseline, or <100 mm Hg systolic blood pressure), a vasopressor (e.g., ephedrine, 10 mg given intravenously) will typically restore maternal blood pressure and uterine blood flow.

PAIN PATHWAYS

The pain pathways of parturition are shown in Figure 8-17.

ADVERSE EFFECTS OF LABOR PAIN

Maternal hyperventilation during contractions causes respiratory alkalosis that results in (1) a shift of the oxyhemoglobin dissociation curve to the left, (2) increased affinity of maternal hemoglobin for oxygen, and (3) decreased oxygen offloading to the fetus. The cyclical nature of contraction pain may cause a hyperventilation-hypoventilation syndrome whereby the mother blows off so much carbon dioxide during a contraction that she **hypoventilates between contractions** and may even become mildly hypoxemic between contractions. This syndrome is exacerbated by systemic narcotics because they do not adequately relieve the pain of the contraction but add to the respiratory depression between contractions. **Hypoxemia between contractions** may be attenuated by providing supplemental oxygen. Finally, **labor pain results in increased levels of circulating catecholamines**. The α-adrenergic effects of the catecholamines may reduce uterine blood flow, whereas the β_2-adrenergic effects may impair uterine contractility.

OPTIONS FOR LABOR PAIN RELIEF

Nonpharmacologic methods include education and psychoprophylaxis (Lamaze method), emotional support, back massage, hydrotherapy, biofeedback, transcutaneous electrical nerve stimulation (TENS), acupuncture, and hypnosis (hypnobirthing). Scientific assessment of these methods has yielded inconsistent results. **Acupuncture decreases pain in most studies**. These techniques tend to work best early in the first stage of labor when the pain is least intense and may decrease pharmacologic use at that time.

Pharmacologic treatment options include parenteral narcotics, regional analgesia (epidural, spinal, combined spinal-epidural, paracervical, caudal, and pudendal nerve blocks), and inhalational analgesia.

Parenteral narcotics have very limited efficacy for the relief of labor pain. They work best in the early first stage when the pain is primarily visceral and less intense. **All opioids readily cross the placental barrier** and may cause neonatal respiratory depression depending on the dose and timing relative to delivery. They may also cause decreased fetal heart rate variability (not necessarily due to fetal acidosis) and impair neonatal breastfeeding. **Fentanyl** and **nalbuphine** have the shortest neonatal half-lives of the commonly used parenteral narcotics.

Neuraxial analgesia (medication injected into the spinal column) is undoubtedly the most effective form of labor pain relief. **Lumbar epidural analgesia is the most common form of neuraxial analgesia used to treat labor pain,** and its use has been steadily increasing to 60% nationally. It may be used to provide pain relief for the first and second stages of labor, and, by

BOX 8-1 *Contraindications to Regional Anesthesia*

Absolute Contraindications
- Patient refusal
- Coagulopathy
- Infection at needle insertion site
- Severe hypovolemia with ongoing blood loss

Relative Contraindications (Selected)
- Prior back surgery (including Harrington rod placement)
- Certain cardiac lesions, especially aortic stenosis
- Increased intracranial pressure

injecting a higher concentration of local anesthetic, the block may be intensified and extended to provide surgical anesthesia for cesarean delivery or postpartum tubal ligation. There is no fixed cervical dilation at which it is appropriate to provide epidural analgesia as long as the patient is having regular, painful contractions. Modern epidural management includes an initial bolus of local anesthetic (bupivacaine, ropivacaine, or lidocaine) and narcotic (fentanyl or sufentanil) to achieve a T10 sensory level, followed by an infusion of a dilute solution of the same agents until delivery. Pain during the first stage of labor is conducted along the sympathetic fibers, entering the spinal cord between T10 and L2. Dilute solutions can be used that permit ambulation, or the "walking epidural." **The goal is to avoid motor block** to minimize any adverse effects on maternal expulsive efforts in the second stage.

A **pudendal nerve block** anesthetizes somatic afferent nerve fibers entering the spinal cord at sacral segments S2 to S4. It **is usually effective at relieving the perineal pain of the second stage of labor**, along with the pain of episiotomy and episiotomy repair. It does not affect the ongoing pain of uterine contractions.

ANESTHESIA FOR CESAREAN DELIVERY

The type of anesthesia selected for cesarean delivery is determined by the urgency of the surgery, the presence or absence of a preexisting epidural catheter for labor, and the patient's medical condition, pregnancy-related complications, and presence of any contraindications to regional anesthesia. Absolute and relative contraindications to regional anesthesia are listed in Box 8-1. All patients requiring anesthesia for surgery must have an airway examination regardless of how urgent the surgery is. A brief history must also be elicited. **If the history or the physical examination suggests that the intubation will be difficult** (Box 8-2), **the patient must have a regional anesthetic or an awake intubation, or the operation must be started under local anesthesia.**

All patients are premedicated with a nonparticulate antacid. Routine monitors are placed, including noninvasive blood pressure monitors, electrocardiograph, and pulse oximeter, and adequate left uterine

BOX 8-2   *Factors Suggesting Difficult Intubation*

- Obesity, short neck
- Neck flexion-extension limitations at atlanto-occipital joint
- Short chin-hyoid distance (receding chin)
- Limited mouth opening
- Poor dentition, buck teeth
- Excess oropharyngeal tissues (want to see uvula and tonsillar pillars)
- Large tongue

TABLE 8-7

CAUSES OF ANESTHETIC-RELATED MATERNAL DEATHS IN THE UNITED STATES, 1979-1990

Causes	Anesthesia Deaths (%)
Airway problems	
Aspiration	23
Induction, intubation problems	12
Inadequate ventilation	12
Respiratory failure	2
Local anesthetic toxicity	13
High spinal, epidural	9
Cardiac arrest	23
Overdosage	1
Anaphylaxis	1

TABLE 8-8

COMPARISON OF SPINAL AND EPIDURAL ANESTHESIA

Spinal	Epidural
ADVANTAGES	
Faster	Can tailor duration to need
Technically easier	Lower chance of postdural puncture headache
More reliable	Slower onset
Defined end point	Beneficial in patients with cardiac and hypertensive disorders
Minimal chance of patchy block	Faster offset
Denser block	Discharge to room sooner
Lower drug exposure for mother and fetus	
No chance of systemic toxicity	
DISADVANTAGES	
Defined (limited) duration	Slower onset
Higher chance of postdural puncture headache (limited by use of small-bore, pencil-point needles)	Higher risk for systemic toxicity due to accidental intravenous injection
	Risk for high spinal due to inadvertent intrathecal or subdural injection
	Risk for "patchy block" due to inadequate or asymmetrical dermatomal spread

displacement must be instituted. Supplemental oxygen is provided. A crystalloid preload (bolus over 30 to 60 minutes) of 10 to 15 mL/kg is given before regional anesthesia.

For elective or urgent cesarean delivery (nonemergency), regional anesthesia is preferred because the airway is maintained. Complications involving loss of the airway are the leading causes of anesthetic-related maternal mortality and are usually associated with general anesthesia. General anesthesia carries a 16-fold higher risk of anesthesia-related maternal mortality compared with regional anesthesia (Table 8-7). Parturients have a higher risk for airway complications than nonpregnant patients because they have (1) an 8 times higher chance of failed intubation, (2) a 60% increased oxygen consumption, (3) a decreased functional residual capacity (FRC) resulting in a lower oxygen store, and (4) an increased risk for aspiration.

If no epidural is in place, a spinal block is frequently used. A comparison of the characteristics of spinal and epidural anesthesia is shown in Table 8-8.

General anesthesia is employed for cesarean delivery in three situations: (1) there is extreme urgency without a preexisting, functional epidural catheter; (2) there is a contraindication to regional anesthesia; or (3) regional anesthesia has failed. When a relative contraindication to regional anesthesia is present, the benefits of regional anesthesia frequently outweigh the risks in the pregnant patient.

The protocol for general anesthesia for cesarean birth includes **oral administration of nonparticulate antacid** (sodium citrate), routine monitoring and **left uterine displacement**, **preoxygenation** for at least four vital capacity breaths, and **rapid sequence induction of anesthesia with cricoid pressure** followed by **intubation to prevent regurgitation and pulmonary aspiration of gastric contents.** Once the correct position of the endotracheal tube has been confirmed by end-tidal CO_2 and auscultation of the lungs, surgery may begin.

Induction agents for general anesthesia include **propofol** (most commonly), **thiopental, etomidate** (when cardiovascular stability is particularly desired), and **ketamine** (for hypovolemic or asthmatic patients). The muscle relaxant used to facilitate intubation is **succinylcholine** (unless contraindicated), owing to its rapid onset and brief duration of action. If contraindicated, vecuronium or rocuronium may be used. **Oxygen delivery is maintained at 50% to 100% until delivery if the baby is stressed.** Nitrous oxide may be added. After induction, a potent inhalational agent is administered and at a modest level (0.5 minimum alveolar concentration [MAC]) to minimize myometrial relaxation. **Narcotics may be administered after the delivery of the baby** to reduce the need for inhalational anesthesia and provide postoperative pain relief. **The patient must be extubated only when fully awake to minimize the risk for aspiration.**

PATIENTS WHO BENEFIT FROM EARLY ANESTHETIC CONSULTATION

General anesthesia can usually be avoided if an epidural catheter is already in place, so it is helpful to identify those patients who are at increased risk for requiring surgery, and those patients who have a normal chance of needing surgery but would pose an especially high anesthetic risk. Patients who are at increased risk for emergency surgery may be advised to get a preemptive epidural catheter early to avoid the risks of a crash cesarean under general anesthesia (e.g., breech presentation, multiple gestation, prematurity, macrosomia, poor fetal heart rate tracing, severe preeclampsia, morbid obesity). These fetuses may also benefit from the improved uterine blood flow and controlled delivery that epidural analgesia allows.

Mothers who are at particularly high anesthetic risk should receive a prelabor consultation for significant preexisting medical conditions (e.g., difficult airway; see Box 8-2); significant respiratory, cardiac, or neurologic disease; spinal surgery; and suspected or known susceptibility to malignant hyperthermia.

Unintended Consequences of Regional Anesthesia or Analgesia

Patients who receive epidural analgesia for labor pain have a similar duration of the first stage of labor, but the second stage may be prolonged by 15 minutes on average. Theoretically, a prolongation of the second stage could arise from effects of the release of endogenous oxytocin, prostaglandin F_{2a}, and other hormones responsible for the propagation of labor. Prolongation of the second stage could also be due to **impaired ability to push** (unlikely as long as motor block is avoided by appropriate adjustment of the epidural infusion), or **decreased maternal urge to push** due to sensory blockade. The latter can usually be overcome by appropriate coaching and decreasing or halting the epidural infusion.

Other side effects and complications of regional anesthesia or analgesia include fever (0.5°C increased body temperature), headache, and backache. The association with maternal fever may be due to (1) an alteration in the thermoregulatory threshold, (2) interference with peripheral thermoreceptor input to the central nervous system, (3) shifting heat calories from the core to the periphery by vasodilation, or (4) an imbalance between maternal heat production and loss (decreased hyperventilation, decreased lower body sweating, increased shivering).

The risk for headache is about 1% to 2% with spinal anesthesia, and it is lower with an epidural (less than 1%). It occurs when there is an unintended dural puncture ("wet tap"). **Postdural puncture headaches are self-limited, usually resolving within 5 to 7 days.** Cerebrospinal fluid leaks through the hole in the dura, resulting in low intracranial pressure. **The hallmark is a severe *positional* headache**—little or no headache supine, sudden onset of severe headache when sitting upright or standing. The dural hole will heal in about 1 week or can be sealed with an epidural blood patch. Symptomatic treatment includes narcotics, nonsteroidal antiinflammatory drugs, caffeine, sumatriptan, and abdominal binder.

There appears to be no association between new-onset, long-term back pain and labor epidural analgesia. The risk for new, chronic back pain in parturients is high (up to 47%) whether or not they have had an epidural.

◼ Resuscitation of the Newborn

Improved surveillance using antenatal and intrapartum fetal heart rate monitoring, real-time ultrasonography, amniocentesis, and umbilical artery Doppler assessments has allowed the clinician to recognize the fetus at risk who may need special care at birth. The goals of an organized approach to neonatal resuscitation are to reverse any intrauterine hypoxia and to prevent postnatal asphyxia, which may result in acute major organ damage and lifelong handicaps.

◼ Preparation for Extrauterine Life

Prematurity is the leading cause of poor neonatal outcome because the fetus has not yet progressed through complete stages of anatomic development and biochemical maturation. Even the fetus delivered at term undergoes changes before and with the onset of labor.

During pregnancy, fetal thyroxine (T_4) is converted to reverse triiodothyronine (rT_3), which is metabolically inactive. **Several days before the onset of term labor, cortisol levels increase in the fetus and induce a change in thyroid hormone dynamics. Cortisol induces the enzyme system, allowing the conversion of T_4 to triiodothyronine (T_3), which is metabolically more active and necessary for neonatal thermogenesis.** At birth, there is a surge of thyroid-stimulating hormone (TSH), and at no time during life does this hormone reach such high levels as it does 30 minutes after birth. This is followed by a hyperthyroid neonatal state for several days, which is necessary for the newborn to maintain its body temperature.

A second change that occurs with the onset of labor is a change in fetal breathing activity. Fetal breathing, as observed by real-time ultrasonography, is rarely observed once labor is established. This is thought to be associated with a decrease in pulmonary fluid dynamics that may be important for the onset of respiration after delivery and the retention of surfactant in the lungs.

Finally, labor is a stress to the fetus that stimulates the release of catecholamines. This may be responsible for the mobilization of glucose, lung fluid absorption, alterations in the perfusion of organ systems, and, possibly, the onset of respiration. Only at times of severe stress later in life are catecholamine levels as high as those at birth.

ETIOLOGY OF NEONATAL CARDIORESPIRATORY DEPRESSION

At term, 1% of infants require vigorous resuscitation (positive pressure ventilation for more than 1 minute). At earlier stages of gestation, almost all infants require some type of supportive care.

FACILITATING NEONATAL ADAPTATION

The physician performing the delivery should delegate the responsibility for neonatal resuscitation. All nurses working in the delivery room should be trained in techniques of neonatal assessment and resuscitation. If risk factors increase the likelihood of delivering a depressed infant, a pediatrician trained in neonatal resuscitation should be summoned.

Following delivery of a normal newborn, the following important steps should occur:

1. Clear the Airway

Descent through the birth canal causes compression of the chest wall, resulting in the discharge of fluid from the mouth and nose. When the head emerges from the vagina, the physician should use a towel to remove secretions from the face. In addition, a bulb suction may be used to aspirate secretions from the oropharynx. **Initially, the bulb suction should not be used to suction the nose because nasal stimulation may initiate a gasp and cause bradycardia from a vagal reflex.** If a moderate amount of meconium is present, placing a nasal tracheal catheter into the oropharynx and applying suction before delivering the body is thought to decrease the risk for meconium aspiration. **If meconium is present and the baby is not vigorous (>100 heart rate, strong respiratory effort, and good muscle tone), intubation should be performed to suction the trachea after suction of the mouth.**

2. Dry the Newborn

An important part of neonatal adaptation is the initiation of nonshivering thermogenesis. Excessive cooling from exposure of the wet skin is detrimental to all preterm infants and to depressed full-term infants. The newborn should be placed in a preheated environment, and the physician should dry off the infant with a towel

before cutting the cord. This also serves to stimulate the onset of respiration.

3. Clamp the Cord

The umbilical arteries usually close spontaneously within 45 to 60 seconds of birth, whereas the umbilical vein remains patent for 3 to 5 minutes or longer. Delayed cord clamping significantly increases the neonatal blood volume, which increases the likelihood of neonatal jaundice and tachypnea. **The ideal time for clamping the cord is 20 to 30 seconds after birth.**

4. Ensure Onset of Respiration

The onset of respiration is normally within a few seconds of birth. If respiration has not commenced at 30 seconds of life or the heart rate is less than 100, positive pressure ventilation with oxygen should be started. If resuscitation is started with less than 100% oxygen and there is no improvement within 90 seconds of birth, oxygen should be increased to 100%.

5. Correct Surfactant Deficiency

For the premature infant, surfactant deficiency is the basic defect responsible for the development of the respiratory distress syndrome. Exogenous surfactant replacement varies from synthetic surfactant to modified or unmodified extracts of natural surfactant. These substances can be given by tracheal injection at birth to prevent the respiratory distress syndrome, or they can be given after the syndrome has developed to reduce its severity and prevent mortality.

◼ Apgar Score

The Apgar score is an excellent tool for assessing the overall status of the newborn soon after birth (1 minute) and after a 5-minute period of observation (Table 8-9). A normal Apgar score is 7 or greater at 1 minute and 9 or 10 at 5 minutes.

◼ Resuscitation of the Asphyxiated Infant

During the past 15 years, increasing emphasis has been placed on transferring the mother with a high-risk pregnancy to a tertiary care regional center before labor, rather than transferring the sick neonate after delivery.

Ideally, at the time of delivery, **a segment of cord should be doubly clamped to allow blood gas determinations** on cord arterial and venous blood. These serve as a baseline to assess the severity of the neonatal hypoxia and acidosis.

A stepwise sequence of procedures is necessary to enable a smooth transition to a normal metabolic state (Figure 8-18).

TABLE 8-9

APGAR SCORE FOR DETERMINING CONDITION OF A NEWBORN INFANT

Sign	Score		
	0	1	2
1. Heart rate	Absent	<100 beats/min	>100 beats/min
2. Respiratory effort	Absent	Slow, weak cry	Good, strong cry
3. Muscle tone	Limp	Some flexion of extremities	Active motion
4. Reflex irritability (response to stimulation of sole of foot)	None	Grimace	Strong cry
5. Color	Pale, blue	Body, pink; extremities, blue	Completely pink

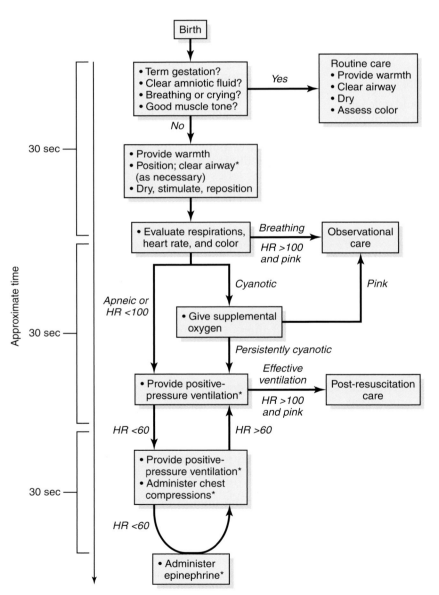

FIGURE 8-18 A time-based approach to the possible resuscitation of a normal and apneic or cyanotic newborn. (*Used with permission of the American Academy of Pediatrics: Summary of Major Changes to the 2005 AAP/AHA Emergency Cardiovascular Care Guidelines for Neonatal Resuscitation: Translating Evidence-Based Guidelines to the NRP. Vol 15, No. 2, Fall/Winter 2005.*)

*Endotracheal intubation may be considered at several steps.

1. ESTABLISH AN AIRWAY

In any infant with a high likelihood of asphyxia, suctioning of the airway should be initiated **after the delivery of the head**. The asphyxiated neonate usually has meconium present in the upper airway, which may be cleared with an oral suction catheter (De Lee trap) before delivery of the shoulders. **Immediately following the delivery, an endotracheal tube should be inserted** to remove thick mucus or meconium from the trachea and upper airway, unless the infant is vigorous (see earlier).

2. INITIATE BREATHING

With an established airway, either bag-mask ventilation or ventilation through an endotracheal tube should be initiated to deliver 100% oxygen to the lungs at a rate of 40 to 60 breaths/minute. Usually, the heart rate increases rapidly after the apnea is corrected, and intermittent bag-mask ventilation with supplemental oxygen can be given until spontaneous respiration commences. In premature infants (<32 weeks), oxygen 100% or less should be commenced and titrated to an oxygen saturation in the infant of 90% to 95%.

3. ENSURE CARDIAC PERFORMANCE

If cardiac performance is poor (heart rate less than 60 beats/minute after 30 seconds of positive pressure ventilation with 100% oxygen), external cardiac massage should be initiated. **The best technique for cardiac massage in the newborn is to compress the lower third of the sternum with two fingers.** A compression should occur every half second, with an interposed ventilation after every third compression (3:1 ratio), resulting in 90 chest compressions and 30 ventilations per minute. The middle and index finger are usually used. The sternum should be depressed to a depth of about one third the anterior-posterior diameter of the chest, typically 2 to 2.5 cm in a full-term infant and 1.5 to 2.0 cm in a preterm neonate. Cardiac arrest is rare. **If cardiac massage and artificial ventilation are not successful in reestablishing cardiac function, an endotracheal or intravenous injection of a dilute solution of epinephrine must be given.** When the heart rate is above 60 beats/minute, sternal compression may be discontinued while ventilation is continued.

4. CORRECT BIOCHEMICAL ABNORMALITIES
Acidosis

In the case of a very sick newborn, an umbilical arterial catheter is placed and blood gas analyses are obtained to monitor the severity of the acidosis and the effectiveness of the resuscitation. Severe acidosis can be corrected by the infusion of sodium bicarbonate if ventilation is adequate.

Anemia

On rare occasions, the newborn may have abnormal perfusion secondary to blood loss (e.g., from vasa previa, abruptio placentae, or a fetomaternal transfusion), which can be corrected only by immediate transfusion with blood (packed red blood cells). A solution of normal saline or lactated Ringer's can be used to temporarily maintain an adequate vascular volume.

Narcotic Depression

Respiratory depression secondary to medication is unusual with the increased use of conduction anesthesia. If neonatal respiratory depression from excessive use of narcotics is suspected, naloxone (Narcan) is an effective antidote. It is just as effective and more easily administered intramuscularly than intravenously. Table 8-10 lists the drugs that are commonly used in resuscitation and their dosages.

Hypoglycemia

Hypoglycemia can also contribute to unsuccessful resuscitation, especially in infants with intrauterine growth retardation or those with diabetic mothers. Glucose administration should be considered after the other issues have been addressed. **The use of high concentrations of glucose (e.g., 25% to 50%) is contraindicated in asphyxiated newborns because the glucose is converted to lactic acid in the absence of oxygen, which may increase the likelihood of brain damage. Concentrated glucose solutions may also cause brain swelling. If glucose is required, its concentration should not exceed 10%.**

Evaluate Other Factors

Following a systematic resuscitative effort, other contributing factors must be identified if cardiorespiratory depression persists. **Hypothermia** is one of the most critical aggravating factors, and temperature control must be continuously supported. A **pneumothorax** is not uncommon following a difficult resuscitation. It must be recognized promptly and decompressed with a chest tube. Also, a **diaphragmatic hernia** can result in the displacement of the stomach, bowel, or both into the thoracic cavity. Decreased breath sounds and failure to improve pulmonary function should alert the team to this possibility.

Neonatal Respiratory Failure

Neonates in imminent danger of death from a narrow range of conditions causing hypoxemia and respiratory distress not responsive to conventional forms of therapy are candidates for **extracorporeal membrane oxygenation** (ECMO). Infants with a congenital diaphragmatic hernia, severe meconium aspiration, or other forms of persistent pulmonary hypertension have been saved

TABLE 8-10

DRUGS USED TO RESUSCITATE THE NEONATE

Medication	Concentration to Administer	Preparation	Dosage, Route	Rate, Precautions

Epinephrine	1:10,000	1 mL	0.01-0.03 mg/kg
			0.1-0.3 mL/kg
			    IV or ET
				Give rapidly
				May dilute with normal
				    saline to 1-2 mL if
				    giving ET
				May give up to 3 times
				    IV dose if via ET

Volume expanders	PRBC Normal saline Ringer's lactate	40 mL	10 mL/kg IV	Give over 5-10 min Give by syringe or IV drip

Sodium bicarbonate	0.5 mEq/mL (4.2% solution)	20 mL or two 10-mL prefilled syringes	2 mEq/kg IV only
			    (4 mL/kg)
				Give slowly, over at least
				    2 min
				Give only if infant is being
				    effectively ventilated

Naloxone hydrochloride	0.4 mg/mL	1 mL	0.1 mg/kg (0.25 mL/kg) IV, ET, IM, SC 0.1 mg/kg (0.1 mL/kg) IV, ET, IM, SC	Give rapidly Acceptable

ET, endotracheal; IM, intramuscular; IV, intravenous; SC, subcutaneous.

using this procedure performed in selected regional centers. Data concerning long-term outcome of infants treated with extracorporeal membrane oxygenation remain limited. **Carotid artery with or without jugular vein ligation, prolonged anticoagulation, and long-term circulatory bypass are necessary with this procedure, and concerns exist about their long-term consequences.**

LONG-TERM OUTCOME

Low birth weight (<2500 g), whether the result of prematurity or intrauterine growth restriction, is an independent risk factor for cerebral palsy. By contrast, for infants weighing more than 2500 g, Apgar scores less than or equal to 3 at 5 minutes are generally not associated with an increased risk for cerebral palsy, provided there is no associated obstetric complication. If both a low Apgar score and an obstetric complication such as severe fetal distress or chorioamnionitis are present, there is an increased risk for cerebral palsy.

SUGGESTED READING

American College of Obstetricians and Gynecologists: ACOG Practice Bulletin No. 36: Obstetric anesthesia and analgesia. Obstet Gynecol 100:177-191, 2002.

American Society of Anesthesiologists: Practical guidelines for obstetrical anesthesia. Amended October 18, 2006. Available at: http:www.asahq.org/publicationsandservices/Obguide.pdf.

Hawkins JL, Kooin LM, Palmer SK, Gibbs CP: Anesthesia-related deaths during obstetric delivery in the United States 1979-1990. Anesthesiology 86:277-284, 1997.

Jönsson ER, Elfaghi I, Rydhström H, Herbst A: Modified Ritgen's maneuver for anal sphincter injury at delivery: A randomized controlled trial. Obstet Gynecol 112:212-217, 2008.

2005 AAP/AHA Guidelines for Neonatal Resuscitation. Available at: http://www.C2005.org.

Chapter 9

Fetal Surveillance during Labor

RICHARD A. BASHORE • BRIAN J. KOOS

Fetal surveillance during labor is an essential element of good obstetric care. **On the basis of antepartum maternal history, physical examination, and laboratory data, 20% to 30% of pregnancies may be designated high risk, and 50% of perinatal morbidity and mortality occurs in this group.** However, the remaining 50% occurs in pregnancies that are considered to be normal at the onset of labor.

▨ Methods of Monitoring Fetal Heart Rate

AUSCULTATION OF FETAL HEART RATE

The time-honored technique of evaluating the fetus during labor has been auscultation of the fetal heart. Optimally, auscultation of the fetal heart is performed every 15 minutes after a uterine contraction during the first stage of labor, and at least every 5 minutes in the second stage of labor. **Some studies have suggested that intermittent auscultation of the fetal heart is comparable to continuous electronic monitoring in terms of neonatal outcome,** if performed at the intervals stated above with a 1:1 patient-to-nurse ratio.

CONTINUOUS ELECTRONIC FETAL MONITORING

Electronic fetal monitoring (EFM) during labor was developed to detect fetal heart rate (FHR) patterns that were frequently associated with delivery of infants in a depressed condition. It was reasoned that early recognition of changes in heart rate patterns that may be associated with such fetal conditions as hypoxia and umbilical cord compression would serve as a warning to enable the physician to intervene and prevent fetal death in utero or irreversible brain injury.

EFM allows continuous reporting of the FHR and uterine contractions (FHR-UC) by means of a monitor that prints results on a two-channel strip chart recorder. **Uterine contractions result in a reduction in blood flow to the placenta, which can cause decreased fetal oxygenation and corresponding alterations in the FHR. The FHR-UC record can be obtained using external transducers** that are placed on the maternal abdomen. This technique is used in early labor. **Internal monitoring** is carried out by placing a spiral electrode onto the fetal scalp to monitor heart rate and placing a plastic catheter transcervically into the amniotic cavity to monitor uterine contractions (Figure 9-1). To carry out this technique, the fetal membranes must be ruptured, and the cervix must be dilated to at least 2 cm.

Internal monitoring gives better FHR tracings because the rate is computed from the sharply defined R-wave peaks of the fetal electrocardiogram, whereas with the external technique, the rate is computed from the less precisely defined first heart sound obtained with an ultrasonic transducer. The internal uterine catheter allows precise measurement of the intensity of the contractions in millimeters of mercury, whereas the external tocotransducer measures only frequency and duration, not intensity.

In the clinical setting, internal and external techniques are often combined by using a scalp electrode for precise heart rate recording and the external tocotransducer for contractions. This approach minimizes possible side effects from invasive internal monitoring.

▨ Etiology of Hypoxia, Acidosis, and Fetal Heart Rate Changes

The developing fetus presents a paradox. Its arterial blood oxygen tension is only 25 ± 5 mm Hg compared with adult values of about 100 mm Hg. The rate of

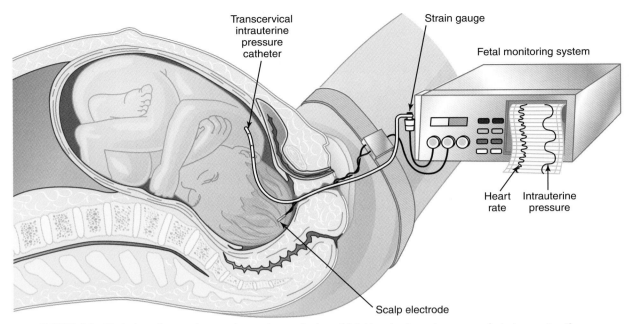

Transcervical intrauterine pressure catheter

Strain gauge

Fetal monitoring system

Heart rate Intrauterine pressure

Scalp electrode

FIGURE 9-1 Technique for continuous electronic monitoring of fetal heart rate and pressure of uterine contractions.

oxygen consumption, however, is twice that of the adult per unit weight, and its oxygen reserve is only enough to meet its metabolic needs for 1 to 2 minutes. Blood flow from the maternal circulation, which supplies the fetus with oxygen through placental exchange of respiratory gases, is momentarily interrupted during a contraction. **A normal fetus can withstand the temporary reduction in blood flow to the placenta without suffering from hypoxia because sufficient oxygen exchange occurs during the interval between contractions.**

Under normal circumstances, the FHR is determined by the atrial pacemaker. Modulation of the rate occurs physiologically through innervation of the heart by the vagus (decelerator) and sympathetic (accelerator) nerves. **A fetus whose oxygen supply is marginal cannot tolerate the stress of contractions and will become hypoxic.** Under hypoxic conditions, chemoreceptors and baroreceptors in the peripheral arterial circulation of the fetus influence the FHR by giving rise to contraction-related or periodic FHR changes. Hypoxia, when sufficiently severe, will also result in anaerobic metabolism, resulting in the accumulation of pyruvic and lactic acid and causing fetal acidosis. **The degree of fetal acidosis can be measured by sampling blood from the presenting part. The pH of fetal scalp blood normally varies between 7.25 and 7.30. Values below 7.20 are considered to be abnormal but not necessarily indicative of fetal compromise.** Clinical and experimental data indicate that fetal death occurs when 50% or more of the transplacental oxygen exchange is interrupted.

Fetal oxygenation can be impaired at different anatomic locations within the uteroplacental-fetal circulatory loop. For example, impairment of oxygen transportation to the **intervillous space** may occur as a result of maternal hypertension or anemia; oxygen diffusion may be impaired in the **placenta** because of infarction or abruption; or the oxygen content in the fetal blood may be impaired because of **hemolytic anemia** in Rh-isoimmunization. Figure 9-2 summarizes the clinical conditions that may be associated with fetal distress during labor.

FETAL HEART RATE PATTERNS

The assessment of the FHR depends on an evaluation of the baseline pattern and the periodic changes related to uterine contractions.

Baseline Assessment

This requires determination of the rate (in beats per minute) and the variability. Normal and abnormal rates are listed in Table 9-1. Baseline variability can be divided into short-term and long-term intervals. These are described as follows:

1. **Short-term or beat-to-beat variability.** This reflects the interval between either successive fetal electrocardiogram signals or mechanical events of the cardiac cycle. **Normal short-term variability fluctuates between 5 and 25 beats/minute.** Variability below 5 beats/minute is considered to be potentially abnormal. When associated with decelerations,

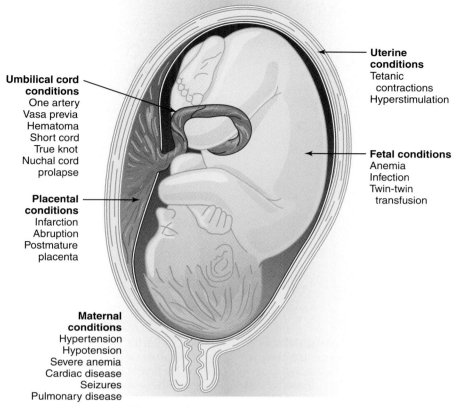

Uterine conditions
Tetanic
 contractions
Hyperstimulation

Umbilical cord conditions
One artery
Vasa previa
Hematoma
Short cord
True knot
Nuchal cord
 prolapse

Fetal conditions
Anemia
Infection
Twin-twin
 transfusion

Placental conditions
Infarction
Abruption
Postmature
 placenta

Maternal conditions
Hypertension
Hypotension
Severe anemia
Cardiac disease
Seizures
Pulmonary disease

FIGURE 9-2   Clinical conditions associated with fetal distress in labor.

a variability of less than 5 beats/minute usually indicates severe fetal distress.
2. **Long-term variability.** These fluctuations may be described in terms of the frequency and amplitude of change in the baseline rate. **The normal long-term variability is 3 to 10 cycles per minute.** Variability is physiologically decreased during the state of quiet sleep of the fetus, which usually lasts for about 25 minutes until transition occurs to another state.

Periodic Fetal Heart Rate Changes

These are changes in baseline FHR related to uterine contractions. The responses to uterine contractions may be categorized as follows:
1. **No change.** The FHR maintains the same characteristics as in the preceding baseline FHR.
2. **Acceleration.** The FHR increases in response to uterine contractions. This is a normal response.
3. **Deceleration.** The FHR decreases in response to uterine contractions. Decelerations may be *early, late, variable,* or *mixed.* All except early decelerations are abnormal.

TABLE 9-1	
BASELINE FETAL HEART RATES	
Rate	**Beats/Minute**
Normal	120-160
Abnormal	
Tachycardia	>160
Bradycardia	<120

Types of Patterns

EARLY DECELERATION (HEAD COMPRESSION). This pattern usually has an onset, maximum fall, and recovery that are coincident with the onset, peak, and end of the uterine contraction (Figure 9-3). The nadir of the FHR coincides with the peak of the contraction. This pattern is seen when engagement of the fetal head has occurred. **Early decelerations are not thought to be associated with fetal distress.** The pressure on the fetal head leads to increased intracranial pressure that elicits a vagal response similar to the Valsalva maneuver in the adult. The vagal reflex can be abolished by the administration of atropine, but this approach is not used clinically.

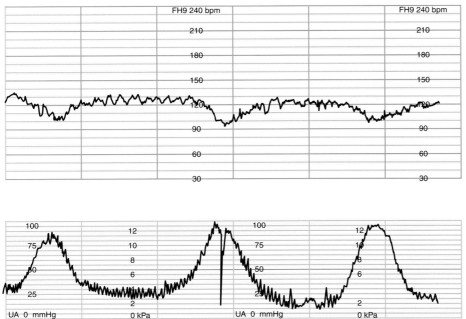

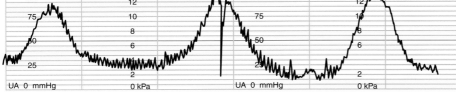

FIGURE 9-3   Early deceleration on electronic fetal monitoring tracing. Note that the deceleration starts and ends with the uterine contraction. Good beat-to-beat variability is demonstrated.

LATE DECELERATION (UTEROPLACENTAL INSUFFICIENCY). This pattern has an onset, maximal decrease, and recovery that are shifted to the right in relation to the contraction (Figure 9-4). The severity of late decelerations is graded by the magnitude of the decrease in FHR at the nadir of the deceleration (Table 9-2). Fetal hypoxia and acidosis are usually more pronounced with severe decelerations. Severe repetitive late decelerations usually indicate fetal metabolic acidosis, low arterial pH, and increased base deficit values. The partial pressure of carbon dioxide (PCO_2) in the fetal blood is usually in the normal range, and the fetal blood oxygen partial pressure (PO_2) is only slightly below normal because of the Bohr effect—the shift to the left of the oxygen dissociation curve caused by the acidosis.

VARIABLE DECELERATION (CORD COMPRESSION). This pattern has a variable time of onset and a variable form and may be nonrepetitive. Variable decelerations are caused by umbilical cord compression. Partial or complete compression of the cord causes a sudden increase in blood pressure in the central circulation of the fetus. The bradycardia is mediated by baroreceptors and is a reflex resulting in a rapid drop in heart rate and, depending upon duration, quickly returns to baseline. This reflex can be abolished or ameliorated by atropine (e.g., chemical vagotomy), although this approach is not used clinically. Fetal blood gases indicate respiratory acidosis with a low pH and high CO_2. When cord compression has been prolonged, hypoxia is also present, showing a picture of combined respiratory and metabolic acidosis in fetal blood gases.

The severity of variable decelerations is graded by their duration (see Table 9-2). When the FHR falls below 80 beats/minute during the nadir of the deceleration, there is usually a loss of the P wave in the fetal electrocardiogram, indicating a nodal rhythm or a second-degree heart block.

COMBINED OR MIXED PATTERNS. These patterns may be difficult to define and may exhibit characteristics of any of the aforementioned patterns.

DECREASED BEAT-TO-BEAT VARIABILITY. A flat baseline can be the result of several conditions: fetal acidosis, quiet sleep state, or maternal sedation with drugs.

▧ *Strategies for Intervention*

A normal FHR pattern on the electronic monitor indicates a greater than 95% probability of fetal well-being. Abnormal patterns, or nonreassuring patterns, may occur in the absence of fetal distress. The false-positive rate (i.e., good Apgar scores and normal fetal acid-base status in the presence of abnormal FHR patterns) is as high as 80%. Therefore, **electronic fetal monitoring is a screening rather than a diagnostic technique.** Failure to appreciate this limitation may lead to inappropriate intervention and contribute to a high rate of cesarean deliveries.

Strategies for intervention always depend on the clinical circumstances. When abnormal FHR patterns are seen, the first step should be a search for the

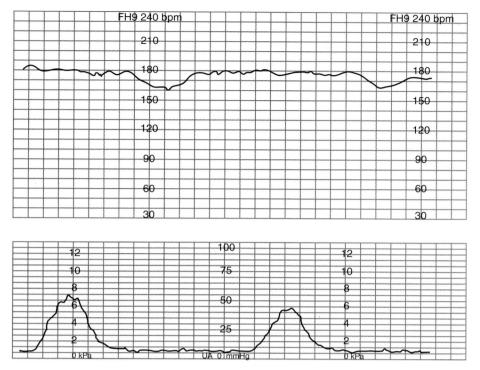

FIGURE 9-4 Late decelerations on electronic fetal monitoring tracing as would be recorded with a severely distressed fetus. Note the fetal tachycardia, decreased beat-to-beat heart rate variability, and the late decelerations (*upper panel*). Uterine contractions are recorded in the lower panel.

TABLE 9-2

PRINCIPLES OF GRADING LATE AND VARIABLE DECELERATIONS			
	Grading Criteria		
	Mild	*Moderate*	*Severe*
Late deceleration: amplitude of drop in fetal heart rate	<15 beats/ min	15-45 beats/ min	>45 beats/min
Variable deceleration: duration of deceleration	<30 sec	30-60 sec	>60 sec

Data from Kubli FW, Hon EH, Khazin AF, et al: Observations on heart rate and pH in the human fetus during labor. Am J Obstet Gynecol 104:1190, 1969.

underlying cause. When the cause is identified, such as maternal hypotension, steps should be taken to correct the problem. **In general, a term-sized fetus tolerates ominous fetal heart patterns better than a preterm fetus.** A fetus with additional risk factors, such as intrauterine infection from chorioamnionitis, may deteriorate sooner than a fetus in a normal parturient. Other considerations in the management of fetal distress include the maternal condition and the stage of labor.

VARIABLE DECELERATIONS

The most frequently encountered abnormal FHR pattern is that of variable decelerations. A change in maternal position to the right or left side generally relieves fetal pressure on the cord and abolishes the decelerations. One hundred percent **oxygen** should be given by face mask to the mother. If the pattern is persistent, placing the mother in the Trendelenburg position or elevating the presenting part by vaginal examination may be tried. If an oxytocic infusion is running, it should be discontinued. A tocolytic agent such as **terbutaline** may also be used to diminish uterine activity.

Variable decelerations of severe degree are most frequently seen during the second stage of labor, with the patient pushing during uterine contractions. **Amnioinfusion, which is the replacement of amniotic fluid with normal saline infused through a transcervical intrauterine pressure catheter, has been reported to decrease both the frequency and severity of variable decelerations.** Amnioinfusion results in reduced cesarean deliveries for fetal distress and fewer low Apgar scores at birth without apparent maternal or fetal distress. The use of a double-lumen uterine catheter is recommended because it allows a continuous infusion while simultaneously measuring uterine tone to guard against overdistention from excessive fluid accumulation.

If cervical dilation and station permit, the safest intervention for compression of the umbilical cord is assisted vaginal delivery. Cesarean delivery is indicated for severe, repetitive decelerations and an FHR tracing indicative of developing acidosis. Another circumstance that may require intervention is a prolonged deceleration. This condition occurs when the FHR falls to 60 to 90 beats/minute for more than 2 minutes.

NONREACTIVE FETAL HEART RATE TRACING

A nonreactive tracing with loss of FHR accelerations and lack of beat-to-beat variability needs further evaluation because it may be associated with fetal acidosis. By placing an artificial larynx with 120 dB of sound on the maternal abdomen in the vicinity of the vertex, **acoustic stimulation can be used to try to induce FHR accelerations.** A response of greater than 15 beats/minute lasting at least 15 seconds always ensures the absence of fetal acidosis. Conversely, the likelihood of acidosis in the fetus who fails to respond to such stimulation is about 50%.

LATE DECELERATIONS

Late decelerations of the FHR are most commonly seen in pregnancies associated with uteroplacental insufficiency. The following steps should be taken in rapid succession:

1. **Change the maternal position from supine to left or right lateral.** The supine hypotension syndrome is caused by compression of the vena cava and aorta by the heavy uterus, leading to lowering of maternal cardiac output and underperfusion of the placenta. In addition, the weight of the term uterus can compress the internal and external iliac vessels, resulting in poor perfusion of the uterus and fetal bradycardia. When this occurs, the femoral pulse cannot be palpated on the affected side. This is called the **Posiero effect.**
2. **Give oxygen by face mask.** This can increase fetal PO_2 by 5 mm Hg.
3. **Stop any oxytocic infusion** to exclude uterine hyperstimulation
4. **Inject intravenously a bolus of a tocolytic drug** (e.g., magnesium sulfate, 2.0 g, or terbutaline, 0.25 mg) to relieve uterine tetany.
5. **Monitor maternal blood pressure** to exclude hypotensive episodes that can occur as a consequence of epidural analgesia.
6. **Notify personnel that operative delivery may be necessary.**

When late decelerations persist for more than 30 minutes despite these resuscitative efforts and the FHR pattern suggests developing acidosis, operative delivery is indicated.

FETAL TACHYCARDIA

As a baseline change, tachycardia is not a very reliable sign of fetal distress. In general, fetal tachycardia occurs to improve placental circulation when the fetus is stressed. Brief periods of tachycardia (15 to 30 minutes) are usually associated with excessive oxytocic augmentation of labor, after which the heart rate returns to baseline when the augmentation is discontinued. **Prolonged periods of tachycardia are usually associated with elevated maternal temperature or an intrauterine infection,** which should be ruled out. The fetal tachycardia improves perfusion of the placenta to allow a greater exchange of excess heat to the mother's circulation (placenta acts as a radiator). The acid-base status is usually normal.

Meconium

The presence of meconium in the amniotic fluid may be a sign of fetal distress. Classification of meconium into early and late passage facilitates a clearer understanding of its importance.

Early passage occurs any time before rupture of the membranes and is classified as light or heavy, based on its color and viscosity. Light meconium is lightly stained yellow or greenish amniotic fluid. Heavy meconium is dark green or black and is usually thick and tenacious. Light passage is not associated with poor outcome. Heavy passage is associated with lower 1- and 5-minute Apgar scores and is associated with the risk for meconium aspiration.

Late passage usually occurs during the second stage of labor, after clear amniotic fluid has been noted earlier. Late passage, which is most often heavy, is usually associated with some event (e.g., umbilical cord compression or uterine hypertonus) late in labor that causes fetal distress.

A decrease in meconium-related respiratory complications in the infants of patients who receive amnioinfusion has been reported, presumably as a result of the dilutional effect of the infused fluid. A common technique is to infuse a bolus of up to 800 mL of normal saline at a rate of 10 to 15 mL/minute over a period of 50 to 80 minutes through an intrauterine catheter. This is followed by a maintenance dose of 3 mL/minute until delivery. Overdistention of the uterine cavity can be avoided by maintaining the baseline uterine tone in the normal range and at less than 20 mm Hg.

Fetal Blood Sampling

Fetal scalp blood sampling for pH determination has been used when clinical parameters, such as heavy meconium, are present or when FHR patterns are suggestive of acidosis, but is not the standard of practice in many centers. **Fetal scalp pH correctly predicts neonatal outcome in 82% of cases as determined by the Apgar score. The false-positive rate is about 8% and** the false-negative rate about 10%. Blood is obtained from the fetus by placing an amnioscope transvaginally against the fetal skull (Figure 9-5). Cervical mucus is removed with cotton swabs. Silicone grease is applied to the skull for blood bead formation. A 2 × 2-mm lancet is used for a stab incision, and a drop of blood is aspirated into a long heparinized capillary tube.

UMBILICAL CORD BLOOD SAMPLING

The Apgar scoring system has been classically used to assess the newborn condition. Over time, however, the Apgar score has come to be used inappropriately to define asphyxia, which is a misapplication, because many other conditions (e.g., prematurity, maternal drug administration) can result in low scores that are not reflective of asphyxia. **Asphyxia implies hypoxia of sufficient degree to cause metabolic acidosis. Thus, the Apgar score alone cannot be used to define asphyxia.** A more appropriate tool for defining this condition is assessment of the fetal and neonatal acid-base status. Normal ranges for these indices are given in Table 9-3. One reasonable protocol for umbilical cord blood pH and blood gas analysis is as follows:

1. Doubly clamp a segment of umbilical cord immediately after birth in all preterm deliveries and in term deliveries in which fetal distress is suspected and in cases in which the 1- or 5-minute APGAR score is low (<7).
2. If a specimen cannot be obtained from the umbilical artery, obtain a specimen from an artery on the chorionic surface of the placenta.

Ultrasonic Doppler velocimetry, for blood flow measurements in umbilical and fetal blood vessels, and **percutaneous umbilical blood sampling** (PUBS) have been used antepartum, but are generally not feasible methods for labor management.

Newborn cerebral dysfunction, manifested as seizures and attributable to true birth asphyxia, does not seem to occur unless the Apgar score at 5 minutes is 3 or less, the umbilical artery blood pH is less than 7, and resuscitation is necessary at birth. The later onset of cerebral palsy can occur without these abnormalities and may be attributed to untoward events occurring earlier in the pregnancy or intrapartum infection in which various cytokines can affect the fetal brain. The impact of lesser degrees of asphyxia, as measured by the Apgar score and acid-base status at birth, requires further study. Figure 9-6 is an algorithm for the management of abnormal heart rate tracings during fetal monitoring.

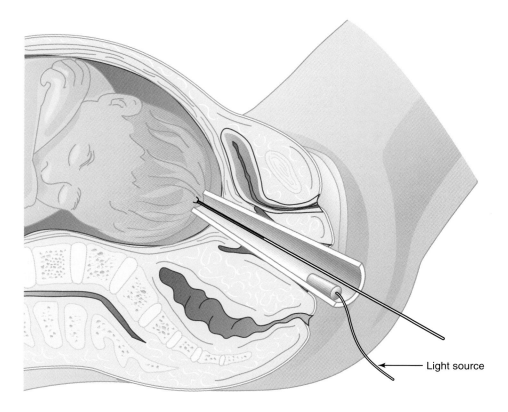

FIGURE 9-5 Technique of fetal scalp blood sampling with an amnioscope still used in many centers. After making a small stab incision in the fetal scalp, the blood is drawn off through a long capillary tube.

Light source

TABLE 9-3

NORMAL RANGES FOR FETAL SCALP AND CORD BLOOD INDICES

Blood	pH	PCO_2 (mm Hg)	PO_2 (mm Hg)	Base Deficit (mEq/L)
SCALP BLOOD				
Early labor	7.34-7.38	43-57	20-24	(−0.2)-(0.4)
Active phase	7.34-7.40	36-54	20-24	(−2.0)-(0.0)
Complete cervical dilation	7.26-7.42	36-60	20-24	(−3.3)-(−0.3)
CORD BLOOD				
Artery	7.22-7.34	32-64	14-22	(−7.8)-(−2.2)
Vein	7.29-7.41	25-53	23-35	(−6.2)-(−1.8)

Data from Hobel CJ: Intrapartum clinical assessment of fetal distress. Am J Obstet Gynecol 110:336, 1971.

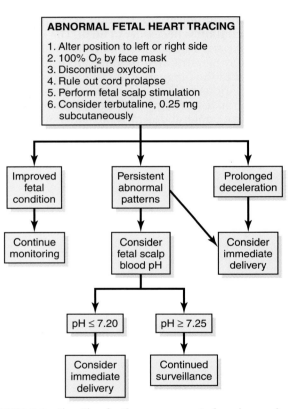

FIGURE 9-6   Algorithm for the management of an abnormal heart tracing during fetal monitoring.

▓ *Complications of Fetal Monitoring*

The introduction of a catheter into the uterine cavity and application of a scalp electrode may cause a slight increase in the incidence of maternal infection, but length of labor, rupture of the membranes, and the number of vaginal examinations are of much greater importance in this regard. **The incidence of fetal scalp abscesses and soft tissue injuries from electrode applications is less than 5%.** Scalp abscesses are managed

by opening the intradermal vesicle to allow drainage. Always consider herpes simplex virus as a cause of the lesion in patients with a history of recurrent vaginal or labial herpes. These small abscesses heal without the need for antibiotic therapy. Spread of the infection into adjacent tissues is rare.

The incidence of scalp abscesses from microblood sampling is less frequent than infection from electrode application. After fetal scalp blood sampling, a cotton swab should always be applied throughout the next uterine contraction and the puncture site inspected for hemostasis during the second contraction. If these precautions are followed, hemorrhage does not occur with scalp blood sampling.

▓ *Controversies about Fetal Monitoring in the Diagnosis and Treatment of Fetal Distress*

After more than 35 years of routine use of electronic monitoring for assessing FHR in labor, there is still no conclusive evidence of its advantage in long-term fetal outcome. **In 12 prospective, randomized, controlled trials involving more than 55,000 infants worldwide, EFM appears to have little documented benefit over intermittent auscultation with respect to perinatal mortality and long-term neurologic outcome.** The increase in the rate of cesarean deliveries in the United States and elsewhere during recent decades has not been reflected in a decrease in the incidence of cerebral palsy.

The prevalence of intrapartum fetal asphyxia is of the order of 2%. Most of these children have no evidence of brain damage.

When the decision has been made to monitor the FHR, the particular method used can be left to the woman and her obstetrician. Both intermittent and continuous monitoring of the heart rate are regarded as acceptable by the American College of Obstetricians and Gynecologists. Either method will have a similar outcome in terms of the overall incidence of long-term neurologic damage, including **cerebral palsy. Intrapartum events appear to play only a small part in the overall incidence of this disorder**. Newer methods must be introduced to determine the actual prenatal event, or unrecognized intrapartum event (e.g., chorioamnionitis), that leads to cerebral palsy.

Despite the "intensive obstetrics" of the past 30 years, with increasing attention directed to prenatal care, reduction of birth trauma, and greater use of cesarean birth for high-risk deliveries, the frequency of cerebral palsy has remained unchanged at about 2 cases per 1000 term infants. There is a pressing need to inform the public, as well as the medical profession, that cerebral palsy is probably not caused by events during labor, and that the cause in most cases remains unknown.

The current technical approaches to fetal assessment are likely to remain. There are many common conditions in obstetrics in which evaluation of uterine contractility is of primary interest to the physician, with FHR being of secondary significance. Among the indications for contraction measurements are arrest disorders of labor. In patients who undergo induction of labor for maternal or fetal reasons, the contraction response to oxytocic stimulation can be quantified in Montevideo units, which many physicians prefer to palpation of the uterus.

Until new concepts for monitoring are validated, the type of fetal monitoring needs to take into consideration the wishes of the informed patient, the capabilities of the nursing service to carry out monitoring, and the requirements of the physician managing the labor.

SUGGESTED READING

American College of Obstetricians and Gynecologists: ACOG Practice Bulletin. Intrapartum Fetal Heart Rate Monitoring. Obstet Gynecol 106:1453-1461, 2005.

Liston R, Sawchuck D, Young D: Society of Obstetricians and Gynecologists of Canada: British Columbia Perinatal Health Program. Fetal health surveillance guideline: Antenatal and intrapartum consensus. [Erratum in: J Obstet Gynaecol Can 29:909, 2007.] J Obstet Gynaecol Can 29:S3–S56, 2007.

Olagundoye V, Black R, Mackenzie IZ: Impact of the severity of fetal distress on decision-to-delivery intervals for assisted vaginal delivery. J Obstet Gynaecol 28:51-55, 2008.

Parer JT, Ideda T: A framework for standardized management of intrapartum fetal heart rate patterns. Am J Obstet Gynecol 197:26e1-26e6, 2007.

Wilson RD: Fetal health surveillance guideline: Antenatal and intrapartum consensus. J Obstet Gynaecol Can 29:912, 2007.

Chapter 10

Obstetric Hemorrhage and Puerperal Sepsis

MATTHEW KIM • ROBERT H. HAYASHI • JOSEPH C. GAMBONE

The most common causes of maternal death are hemorrhage, embolism, hypertensive disease, and infection. In this chapter, the problems of obstetric hemorrhage and infection are considered. These conditions are associated not only with potential maternal and fetal mortality but also with significant morbidity and prolonged hospitalization.

Antepartum Hemorrhage

It is critical for the well-being of both the mother and the fetus that the patient who presents with third-trimester bleeding be evaluated and managed emergently. The differential diagnosis of third-trimester bleeding is listed in Box 10-1.

INITIAL EVALUATION

If a patient is bleeding profusely, a team approach to the assessment and management should be instituted to establish hemodynamic stability. This team should include an obstetrician, an anesthesiologist, and nurses who are knowledgeable about the management of the critically ill patient. At least two large-bore peripheral intravenous lines should be placed because this allows for the most rapid replacement of fluid and blood volume. A central venous pressure line, or preferably a Swan-Ganz catheter, is helpful in the management of hypovolemic shock.

The vital signs and amount of bleeding should be checked immediately, as should the patient's mental status. Medical history should be checked for known bleeding disorders or liver disease, which predisposes to coagulopathy. **A pelvic examination should not be performed until placenta previa has been excluded by ultrasonography.** Once placenta previa has been excluded, a sterile speculum examination can be safely done to rule out genital tears or lesions (e.g., **cervical cancer**) that may be responsible for the bleeding. If none are identified, a digital examination may be performed to determine whether cervical dilation is present.

A complete blood count should be obtained and compared with previous evaluations to help assess the amount of blood loss, although acute blood loss may not be reflected in the hemoglobin level until homeostasis has been reestablished. An assessment of the patient's coagulation profile should be done by obtaining a platelet count, serum fibrinogen level, prothrombin time, and partial thromboplastin time. Additionally the patient should be typed and crossmatched for at least 4 units of blood (packed cells). A rapid but subjective method to test for coagulopathy is to partially fill a red-topped tube with blood. If a clot does not form, or once formed does not stay clotted, the patient most likely has disseminated intravascular coagulopathy (DIC).

An important and accurate method for determining the cause of third-trimester bleeding is ultrasonography. This evaluation should include not only the location and extent of the placenta but also an assessment of gestational age, an estimate of fetal weight, a determination of the fetal presentation, and a screening for fetal anomalies. Uterine activity and the fetal heart rate should be assessed with a monitored strip to rule out labor and establish fetal well-being.

Abnormal Placentation

The incidence of placenta previa, the most common type of abnormal placentation, is 0.5%. Bleeding from a placenta previa accounts for about 20% of all cases of antepartum hemorrhage. Seventy percent of patients with placenta previa present with painless vaginal bleeding in the third trimester, 20% have contractions

BOX 10-1   *Causes of Antepartum Bleeding*

Common
Placenta previa
Abruptio placentae
Preterm labor

Uncommon
Uterine rupture
Fetal (chorionic) vessel rupture
Cervical or vaginal lacerations
Cervical or vaginal lesions, including cancer
Congenital bleeding disorder
Unknown (by exclusion of the above)

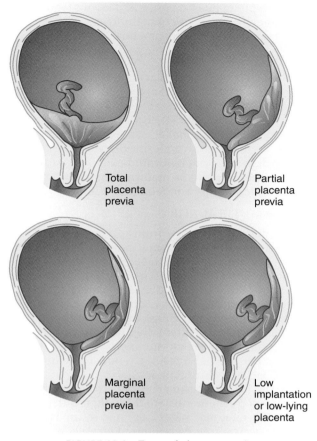

FIGURE 10-1   Types of placenta previa.

associated with bleeding, and 10% have the diagnosis made incidentally by ultrasonography or at term.

PREDISPOSING FACTORS

Factors that have been associated with a higher incidence of placenta previa include (1) **multiparity,** (2) **increasing maternal age,** (3) **prior placenta previa,** and (4) **multiple gestation.** Patients with a placenta previa have a 4% to 8% risk for having placenta previa in a subsequent pregnancy.

CLASSIFICATION

Placenta previa is classified according to the relationship of the placenta to the internal cervical os (Figure 10-1). **Complete placenta previa** implies that the placenta totally covers the cervical os. A complete placenta previa may be central, anterior, or posterior, depending on where the center of the placenta is located relative to the os. **Partial placenta previa** implies that the placenta partially covers the internal cervical os. **A marginal placenta previa** is one in which the edge of the placenta extends to the margin of the internal cervical os.

DIAGNOSIS

The classic presentation of placenta previa is painless vaginal bleeding in a previously normal pregnancy. The mean gestational age at onset of bleeding is 30 weeks, with one third presenting before 30 weeks. Placenta previa is almost exclusively diagnosed today by ultrasonography. Between 4% and 6% of patients have some degree of placenta previa on ultrasonic examination before 20 weeks' gestation. With the development of the lower uterine segment, a relative upward placental migration occurs, with 90% of these resolving by the third trimester. Complete placenta previa is the least likely to resolve, with only 10% of cases resolving by the third trimester. **When placenta previa is diagnosed in the second trimester, a repeat sonogram is indicated at 30 to 32 weeks for follow-up evaluation.**

   Transabdominal ultrasonography has an accuracy of 95% for placenta previa detection. If the placenta is implanted posteriorly and the fetal vertex is low, the lower margin of the placenta may be obscured and the diagnosis of placenta previa missed. **Transvaginal ultrasonography can accurately diagnose placenta previa in virtually all cases.**

MANAGEMENT

Once the diagnosis of placenta previa is established, management decisions depend on the gestational age of the fetus and the extent of the vaginal bleeding. **With a preterm pregnancy, the goal is to attempt to obtain fetal maturation without compromising the mother's health.** If bleeding is excessive, delivery must be accomplished by cesarean birth regardless of gestational age. When the bleeding episode is not profuse or repetitive, the patient is managed expectantly in the hospital on bed rest. With expectant management, 70% of patients will have recurrent vaginal bleeding before completion of 36 weeks' gestation and will require delivery. **If the patient reaches 36 weeks, fetal lung maturity should be determined by amniocentesis and the patient delivered by cesarean birth if the fetal lungs are mature.** Elective delivery is preferable because spontaneous labor places the mother at greater risk for hemorrhage and the fetus at risk for hypovolemia and anemia.

LOW-LYING PLACENTA

A patient with a low-lying placenta, when the placental margin is within 2 cm of the endocervical os, may present in the same way as a patient with placenta previa. It may be difficult to distinguish a low-lying placenta from a marginal placenta previa, but a transvaginal ultrasound is typically diagnostic. **Although vaginal delivery is not contraindicated, the same level of monitoring should be maintained for maternal hemodynamic stability and fetal well-being.**

MATERNAL-FETAL RISKS

The maternal mortality from placenta previa has dropped precipitously during the past 60 years from 30% to less than 1%. This has primarily been the result of the liberal use of cesarean delivery and careful expectant management. **The rare maternal death is generally associated with complications of cesarean or uncontrolled hemorrhage from the placental site. The lower uterine segment does not contract well, especially after a lower uterine incision from cesarean delivery.** DIC may also result if a massive hemorrhage or an associated abruption occurs.

The risk for antepartum or intrapartum hemorrhage, or both, is a constant threat to the patient with placenta previa. Bleeding may be exacerbated by an associated placenta accreta or uterine atony. **Placenta accreta implies an abnormal attachment of the placenta through the uterine myometrium as a result of defective decidual formation (absent Nitabuch's layer).** This abnormal attachment may be superficial (**accreta**), or the placental villi may invade partially through the myometrium (**increta**) or extend to the uterine serosa (**percreta**). **Two thirds of patients with this complication require hysterectomy.** Patients with a history of uterine surgery are at greatest risk for developing an accreta. In fact, **those with a prior cesarean delivery have a 25% risk.**

Placenta previa predisposes to preterm delivery, which poses the greatest risk to the fetus. As a result of advances in obstetric and neonatal care, the perinatal mortality rate (PMR) for premature infants has declined over the past decade. **The incidence of malpresentation with placenta previa is 30%, presumably owing to the mass effect and distortion of the lower uterine segment.**

▇ Abruptio Placentae

Abruptio placentae, or premature separation of the normally implanted placenta, complicates 0.5% to 1.5% of all pregnancies (1 in 120 births). Abruption severe enough to result in fetal death occurs in 1 per 500 deliveries.

> BOX 10-2   *Risk Factors for Abruptio Placentae*
>
> Maternal hypertension
> Placental abruption in a prior pregnancy
> Trauma
> Polyhydramnios with rapid decompression
> Premature rupture of membranes
> Short umbilical cord
> Tobacco use
> Folate deficiency

PREDISPOSING FACTORS

Factors associated with an increased incidence of abruption are noted in Box 10-2. The most common of these risk factors is **maternal hypertension**, either chronic or as a result of preeclampsia. The risk for recurrent abruption is high: 10% after one abruption and 25% after two.

PATHOPHYSIOLOGY

Placental separation is initiated by hemorrhage into the decidua basalis with formation of a decidual hematoma. The resulting separation of the decidua from the basal plate predisposes to further separation and bleeding as well as to compression and destruction of placental tissue. The inciting cause of placental separation is unknown. It may be due to an inherent weakness or anomaly in the spiral arterioles. Blood may either dissect upward toward the fundus, resulting in a **concealed hemorrhage,** or extend downward toward the cervix, resulting in an external or **revealed hemorrhage.**

DIAGNOSIS AND MANAGEMENT

Clinically, the diagnosis of a placental abruption is entertained if a patient presents with painful vaginal bleeding in association with uterine tenderness, hyperactivity, and increased tone. The signs and symptoms of placental abruption are, however, variable. The most common finding is vaginal bleeding, seen in 80% of cases. **Abdominal pain and uterine tenderness are present in 66% of cases, fetal distress in 60%, uterine hyperactivity and increased uterine tone in 34%, and fetal demise in 15%.**

The diagnosis of placental abruption is made clinically. **Ultrasonography may detect only 2% of abruptions.** Because placental abruption may coexist with a placenta previa, the reason for doing an initial ultrasonic examination is to exclude the previa.

Management of the patient with an abruption includes careful maternal hemodynamic and fetal monitoring, serial evaluation of the hematocrit and coagulation profile, and delivery. **Intensive monitoring of both the mother and the fetus is essential** because rapid deterioration of the condition of either one can occur. Blood products for replacement should always be available, and a large-bore (16- to 18-gauge) intravenous line must be secured. Red blood cells should be given liberally if indicated. **In the setting of placental abruption, the use of tocolytics or uterine relaxants is not advised**. Uterine tone must be maintained to control bleeding following delivery, or at least to control the bleeding sufficiently to allow a safe hysterectomy to be performed, if necessary.

MATERNAL-FETAL RISKS

Abruption places the fetus at significant risk for hypoxia and, ultimately, death. **The perinatal mortality rate due to placental abruption is 35%,** and the condition accounts for 15% of third-trimester stillbirths. Fifteen percent of live-born infants have significant neurologic impairment.

Placental abruption is the most common cause of DIC in pregnancy. This results from release into the maternal circulation of thromboplastin from the disrupted placenta and subplacental decidua, causing a consumptive coagulopathy. Clinically significant DIC complicates 20% of cases and is most commonly seen when the abruption is massive or fetal death has occurred. **Hypovolemic shock and acute renal failure due to massive hemorrhage may be seen with a severe abruption if hypovolemia is left uncorrected.** Sheehan's syndrome (amenorrhea as a result of maternal postpartum pituitary necrosis) may be a delayed complication resulting from coagulation within the portal system of the pituitary stalk.

■ *Uterine Rupture*

Uterine rupture implies complete separation of the uterine musculature through all of its layers, ultimately with all or a part of the fetus being extruded from the uterine cavity. The overall incidence is 0.5%.

Uterine rupture may be spontaneous, traumatic, or associated with a prior uterine scar, and it may occur during or before labor or at the time of delivery. **A prior uterine scar is associated with 40% of cases.** With a prior lower-segment transverse incision, the risk for rupture is less than 1%, whereas **the risk with a high vertical (classical) scar is 4% to 7%.** Sixty percent of uterine ruptures occur in previously unscarred uteri.

DIAGNOSIS AND MANAGEMENT

The signs and symptoms of uterine rupture are highly variable. **Typically, rupture is characterized by the sudden onset of intense abdominal pain and some vaginal bleeding.** Impending rupture may be heralded by hyperventilation, restlessness, agitation, and tachycardia. After the rupture has occurred, the patient may be free of pain momentarily and then complain of diffuse pain thereafter. The most consistent clinical finding is an abnormal fetal heart rate pattern. The patient may or may not have vaginal bleeding, and if it occurs, it can range

from spotting to severe hemorrhage. **The presenting part may be found to have retracted on pelvic examination, and fetal parts may be more easily palpated abdominally.** Abnormal contouring of the abdomen may be seen. Fetal distress develops commonly, and fetal death or long-term neurologic sequelae may occur in 10% of cases.

A high index of suspicion is required, and immediate laparotomy is essential. **In most cases, total abdominal hysterectomy is the treatment of choice,** although débridement of the rupture site and primary closure may be considered in women of low parity who desire more children.

MATERNAL-FETAL RISK

Delay in management places both mother and child at significant risk. The major risk to the mother is hemorrhage and shock. Although **the associated maternal mortality rate is now less than 1%,** if the mother is left untreated, she will almost certainly die. For the fetus, rapid intervention will minimize morbidity and mortality. **The associated fetal mortality rate is still about 30%.**

■ *Fetal Bleeding*

Rupture of a fetal umbilical vessel complicates 0.1% to 0.8% of pregnancies. The diagnosis of fetal bleeding is made by performing an Apt test. After obtaining blood from the vagina and putting it into a red-topped test tube, tap water is added. The water will lyse blood cells and release hemoglobin. Adding 1 mL of KOH results in a brown discoloration when the hemoglobin is maternal. If the blood is fetal in origin, the color of the fluid will remain red because the fetal hemoglobin will not be denatured by the KOH. **Fetal bleeding often results when the cord insertion is velamentous,** implying that the vessels of the cord insert between the amnion and chorion away from the placenta. The incidence of velamentous cord insertion varies from 1% in singleton pregnancies to 10% in twins and 50% in triplets. If the unprotected vessels pass over the cervical os, this is termed a **vasa previa.** The incidence of vasa previa is 1 in 5000 pregnancies. Velamentously inserted vessels need not pass over the os to rupture, although the risk for rupture is greatest with a vasa previa. Rupture of a fetal vessel necessitates immediate abdominal delivery. **Vasa previa alone carries a perinatal mortality rate of 50%, which increases to 75% if the membranes rupture.**

■ *Postpartum Hemorrhage*

Postpartum hemorrhage is defined as blood loss in excess of 500 mL at the time of vaginal delivery. There is normally a greater blood loss **following cesarean**

delivery; therefore, **blood loss in excess of 1000 mL** is considered a postpartum hemorrhage in these patients. The excessive blood loss usually occurs in the immediate postpartum period but can occur slowly over the first 24 hours. **Delayed postpartum hemorrhage can occasionally occur, with the excessive bleeding commencing more than 24 hours after delivery.** This is usually a result of subinvolution of the uterus and disruption of the placental site "scab" several weeks postpartum, or of the retention of placental fragments that separate several days after delivery. **Postpartum hemorrhage occurs in about 4% of deliveries.**

ETIOLOGY

Most of the blood loss occurs from the myometrial spiral arterioles and decidual veins that previously supplied and drained the intervillous spaces of the placenta. As the contractions of the partially empty uterus cause placental separation, bleeding occurs and continues until the uterine musculature contracts around the blood vessels and acts as a physiologic-anatomic ligature. Failure of the uterus to contract after placental separation (**uterine atony**) leads to excessive placental site bleeding. Other causes of postpartum hemorrhage are listed in Box 10-3.

BOX 10-3   *Causes of Postpartum Hemorrhage*

Uterine atony
Genital tract trauma
Retained placental tissue
Low placental implantation
Uterine inversion
Coagulation disorders
Abruptio placentae
Amniotic fluid embolism
Retained dead fetus
Inherited coagulopathy

BOX 10-4   *Factors Predisposing to Postpartum Uterine Atony*

Overdistention of the uterus
Multiple gestations
Polyhydramnios
Fetal macrosomia
Prolonged labor
Oxytocic augmentation of labor
Grand multiparity (a parity of five or more)
Precipitous labor (lasting <3 hr)
Magnesium sulfate treatment of preeclampsia
Chorioamnionitis
Halogenated anesthetics
Uterine leiomyomas

UTERINE ATONY

Most postpartum hemorrhages (75% to 80%) are due to uterine atony. The factors predisposing to postpartum uterine atony are listed in Box 10-4.

GENITAL TRACT TRAUMA

Trauma during delivery is the second most common cause of postpartum hemorrhage. During vaginal delivery, lacerations of the cervix and vagina may occur spontaneously, but they are more common following the use of forceps or a vacuum extractor. The vascular beds in the genital tract are engorged during pregnancy, and bleeding can be profuse. Lacerations are particularly prone to occur over the perineal body, in the periurethral area, and over the ischial spines along the posterolateral aspects of the vagina. The cervix may lacerate at the two lateral angles while rapidly dilating in the first stage of labor. Uterine rupture may occasionally occur. At the time of delivery by low transverse cesarean, an inadvertent lateral extension of the incision can damage the ascending branches of the uterine arteries; an extension inferiorly can damage the cervical branches of the uterine artery.

RETAINED PLACENTAL TISSUE

In about half of patients with delayed postpartum hemorrhage, placental fragments are present when uterine curettage is performed with a large curette. Bleeding occurs as the uterus is unable to maintain a contraction and involute normally around a retained placental tissue mass.

LOW PLACENTAL IMPLANTATION

Low implantation of the placenta can predispose to postpartum hemorrhage because the relative content of musculature in the uterine wall decreases in the lower uterine segment, which may result in insufficient control of placental site bleeding. Verifying a completely evacuated lower genital tract, a fully drained bladder and use of uterotonic agents such as pitocin, methylergonovine, or prostaglandin agents is usually sufficient. If bleeding continues, surgical management must be considered.

COAGULATION DISORDERS

Peripartum coagulation disorders are high-risk factors for postpartum hemorrhage but fortunately are quite rare.

Patients with **thrombotic thrombocytopenia** have a rare syndrome of unknown etiology characterized by thrombocytopenic purpura, microangiopathic hemolytic anemia, transient and fluctuating neurologic signs, renal dysfunction, and a febrile course. In pregnancy, the disease is usually fatal. An **amniotic fluid embolus** is also rare and is associated with an 80% mortality rate. This syndrome is characterized by a fulminating consumption coagulopathy, intense bronchospasm, and vasomotor collapse. It is triggered by an intravascular infusion of a significant amount of amniotic fluid during a tumultuous or rapid labor in the presence of ruptured membranes. During the process of **placental abruption,** a small amount of amniotic fluid may leak into the vascular system, and the thromboplastin in the amniotic fluid may trigger a consumption coagulopathy. Patients with **idiopathic thrombocytopenic purpura** have platelets with abnormal function or a shortened life span. This causes thrombocytopenia and a tendency to bleed. Circulating antiplatelet antibodies of the IgG type may occasionally cross the placenta and result in fetal and neonatal thrombocytopenia as well. **Von Willebrand's disease** is an inherited coagulopathy characterized by a prolonged bleeding time due to factor VIII deficiency. During pregnancy, these patients are likely to have a decreased bleeding diathesis because pregnancy elevates factor VIII levels. In the postpartum period, they are susceptible to delayed bleeding as factor VIII levels fall.

UTERINE INVERSION

Uterine inversion is the "turning inside-out" of the uterus in the third stage of labor. It is quite rare, occurring in only about 1 in 20,000 pregnancies. Just after the second stage, the uterus is somewhat atonic, the cervix open, and the placenta attached. **Improper management of the third stage of labor can cause an iatrogenic uterine inversion.** If the inexperienced physician exerts fundal pressure while pulling on the umbilical cord before complete placental separation (particularly with a fundal implantation of the placenta), uterine inversion may occur. As the fundus of the uterus moves through the vagina, the inversion exerts traction on peritoneal structures, which can elicit a profound vasovagal response. The resulting vasodilation increases bleeding and the risk for hypovolemic shock. **If the placenta is completely or partially separated, the uterine atony may cause profuse bleeding, which compounds the vasovagal shock.**

Obstetric Shock

Hypotension without significant external bleeding may occasionally develop in an obstetric patient. This condition is called obstetric shock. **The causes of obstetric shock include concealed hemorrhage, uterine inversion, and amniotic fluid embolism.**

An improperly sutured episiotomy can lead to a concealed postpartum hemorrhage. If the first suture at the vaginal apex of the episiotomy incision does not incorporate the cut and retracted arterioles, they can continue to bleed, creating a hematoma that can dissect cephalad into the retroperitoneal space. This may cause shock without external evidence of blood loss. **A soft tissue hematoma, usually of the vulva, may occur** following delivery in the absence of any laceration or episiotomy and may also contribute to occult blood loss.

DIFFERENTIAL DIAGNOSIS

Identification of the cause of postpartum hemorrhage requires a systematic approach. The fundus of the uterus should be palpated through the abdominal wall to determine the presence or absence of **uterine atony.** Next, a quick but thorough inspection of the vagina and cervix should be performed to ascertain whether any **lacerations** may be compounding the bleeding problem. Any uterine inversion or **pelvic hematoma** should be excluded during the pelvic examination. If the cause of bleeding has not been identified, **manual exploration of the uterine cavity** should be performed, under general anesthesia if necessary. With fingertips together, a gloved hand is slipped through the open cervix, and the hand is inserted into the uterus. The endometrial surface is palpated carefully to identify any retained products of conception, uterine wall lacerations, or partial uterine inversion. If no cause for the bleeding is found, a **coagulopathy** must be considered.

Management of Postpartum Hemorrhage and Obstetric Shock

The first steps toward good management are the identification of patients at risk for postpartum hemorrhage and the institution of prophylactic measures during labor to minimize the possibility of maternal mortality. Patients with any predisposing factors for postpartum hemorrhage, including a history of postpartum hemorrhage, should be screened for anemia and atypical antibodies to ensure that an adequate supply of type-specific blood is available. An intravenous infusion through a large-bore needle or catheter should be started before delivery, and blood should be held in the laboratory for possible crossmatching.

During the diagnostic workup of an established hemorrhage, the patient's vital signs must be monitored closely. Multiple units of packed red blood cells must be typed and crossmatched and intravenous crystalloids (such as normal saline or lactated Ringer's solution) infused to restore intravascular volume. **Resuscitation with normal saline usually requires a volume of 3 times the estimated blood loss.**

UTERINE ATONY

If uterine atony is determined to be the cause of the postpartum hemorrhage, a rapid continuous intravenous infusion of dilute oxytocin (40 to 80 U in 1 L of normal saline) should be given to increase uterine tone. If the uterus remains atonic and the placental site bleeding continues during the oxytocic infusion, **ergonovine maleate or methylergonovine,** 0.2 mg, may be given intramuscularly. The ergot drugs are contraindicated in patients with hypertension because the pressor effect of the drug may increase blood pressure to dangerous levels.

Analogues of prostaglandin $F_{2\alpha}$ given intramuscularly are quite effective in controlling postpartum hemorrhage caused by uterine atony. The 15-methyl analogue (Hemabate) has a more potent uterotonic effect and longer duration of action than the parent compound. The expected time of onset of the uterotonic effect when the 15-methyl analogue (0.25 mg) is given intramuscularly is 20 minutes, whereas when injected into the myometrium, it may take up to 4 minutes.

Failing these pharmacologic treatments, **a bimanual compression and massage of the uterine corpus may control the bleeding and cause the uterus to contract.** Although **packing the uterine cavity is not widely practiced,** it may occasionally control postpartum hemorrhage and obviate the need for surgical intervention. Alternatively, a **large-volume balloon catheter** has been developed that performs a similar function while maintaining a channel into the uterine cavity, allowing further bleeding to be monitored.

If uterine bleeding persists in an otherwise stable patient, she can be transported to the angiocatheterization laboratory, where radiologists can **place an angiocatheter into the uterine arteries for injection of thrombogenic materials to control blood flow and hemorrhaging.**

Operative intervention is a last resort. If the patient has completed her childbearing, a **supracervical or total abdominal hysterectomy** is definitive therapy for intractable postpartum hemorrhage caused by uterine atony. When reproductive potential is important to the patient, **ligation of the uterine arteries** adjacent to the uterus will lower the pulse pressure. This procedure is more successful in controlling placental site hemorrhage and is easier to perform than bilateral hypogastric artery ligation.

GENITAL TRACT TRAUMA

When postpartum hemorrhage is related to genital tract trauma, surgical intervention is necessary. When repairing genital tract lacerations, **the first suture must be placed well above the apex of the laceration to incorporate any retracted bleeding arterioles into the ligature.** Repair of vaginal lacerations requires good light and good exposure, and the tissues should be approximated without dead space. A running lock suture technique provides the best hemostasis (Figure 10-2). **Cervical lacerations need not be sutured unless they are actively bleeding.** Large, expanding hematomas of the genital tract require surgical evacuation of clots and a search for bleeding vessels that can be ligated, then packed for hemostasis. Stable hematomas can be observed and treated conservatively. A retroperitoneal hematoma generally begins in the pelvis. If the bleeding

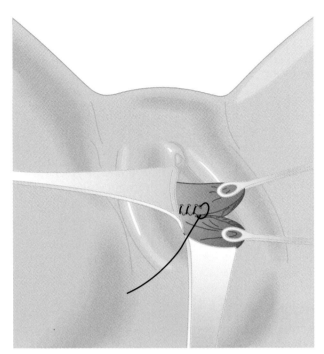

FIGURE 10-2 Suturing a cervical laceration. The first suture must be placed above the apex of the laceration.

cannot be controlled from a vaginal approach, a laparotomy and bilateral hypogastric artery ligation may be necessary.

The **intraoperative laceration of the ascending branch of the uterine artery** during delivery through a low transverse incision can be easily controlled by the placement of a large suture ligature through the myometrium and broad ligament below the level of the laceration. A **uterine rupture** usually necessitates subtotal or total abdominal hysterectomy, although small defects may be repaired.

RETAINED PRODUCTS OF CONCEPTION

When the placenta cannot be delivered in the usual manner, **manual removal** is necessary (Figure 10-3). This should be performed urgently if bleeding is profuse. Otherwise, it is reasonable to delay 30 minutes to await spontaneous separation. General anesthesia may be required. Following manual removal of the placenta or placental remnants, the uterus should be scraped with a large curette.

UTERINE INVERSION

The management of a uterine inversion requires quick thinking. The patient rapidly goes into shock, and **immediate intravascular volume expansion with intravenous crystalloids is required.** An anesthesiologist should be present. When the patient's condition

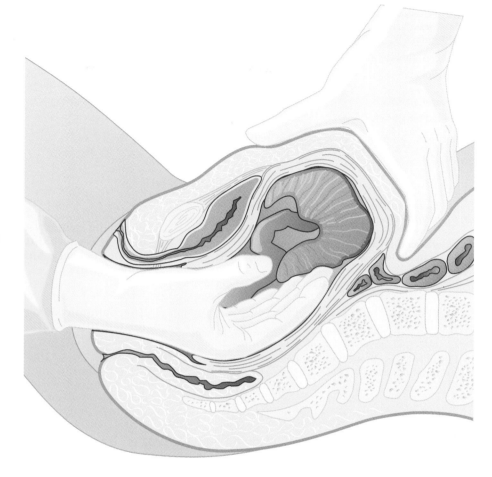

FIGURE 10-3   Manual removal of the placenta. The abdominal hand provides counterpressure on the uterine fundus against the shearing force of the fingers in the uterus.

is stable, the partially separated placenta should be completely removed and an attempt made to replace the uterus by placing a cupped hand around the fundus and elevating it in the long axis of the vagina. If this is unsuccessful, a further attempt should be made using **IV nitroglycerin** (100 μg) **or general anesthesia to relax the uterine muscle.** Once replaced, a dilute oxytocin infusion should be started to cause the uterus to contract before removing the intrauterine hand. **Rarely, the uterus cannot be replaced from below, and a surgical procedure may be required.** At laparotomy, a vertical incision should be made through the posterior portion of the cervix to incise the constriction ring and allow the fundus to be replaced into the peritoneal cavity. Suturing of the cervical incision completes this procedure.

AMNIOTIC FLUID EMBOLUS

The principal objectives of treatment for amniotic fluid embolism are to support the respiratory system, correct the shock, and replace the coagulation factors. This type of embolism requires immediate cardiopulmonary resuscitation, usually with mechanical ventilation; rapid volume expansion with an electrolyte solution; positive inotropic cardiac support; placement of a bladder catheter to monitor urine output; correction of the red cell deficit by transfusion with packed red blood cells; and reversal of the coagulopathy with the use of platelets, fibrinogen, and other blood components.

COAGULOPATHY

When postpartum hemorrhage is associated with coagulopathy, the specific defect should be corrected by the infusion of blood products, as outlined in Table 10-1 and Box 10-5. **Patients with thrombocytopenia require platelet concentrate infusions; those with von Willebrand's disease require factor VIII concentrate or cryoprecipitate.**

A packed red cell infusion is given to a patient who has bled enough to drop the circulating red cell population sufficiently to compromise the delivery of oxygen to the tissues. Therefore, institution of blood transfusion is best judged by symptoms of oxygen deprivation

TABLE 10-1

BLOOD PRODUCTS USED TO CORRECT COAGULATION DEFECTS		
Blood Product	**Volume (mL) in 1 Unit***	**Effect of Transfusion**
Platelet concentrate	30-40	Increases platelet count by about 20,000 to 25,000
Cryoprecipitate	15-25	Supplies fibrinogen, factor VIII, and factor XIII (3-10 times more concentrated than the equivalent volume of fresh plasma)
Fresh-frozen plasma	200	Supplies all factors except platelets (1 g of fibrinogen)
Packed red blood cells	200	Raises hematocrit 3%-4%

*Quantity obtained from 1 Unit (500 mL) of fresh whole blood.

BOX 10-5   *Laboratory Evaluation of Disseminated Intravascular Coagulation*

- **Platelet count** (normal range = 150-450 × 10^9/L): 1 unit of platelets will raise the platelet count by 5-10 × 10^9/L
- **Plasma fibrinogen** (normal range = 175-600 mg/dL): fresh frozen plasma (FFP): 1 unit = 1 g of fibrinogen; 4 units of FFP will raise the plasma fibrinogen by 5-10 mg/dL
- **Cryoprecipitate:** 1 bag = 0.25 g of fibrinogen; 16 bags raise the plasma fibrinogen by 5-10 mg/dL
- **Fibrin split products:** normal range = <0.05 μg/mL (D-dimer method)

rather than by some empirical hemoglobin level. No important physiologic impairment has been noted at hemoglobin levels as low as 6 to 8 g/dL (hematocrit, 18% to 24%). **In general, a 1-U transfusion of packed red blood cells will increase the hemoglobin level by 1 g/dL (and the hematocrit by 3% to 4%).**

Massive blood replacement (when total blood volume is replaced in a 24-hour period) may be associated with thrombocytopenia, prolonged prothrombin time (PT), and hypofibrinogenemia. Thrombocytopenia is the most common abnormality, so platelet transfusion following determination of a low platelet count is not an uncommon scenario. Fresh frozen plasma may be transfused for prolonged PT or hypofibrinogenemia.

■ *Puerperal Sepsis*

Puerperal sepsis still accounts for significant postpartum maternal morbidity and mortality. **Patients with a puerperal genital tract infection are susceptible to the development of septic shock, pelvic thrombophlebitis, and pelvic abscess.**

Following a vaginal delivery, about 6% to 7% of women demonstrate febrile morbidity, defined as a temperature of 100.4°F (38°C) or higher that occurs for more than 2 consecutive days (exclusive of the first postpartum day) during the first 10 postpartum days. **Following primary cesarean delivery, the incidence of febrile morbidity is about twice that following vaginal delivery. Most of these fevers are caused by endometritis.**

ETIOLOGY

The pathophysiology of puerperal sepsis is closely related to the various microbial inhabitants of the vagina and cervix. The vaginal flora during gestation resembles the nonpregnant state, although there is a trend toward isolating more *Mycoplasma genitalis* and anaerobic streptococci in the last trimester. **Potentially pathogenic organisms can be cultured from the vagina in about 80% of pregnant women. These organisms include enterococci, hemolytic and nonhemolytic streptococci, anaerobic streptococci, enteric bacilli, pseudodiphtheria bacteria, and *Neisseria* species other than *N. gonorrhoeae*.** Excessive overgrowth of these organisms during pregnancy is inhibited by the acidity of the vagina (pH 4 to 5), primarily as a result of the production of lactic acid by the lactobacilli.

The uterine cavity is normally free of bacteria during pregnancy. After parturition, the pH of the vagina changes from acidic to alkaline because of the neutralizing effect of the alkaline amniotic fluid, blood, and lochia, as well as the decreased population of lactobacilli. This change in pH favors an increased growth of aerobic organisms. About 48 hours postpartum, progressive necrosis of the endometrial and placental remnants produces a favorable intrauterine environment for the multiplication of anaerobic bacteria.

About 70% of puerperal infections are caused by anaerobic organisms. Most of these are anaerobic cocci (*Peptostreptococcus, Peptococcus,* and *Streptococcus*), although mixed infections with *Bacteroides fragilis* are encountered in up to one third of cases. **Of the aerobic organisms, *Escherichia coli* is the most common pathogen,** followed by enterococci. Puerperal infection from clostridia is rare.

Intrauterine staphylococcal infection is rare. This organism is frequently responsible for infection of perineal wounds and abdominal incisions. *Trichomonas vaginalis* and *Candida albicans* are frequent inhabitants of the vagina, but no connection with puerperal sepsis has been established. *Mycoplasma* **organisms have been shown to contribute to puerperal endometritis.**

PREDISPOSING FACTORS

Predisposing factors for the development of a puerperal genital tract infection are shown in Box 10-6.

After delivery, the placental site vessels are clotted off, and there is an exudation of lymph-like fluid along with massive numbers of neutrophils and other white cells to form the lochia. Vaginal microorganisms readily enter the uterine cavity and may become pathogenic at the placental site, depending on such variables as the size of the inoculum, the local pH, and the presence or absence of devitalized tissue. The latter may include tissue incorporated in the suture line of a cesarean incision.

The normal body defense mechanisms usually prevent any progressive infection, but a breakdown of these defenses allows the bacteria to invade the myometrium. Further invasion into the lymphatics of the parametrium can cause lymphangitis, pelvic cellulitis, and the possibility of widespread infection from septic emboli.

Endomyoparametritis is a potentially life-threatening condition. It commonly begins with retention of secundines (placental and amniochorionic membrane fragments) that block the normal lochial flow, allowing accumulation of intrauterine lochia, which in turn changes the local pH and acts as a culture medium for bacterial growth. Unless normal lochial flow is established, bacterial invasion progresses.

CLINICAL FEATURES

Puerperal infection presents with a rising fever and increasing uterine tenderness on postpartum day 2 or 3. With the development of parametritis (pelvic cellulitis),

the temperature elevation will be sustained, and signs of pelvic peritonitis may develop. Erratic temperature fluctuations and severe chills suggest bacteremia and dissemination of septic emboli, with the particular likelihood of spread to the lungs.

When the usual relative pelvic venous stasis is combined with a large inoculum of pathogenic anaerobic bacteria, a pelvic vein thrombophlebitis is likely to develop, usually on the right side of the pelvis. **The clinical picture of pelvic thrombophlebitis is characterized by a persistent spiking fever for 7 to 10 days after delivery, despite antibiotic therapy.**

DIAGNOSIS

Evaluation of a febrile postpartum patient should include a careful history and physical examination. Extrapelvic causes of fever, such as breast engorgement, mastitis, aspiration pneumonia, atelectasis, pyelonephritis, thrombophlebitis, or wound infection, should be excluded.

Although a pelvic examination is generally not helpful in diagnosing pelvic thrombophlebitis, it may allow the palpation of tender, thrombosed, and edematous ovarian, parauterine, or iliac veins. An abdominal pelvic computed tomography scan or ultrasonogram may be helpful. This diagnosis is usually made by exclusion, however, and by the prompt regression of fever following commencement of heparin anticoagulant therapy.

Before the institution of antibiotic therapy for puerperal endometritis, aerobic and anaerobic cultures should be obtained from the blood, endocervix, and uterine cavity, and a catheterized urine specimen obtained for culture.

MANAGEMENT

A febrile puerperal patient with cessation of lochial flow should undergo a pelvic examination and removal of any secundines that may be occluding the cervical os.

The antibiotic treatment of puerperal infection usually follows two major principles. **First, early antibiotic treatment should be instituted** to confine and then eliminate the infectious process. **Second, the antibiotics should provide anaerobic coverage** because these organisms are involved in 70% of puerperal infections. Antibiotics should be continued for at least 48 hours after the patient becomes afebrile. Anaerobic organisms especially require prolonged chemotherapy for elimination.

Broad-spectrum antibiotics, such as ampicillin and the cephalosporins, are effective first-line drugs for mild and moderate cases of puerperal infection. When the infection is moderate to severe, a penicillin-aminoglycoside combination has traditionally been used as first-line therapy. The major pelvic pathogen resistant to this combination is *Bacteroides* *fragilis,* which is usually sensitive to clindamycin. **The use of clindamycin with either an aminoglycoside or ampicillin will provide the best first-line coverage.**

When pelvic thrombophlebitis or thromboembolism is suspected or clinically diagnosed, unfractionated heparin therapy should be instituted to increase the clotting time (Lee-White method) or activated prothrombin time to 2 to 3 times normal. Only 2 to 3 weeks of anticoagulant therapy are needed for uncomplicated pelvic thrombophlebitis. Patients with femoral thrombophlebitis require 4 to 6 weeks of heparin therapy followed by the administration of oral anticoagulants for a few months.

If the patient does not respond to heparin therapy and the clinical course is one of unrelenting fever and pelvic tenderness, a diagnosis of **pelvic abscess** must be considered. Diagnosis is made by pelvic examination and confirmed by pelvic ultrasonography or computed tomography scan. The finding of a tender, pelvic parametrial mass suggests an abscess. Ultrasonography will confirm that the mass is fluid-filled rather than solid. **The presence of a pelvic abscess requires surgical drainage.**

SUGGESTED READING

Adesiyun AG: Septic postpartum uterine inversion. Singapore Med J 48:943-945, 2007.

American College of Obstetricians and Gynecologists: Postpartum hemorrhage: ACOG Practice Bulletin No. 76. Obstet Gynecol 108:1039-1047, 2006.

Castagnola DE, Hoffman MK, Carlson J, Flynn C: Necrotizing cervical and uterine infection in the postpartum period caused by group A streptococcus. Obstet Gynecol 111:533-535, 2008.

Dane B, Dane C: Maternal death after uterine rupture in an unscarred uterus: A case report. J Emerg Med 2008 Mar 31 (Epub ahead of print).

Maharaj D: Puerpueral pyrexia: A review. Parts 1 and 2. Obstet Gynecol Surv 62:393-406, 2007.

Papathanasiou K, Tolikas A, Dovas D, et al: Ligation of internal iliac artery for severe obstetric and pelvic hemorrhage: 10 Year experience with 11 cases is a university hospital. J Obstet Gynaecol Res 28:183-184, 2008.

Chapter 11

Uterine Contractility and Dystocia

RICHARD A. BASHORE • DOTUN OGUNYEMI • ROBERT H. HAYASHI

Although the definition of **dystocia** is **"difficult childbirth,"** the term is used interchangeably with **dysfunctional labor** and characterizes labor that does not progress normally. The problem may be caused by (1) **abnormalities of the "powers": ineffective uterine expulsive forces;** (2) **abnormalities of the "passenger": abnormal fetal lie, malpresentation, malposition, or fetal anatomic defects;** or (3) **abnormalities of the "passage": maternal bony pelvic contractures, resulting in mechanical interference with the passage of the fetus through the birth canal.** The cause or causes of abnormal labor should be determined as accurately as possible so that an effective and safe management plan can be developed.

▨ Physiologic Changes of Labor

The pregnant uterus is a large smooth muscle organ consisting of billions of smooth muscle cells. Each smooth muscle cell becomes a contractile element when the intracellular ionic calcium concentration increases to trigger an enzymatic process that results in the formation of the actin-myosin element. Stimulation of oxytocin or prostaglandin receptors on the plasma membrane further activates the formation of the actin-myosin element.

Contractions occur in localized areas of the uterus during gestation, but during parturition, the entire uterus contracts in an organized way to empty itself. These coordinated smooth muscle contractions occur as a result of the involvement and action of special gap junction structures. **Gap junctions are protein structures that form along the interface of two smooth muscle cell membranes and that act by promoting the movement of action potentials throughout the myometrium.**

During labor, two distinct segments of the uterus are formed. The **upper segment** actively contracts and retracts to expel the fetus while the **lower segment**, along with the dilating cervix, becomes thinner and passive and is referred to as the lower uterine segment (LUS). A physiologic retraction ring forms at the interface between the two segments. With obstructed labor, the thinning of the LUS becomes very pronounced and is called the **pathologic retraction ring of Bandl,** and if the obstruction is not relieved, uterine rupture may occur.

The pregnant cervix contains collagen, smooth muscle, and ground substance and must be structurally altered from a firm, intact sphincter to a soft, pliable, dilatable structure through which the products of conception can pass at the appropriate time. **These structural changes are the result of collagenolysis and increased hyaluronic acid, with a decrease in dermatan sulfate, which favors increased water content.** These changes probably occur in response to an increase in the estrogen-to-progesterone ratio, prostaglandin E_2, and enzymatic remodeling of cervical tissue.

▨ Normal Labor

Labor is diagnosed by regular, painful uterine contractions that increase in frequency and intensity with progressive cervical effacement or dilation.

The early part, or **latent phase,** of labor is involved with softening and effacement of the cervix with minimal dilation. This is followed by a more rapid rate of cervical dilation, known as the **active phase of labor,** which is **further divided into the acceleration (maximal slope) and deceleration phases.** The descent of the fetal presenting part usually begins during the active phase of labor, then progresses at a more rapid rate toward

139

the end of the active phase and continues after the cervix is completely dilated. A useful method for assessing the progress of labor and detecting abnormalities in a timely manner is to plot the rate of cervical dilation and descent of the fetal presenting part (Figure 11-1).

Normal cervical dilation and descent of the fetus take place in a progressive manner and occur within a well-defined time period. Dysfunctional labor occurs when rates of dilation and descent exceed these time limits. The phase of labor during which the abnormality occurs and the configuration of the abnormal labor curve may indicate the potential causes for the abnormal labor.

■ Abnormalities of the Latent Phase of Labor

The normal limits of the latent phase of labor extend up to 20 hours for nulliparous patients and up to 14 hours for multiparous patients. A latent phase that exceeds these limits is considered prolonged and may be caused by dysfunctional labor, premature or excessive use of sedatives or analgesics, fetal malpositions, or fetal size. A long, closed, firm cervix requires more time to efface and to undergo early dilation than does a soft, partially effaced cervix, but it is doubtful that a cervical factor alone causes a prolonged latent phase. **Many patients who appear to be developing a prolonged latent phase are shown eventually to be in false labor or prelabor, with no progressive dilation of the cervix.**

The outcome of a prolonged latent phase is generally favorable for both the mother and the fetus, provided that no other abnormalities of labor subsequently occur.

MANAGEMENT

A prolonged latent phase caused by premature or excessive use of sedation or analgesia usually resolves spontaneously after the effects of the medication have disappeared. Therapeutic rest with morphine sulfate or an equivalent drug has been shown to be effective in ruling out prelabor; women in true labor wake up in active labor, whereas those in prelabor stop contracting.

If a definite diagnosis of prolonged latent phase of labor is made or there are reasons to expedite delivery, augmentation of labor by oxytocin can be performed. This is accomplished by the addition of 10 U of oxytocin to 1000 mL of intravenous solution for a final concentration of 10 mU of oxytocin to each 1 mL of solution. A number of protocols have been suggested for the infusion of oxytocin. Oxytocin can be given as a low dose, in which the infusion is begun at a rate of 1 to 2 mU/minute and is increased in 1- to 2-mU/minute increments every 15 to 40 minutes until the desired frequency and intensity are obtained, or a maximum of 20 to 40 mU/minute is reached. The higher-dose infusion

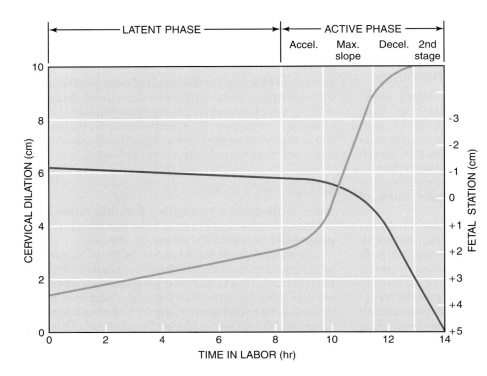

FIGURE 11-1   Graphic plot of cervical dilation (*green*) and descent of the fetal presenting part (*red*) during labor. *(From Cohen WR, Friedman EA [eds]: Management of Labor. Gaithersburg, MD, Aspen Publishers, 1983, p 13.)*

method is begun at a rate of 6 mU/minute, with incremental increases of 6 mU/minute every 15 to 40 minutes until uterine contractions of the desired frequency and intensity are obtained or a maximum of 40 mU/minute is reached.

Amniotomy or artificial rupture of the membranes may be considered as part of the management of the latent phase of labor. An associated risk is an increased incidence of chorioamnionitis.

■ *Abnormalities of the Active Phase of Labor*

When the cervix dilates to about 3 to 4 cm, the rate of dilation progresses more rapidly. Cervical dilation of less than 1.2 cm/hour in nulliparous women and 1.5 cm in multiparous women constitutes a **protraction disorder of the active phase of labor.** During the latter part of the active phase, the fetal presenting part also descends more rapidly through the pelvis and continues to descend through the second stage of labor. A rate of descent of the presenting part of less than 1 cm/hour in nulliparous women and 2 cm/hour in multiparous women is considered to be a **protraction disorder of descent** (Figure 11-2). If a period of 2 hours or more elapses during the active phase of labor without progress in cervical dilation, an **arrest of dilation** has occurred; a period of more than 1 hour without a change in station of the fetal presenting part is defined as an **arrest of descent** (Figure 11-3).

Etiology of active phase abnormalities include inadequate uterine activity, cephalopelvic disproportion, **fetal malposition, or conduction anesthesia.** The maternal pelvis should be evaluated, and the presenting fetal part should also be evaluated under these conditions.

MANAGEMENT

The American College of Obstetricians and Gynecologists (ACOG) recommends the use of oxytocin for all protraction and arrest disorders. Adequate labor (as assessed by intrauterine catheter) is defined as 200 Montevideo units (which is the sum of all the amplitudes of all the contractions in a 10-minute window) for at least 2 hours. Thus, a patient having four contractions in 10 minutes, each with an amplitude of 50 mm Hg, has adequate labor. **Amniotomy should be performed if rupture of membranes has not occurred spontaneously.**

Before deciding to proceed to cesarean delivery in the first stage of labor for abnormal labor progression, it should be ascertained that at least 4 hours of adequate contractions, as defined by 200 Montevideo units, has occurred. In a nullipara with dystocia, continuing labor for 6 to 8 hours is still associated with a high likelihood of vaginal delivery provided that the fetal heart rate is reassuring and there is some labor progress.

A cesarean delivery is indicated if cephalopelvic disproportion is diagnosed.

ACTIVE MANAGEMENT OF LABOR

Active management of labor has been proposed and used in the nulliparous patient as a strategy to lower the incidence of cesarean delivery for dystocia. This

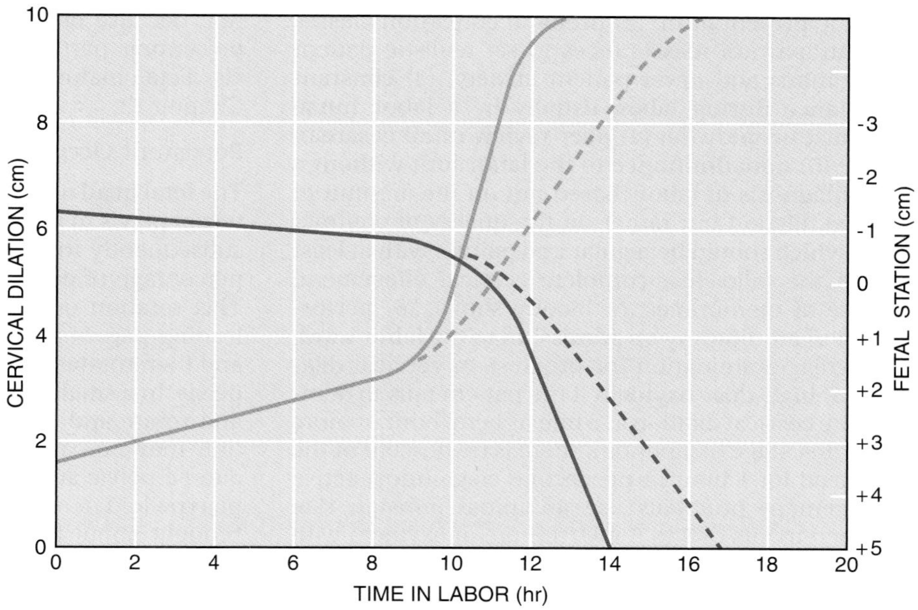

FIGURE 11-2   Normal dilation (*green*) and descent (*red*) curves of normal labor and curves depicting protracted dilation and descent abnormalities of labor. (*Modified from Friedman EA: Labor: Clinical Evaluation and Management, 2nd ed. New York, Appleton-Century-Crofts, 1978, p 65.*)

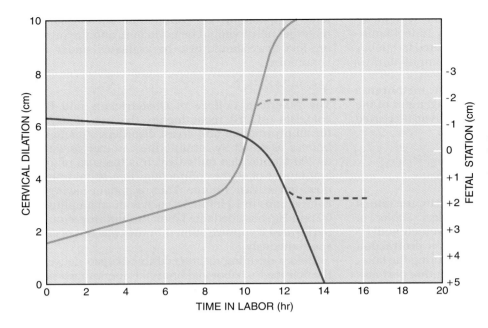

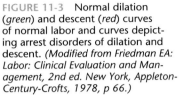

FIGURE 11-3   Normal dilation (*green*) and descent (*red*) curves of normal labor and curves depicting arrest disorders of dilation and descent. *(Modified from Friedman EA: Labor: Clinical Evaluation and Management, 2nd ed. New York, Appleton-Century-Crofts, 1978, p 66.)*

approach was initiated in the 1960s at the National Maternity Hospital in Dublin, where the rate of cesarean deliveries is relatively low. Published studies of this approach in institutions in the United States and Canada have been controversial with respect to the lowering of cesarean birth rates, but all studies have reported decreased length of labor in general when active management of labor is employed.

The criteria and components of this program are as follows: (1) **nulliparous pregnant patient with spontaneous onset of labor and a singleton fetus in a cephalic presentation;** (2) **prenatal education classes** and intrapartum reassurances to set realistic patient expectations and lower patient anxiety; (3) **constant attendance during labor, usually by a labor nurse specialist or midwife;** (4) **peer review of all cesarean births;** (5) **nonadmittance to the labor unit without a clear diagnosis of labor** (based not on the amount of cervical dilation but rather on the quality of contractions, which should be regular and painful with at least one of the following: complete cervical effacement, rupture of membranes, or bloody show); (6) **performance of amniotomy on admission to the labor ward;** (7) regular examination for progress in cervical dilation; (8) **high-dose oxytocin** if the patient fails to demonstrate cervical dilation at a rate of 1 cm/hour or more in the first stage of labor or if there is no descent of the fetal head for 1 hour in the second stage (most active management protocols use an initial infusion rate and increments of 4 to 6 mU/minute of oxytocin with only 15 minutes between increments to a maximum of 40 mU/minute); and (9) **peer review of outcomes.**

Many active management of labor programs have reported no compromise of perinatal outcomes and no cases of uterine rupture.

DYSTOCIA CAUSED BY ABNORMAL PRESENTATION AND POSITION

Presentations other than vertex and positions other than occipitoanterior (OA) are considered to be abnormal in the laboring patient. Disorders of the dilation and descent phases of labor occur with increased frequency in cases of abnormal presentation or position because of the altered relationship between the presenting part of the fetus and the maternal pelvis. Fetal malpresentations are discussed further in Chapter 13.

Persistent Occipitotransverse Position

The fetal head normally enters and engages in the maternal pelvis in an occipitotransverse (OT) position. It subsequently rotates to an OA position or, in a small percentage of cases, to an occipitoposterior position. This rotation occurs because the head flexes as the leading part of the vertex encounters the pelvic floor and then rotates to adjust to the shape of the gynecoid pelvis. In a small number of cases, the head fails to flex and rotate and persists in an OT position. This position may be caused by cephalopelvic disproportion; altered pelvic architecture, such as in a patient with a platypelloid or android pelvis; or a relaxed pelvic floor, brought about by epidural anesthesia or multiparity. The diagnosis of a persistent OT position may be difficult at times, owing to the obscuring of suture lines and

fontanelles by the excessive molding and caput formation that often accompany this abnormal position.

A persistent OT position with arrest of descent for a period of 1 hour or more is known as transverse arrest. Arrest occurs because of the deflexion that accompanies the persistent OT position, resulting in the larger occipitofrontal diameter (11 cm) becoming the presenting diameter. Until the head undergoes flexion and rotation, further descent cannot take place. Transverse arrest commonly occurs with the vertex at a +1 to +2 station.

The management of transverse arrest at a +1 to +2 station is complex, in part, because at these stations the widest part of the fetal head is at or above the level of the ischial spines. If the midpelvis is compromised, cesarean delivery is indicated. If the pelvis is judged to be of normal size and the fetus is not macrosomic, oxytocic stimulation of labor may be appropriate if uterine contractions are inadequate.

Manual rotation using the fingers of the examiner's hand or forceps rotation using Kielland forceps may be indicated if the pelvis is of normal size and shape. **Forceps rotation and delivery of a persistent OT position at a +1 to +2 station is now referred to as a low forceps procedure. However, because of the marked degree of molding and caput formation that usually occurs in this circumstance, the bony part of the fetal vertex may be at a +1 station even though the scalp may be visible at the introitus. Thus, what appears to be an uncomplicated low forceps operation may actually be a more difficult midforceps procedure.** One method for avoiding this problem is to clinically evaluate the relationship between the fetal head and the sacrum. If the fetal head fills the hollow of the sacrum, the biparietal diameter is usually at or below the spines, and an attempt at forceps delivery can be considered.

Persistent Occipitoposterior Position

The head generally rotates from OT to OA during the descent through the maternal pelvis. Even if the head initially rotates to an occipitoposterior position, most fetuses will eventually rotate spontaneously during labor to OA, leaving only a small percentage (5% to 15%) of fetuses with a persistent OP position.

The course of labor in the presence of a persistent OP position is usually normal except for a tendency for the second stage to be prolonged (>2 hours). It is also associated with considerably more discomfort. As with the persistent OT position, the fetal head may become markedly molded with extensive caput formation, which may cause difficulty in diagnosing its correct station and position. **Observation of a prolonged second stage of labor is appropriate, provided that labor continues to be progressive, and the fetal heart rate is normal.**

Delivery of the head may occur spontaneously in the OP position, but if the perineum provides undue resistance to delivery, a low forceps-assisted delivery may be required (e.g., using Simpson's forceps). In the past a Kielland forceps rotation was usually performed, but because of a lack of experience and training, **fetuses in the OP position are usually now delivered without rotation. Use of a vacuum extractor with a cup designed for a safe and secure posterior application may be performed.** Sometimes the head will rotate, but it will usually deliver in the OP position. A wide mediolateral episiotomy may be required to lessen the resistance of the outlet to the delivery of the fetal head.

DYSTOCIA CAUSED BY ABNORMALITIES OF FETAL STRUCTURE

Macrosomia and Shoulder Dystocia

The ACOG defines macrosomia as a fetus weighing 4500 g or more. Large for gestational age is defined as birth weight equal to or above the 90th percentile of fetal weight for a given gestational age. Macrosomia is associated with genetic determinants, maternal diabetes, prepregnancy weight, weight gain during pregnancy, multiparity, male sex, gestational age greater than 40 weeks, ethnicity, maternal birth weight, maternal height, and maternal age. **Maternal morbidity associated with macrosomia includes labor dystocia, shoulder dystocia, and genital trauma, with a corresponding increase in the cesarean delivery rate. There is also an increase in postpartum hemorrhage and puerperal infection.** There is increased perinatal morbidity resulting from dystocia and birth trauma, especially shoulder dystocia.

An accurate estimate of fetal weight is elusive. **Errors in the estimation of macrosomia by ultrasound may be up to 50%.** Prospective studies have shown that clinical estimates by physicians or patients are as inaccurate as ultrasonic assessments. Suspected macrosomia alone is not an indication for cesarean delivery or induction of labor. Induction of labor has not been shown to improve fetal or maternal outcome. Because the risk for shoulder dystocia and possible fetal injury increases significantly as the upper extremes of fetal weight are reached, however, ACOG recommends cesarean delivery for an estimated fetal weight of 5000 g or more in women **without** diabetes, and 4500 g or more in women **with** diabetes.

Although the mean duration of labor is prolonged for excessively large fetuses, **it is not unusual to encounter unexpected shoulder dystocia after a labor that has been entirely normal up to the moment of delivery.**

Shoulder dystocia means difficult delivery of the shoulder. It has been defined as delivery of the shoulder requiring the use of procedures in addition to gentle downward traction on the fetal head or a prolonged

head-to-body delivery interval of more than 60 seconds.

Shoulder dystocia depends on the size of the maternal pelvis in relation to the size of the fetus **and occurs from impaction of the shoulder on the pubic symphysis anteriorly or the sacral promontory posteriorly. The most important risk factors for shoulder dystocia are fetal macrosomia and maternal diabetes.** Others include obesity, multiparity, post-term gestation, short stature, previous history of macrosomic birth, and previous history of shoulder dystocia. During labor, risk factors include labor induction, epidural analgesia, prolonged labor, and operative vaginal delivery.

The major neonatal complication is the occurrence of Erb's palsy, which can be caused by excessive traction on the brachial plexus by the delivery attendant. This is an important cause of malpractice in obstetrics. If Erb's palsy occurs on the posterior shoulder, the damage could not have been caused by excessive traction, but was most likely caused by abnormalities of the sacral promontory applying pressure on the brachial plexus before delivery. Other neonatal complications include **Klumpke's palsy,** clavicular fracture, humeral fracture, hypoxia, brain injury, and death. Maternal complications include genital tract lacerations and postpartum hemorrhage.

Shoulder dystocia is recognized at delivery by retraction of the fetal head, which is called the *turtle sign.* Shoulder dystocia is not overcome by traction on the fetal head but, instead, by one or more maneuvers designed to displace the anterior shoulder from behind the symphysis pubis. **An initial maneuver is suprapubic pressure,** which involves lateral pressure only with the hand over the maternal suprapubic region in an effort to guide the anterior shoulder under or away from the symphysis pubis. **McRoberts' maneuver** may also be employed as an initial or second procedure. In McRoberts' maneuver, the maternal thighs are sharply flexed against the maternal abdomen to reduce the angle between the sacrum and spine, thus freeing the impacted shoulder. If this is not successful, **pressure is applied with the operator's fingers against the scapula of the posterior shoulder in an attempt to rotate (corkscrew, Woods maneuver) the posterior shoulder upward until it becomes the anterior shoulder.** If this maneuver does not correct the problem, **a hand is inserted into the vagina, and the posterior arm is grasped and pulled across the chest, resulting in delivery of the posterior shoulder and displacement of the anterior shoulder from behind the symphysis pubis.** Fracture of the humerus may result from this maneuver, but the bone heals quickly in the neonate. Putting the patient on all fours (knee-chest position) may also be considered because the downward pull of gravity may disimpact the shoulder. **If none of these maneuvers is successful,** one or both clavicles must be fractured, preferably by pressure on the clavicle directed away from the pleural cavity to prevent traumatic puncture of the lungs.

A maneuver has been described, attributed to **Zavanelli,** to manage shoulder dystocia that is not corrected successfully by the methods already described. In this last-resort procedure, the fetal head is manually returned to its prerestitution position, and then slowly replaced into the vagina by steady upward pressure against the head. Delivery is subsequently accomplished by cesarean birth. A uterine relaxant may be required to carry out this procedure.

Developmental Abnormalities

Localized abnormalities of fetal anatomy may lead to dystocia. **Internal hydrocephalus** may cause enlargement of the fetal head to the extent that vaginal delivery is not possible. The diagnosis is usually made by ultrasonography performed because of the clinical suspicion, or it may appear as an unexpected finding on ultrasonography performed for other indications.

Several options are available for the delivery of the fetus with hydrocephalus. **Excessive cerebrospinal fluid may be removed** by inserting a needle directly into the ventricular space through the dilated cervix during labor, or transabdominally under ultrasonic guidance before or during labor. **Alternatively, the fetus may be delivered by cesarean birth** to avoid the risk for infection, which can result from transvaginal or transabdominal drainage.

Intrauterine shunting of the fetal ventricular system into the amniotic fluid compartment is an experimental procedure that has not been shown to have the long-term benefits to justify its performance.

The accumulation of **ascites** in the fetal abdomen or **enlargement of fetal organs, such as the bladder or liver, may result in unexpected dystocia (due to an enlarged fetal abdomen) after the fetal head has been delivered. Ascites usually occurs as part of hydrops, which is defined as fetal fluid retention in two of the following sites: skin, abdomen, pericardial cavity, or pleural cavity. Immune hydrops is usually caused by Rhesus disease, while nonimmune hydrops may be caused by congenital infections, chromosomal abnormalities, or fetal arrhythmias.** If any of the above conditions is present, careful ultrasonic evaluation before or during labor should be performed to identify excessive enlargement of the fetal abdomen. Ascitic fluid or urine from a massively enlarged bladder may be removed by transabdominal drainage with a needle before vaginal delivery. Cesarean delivery may be indicated if the fetal abdomen cannot be sufficiently decompressed.

A defect in the fetal lumbosacral vertebrae may result in the protrusion of a meningeal sac (**meningocele**) or a sac containing spinal cord (**meningomyelocele**). These defects are usually detected as a result of abnormal serum or amniotic fluid alpha-fetoprotein values or by ultrasonography. If the sac is large, abdominal delivery is advisable to avoid dystocia or rupture of the sac and potential infection. If the sac is small and is covered by fetal skin, as reflected by a normal alpha-fetoprotein value, vaginal delivery may be appropriate.

Other potential causes of fetal dystocia include a very large fetal **sacrococcygeal teratoma, conjoined twins, and locked preterm twins when twin A is breech and twin B is vertex and they enter the pelvis at the same time.**

DYSTOCIA CAUSED BY MATERNAL PELVIC ABNORMALITIES

Cephalopelvic disproportion (CPD) exists if the maternal bony pelvis is not of sufficient size and of appropriate shape to allow the passage of the fetal head. This problem may occur as a result of contraction of one of the planes of the pelvis. Relative CPD may exist with a normal pelvis, if the fetal head is excessively large or if it is in an abnormal position. Contraction of the maternal pelvis may occur at the level of the inlet or midpelvis, but **contraction of the outlet is extremely unusual** unless it is found in association with a midpelvic contraction (see Chapter 8).

Cephalopelvic disproportion at the level of the pelvic inlet causes a failure of descent and engagement of the head. The finding of an unengaged head in a nulliparous patient at the start of labor indicates an increased likelihood of CPD at the pelvic inlet, but an unengaged fetal head in a multiparous patient in labor is not an unusual occurrence. Relative CPD can occur in the multiparous patient (the "multip trap"), however, and should be kept in mind.

The management of a nulliparous patient with an unengaged fetal head in labor should begin with a careful clinical evaluation of the maternal pelvis. If the pelvis is clinically adequate, expectant management with observation of the labor pattern is appropriate. If uterine contractions are ineffective, oxytocic stimulation of labor may be considered.

The occurrence of CPD at the level of the midpelvis occurs more frequently than inlet dystocia because the capacity of the midpelvis is smaller than that of the inlet and also because deflection or positional abnormalities of the fetal head are more likely to occur at that level. The occurrence of bony dystocia at the level of the midpelvis is usually indicated by an arrest of descent of the head at a +1 to +2 station. With CPD and arrest of descent, application of the head to the cervix is poor, resulting in the loss of part of the force needed for cervical dilation. Thus, CPD may be associated with a protracted or expected rate of cervical dilation before an arrest of descent is apparent.

DYSTOCIA CAUSED BY CONDUCTION ANESTHESIA

The use of epidural anesthesia for pain control during the first stage of labor has gained wide acceptance. Refinement of the epidural technique has allowed a segmental block and titratable continuous infusion of narcotics and local anesthetics to better tailor pain control, with less interference with the process of labor (see Chapter 8).

Current evidence suggests that **epidural analgesia does not increase the primary cesarean delivery rate,** but it may be associated with increased need for oxytocin augmentation, prolonged first and second stages of labor, and operative vaginal delivery.

SUGGESTED READING

American College of Obstetricians and Gynecologists: Shoulder dystocia. ACOG Practice Bulletin No. 40. Washington, DC, 2002.

American College of Obstetricians and Gynecologists: Vaginal birth after previous cesarean section. ACOG Practice Bulletin No. 54. Washington, DC, 2004.

Gottlieb AG, Galan HL: Shoulder dystocia: An update. Obstet Gynecol Clin North Am 34:501-531, xii, 2007.

Lowe NK: A review of factors associated with dystocia and cesarean section in nulliparous women. J Midwifery Womens Health 52:216-228, 2007.

Shields SG, Ratcliffe SD, Fontaine P, Leeman L: Dystocia in nulliparous women. Am Fam Physician 75:1671-1678, 2007.

Chapter 12

Obstetric Complications
PRETERM LABOR, PROM, IUGR, POSTTERM PREGNANCY, AND IUFD

CALVIN J. HOBEL

◾ *Preterm Labor*

Worldwide, preterm labor and delivery are major causes of perinatal morbidity and mortality. **Although fewer than 12% of all infants born in the United States are preterm, their contribution to neonatal morbidity and mortality ranges from 50% to 70%.** The medical and economic impact of preterm delivery is significant, and major goals of obstetric care are to reduce the incidence of the condition and to increase the gestational age of infants whose preterm births are unavoidable.

DEFINITION AND INCIDENCE

Preterm birth is usually defined as one occurring after 20 weeks and before 37 completed weeks of gestation. Labor that occurs between these gestational ages is defined as preterm labor. Internationally, the lower boundary defining preterm birth varies between 20 and 24 weeks.

Preterm births in the United States have increased from 9.8% in 1981 to 12.7% in 2005. Between 1988 and 2004, the mortality rate for white infants declined by 55% to 5.7 infant deaths per 1000 live births, and the mortality rate for black infants declined by 45% to 13.6. In the past 10 years, the decline in infant mortality for both races has been less than anticipated. **Because prematurity is the leading cause of infant mortality, the prevention of prematurity has become a high priority.**

ETIOLOGY AND RISK FACTORS

The estimated causes of preterm birth are listed in Table 12-1. **Private patients have a much higher proportion of spontaneous preterm labor, whereas black** patients in public institutions have a higher proportion of deliveries due to PPROM.

Attempts have been made to define further the spontaneous preterm labor subgroup. Some experts now believe this may be caused by undiagnosed conditions of placental, infectious, immunologic, uterine, or cervical origin. **Recently, genetic thrombophilias have been shown to account for a significant proportion of the uteroplacental problems leading to intrauterine growth restriction (IUGR) and preeclampsia**, the two major reasons for the early induction of labor to avoid fetal death. In the past 10 years, closer surveillance of high-risk pregnancies has led to earlier delivery and an increase in late preterm deliveries (between 34 and 37 weeks), a major contribution to the increasing preterm birth rate.

Another reason for the increasing incidence of preterm birth is that more women are postponing childbirth as a lifestyle choice. This is associated with a greater risk for infertility and therefore greater use of assisted reproductive technologies (ART), which are associated with multiple gestations and increased risk for preterm birth. A variety of socioeconomic, psychosocial, and medical conditions have been found to carry an increased risk for preterm delivery in these women who postpone childbearing.

Socioeconomic Factors

In the United States, the incidence of preterm deliveries in the black population is twice as high as that in the white population. This factor cannot be viewed as a single entity but probably encompasses other characteristics of the population, such as poor access to and procurement of antenatal care, high stress levels, poor nutritional status, and the possibility of genetic differences.

TABLE 12-1

ETIOLOGY OF PRETERM BIRTH

Cause	Estimated Percentage of Preterm Births
Spontaneous preterm labor	35-37
Multiple pregnancies*	12-15
Preterm premature rupture of membranes (PPROM)	12-15
Pregnancy-associated hypertension	12-14
Cervical incompetence or uterine anomalies	12-14
Antepartum hemorrhage	5-6
Intrauterine growth restriction (IUGR)	4-6

*Increasing proportion due to advancing maternal age and assisted reproductive technologies (ART).

Medical and Obstetric Factors

When one preterm birth has occurred, the relative risk for preterm delivery in the next pregnancy is 3.9, and the risk increases to 6.5 with two previous preterm deliveries.

Second-trimester abortions seem to carry an increased risk for subsequent preterm delivery, especially if a previous preterm birth has also occurred. The risk associated with induced first-trimester abortions is controversial. **Repeated spontaneous first-trimester abortions,** however, do **increase the risk.**

Other medical and obstetrical factors include bleeding in the first trimester, urinary tract infections, multiple gestation, uterine anomalies, polyhydramnios, and incompetent cervix.

Recently, attention has been directed toward maternal employment, physical activity, nutritional status, genital tract infections, stress, and anxiety as major risk factors for preterm birth.

PREVENTION

"Group education" has been shown to decrease preterm birth. All at-risk patients, together with a healthcare provider, should discuss how to adjust personal behaviors and lifestyles to decrease the risk.

Four potential pathways leading to preterm delivery have been identified:
1. Infection (cervical)
2. Placental-vascular
3. Psychosocial stress and work strain (fatigue)
4. Uterine stretch (multiple gestations)

Infection-Cervical Pathway

Bacterial vaginosis has been shown to be associated with preterm delivery, independent of other recognized risk factors. **Treatment of bacterial vaginosis has reduced the incidence of preterm delivery.** In addition, treating women in preterm labor with antibiotics significantly prolongs the time from the onset of treatment to delivery, compared with that in patients who do not receive antibiotics. Thus, addressing the issue of these relatively asymptomatic infections is an important strategy for preventing preterm birth.

There is a link between vaginal-cervical infections and progressive changes in the cervical length, as measured by vaginal ultrasonography. The relative risk for preterm birth increases significantly from 2.4 for a cervical length of 3.5 cm (50th percentile) to 6.2 for a length of 2.5 cm (10th percentile). Short cervices appear to be more common in women who have had prior preterm births and pregnancy terminations.

The most recent test to be developed is cervical and vaginal fetal fibronectin. This substance is a basement membrane protein produced by the fetal membranes. When the fetal membranes are disrupted, as with repetitive uterine activity, shortening of the cervix, and in the presence of infection, fibronectin is secreted into the vagina and can be tested. **A positive fetal fibronectin test at 22 to 24 weeks predicts more than half of the spontaneous preterm births that occur before 28 weeks.** A positive test for fetal fibronectin is significantly associated with a short cervix, vaginal infections, and uterine activity. A negative test is the best predictor of a low risk for preterm delivery.

Placental-Vascular Pathway

The placental-vascular pathway begins early in pregnancy at the time of implantation, when there are important changes taking place at the placental-decidual-myometrial interface. First, there are important immunologic changes, with a switch from a T_H1 type of immunity, which may be embryotoxic, to T_H2 antibody profile, in which blocking antibody production is thought to prevent rejection. At the same time, the trophoblasts are invading the spiral arteries of the decidua and myometrium, thus assuring that a low-resistance vascular connection is established. Alterations in both of these early changes are thought to play an important role in the pathophysiology of poor fetal growth, an important component of preterm birth (indicated and spontaneous), fetal growth restriction, and preeclampsia.

Stress-Strain Pathway

Both mental (cognitive) and work-related stress and strain are postulated to initiate a stress response that increases release of cortisol and catecholamines. Cortisol from the adrenal gland initiates early placental corticotrophin-releasing hormone (CRH) gene expression, and elevated levels of CRH are known to initiate labor at term. Catecholamines released during the stress response not only affect blood flow to the uteroplacental unit but also cause uterine contractions (norepinephrine). Poor nutrition in the form of reduced calories or abnormal patterns of intake (fasting) are known stressors and have been associated with a significantly increased risk for preterm birth. **In support of the stress pathway are the studies that have shown that the rate of change of CRH, a mediator of the stress response, increases significantly in the weeks before the onset of preterm labor.** Stress reduction and improved nutrition are the only current interventions that can be applied to this pathway.

Uterine Stretch Pathway

Uterine stretch as a result of increasing volume during normal and abnormal gestations is an important physiologic mechanism that facilitates the process of emptying the uterus. This pathway is common in patients with **polyhydramnios** and those with **multiple gestations**, both of which have an increased risk for preterm birth.

DIAGNOSIS

The diagnosis of preterm labor occurring between 20 and 37 weeks is based on the following criteria in patients with ruptured or intact membranes: (1) **documented uterine contractions** (four per 20 minutes) and (2) **documented cervical change** (cervical effacement of 80% or cervical dilation of 2 cm or more). Uterine contractions are not a good predictor of preterm labor, but cervical changes are.

MANAGEMENT

Provided that membranes are not ruptured and there is no contraindication to a vaginal examination (e.g., placenta previa), **an initial assessment must be done to ascertain cervical length and dilation and the station and nature of the presenting part.** The patient should also be evaluated for the presence of any underlying correctable problem, such as a urinary tract or vaginal infection. She should be placed in the lateral decubitus position (taking the weight of the uterus off the great vessels and improving blood flow to the uterus), monitored for the presence and frequency of uterine activity, and reexamined for evidence of cervical change after an appropriate interval, unless she already meets the preceding criteria for preterm labor. During the period of observation, either oral or parenteral hydration should be initiated.

With adequate hydration and bed rest, uterine contractions cease in about 20% of patients. These patients, however, remain at high risk for recurrent preterm labor.

Because of the role of cervical colonization and vaginal infection in the etiology of preterm labor and premature rupture of membranes, **cultures should be taken for group B streptococcus.** Other organisms

that may be important are *Ureaplasma, Mycoplasma,* and *Gardnerella vaginalis.* The latter is associated with bacterial vaginosis, a diagnosis that can be made by the presence of three of four clinical signs (vaginal pH > 4.5, amine odor after addition of 10% potassium hydroxide [KOH], and presence of clue cells or milky discharge).

Antibiotics should be administered to patients who are in preterm labor. For patients who are not allergic to penicillin, a 7-day course of ampicillin, erythromycin, or both can be given. Those allergic to penicillin can be given clindamycin.

Once the diagnosis of preterm labor has been made, the following laboratory tests should be obtained: complete blood cell count, random blood glucose level, serum electrolyte levels, urinalysis, and urine culture and sensitivity. An ultrasonic examination of the fetus should be performed to assess fetal weight, document presentation, assess cervical length, and rule out the presence of any accompanying congenital malformation. The test may also detect an underlying etiologic factor, such as twins or a uterine anomaly.

If the patient does not respond to bed rest and hydration, tocolytic therapy is instituted, provided there are no contraindications. Measures implemented at 28 weeks should be more aggressive than those initiated at 35 weeks. Similarly, a patient with advanced cervical dilation on admission requires more aggressive management than one whose cervix is closed and minimally effaced.

UTERINE TOCOLYTIC THERAPY

It is assumed that physiologic events leading to the initiation of labor also occur in preterm labor. The pharmacologic agents presently being used all seem to inhibit the availability of calcium ions, but they may also exert a number of other effects. The agents currently used and their dosages are presented in Box 12-1.

Magnesium Sulfate

In the United States, magnesium sulfate is frequently the drug of choice for initiating tocolytic therapy. Magnesium acts at the cellular level by competing with calcium for entry into the cell at the time of depolarization. Successful competition results in an effective decrease of intracellular calcium ions, resulting in myometrial relaxation.

Although magnesium levels required for tocolysis have not been critically evaluated, it appears that the levels needed may be higher than those required for prevention of eclampsia. Levels from 5.5 to 7.0 mg/dL appear to be appropriate. These can be achieved using the dosage regimen outlined in Box 12-1. **After the loading dose is given, a continuous infusion is maintained, and plasma levels should be determined until therapeutic levels are reached.** The drug should be continued at therapeutic levels until contractions

Magnesium Sulfate

Solution: Initial solution contains 6 g (12 mL of 50% $MgSO_4$) in 100 mL of 5% dextrose. Maintenance solution contains 10 g (20 mL of 50% $MgSO_4$) in 500 mL of 5% dextrose

Initial dose: 6 g over 15-20 min, parenterally

Titrating dose: 2 g/hr until contractions cease; follow serum levels (5-7 mg/dL); maximal dose, 4 g/hr

Maintenance dose: Maintain dose for 12 hr, then 1 g/hr for 24-48 hr

Nifedipine

Preparation: Oral gelatin capsules of 10 or 20 mg

Loading dose: 30 mg; if contractions persist after 90 min, give an additional 20 mg (second dose); if labor is suppressed, a maintenance dose of 20 mg is given orally every 6 hr for 24 hr and then every 8 hr for another 24 hr.

Failure: If contractions persist 60 min after the second dose, treatment should be considered a failure.

Prostaglandin Synthetase Inhibitors

Short-term use only

---

cease unless the labor progresses. Because magnesium is excreted by the kidneys, adjustments must be made in patients with an abnormal creatinine clearance. **Once successful tocolysis has been achieved, the infusion is continued for at least 12 hours, and then the infusion rate is weaned over 2 to 4 hours and then discontinued.** In high-risk patients (advanced cervical dilation or continued labor in very-low-birth-weight cases), the infusion can be continued until the fetus has been exposed to glucocorticoids to enhance lung maturity.

A common minor side effect of magnesium therapy is **a feeling of warmth and flushing on first administration. Respiratory depression** is seen at magnesium levels of 12 to 15 mg/dL, and **cardiac conduction defects and arrest** are seen at higher levels.

In the fetus, plasma magnesium levels approach those of the mother, and a low plasma calcium level may also be demonstrated. The neonate may show some loss of muscle tone and drowsiness, resulting in a lower Apgar score. These effects are prolonged in the preterm neonate because of the decrease in renal clearance.

Long-term parenteral magnesium therapy has been used for control of preterm labor in selected patients. An important side effect seems to be loss of calcium, and it may be important in such patients to institute calcium therapy on a prophylactic basis.

Nifedipine

Nifedipine as an oral agent is very effective in suppressing preterm labor with minimal maternal and fetal side effects. It works by inhibiting the slow, inward current of calcium ions during the second phase of the action potential of uterine smooth muscle cells **and may gradually replace intravenous magnesium sulfate.** The only side effects are headache, cutaneous flushing, hypotension, and tachycardia. The latter two side effects can be partially avoided by making certain the patient is well hydrated and by the use of support stockings, such as TED (antiembolism) hose.

Prostaglandin Synthetase Inhibitors

Prostaglandins induce myometrial contractions at all stages of gestation, both in vivo and in vitro. Because prostaglandins are locally synthesized and possess a relatively short half-life, prevention of their synthesis within the uterus could abort labor. **These agents are used on a short-term basis** in special circumstances when prostaglandin production may be the inciting factor in preterm labor, such as with the presence of uterine fibroids. In the United States, **indomethacin is the most commonly used prostaglandin inhibitor; it can be administered both orally and rectally, with some slight delay in absorption from rectal administration as compared with the oral route.** Peak serum levels of indomethacin occur 1.5 to 2 hours after oral administration. Excretion of the intact drug occurs in maternal urine. It can result in oligohydramnios and premature closure of the fetal ductus arteriosus, which in turn may lead to neonatal pulmonary hypertension and cardiac failure. In addition, **indomethacin decreases fetal renal function, and indomethacin-exposed infants have a greater risk for necrotizing enterocolitis, intracranial hemorrhage, and patent ductus arteriosus.** Short-term use may be acceptable, but if patients are given indomethacin, the fetus should be evaluated with ultrasonography for ductus arteriosus flow.

Oxytocin Receptor Antagonists

Atosiban was the first oxytocin receptor antagonist developed. It binds to receptors in the myometrium and other gestational tissues, preventing the oxytocin-induced increase in inositol triphosphate, the messenger that increases intracellular calcium and causes myometrial contractions and upregulation of prostaglandin production. **These agents are not approved for use in the United States.**

Combined Therapy

Combined therapy, using a combination of nifedipine and prostaglandin synthetase inhibitors, is being explored in countries such as Australia, Canada, and Europe.

Efficacy of Tocolytic Therapy

Although the advent of tocolytic agents has failed to decrease preterm births in large population studies, their use has improved neonatal survival, decreased respiratory distress syndrome (RDS), and increased the birth weight of infants. The benefit of measures to postpone delivery beyond 34 weeks' gestational age is under investigation.

Antibiotic Therapy

A number of studies have advocated the use of antibiotic prophylaxis in patients with preterm labor. Such patients may have a higher incidence of **subclinical chorioamnionitis** than previously thought.

Diagnostic amniocentesis in patients with idiopathic preterm labor has identified about 15% whose amniotic cavity is colonized with pathogens. It is reasonable to assume that a proportion of the remaining cases will have bacteria in the decidual cell space between the chorion and the myometrium. Thus **the use of prophylactic antibiotics in women with preterm labor may prevent the progression of a subclinical infection to clinical amnionitis.**

Contraindications to Tocolytic Therapy

Contraindications include **severe preeclampsia, severe bleeding from placenta previa or abruptio placentae, chorioamnionitis, intrauterine growth restriction, fetal anomalies incompatible with life, and fetal demise.** Because of the low success rate, advanced cervical dilation may also preclude tocolytic therapy, although therapy may delay delivery sufficiently for glucocorticoid administration to accelerate fetal lung maturity. Management of patients should be individualized, and even if the patient's cervix is dilated 6 cm and she is having infrequent contractions, it is advisable to employ tocolysis and administer glucocorticoid therapy.

USE OF GLUCOCORTICOIDS FOR FETAL PULMONARY MATURATION

Antenatal corticosteroid therapy for fetal pulmonary maturation reduces mortality and the incidence of RDS and intraventricular hemorrhage (IVH) in preterm infants. These benefits extend to a broad range of gestational ages (24 to 34 weeks) and are not limited by gender or race. **Treatment consists of 2 doses of 12 mg of betamethasone, given intramuscularly 24 hours apart, or 4 doses of 6 mg of dexamethasone, given intramuscularly 12 hours apart.** Optimal benefit begins 24 hours after initiation of therapy and lasts 7 days. Because treatment with corticosteroids for less than 24 hours is still associated with significant reductions in neonatal mortality, RDS, and IVH, antenatal corticosteroids should be given unless immediate delivery is anticipated.

LABOR AND DELIVERY OF THE PRETERM INFANT

A certain number of patients will not respond to tocolytic therapy. The goal in these patients is to conduct both labor and delivery in an optimal manner so as not to contribute to the morbidity or mortality of the preterm infant. All parameters for assessing gestational age and fetal weight must be considered. **With modern neonatal care, the lower limit of potential viability is 24 weeks or 500 g, although these limits vary with the expertise of the neonatal intensive care unit.**

Fetal heart rate patterns that are relatively innocuous in the term fetus may indicate a more ominous outcome for the preterm fetus. **Continuous fetal heart monitoring and prompt attention to abnormal fetal heart rate patterns are extremely important.** Acidosis at birth adversely affects respiratory function by destroying surfactant and delaying its release.

With a vertex presentation, vaginal delivery is preferred, independent of gestational age, provided that fetal acidosis and delivery trauma are avoided. **Use of outlet forceps and an episiotomy to shorten the second stage are advocated.** Some reports recommend cesarean delivery of the very-low-birth-weight baby.

About 23% of infants present as a breech at 28 weeks, compared with about 4% at term. This presentation carries an increased risk for cord prolapse or compression. In addition, cervical entrapment of the aftercoming fetal head may occur at delivery because, before term, the head is proportionally larger than the buttocks. **For the breech fetus estimated at less than 1500 g, neonatal outcome is improved by cesarean birth.**

Premature Rupture of the Membranes

DEFINITION AND INCIDENCE

Premature rupture of the membranes (PROM) is defined as amniorrhexis (spontaneous rupture of membranes as opposed to amniotomy) before the onset of labor at any stage of gestation. PPROM should be used to define those patients who are preterm with ruptured membranes, whether or not they have contractions.

ETIOLOGY AND RISK FACTORS

The etiology of PROM remains unclear, but a variety of factors are purported to contribute to its occurrence, including vaginal and cervical infections, abnormal membrane physiology, incompetent cervix, and nutritional deficiencies.

DIAGNOSIS

Diagnosis of PROM is based on the history of vaginal loss of fluid and confirmation of amniotic fluid in the vagina. Episodic urinary incontinence, leukorrhea, or loss of the mucous plug must be ruled out. Management of the patient presenting with this history depends on the gestational age. **Because of the risk for introducing infection and the usually long latency period from the time of examination until delivery, the examiner's hands should not be inserted into the vagina of a patient who is not in labor, whether preterm or term.** A sterile vaginal speculum examination should be performed to confirm the diagnosis, to assess cervical dilation and length, and if the patient is preterm, to obtain cervical cultures and amniotic fluid samples for pulmonary maturation tests.

On examination, pooling of amniotic fluid in the posterior vaginal fornix can usually be seen. A Valsalva maneuver or slight fundal pressure may expel fluid from the cervical os, which is diagnostic of PROM. **Confirmation of the diagnosis can be made by (1) testing the fluid with Nitrazine paper, which will turn blue in the presence of the alkaline amniotic fluid, and (2) placing a sample on a microscopic slide, air drying, and examining for ferning.** False-positive Nitrazine test results occur in the presence of alkaline urine, blood, or cervical mucus. In the presence of blood, which is usually seen in patients who are also in early labor, the pattern may appear to be skeletonized, and a distinct ferning may not be seen. As in the case of preterm labor with intact membranes, a complete ultrasonic examination should be carried out to rule out fetal anomalies and to assess gestational age and amniotic fluid volume.

MANAGEMENT

General Considerations

An intact amniotic sac serves as a mechanical barrier to infection, but in addition, amniotic fluid has some bacteriostatic properties that may play a role in preventing chorioamnionitis and fetal infections. Intact membranes are not an absolute barrier to infection because bacterial colonization still occurs in the decidual space and membrane interface in 10% of patients in term labor and in up to 25% of patients in preterm labor.

For preterm fetuses with PPROM, the risks associated with preterm delivery must be balanced against the risks for infection and sepsis that may make in utero existence even more problematic. For the mother, the risks include not only the development of chorioamnionitis but also the possibility of failed induction in the presence of an unfavorable cervix, resulting in subsequent cesarean birth.

Management is dictated to a large extent by the gestational age at the time of membrane rupture, although **the quantity of amniotic fluid remaining after PPROM may be as important as gestational age in determining pregnancy outcome.**

Ultrasonic definition of oligohydramnios has been standardized. Objective criteria include measurement of the vertical axis of amniotic fluid present in four quadrants, the total being called the **amniotic fluid index (AFI).** A value of less than 5 cm is considered abnormal.

Oligohydramnios associated with PROM in the fetus at less than 24 weeks' gestation may lead to the development of pulmonary hypoplasia. Factors that may be responsible include fetal crowding with thoracic compression, restriction of fetal breathing, and disturbances of pulmonary fluid production and flow. The duration of membrane rupture is an important consideration. Constraints placed on fetal movements in utero can also result in a variety of positional skeletal abnormalities, such as talipes equinovarus.

If PROM occurs at 36 weeks or later and the condition of the cervix is favorable, labor should be induced after 6 to 12 hours if no spontaneous contractions occur. In the presence of an unfavorable cervical condition with no evidence of infection, it is reasonable to wait 24 hours before induction of labor to decrease the risk for failed induction and maternal febrile morbidity. The following discussion applies when premature membrane rupture occurs before 36 weeks' gestational age.

Laboratory Tests

In addition to the laboratory tests obtained for the patient in preterm labor, sufficient amniotic fluid can usually be obtained from the vaginal pool for pulmonary maturation studies. Because of the higher incidence of chorioamnionitis in association with PROM, amniotic fluid should also be examined with Gram stain and culture.

Conservative Expectant Management

Conservative management applies to the care of patients with PPROM who are observed with the expectation of prolonging gestation. **Because the risk for infection appears to increase with the duration of membrane rupture, the goal of expectant management is to continue the pregnancy until the lung profile is mature.** Careful surveillance must be maintained to diagnose chorioamnionitis at an early enough stage to minimize fetal and maternal risks. In its fulminant state, chorioamnionitis is associated with a high maternal temperature and a tender, sometimes irritable, uterus.

In cases of subclinical infection, diagnosis and treatment may be delayed. A combination of factors should alert the clinician to the possibility of chorio-amnionitis, including maternal temperature greater than 100.4°F (38°C) in the absence of any other site of infection, fetal tachycardia, a tender uterus, and uterine irritability on nonstress testing.

The presence of bacteria by Gram stain or culture of amniotic fluid obtained at amniocentesis correlates with subsequent maternal infection in about 50% of cases and with neonatal sepsis in about 25%. The presence of white blood cells alone in amniotic fluid is less predictive of infection. The decision to perform amniocentesis is based on the gestational age, the presence of early signs of infection, and the AFI as measured by real-time ultrasonography. Recently investigators have described elevation of inflammatory cytokines in the amniotic fluid and fetal circulation in preterm infants who subsequently developed chronic lung disease during the neonatal period. A similar response may be associated with a greater risk for damage to the preterm baby's brain, thus increasing the risk for cerebral palsy. Thus the management of patients with PROM is critical for the prevention of neonatal morbidity.

Ampicillin or erythromycin significantly prolongs the interval to delivery in patients with PPROM. The neonates delivered from patients receiving prophylaxis also have less morbidity.

Management of Chorioamnionitis

Once chorioamnionitis is diagnosed, antibiotic therapy should be delayed only until appropriate cultures have been taken. Ampicillin and gentamycin in combination are the drugs of choice. In the penicillin-sensitive patient, cephalosporins may be indicated, noting the 12% incidence of crossover sensitivity. Once antibiotics have been started, labor should be induced. **If the condition of the cervix is unfavorable and there is evidence of fetal involvement, it may be necessary to perform a cesarean delivery.**

The presence of active genital herpes is an important concern in the presence of ruptured membranes. Herpes infection at a site remote from the cervix and vagina is probably not associated with an increased risk for fetal infection, so the site of infection should be taken into consideration before recommending immediate cesarean delivery.

Tocolytic Therapy

The use of tocolytics to control preterm labor in patients with PROM is controversial. The arguments against their use are that they may mask evidence of maternal infection (e.g., tachycardia) and that contractions associated with the membrane rupture may be indicative of uterine infection. Arguments for their use are that PROM is sometimes initially associated with evidence of uterine contractions, and time is gained for

pulmonary maturation. **In the presence of infection, tocolysis is usually unsuccessful.**

Use of Corticosteroids

There is a decreased incidence of RDS in infants who are born with PPROM 16 to 72 hours after membrane rupture, presumably owing to the endogenous release of corticosteroids from the stress of decreased amniotic fluid. Perhaps for this reason, the National Institutes of Health (NIH) guidelines for glucocorticoid therapy recommend they be given to patients with PPROM only up to 32 weeks' gestation, rather than up to 34 weeks' gestation, when membranes are intact.

Outpatient Management

After inpatient observation for 2 to 3 days without any evidence of infection, outpatient management can be considered in an attempt to reduce the incidence of late preterm births (34 to 37 weeks). **To be eligible for such management, the patient should be reliable, fully informed regarding the risks involved, and prepared to participate in her own care.** The fetus should be presenting as **a vertex**, and the **cervix should be closed** to minimize the chance of cord prolapse. At home, restricted physical activity is advised, no coital activity should occur, and the patient must monitor her temperature at least 4 times per day. Instructions should be given to return immediately if the temperature exceeds 100°F (37.8°C).

The patient should be seen weekly, at which time her temperature should be taken, nonstress testing performed after 28 weeks, and the baseline fetal heart rate and AFI evaluated. Ultrasonic evaluation of fetal growth should also be carried out every 2 weeks. **Any patient with oligohydramnios is not a candidate for outpatient management.**

Labor and Delivery

The same considerations discussed under preterm labor apply to patients with PROM. The decrease in amniotic fluid that is sometimes seen can result in early cord compression and the presence of variable fetal heart decelerations. This is true of both vertex and breech presentations; therefore, there is a necessity for abdominal delivery in a large number of cases unless fluid replacement can be instituted by amnioinfusion.

■ Tests of Pulmonary Maturity

By far, the major determinant of successful extra-uterine existence is the ability of the neonate to maintain successful oxygenation. Pulmonary maturation involves changes in pulmonary anatomy in addition to alterations of physiologic and biochemical parameters. Beginning at about 24 weeks, the terminal bronchioles divide into three or four respiratory bronchioles. Type II pneumocytes, which are important in surfactant synthesis, begin to proliferate during this phase.

Surfactant is required for successful lung function in the fetus and is a complex mixture of phospholipids, neutral lipids, proteins, carbohydrates, and salts. It is important in decreasing alveolar surface tension, maintaining alveoli in an open position at a low internal alveolar diameter, and decreasing intraalveolar lung fluid. **Synthesis takes place in the type II pneumocytes by incorporation of choline, and significant recycling seems to occur by resorption and secretion.**

Initially, the important phospholipid was thought to be phosphatidylcholine (lecithin), but it is apparent that other components, such as phosphatidylinositol (PI) and phosphatidylglycerol (PG), are also important. These substances are produced and secreted in increasing amounts as gestation advances, and the continued egress of tracheal fluid into the amniotic fluid results in their increasing presence near term.

Measurement of these substances in the amniotic fluid obtained by amniocentesis allows prediction of the risk for development of RDS in the neonate. Lecithin (L) levels increase rapidly after 35 weeks' gestation, whereas sphingomyelin (S) levels remain relatively constant after this gestational age. The lecithin and sphingomyelin concentrations are measured by thin-layer chromatography and are expressed as the L/S ratio. The presence of blood or meconium in the amniotic fluid will affect the L/S ratio; meconium will decrease it, and blood will normalize it to a value of 1.4.

LUNG PROFILE

Using two-dimensional thin-layer chromatography, both PG and PI can be measured. Along with the L/S ratio, these make up the lung profile. RDS is rare when the L/S ratio is greater than 2 and PG is present, whereas when the L/S ratio is less than 2 and no PG is present, more than 90% of infants develop RDS. **When the L/S ratio indicates pulmonary immaturity (L/S < 2), but PG is present, fewer than 5% of infants develop RDS.** The lung profile offers a more reliable predictor of pulmonary maturity, especially in infants of diabetic mothers. Other advantages of using PG are that contamination with vaginal secretions or blood, as occurs in cases of ruptured membranes and vaginal pool sampling, does not interfere with the detection of PG.

RAPID TESTS FOR FETAL LUNG MATURITY

A rapid test to assess fetal lung maturity, which could then be followed up with the more standard tests, provides a very useful clinical tool. One such test is the **lamellar body number density (LBND) assessment,** performed using an electronic cell counter (Coulter), which is gaining increased interest and use. This test can be completed within 2 hours by any hospital clinical laboratory. Normal ranges have been developed and depend on the individual laboratory (maturity ≥ 46,000 μL LBND), and the sensitivity and predictive value are as good as if not better than the standard L/S ratio.

▓ *Surfactant Therapy*

RDS in preterm infants is caused by a lack of surfactant. Production of surfactant by type II pneumocytes may be induced by corticosteroids and thyroid-releasing hormone, but many premature infants still develop RDS. Several human studies using instillation of surfactant into the pulmonary tree immediately after delivery have shown dramatic improvements in lung mechanics and the survival of infants. A wide variety of surfactant preparations are now available, including synthetic surfactants and surfactants derived from animal sources.

▓ *Intrauterine Growth Restriction*

Intrauterine growth restriction (IUGR) by definition occurs when the birth weight of a newborn infant is below the 10th percentile for a given gestational age. The terms small for gestational age (SGA) and IUGR, should not be used synonymously. SGA merely indicates that a fetus or neonate is below a defined reference range of weight for a gestational age, whereas IUGR refers to a small group of fetuses or neonates whose growth potential has been limited by pathologic processes in utero, with resultant increased perinatal morbidity and mortality. **Growth-restricted fetuses are particularly prone to problems such as meconium aspiration, asphyxia, polycythemia, hypoglycemia, and mental retardation, and they are at greater risk for developing adult-onset conditions such as hypertension, diabetes. and atherosclerosis.**

ETIOLOGY

The causes of IUGR can be grouped into three main categories: maternal, placental, and fetal. Combinations of these are frequently found in pregnancies with IUGR.

Maternal

Maternal causes include poor nutritional intake, cigarette smoking, drug abuse, alcoholism, cyanotic heart disease, and pulmonary insufficiency. In recent years, the **antiphospholipid syndrome** (autoantibody production) has been identified as a cause of IUGR in some women, both with and without hypertension. Antiphospholipid antibodies such as lupus-like anticoagulant and anticardiolipin antibodies are autoimmune (acquired) conditions, which contribute to the formation of vascular lesions in both the uterine and the placental vasculature that may result in impaired fetal growth and demise. Recently, several **hereditary thrombophilias** have been identified, which have been associated with a greater risk for IUGR, abruption, and preeclampsia. These conditions result in vascular lesions within the spinal arteries supplying the placenta. Identification and treatment with low-dose heparin and low-dose aspirin have been shown to reduce the risk for IUGR.

Placental

This category is representative of circumstances in which there is inadequate substrate transfer because of placental insufficiency. **Conditions that lead to this state include essential hypertension, chronic renal disease, and pregnancy-induced hypertension.** If the latter occurs late in pregnancy and is not accompanied by chronic vascular or renal disease, significant IUGR is unlikely to occur. A small fraction of IUGR cases may be attributed to placental or cord abnormalities (e.g., velamentous cord insertion).

Fetal

In this case, inadequate or altered substrate is present. Examples of fetal causes include **intrauterine infection** (listeriosis and TORCH [*t*oxoplasmosis, *o*ther infections, *r*ubella, *c*ytomegalovirus infection, and *h*erpes simplex] agents) and **congenital anomalies.**

CLINICAL MANIFESTATIONS

Two types of fetal growth restriction have been described: symmetrical and asymmetrical. In fetuses with symmetrical growth restriction, growth of both the head and the body is inadequate. The head-to-abdominal circumference ratio may be normal, but the absolute growth rate is decreased. Symmetrical growth restriction is most commonly seen in association with intrauterine infections or congenital fetal anomalies. **When asymmetrical growth restriction occurs, usually late in pregnancy, the brain is preferentially spared at the expense of abdominal viscera.** As a result, the head size is proportionally larger than the abdominal size. The liver and fetal pancreas undergo the most dramatic anatomic and biochemical changes, and these changes are now thought to play an important role in programming the fetus for a greater risk for obesity and diabetes later in life (see Chapter 1).

DIAGNOSIS

Growth restriction may go undiagnosed unless the obstetrician establishes the correct gestational age of the fetus (Box 12-2), identifies high-risk factors from the obstetric database, and serially assesses fetal growth by fundal height or ultrasonography. **Fetal or neonatal IUGR is usually defined as weight at or below the 10th percentile for gestational age.**

BOX 12-2 *Factors Evaluated in Dating a Pregnancy*

- Accuracy of the date of the last normal menstrual period
- Evaluation of uterine size on pelvic examination in the first trimester
- Evaluation of uterine size in relation to gestational age during subsequent antenatal visits (concordance or size-for-dates discrepancy)
- Gestational age when fetal heart tones were first heard using a Doppler ultrasonic device (usually at 12-14 wk)
- Date of quickening (usually 18-20 wk in a primigravida and 16-18 wk in a multigravida)
- Sonographic measurement of fetal length (crown-rump) in first trimester (most accurate)

Serial uterine fundal height measurements should serve as the primary screening tool for IUGR. A more thorough sonographic assessment should be undertaken when (1) the fundal height lags more than 3 cm behind a well-established gestational age or (2) the mother has a high-risk condition such as preexisting hypertension; chronic renal disease; advanced diabetes with vascular involvement; preeclampsia; viral disease; addiction to nicotine, alcohol, or hard drugs; or the presence of serum lupus anticoagulant or antiphospholipid antibodies.

Recently, interest has focused on the prediction of patients at risk for IUGR at mid-pregnancy. Patients with abnormal triple screens (alpha-fetoprotein, human chorionic gonadotropin [hCG], and estriol [E3]) who do not have abnormal fetuses by ultrasound and amniocentesis may be at risk for IUGR. In addition, elevations of umbilical artery and uterine artery Doppler assessments (increased resistance) as early as mid-pregnancy are associated with a greater risk for IUGR as pregnancy progresses.

At present, a number of sonographic parameters are used to diagnose IUGR: (1) biparietal diameter (BPD), (2) head circumference, (3) abdominal circumference (Figure 12-1), (4) head-to-abdominal circumference ratio, (5) femoral length, (6) femoral length–to–abdominal circumference ratio, (7) amniotic fluid volume, (8) calculated fetal weight, and (9) umbilical and uterine artery Doppler. Of these, the abdominal circumference is the single most effective parameter for predicting fetal weight because it is reduced in both symmetrical and asymmetrical IUGR. Most formulas for estimating fetal weight incorporate two or more parameters to reduce the variance of measurements.

During advancing gestation, the head circumference remains greater than the abdominal circumference until about 34 weeks, at which point the ratio approaches 1 (Figure 12-2). **After 34 weeks, the normal pregnancy is associated with an abdominal circumference that**

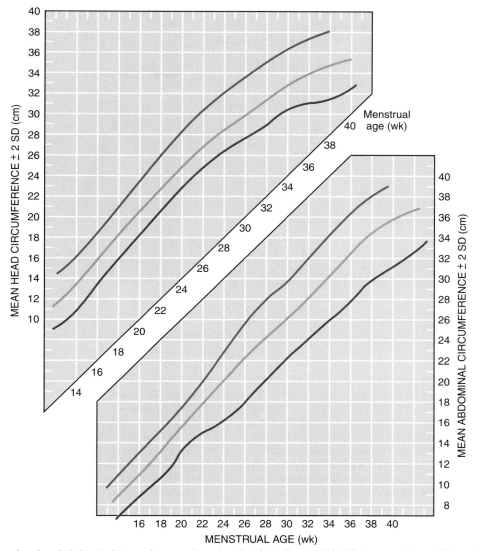

FIGURE 12-1   Mean head and abdominal circumferences (*green*) with 5th (*red*) and 95th (*blue*) percentile confidence limits between 16 and 40 weeks' menstrual age. (*Adapted from Campbell S, Griffin D, Roberts A, et al: Early prenatal diagnosis of abnormalities of the fetal head, spine, limbs, and abdominal organs. In Orlandi C, Polani PE, Bovicelli L [eds]: Recent Advances in Prenatal Diagnosis: Proceedings of the First International Symposium on Recent Advances in Prenatal Diagnosis, Bologna, September 15-16, 1980. New York, John Wiley & Sons, 1980.*)

is greater than the head circumference. When asymmetrical growth restriction occurs, usually in the third trimester, the BPD is essentially normal, whereas the ratio of head to abdominal circumference is abnormal. **With symmetrical growth restriction, the head-to-abdominal circumference ratio may be normal**, but the absolute growth rate is decreased, and estimated fetal weight is reduced.

From 50% to 90% of infants with manifestations of IUGR at birth can be identified with serial prenatal ultrasonography. The accuracy depends on the quality of the assessments, the criteria used for diagnosis, and

the effect of interventions applied when this diagnosis is made. For example, it is not unusual to observe an improvement in fetal growth after interventions such as work stoppage, bed rest, dietary modification, and curtailment of the use of tobacco, hard drugs, and alcohol.

It is worthwhile to plot out each serial measurement on a standard growth curve. For example, a fetus measuring near the 10th percentile in mid-gestation may continue to grow along that curve (SGA) or, conversely, may fall well below the 10th percentile (IUGR) later in pregnancy.

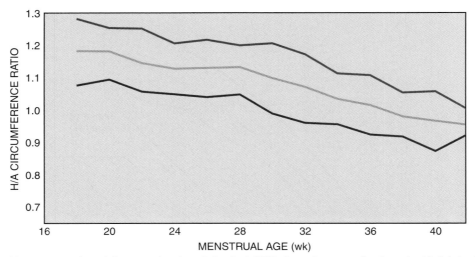

FIGURE 12-2   Graphic representation of the mean head-to-abdominal (H/A) circumference ratios (*green*) with 5th (*red*) and 95th (*blue*) percentile confidence limits from 17 to 42 weeks' menstrual age. *(From Campbell S, Thomas A: Ultrasound measurement of the fetal head to abdominal circumference ratio in the assessment of growth retardation. Br J Obstet Gynaecol 84:165, 1977.)*

MANAGEMENT

Prepregnancy

An important part of preventive medicine is to anticipate risks that can be modified before a woman becomes pregnant. Improving nutrition and stopping smoking are two approaches that should improve fetal growth in women who are underweight, who smoke, or both. **For women with antiphospholipid antibodies associated with the delivery of a prior IUGR infant, low-dose aspirin (81 mg/day) in early pregnancy may reduce the likelihood of recurrent IUGR.** For patients with one of the hereditary thrombophilias, low-dose heparin (5000 U twice daily) with or without low-dose aspirin has also been shown to reduce the risk for recurrent IUGR.

Antepartum

Once a fetus has been identified as having decreased growth, attention should be directed toward modifying any associated factors that can be changed. Because **poor nutrition and smoking** exert their main effects on birth weight in the latter half of pregnancy, cessation of smoking and improved nutrition can have a positive impact. The working woman who becomes fatigued is more likely to have a low-birth-weight infant. Work leave, or in some cases of maternal disease, hospitalization, will increase uterine blood flow and may improve the nutrition of the fetus at risk.

   The objective of clinical management is to expedite delivery before the occurrence of fetal compromise, but after fetal lung maturation has been achieved. This requires regular fetal monitoring with a twice-weekly nonstress test (NST) and biophysical profile. Most institutions use a modified biophysical profile that includes an NST and AFI. The oxytocin challenge test (OCT) is rarely used because its false-positive rate approaches 50%.

   Fetuses clinically suspected of IUGR could be approached as follows:
1. For cases in which results of fetal monitoring are normal and ultrasonic findings strongly suggest normal growth, no clinical intervention is warranted.
2. **For cases in which ultrasonic findings strongly suggest IUGR, with or without abnormal fetal surveillance, delivery is indicated at gestational ages of 34 weeks or later, or at any reasonable gestational age if pulmonary maturity is documented.** In the presence of severe oligohydramnios, amniocentesis may not be safe or feasible. Delivery should be strongly considered without assessing lung maturity because these fetuses are at great risk for asphyxia, and the stress associated with IUGR usually accelerates fetal pulmonary maturity.
3. For those cases in which ultrasonic findings are equivocal for IUGR, bed rest, fetal surveillance, and serial ultrasonic measurements at 3-week intervals are indicated.

   A simple technique is available whereby a pregnant woman can help in the assessment of fetal well-being. She assesses **fetal movement** (kick counts) each evening while resting comfortably on her left side. If she does not perceive 10 movements in 1 hour, she is instructed to call her healthcare provider to schedule a biophysical assessment. Some providers instruct their patients, irrespective of their risk, to begin a fetal kick count chart during the last trimester of pregnancy.

Doppler-derived umbilical artery systolic-to-diastolic ratios are abnormal in IUGR fetuses. Fetuses with growth restriction tend to have increased resistance to flow and to demonstrate low, absent, or reversed diastolic flow This noninvasive technique can be used to evaluate high-risk patients and may help in the timing of delivery when used in conjunction with the modified biophysical profile (see Chapter 7 for more information about Doppler assessment of fetal well-being).

LABOR AND DELIVERY

IUGR per se is not a contraindication for induction of labor, but there should be a low threshold to perform a cesarean birth because of the poor capacity of the IUGR fetus to tolerate asphyxia. As a result, **during labor, these high-risk patients must be electronically monitored to detect the earliest evidence of fetal distress.**

A combined obstetric-neonatal team approach to delivery is mandatory because of the likelihood of neonatal asphyxia.

After birth, the infant should be carefully examined to rule out the possibility of congenital anomalies and infections. **The monitoring of blood glucose levels is important because the fetuses do not have adequate hepatic glycogen stores, and hypoglycemia is a common finding.** Furthermore, hypothermia is not uncommon in these infants. **Respiratory distress syndrome is more common in the presence of fetal distress** because fetal acidosis reduces surfactant synthesis and release.

PROGNOSIS

The long-term prognosis for infants with IUGR must be assessed according to the varied etiologies of the growth restriction. If infants with chromosomal abnormalities, autoimmune disease, congenital anomalies, and infection are excluded, the outlook for these newborns is generally good. However, the IUGR infant is at greater risk for adult-onset diseases such as hypertension, diabetes, and atherosclerosis (see Chapter 1).

▥ *Postterm Pregnancy*

The prolonged or postterm pregnancy is one that persists beyond 42 weeks (294 days) from the onset of the last normal menstrual period. **Estimates of the incidence of postterm pregnancy range from 6% to 12% of all pregnancies.**

Perinatal mortality is 2 to 3 times higher in these prolonged gestations. Much of the increased risk to the fetus and neonate can be attributed to development of the **fetal postmaturity (dysmaturity) syndrome, which occurs when a growth-restricted fetus remains in utero beyond term.** Occurring in 20% to 30% of postterm pregnancies, **this syndrome is related to the aging and infarction of the placenta,** resulting in placental

insufficiency with impaired oxygen diffusion and decreased transfer of nutrients to the fetus. Some of these fetuses meet the criteria for having IUGR and should not have been allowed to advance to term. If evidence of intrauterine hypoxia is present (such as meconium staining of the umbilical cord, fetal membranes, skin, and nails), perinatal mortality is even further increased.

The fetus with postmaturity syndrome typically has loss of subcutaneous fat, long fingernails, dry and peeling skin, and abundant hair. The 70% to 80% of postdate fetuses not affected by placental insufficiency continue to grow in utero, many to the point of **macrosomia (birth weight greater than 4000 g). This macrosomia often results in abnormal labor, shoulder dystocia, birth trauma, and an increased incidence of cesarean birth.**

ETIOLOGY

The cause of postdate pregnancy is unknown in most instances. Prolonged gestation is common in association with an anencephalic fetus and is probably linked to the lack of a fetal labor-initiating factor from the fetal adrenals, which are hypoplastic in anencephalic fetuses. **Prolonged gestation may also be associated rarely with placental sulfatase deficiency and extrauterine pregnancy.** Paternal genes, as expressed by the fetus, play a role in the timing of birth and the risk for repeating a prolonged pregnancy.

DIAGNOSIS

The diagnosis of postterm pregnancy is often difficult. The key to appropriate classification and subsequent successful perinatal management is the accurate dating of gestation. It is estimated that **uncertain dates are present in 20% to 30% of all pregnancies**; hence, the importance of early and accurate assessment of gestational age cannot be overemphasized.

MANAGEMENT

Antepartum

The appropriate management of prolonged pregnancy revolves around **identification of the low percentage of fetuses with postmaturity syndrome** who are truly at risk for intrauterine hypoxia and fetal demise. When biophysical tests of fetal well-being are available, the time of delivery for each patient should be individualized. **However, if the gestational age is firmly established at 42 weeks, the fetal head is well fixed in the pelvis, and the condition of the cervix is favorable, labor usually should be induced.**

The two clinical problems that remain are (1) patients with good dates at 42 weeks' gestation with an unripe cervix, and (2) patients with uncertain gestational age seen for the first time with a possible or probable diagnosis of prolonged pregnancy.

In the first group of patients, a twice-weekly NST and biophysical profile should be performed. The AFI is an important ultrasonic measurement that should also be used in the management of these patients. The AFI is the sum of the vertical dimensions (in centimeters) of amniotic fluid pockets in each of the four quadrants of the gestational sac. **Delivery is indicated if there is any indication of oligohydramnios (AFI ≤ 5) or if spontaneous fetal heart rate decelerations are found on the NST.** So long as these parameters of fetal well-being are reassuring, labor need not be induced unless the cervical condition becomes favorable, the fetus is judged to be macrosomic, or there are other obstetric indications for delivery.

Some institutions begin weekly testing at 41 weeks to avoid missing the few fetuses who are stressed before 42 weeks. **At 42 weeks' gestation with firm dates, delivery is initiated by the appropriate route, regardless of other factors,** in view of the increasing potential for perinatal morbidity and mortality.

When the patient presents very late in gestation for initial assessment of prolonged pregnancy, but the gestational age is in question and fetal assessment is normal, an expectant approach is often acceptable. The risk of intervention with the delivery of a preterm infant must be considered. The woman herself can participate in the fetal assessment by doing fetal kick counts during the postterm period.

Intrapartum

Continuous electronic fetal monitoring must be employed during the induction of labor. The patient should be encouraged to lie on her left side. **The fetal membranes should be ruptured as early as is feasible in the intrapartum period so that internal electrodes can be applied and the color of the amniotic fluid assessed.** Cesarean birth is indicated for fetal distress. It should not be delayed because of the decreased capacity of the postterm fetus to tolerate asphyxia and the increased risk for meconium aspiration. If meconium is present, neonatal asphyxia should be anticipated, and a neonatal resuscitative team should be present at delivery.

▓ *Intrauterine Fetal Demise*

Intrauterine fetal demise (IUFD) is fetal death after 20 weeks' gestation but before the onset of labor. It complicates about 1% of pregnancies. With the development of newer diagnostic and therapeutic modalities over the past two decades, the management of IUFD has shifted from watchful expectancy to more active intervention.

ETIOLOGY

In more than 50% of cases, the etiology of antepartum fetal death is not known or cannot be determined. Associated causes include hypertensive diseases of pregnancy, diabetes mellitus, erythroblastosis fetalis, umbilical cord accidents, fetal congenital anomalies, fetal or maternal infections, fetomaternal hemorrhage, antiphospholipid antibodies, and hereditary thrombophilias.

DIAGNOSIS

Clinically, fetal death should be suspected when the patient reports the absence of fetal movements, particularly if the uterus is small for date or if the fetal heart tones are not detected using a Doppler device. Because the placenta may continue to produce hCG, a positive pregnancy test does not exclude an IUFD.

Diagnostic confirmation has been greatly facilitated since the advent of ultrasonography. **Real-time ultrasonography confirms the lack of fetal movement and absence of fetal cardiac activity.**

MANAGEMENT

Fetal demise between 14 and 28 weeks allows for two different approaches: watchful expectancy and induction of labor.

Watchful Expectancy

About 80% of patients experience the spontaneous onset of labor within 2 to 3 weeks of fetal demise. The patient's feeling of personal loss and guilt may create such anxiety, however, that this conservative approach may prove unacceptable. Thus, in general, the management of women who fail to go into labor spontaneously is active intervention by induction of labor or dilation and evacuation (D&E).

Induction of Labor

Justifications for such intervention include the **emotional burden** on the patient associated with carrying a dead fetus, the slight possibility of **chorioamnionitis**, and the **10% risk for disseminated intravascular coagulation** when a dead fetus is retained for more than 5 weeks in the second or third trimester.

Vaginal suppositories of prostaglandin E$_2$ (dinoprostone [Prostin E2]) can be used from the 12th to the 28th week of gestation. Dinoprostone is an effective drug with an overall success rate approaching 97%. Although at least 50% of patients receiving dinoprostone experience nausea and vomiting or diarrhea with temperature elevations, these side effects are transient and can be minimized with premedication (i.e., prochlorperazine [Compazine]). **There have been reported cases of uterine rupture and cervical lacerations**, but with properly selected patients, the drug is safe. The maximal recommended dose is a 20-mg suppository every 3 hours until delivery. Dinoprostone use in this range is contraindicated in patients with prior uterine incisions (e.g., cesarean, myomectomy) because of the unacceptable risk for uterine rupture. Furthermore, prostaglandins are contraindicated in patients with a history of bronchial asthma or active pulmonary disease, although the E series drugs act primarily as bronchodilators. **Misoprostol (Cytotec, a synthetic prostaglandin E$_1$ analogue) vaginal tablets** have been found to be quite effective with little or no gastrointestinal side effects, and they are less expensive than dinoprostone.

After 28 weeks' gestation, if the condition of the cervix is favorable for induction and there are no contraindications, misoprostol followed by oxytocin is the treatment of choice.

Monitoring of Coagulopathy

Regardless of the mode of therapy chosen, **weekly fibrinogen levels should be monitored during the period of expectant management, along with a hematocrit and platelet count.** If the fibrinogen level is decreasing, even a "normal" fibrinogen level of 300 mg/dL may be an early sign of consumptive coagulopathy in cases of fetal demise. An elevated prothrombin and partial thromboplastin time, the presence of fibrinogen-fibrin degradation products, and a decreased platelet count may clarify the diagnosis.

If laboratory evidence of mild disseminated intravascular coagulation is noted in the absence of bleeding, delivery by the most appropriate means is recommended. If the clotting defect is more severe or if there is evidence of bleeding, blood volume support or use of component therapy (fresh-frozen plasma) should be given before intervention.

FOLLOW-UP

A search should be undertaken to determine the cause of the intrauterine death. **TORCH (see Table 7-1) and parvovirus studies and cultures for *Listeria* are indicated.** In addition, **all women with a fetal demise** should be tested for the presence of anticardiolipin antibodies. Testing for the hereditary thrombophilias should also be considered. If congenital abnormalities are detected, fetal chromosomal studies and total body radiographs should be done, in addition to a complete autopsy. The autopsy report, when available, must be discussed in detail with both parents. In a stillborn fetus, the best tissue for a chromosomal analysis is the fascia lata, obtained from the lateral aspect of the thigh. The tissue can be stored in saline or Hanks' solution. **A significant number of cases of IUFD are the result of fetomaternal hemorrhage,** which can be detected by identifying fetal erythrocytes in maternal blood **(Kleihauer-Betke test).**

The parents may experience feelings of guilt or anger, which may be magnified when there is an abnormal fetus or genetic defect. Referral to a bereavement support group for counseling is advisable.

Subsequent pregnancies in a woman with a history of IUFD must be managed as high-risk cases.

SUGGESTED READING

American College of Obstetricians and Gynecologists: Antenatal corticosteroid therapy for fetal maturation. ACOG Committee Opinion No 273. Obstet Gynecol 99:871-873, 2002.

American College of Obstetricians and Gynecologists: Evaluation of stillbirths and neonatal deaths. ACOG Committee Opinion No 383. Obstet Gynecol 110:963-966, 2007.

Caritis S: Adverse effects of tocolytic therapy. Br J Obstet Gynaecol 112(Suppl 1):74-88, 2005.

Nardin JM, Carroli G, Alfirevic Z: Combination of tocolytic agents for inhibiting preterm labour (Protocol). Most recent amendment: 22 July 2006. Available at: http://www.thecochranelibrary.com.

National Center for Health Statistics: 2004 Final Nationality Data. March of Dimes Perinatal Data Center, 2007. Available at: http://www.marchofdimes.com/peristats.

Tucker J, McGuire W: Epidemiology of preterm birth. BMJ 329:675-678, 2004.

Chapter 13

Multifetal Gestation and Malpresentation

MARYAM TARSA • THOMAS R. MOORE

■ Multiple Gestation

Multiple gestation is defined as any pregnancy in which two or more embryos or fetuses occupy the uterus simultaneously. It is of utmost importance to recognize multiple gestation as a complication of pregnancy. **Because the mean gestational age of delivery of twins is about 36 weeks, the perinatal mortality and morbidity in multiple gestation exceeds that of singletons disproportionately.** Because of the additional physiologic stresses associated with two fetuses and placentas and a rapidly enlarging uterus, maternal morbidity is also increased.

ETIOLOGY AND CLASSIFICATION OF TWINNING

Multiple gestation occurs as the result of either the splitting of an embryo (i.e., **identical or monozygotic twinning**) or the fertilization of two or more eggs produced in a single menstrual cycle (i.e., **fraternal or dizygotic twinning**). Because **dizygotic twins** arise from separate eggs, they are structurally distinct pregnancies coexisting in a single uterus, each with its own amnion, chorion, and placenta. **Monozygotic twins** arise from cleavage of a single fertilized egg at various stages during embryogenesis, and thus the arrangement of the fetal membranes and placentas will depend on the time at which the embryo divides (Table 13-1). The earlier the embryo splits, the more separate the membranes and placentas will be. If division occurs within the first 72 hours of fertilization, the membranes will be **dichorionic, diamniotic** with a thick, four-layered intervening membrane. If division occurs after 4 to 8 days of development, when the chorion has already formed, **monochorionic, diamniotic** twins will evolve with a thin, two-layer septum. If splitting occurs after 8 days, when both amnion and chorion have already formed, the result will be **monochorionic, monoamniotic** twins residing in a single sac with no septum. Of all monozygotic twins, 30% are dichorionic, diamniotic, and 69% are monochorionic, diamniotic. Only 1% of twins are monoamnionic. Because twins share a sac in this type, without an intervening membrane, the risk for umbilical cord entanglement is high, resulting in a net mortality in these twins of almost 50% (Figure 13-1).

INCIDENCE AND EPIDEMIOLOGY

Twins account for about 3.5% of all U.S. births. The frequency of **monozygotic** twinning, which depends on a very infrequent biologic event (embryo splitting), is constant in all populations studied at about 1 in 250 births. However, **the frequency of dizygotic twinning, which arises from multiple ovulations in the mother, is strongly influenced by family history, ethnicity, and maternal age.** A family history of dizygotic but not monozygotic twins in the maternal pedigree increases the likelihood of dizygotic twinning in subsequent generations. In western Nigeria, twinning occurs in 1 in 22 gestations, whereas in the Native American and Inuit populations, twinning is less than one fifth of that rate.

TABLE 13-1	
RELATIONSHIP BETWEEN TIMING OF CLEAVAGE AND NATURE OF MEMBRANES IN TWIN GESTATIONS	
Time of Cleavage*	**Nature of Membranes**
0-72 hr	Dichorionic, diamniotic
4-8 days	Monochorionic, diamniotic
9-12 days	Monochorionic, monoamniotic

*Time interval between ovulation and cleavage of the egg.

MONOCHORIONIC TWIN PLACENTATION   DICHORIONIC TWIN PLACENTATION

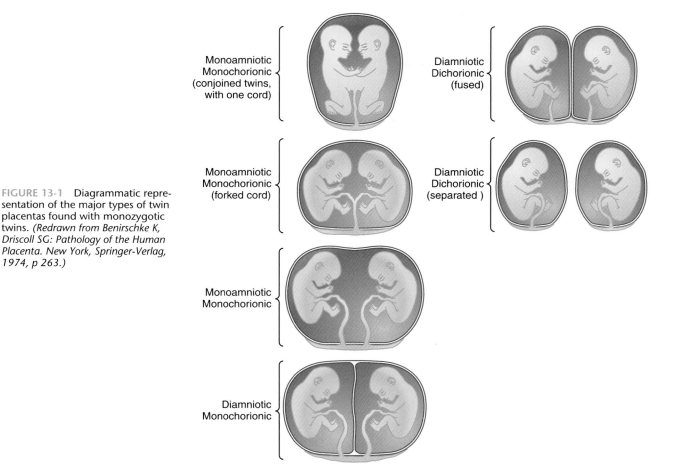

Monoamniotic
Monochorionic
(conjoined twins,
with one cord)

Diamniotic
Dichorionic
(fused)

Monoamniotic
Monochorionic
(forked cord)

Diamniotic
Dichorionic
(separated)

Monoamniotic
Monochorionic

Diamniotic
Monochorionic

FIGURE 13-1   Diagrammatic representation of the major types of twin placentas found with monozygotic twins. *(Redrawn from Benirschke K, Driscoll SG: Pathology of the Human Placenta. New York, Springer-Verlag, 1974, p 263.)*

Twins are twice as common in women over 35 years of age as in women at 25 years of age. Given these statistics, about **two thirds of spontaneously conceived twins are fraternal,** and one third are identical (monozygotic). However, in recent years, the incidence of multizygotic multifetal gestation has increased markedly with the more widespread use of ovulation induction agents and the practice of transferring multiple embryos after in vitro fertilization. The incidence of multiple gestation with the use of clomiphene is about 6% to 8%, and it is about 20% to 30% following gonadotropin therapy.

DETERMINATION OF ZYGOSITY

The prognosis and expected morbidity with twins is strongly dependent on zygosity: monozygotic twins are more likely to involve congenital anomalies, weight discordancy, twin-twin transfusion syndrome (TTTS), neurologic morbidity, premature delivery, and fetal death. Thus, **determination of zygosity is the most important next step after multifetal pregnancy has been first diagnosed.**

Ultrasonographic evaluation of the pregnancy is frequently very helpful in determining zygosity. Imaging of discordant fetal gender confirms a dizygotic gestation. Visualization of a thick amnion-chorion septum is suggestive of dizygotic twins, as is the presence of a "peak" or inverted "V" at the base of the membrane septum (Figure 13-2A). Conversely, in monochorionic gestation, the dividing membrane is fairly thin (Figure 13-2B). Because an early embryonic split can infrequently result in dichorionic, diamniotic twins with separate placentas, these findings are not definitive. Similarly, in rare cases of postzygotic genetic events, monochorionic twins may be gender discordant. **Thus, confident diagnosis of zygosity may require detailed examination of the placenta after delivery.** Thirty percent of twins will be of different sex and are, therefore, dizygotic. Twenty-three percent have monochorionic placentas and are, therefore, monozygotic.

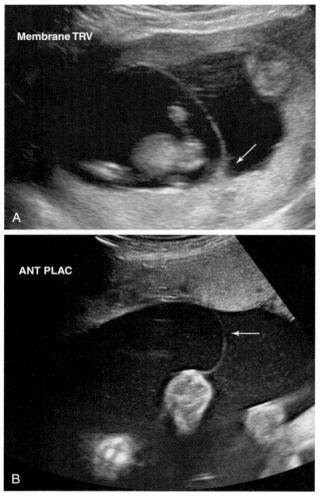

FIGURE 13-2   **A:** Real-time ultrasound with a thick vertical amnion-chorion septum (membrane) separating one twin on the left side from the second twin on the right. The *arrow* points to a "peak or inverted V" suggesting dizygotic twins. **B:** Ultrasound of a thin vertical membrane separating one twin on the left side from the second twin on the right, suggesting a monochorionic gestational sack.

Twenty-seven percent have the same sex, dichorionic placentas, but different blood groupings, and must be, therefore, dizygotic. **Twenty percent have the same sex, dichorionic placentas, and identical blood groupings. For the latter group, further studies, such as human leukocyte antigen (HLA) typing or DNA analysis, allow determination of zygosity.**

ABNORMALITIES OF THE TWINNING PROCESS

Among monozygotic multiple gestations, abnormalities in the twinning process are relatively common and include conjoined twins, interplacental vascular anastomoses, TTTS, fetal malformations, and umbilical cord abnormalities.

Conjoined Twins

If division of the embryo occurs very late (after 13 days, when the embryonic disk has completely formed), cleavage of the embryo will be incomplete, resulting in **conjoined twins.** Fortunately, this is a very rare event, occurring **once in 70,000 deliveries.** Conjoined twins are classified according to the anatomic location of the incomplete splitting: **thoracopagus** (anterior), **pygopagus** (posterior), **craniopagus** (cephalic), or **ischiopagus** (caudal). Most of such twins are thoracopagus. Delivery of conjoined twins frequently requires cesarean delivery, but postnatally, these gestations have a surprisingly optimistic prognosis in many cases. More advanced contemporary imaging has allowed detailed mapping of the shared organs and more successful surgical separation procedures.

Interplacental Vascular Anastomoses

Interplacental vascular anastomoses occur almost exclusively in monochorionic twins at a rate of 90% or more. The most common type is arterial-arterial, followed by arterial-venous and then venous-venous. **Vascular communications between the two fetuses through the placenta may give rise to a number of problems, including abortion, hydramnios, TTTS, and fetal malformations.** Overall, the incidence of both minor and major congenital malformations in twins is twice that in singletons, with the greater incidence of malformations occurring in monochorionic twins.

Twin-Twin Transfusion Syndrome

The presence of unbalanced anastomoses in the placenta (typically arterial-venous connections) leads to a syndrome in which one twin's circulation perfuses the other (i.e., TTTS) in about **10% of monozygotic twins.** In this syndrome, arterial blood from the "donor twin" enters the placenta (through the umbilical artery) and is taken up by the umbilical venous system belonging to the "recipient twin," which results in a net transfer of blood from the donor to the recipient twin. **Fetal complications include hypovolemia, hypotension, anemia, oligohydramnios, and growth restriction in the donor twin, and hypervolemia, hydramnios, hyperviscosity, thrombosis, hypertension, cardiomegaly, polycythemia, edema, and congestive heart failure in the recipient twin.** Both twins are at risk for demise from the circulatory derangement, and the pregnancy is predisposed further for preterm delivery due to uterine overdistention with hydramnios.

TTTS is diagnosed using ultrasound. Typically the donor twin is smaller and may have oligohydramnios, absent bladder, and anemia. The recipient, on the other hand, is larger with possible polyhydramnios, cardiomegaly, and ascites or hydrops (Figure 13-3).

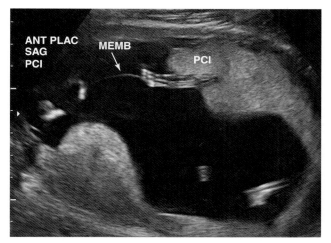

FIGURE 13-3 Ultrasound of a twin-twin transfusion syndrome, with one twin (*upper left*) in an amniotic cavity with a reduced fluid volume and a membrane (memb) separating this fetus from the second twin in an amniotic cavity with an excessive amount of fluid (*right and lower half of scan image*).

Given the poor prognosis of untreated TTTS (about 50% survival of either twin), **treatment with either serial amniocentesis and fluid reduction from the recipient twin's sac or laser photocoagulation of the anastomotic vessels** on the surface of the placenta is performed in specialized centers.

Fetal Malformations

Arterial-arterial placental anastomoses can result in fetal structural malformations. In this situation, the arterial blood from the donor twin enters the arterial circulation of the recipient twin, and the reversed blood flow may cause thrombosis within critical organs or atresias due to trophoblastic embolization. The recipient twin, being perfused in a reverse direction with relatively poorly oxygenated blood, fails to develop normally. This so-called **acardiac twin** typically has no anatomic structures cephalad of the abdomen but often has fully formed lower extremities.

Umbilical Cord Abnormalities

Abnormalities of the umbilical cord occur with a higher frequency in twins and are primarily associated with monochorionic twins. Absence of one umbilical artery occurs in about 3% to 4% of twins, as opposed to 0.5% to 1% of singletons. **The absence of one umbilical artery is significant because in 30% of such cases, it is associated with other congenital anomalies (e.g., renal agenesis).** Marginal and velamentous umbilical cord insertions also occur more frequently in twins and may cause growth abnormalities, particularly in the third trimester.

Retained Dead Fetus Syndrome

It is not unusual for one twin to die in utero remote from term, whereas the remaining twin and the pregnancy continue to be viable. Over time (after 3 weeks or more in pregnancies that have progressed beyond 20 weeks), the **retained dead fetus syndrome can develop, which involves disseminated intravascular coagulopathy in the mother** as a result of transfer of nonviable fetal material with thromboplastin-like activity into her circulation. In such cases, the maternal platelet count and fibrinogen level should be checked once a week to identify possible coagulation abnormalities. The dead fetus is reabsorbed if the demise occurs before 12 weeks' gestation. Beyond this time, the fetus shrinks and becomes dehydrated and flattened (**fetus papyraceus**).

ALTERED MATERNAL PHYSIOLOGIC ADAPTATION WITH MULTIPLE FETUSES

A number of normal maternal physiologic responses to pregnancy are exaggerated with multiple gestation. Whereas in normal pregnancy, maternal blood volume is augmented by 40% (2 L) over the nonpregnant baseline, in twins this increase may be 3 L or more. **The increased blood volume and demand for iron and folate increase the risk for anemia in the mother** and makes the patient less able to tolerate the stresses of infection, labor, and premature labor therapy. **Preeclampsia and gestational hypertension are almost doubled in multifetal gestation.** The increased uterine size associated with multiple fetuses can cause **maternal respiratory embarrassment, orthostatic hypotension due to compression of the vena cava and aorta, and compromise of renal function due to compression of the ureters.**

DIAGNOSIS

Historical factors such as a maternal family history of dizygotic twinning, the use of fertility drugs, a maternal sensation of feeling larger than with previous pregnancies, or a sensation of excessive fetal movements should raise the suspicion of twins. Physical signs, including excessive weight gain, excessive uterine fundal growth, and auscultation of fetal heart rates in separate quadrants of the uterus are suggestive but not diagnostic. An obstetric ultrasound should be performed when multiple gestation is suspected. **The diagnosis of multiple gestation requires a sonographic examination demonstrating two separate fetuses and heart activities and can be made as early as 6 weeks of gestation.**

ANTEPARTUM MANAGEMENT

Because of the high risk for preterm birth, intensive antepartum management schemes are directed at prolonging gestation and increasing birth weight in order to decrease perinatal morbidity and mortality.

Complications of Multiple Gestations

Maternal

Anemia
Hydramnios
Hypertension
Premature labor
Postpartum uterine atony
Postpartum hemorrhage
Preeclampsia
Cesarean delivery

Fetal

Malpresentation
Placenta previa
Abruptio placentae
Premature rupture of the membranes (PROM)
Prematurity
Umbilical cord prolapse
Intrauterine growth restriction (IUGR)
Congenital anomalies
Increased perinatal morbidity
Increased perinatal mortality

The complications of multiple gestation are shown in Box 13-1.

First and Second Trimesters

Between 16 and 22 weeks, the patient is seen every 2 weeks for ultrasonographic cervical length assessment because **incompetent cervix is more common with multiple gestations.** A suture (cerclage) can be placed in the cervix if marked shortening is noted in the absence of contractions, although the benefit of a cervical cerclage has been under scrutiny recently and is the subject of multiple clinical studies with conflicting findings. Adequacy of maternal diet is assessed due to the increased need for overall calories, iron, vitamins, and folate. The Institute of Medicine (IOM) recommends women with twins gain a total of 16.0 to 20.5 kg (35 to 45 lb) during the pregnancy. However, optimal weight gain is somewhat dependent on prepregnancy maternal body mass index (BMI) because obese women (BMI > 30) have better outcomes with less weight gain.

Third Trimester

During the third trimester, **prevention of prematurity is of utmost importance.** The cervix is monitored closely with ultrasonographic measurements for early effacement and dilation that may precede frank premature labor. A cervical length of less than 25 mm at 24 to 28 weeks is associated with doubling of the risk for premature birth. Interventions to prolong the length of twin pregnancy, such as bed rest, serial uterine activity monitoring, hospitalization,

and prophylactic tocolytic therapy, have been carried out but have not been consistently shown to prolong gestation. Nevertheless, most experts use a combination of these therapies, individualized for the patient's circumstances.

Discordant fetal growth, which is signified by one fetus flattening its growth rate, is a cause of morbidity and mortality. Fetal growth is monitored by ultrasound every 4 to 6 weeks beginning at 24 weeks, with additional fetal surveillance (e.g., biophysical testing, nonstress fetal heart rate assessment) when fetal growth falls below the normal curve. **The patient is monitored closely for signs of preeclampsia,** including the development of nondependent edema, urinary protein, and rising arterial blood pressure.

Because twins experience higher rates of stillbirth and growth restriction than singletons, **fetal well-being should be confirmed at least weekly by nonstress testing (NST) or biophysical profile (BPP) from 36 weeks onward,** and earlier in the presence of complications such as intrauterine growth restriction (IUGR), discordant growth, hypertension, or polyhydramnios. The contraction stress test (CST) is particularly useful in cases with IUGR or a nonreactive NST, but because these pregnancies are already predisposed to result in preterm labor, a CST should be used judiciously. The contraction stress test can be used in cases with IUGR or a nonreactive NST, but because these pregnancies are at risk for preterm labor, which could be initiated by a CST, an umbilical artery Doppler assessment should be considered instead.

Intrapartum Management

TREATMENT OF PRETERM LABOR

The treatment of preterm labor is discussed elsewhere, but multiple gestations present special challenges. **Relative contraindications to tocolysis in these pregnancies include a gestational age of 34 weeks or more, growth failure of one or more fetuses, concerning fetal status on biophysical monitoring, and preeclampsia.** Aggressive tocolysis typically involves use of agents with adverse cardiovascular effects in the mother, such as β-mimetics and magnesium sulfate and calcium channel blockers. These agents, particularly when combined with antenatal corticosteroid therapy, have been associated with maternal volume overload and congestive heart failure. Box 13-2 provides a list of necessary prerequisites for the management of labor in pregnancies complicated by multiple gestation.

In the special case of monoamniotic twins, delivery by cesarean birth is usually accomplished by 34 to 36 weeks because of the increased risk for lethal cord entanglement. For diamniotic twin pregnancies, delivery management is outlined later.

BOX 13-2 *Prerequisites for the Intrapartum Management of Multiple Gestation*

A secondary or tertiary care center
A delivery room equipped for immediate cesarean birth, if necessary
A well-functioning large-bore intravenous line (e.g., 16-gauge) for rapid administration of fluids and blood
Blood available for transfusion
The capability to continuously monitor the fetal heart rates simultaneously
An anesthesiologist who is immediately available to administer nitroglycerine or general anesthesia should intrauterine manipulation or cesarean birth be necessary for delivery of the second twin
Two obstetricians scrubbed and gowned for the delivery, one of whom is skilled in intrauterine manipulation and delivery of the second twin
Imaging techniques (i.e., sonography) for determining the precise presentations of the twins
Two pediatricians, one of whom is skilled in the immediate resuscitation of the newborn
An appropriate number of nurses to assist in the delivery and care of the newborn infants

BOX 13-3 *Causes of Perinatal Morbidity and Mortality in Twins*

Respiratory distress syndrome
Birth trauma
Cerebral hemorrhage
Birth asphyxia
Birth anoxia
Congenital anomalies
Stillbirths
Prematurity

VERTEX-VERTEX PRESENTATIONS

To choose the safest route of delivery for mother and babies, the presentations of the fetuses must be accurately known. By convention, the presenting twin is designated as twin A and the second twin as twin B. **Vertex (twin A)-vertex (twin B) presentation occurs most frequently (50% of the time),** followed by vertex-breech, breech-vertex, and breech-breech presentations.

Vertex-vertex twins are managed similarly to a singleton vertex presentation. Both fetal heart rates should be monitored continuously during labor. Oxytocin (Pitocin) can be used to manage hypotonic contractions. After delivery of the first twin, the cord is clamped (identified as twin A) and cut, but cord blood samples are not obtained until the second fetus has been delivered to prevent potential hemorrhage from the undelivered fetus through placental vascular anastomoses. A vaginal examination is then performed to assess the presentation and station of the second twin. If the second twin is still in a vertex presentation, spontaneous delivery is expected. If necessary, forceps or vacuum can be used to assist delivery of a vertex second twin. **Because the second twin is at increased risk for cord prolapse, abruptio placentae, and malpresentation, careful attention to fetal heart monitoring is necessary.**

After delivery of the second fetus, the cord blood samples are obtained, and the placenta is delivered. Care should be taken not to disrupt the fetal membranes because these will often reveal the zygosity of the twins. Following delivery of the placenta, uterine tone should

be closely monitored because the incidence of postpartum atony and hemorrhage is increased in multiple gestations.

MANAGEMENT OF OTHER PRESENTATIONS

Increased risk for fetal injury exists with delivery of a breech fetus. For this reason, **breech-breech and breech-vertex twins are usually delivered by cesarean birth.** When delivery of vertex-breech or vertex-transverse twins is contemplated, informed consent by the mother and skill of the obstetrician are determining factors in choosing between cesarean and vaginal delivery. **Although there is presently no scientific evidence that cesarean birth is superior for the vertex-breech presentation, difficulty in extracting the breech second twin can result in umbilical cord prolapse, head entrapment, neck injury, and asphyxia.** To avoid head entrapment an anesthesiologist can give IV or sublingual nitroglycerine to relex the uterus. Unless the obstetrician is comfortable with managing these problems, planned cesarean is the only reasonable choice.

PERINATAL OUTCOME

The high perinatal mortality rate in twin gestations (30 to 50 per 1000 births), which is about 5 times that in singleton gestations, **is largely attributable to prematurity and congenital anomalies** (Box 13-3). Birth asphyxia is also a significant factor, and thus it is not surprising that second twins have twice the perinatal mortality of first-born twins. **Compared with singletons, death from complications of birth trauma is 4 times more frequent with second-born twins and twice as frequent in first-born twins.** Congenital anomalies and stillbirths account for about one third of the perinatal mortality rate. **Stillbirths occur twice as frequently in twins as in singletons.** Cerebral hemorrhage, asphyxia, and anoxia account for one tenth of the overall perinatal mortality rate.

Twin gestations experience a fourfold increase in cerebral palsy. The increased morbidity in multiple gestations is related to placental, anatomic, and delivery abnormalities. **Low birth weight** (mean birth weight in twins is 2395 g vs. 3377 g for singletons), **prematurity, and IUGR may predispose to permanent brain injury.** The increased frequency of congenital anomalies and injuries during delivery (with both cesarean and vaginal routes) contributes to the increase in suboptimal outcome in newborns from multiple gestations. Postnatally, twins on average are shorter and lighter than singletons of similar birth weight until 4 years of age.

MULTIPLE GESTATION WITH MORE THAN TWO FETUSES

Although higher-order multiple gestations (triplets and higher) can result from embryo splitting and polyovulation, today **the most frequent cause is iatrogenic from the use of ovulation induction agents.** The incidence of spontaneous triplets is 1 in 8000 and that of spontaneous quadruplets 1 in 700,000 births. However, because of the widespread use of assisted reproductive technologies, current estimate of the incidence of triplets is 1 in 3000 births. This rate has tripled in the past two decades.

Prematurity increases as the number of fetuses increases. The average length of gestation is 33 weeks for triplets but only 29 weeks for quadruplets, with mean birth weights 1818 g and 1395 g, respectively. Theoretically, delivery of higher-order multiples can follow the principles outlined above for twins. However, in contemporary practice, almost all high-order multiples are delivered by cesarean birth to decrease the risk for morbidity in these very premature pregnancies. **The perinatal mortality rate for triplets and quadruplets is 50 to 100 per 1000 births, a rate that is twice that of twins.**

Fetal Malpresentation

The term *malpresentation* encompasses any fetal presentation other than vertex, including breech, face, brow, shoulder, and compound presentations. Both fetal and maternal factors contribute to the occurrence of malpresentation. The most common malpresentation is breech.

BREECH PRESENTATION

Breech presentation occurs when the fetal buttocks or lower extremities present into the maternal pelvis. **The incidence of breech presentation is 4% of all deliveries.** Before 28 weeks, about 25% of fetuses are in a breech presentation position. As the fetus grows and occupies more of the uterus, it tends to assume a vertex presentation to accommodate best to the confines and shape of the uterus. By 34 weeks' gestation, most fetuses have assumed the vertex presentation position.

Etiology

The major factor predisposing to breech presentation is prematurity. About 20% to 30% of all singleton breeches are of low birth weight (<2500 g). However, fetal structural anomalies (e.g., hydrocephalus) may restrict the ability of the fetus to present as a vertex. In breech presentations, the incidence of structural anomalies is greater than 6%, or 2 to 3 times that of a vertex. Other etiologic factors include uterine anomalies (e.g., bicornuate uterus), multiple gestation, placenta previa, hydramnios, contracted maternal pelvis, and pelvic tumors that obstruct the birth canal.

Classification

There are three types of breech presentation: **frank, complete, and incomplete or footling** (Figure 13-4). **Frank breech** occurs when both fetal thighs are flexed and both lower extremities are extended at the knees. **A complete breech** has both thighs flexed and one or both knees flexed (sitting in a "squat" position). **An incomplete (or footling) breech** has one or both thighs extended and one or both knees or feet lying below the buttocks. At term, 65% of breech fetuses are frank, 25% are complete, and 10% are incomplete.

Diagnosis

The diagnosis of breech presentation can often be made by the Leopold maneuvers (see Chapter 7, pg 86), in which the firm fetal head is palpated in the fundal region and the softer, smaller breech occupies the lower uterine segment above the symphysis pubis. In a frank breech in labor, the fetal buttocks, anus, sacrum, and ischial tuberosities can be palpated on vaginal examination. With a complete breech, the feet, ankles, and often the buttocks are palpable through the dilated cervix. Vaginal examination of an incomplete breech reveals one or both fetal feet but may require ultrasound for definitive diagnosis.

Pregnancy Management

EXCLUDE FETAL AND UTERINE ANOMALIES. If breech presentation is suspected after 34 weeks, the prenatal records and any prior ultrasonic examinations should be reviewed for the presence of uterine myomas, müllerian anomaly, or fetal structural abnormality. If suspicious, a thorough ultrasonic examination should be performed.

EXTERNAL CEPHALIC VERSION. External cephalic version (ECV) is a procedure in which the obstetrician manually converts the breech fetus to a vertex presentation through external uterine manipulation under ultrasonic guidance. ECV may be considered in a breech presentation at term before the onset of labor. Version is not carried out before 36 to 37 weeks' gestation because of the tendency for the premature fetus to revert

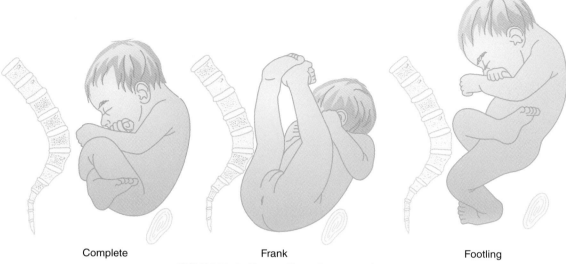

Complete   Frank   Footling

FIGURE 13-4   Types of breech presentation.

spontaneously to a breech presentation. The procedure must be carried out in a hospital that is equipped to perform an emergency cesarean section because of the small risk for placental abruption or cord compression. The patient should have nothing by mouth for 8 hours before the version attempt in case emergency delivery is necessary and should have an intravenous access. **Evidence of uteroplacental insufficiency, placenta previa, nonreassuring fetal monitoring, hypertension, IUGR, or oligohydramnios or a history of previous uterine surgery is a contraindication to external cephalic version.** The immediate success rate of external version is 35% to 76%. Although ECV has shown to decrease the rate of cesarean delivery, perinatal mortality rate has not been affected by this procedure. Only 2% of successful term versions revert to breech.

Labor Management

VAGINAL DELIVERY. Until the publication of randomized trials demonstrating that vaginal breech delivery is associated with increased perinatal mortality compared with planned cesarean birth, vaginal breech deliveries were performed in selected centers in patients who met strict criteria. These criteria are summarized in Box 13-4. **The standard of care now in most practices is to deliver all breeches by cesarean birth** to avoid the potential morbidities of umbilical cord prolapse, head entrapment, birth asphyxia, and birth trauma.

ASSISTED BREECH DELIVERY. Because the breech presentation can present in a setting in which cesarean birth is impossible or unsafe, vaginal delivery of the breech continues to be an important practitioner skill. Once the fetus has delivered spontaneously to the umbilicus

BOX 13-4   *Criteria for Vaginal Delivery of a Breech Presentation*

Fetus must be in a frank or complete breech presentation.
Gestational age should be at least 36 weeks.
Estimated fetal weight should be between 2500 and 3800 g.
Fetal head must be flexed.
Maternal pelvis must be adequately large, as assessed by x-ray pelvimetry,* or tested by prior delivery of a reasonably large baby.
There must be no other maternal or fetal indication for cesarean delivery.
Anesthesiologist must be in attendance.
Obstetrician must be experienced.
Assistant must be scrubbed and prepared to guide the fetal head into the pelvis.

---

*Inlet: anteroposterior (AP) diameter ≥ 11.0 cm; transverse diameter ≥ 10.0 cm. Midpelvis: AP diameter ≥ 11.5 cm; transverse diameter ≥ 10.0 cm.

(Figure 13-5A), gentle downward traction is exerted until the scapulae appear at the introitus (see Figure 13-5B). After delivery of the scapulae, the shoulders are delivered by sweeping each arm in turn across the fetal chest until only the fetal head remains undelivered (see Figure 13-5C). Once the shoulders have been delivered, the head is delivered by manual flexion of the fetal head with one hand flexing the head at the base of the skull while the operator's other hand is applied to the fetal maxilla for downward flexion (see Figure 13-5D). Some obstetricians use Piper forceps routinely because this method has been shown to result in

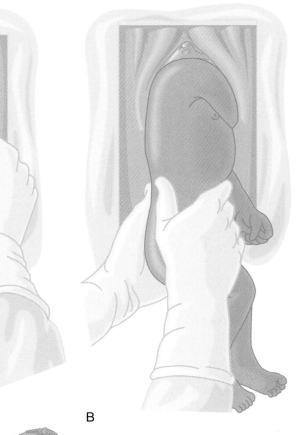

A

B

C

FIGURE 13-5 Partial breech extraction. **A:** After spontaneous delivery to the umbilicus, traction is applied to the infant's pelvis. When the scapulae are visible, rotation of the trunk allows delivery of the anterior shoulder. **B:** Delivery of the anterior shoulder by downward traction. **C:** Delivery of the posterior shoulder by upward traction. The posterior arm is freed digitally by splinting the fetal humerus (*inset*).

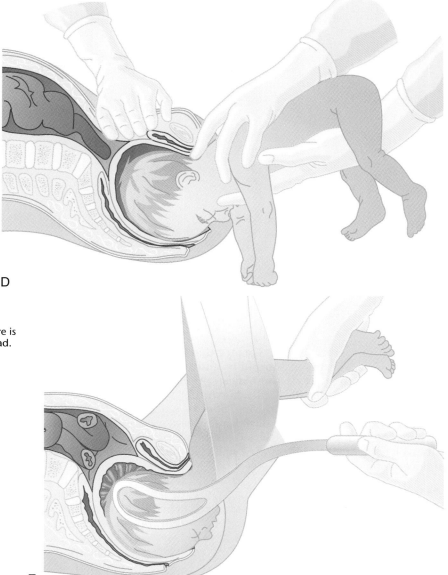

D

FIGURE 13-5, CONT'D **D:** Delivery of the aftercoming head using the Mauriceau-Smellie-Veit maneuver. Abdominal pressure is applied to maintain flexion of the fetal head. **E:** Delivery of the aftercoming head using Piper forceps.

E

delivery of the head with the least amount of trauma to the fetus (see Figure 13-5E).

Cesarean Delivery

During the process of breech vaginal delivery, successively larger parts of the fetus deliver, with the largest part, the fetal head, delivering last. In the very premature infant whose abdomen is much smaller than the head, the lower extremities, abdomen, and trunk may deliver through an incompletely dilated cervix, leaving the fetal head trapped and leading to fetal asphyxia and birth trauma. **Premature breech fetuses are thus preferentially delivered by cesarean birth because of the head-abdominal size disparity.** Cesarean delivery is currently preferred for both preterm and term breech infants, although significant trauma can still occur if care is not taken with delivery of the arms and head.

Complications and Outcome

Even with optimal management, the perinatal mortality of breech fetuses is about 25 per 1000 live births, vs. 12 to 16 per 1000 for nonbreech fetuses. When prematurity and multiple gestations are excluded, the perinatal mortality for breech fetuses is still significantly

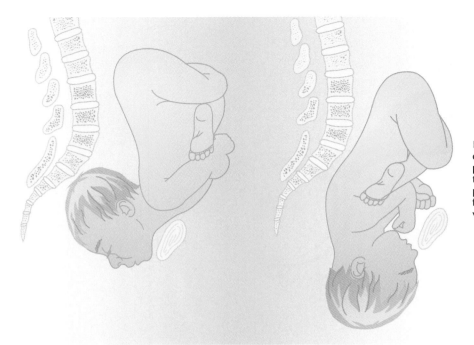

FIGURE 13-6   Spontaneous delivery of a mentum anterior face presentation. Note the flexion of the head under the symphysis pubis. The chin appears first, followed by the nose, brow, vertex, and occiput.

higher than for vertex fetuses. **Factors that contribute to increased perinatal morbidity and mortality include lethal congenital anomalies, prematurity, birth trauma, and asphyxia.** Asphyxia typically results from umbilical cord prolapse during labor or entrapment of the aftercoming head. Birth trauma can occur whenever forceful traction is exerted on the fetus and can involve the brachial plexus **(Erb's palsy)**, pharynx, and liver.

FACE PRESENTATION

Face presentation occurs when the fetal head is hyperextended such that the fetal face, between the chin and orbits, is the presenting part. **The incidence is about 1 in 500 deliveries.**

Etiology

The etiology of face presentation is somewhat enigmatic. During normal vertex delivery, the fetal head is markedly flexed, with the fetal occiput as the leading part. Factors that permit the fetus to enter the pelvis with a markedly extended head include extreme prematurity, high maternal parity, and congenital anomalies such as fetal goiter. In most, however, no etiologic factor is evident.

Diagnosis

The diagnosis of face presentation is usually made at the time of vaginal examination during labor, when the soft tissues of the fetal mouth and nose are noted adjacent to the malar bones and orbital ridges. Face presentation is then confirmed by sonography or by radiography. Because anencephalic fetuses uniformly present face first, **anencephaly should be ruled out when face presentation is suspected.**

Mechanism of Labor

The position of the presenting face is classified according to the location of the fetal chin (mentum). **About 60% of face presentations are mentum anterior at the time of diagnosis**, whereas 15% are mentum transverse and 25% mentum posterior. The mechanism of labor with a face presentation is similar to the vertex presentation in that the longest diameter (mentum to brow) enters the pelvis transversely. As labor proceeds and the face descends to the midplane, internal rotation occurs into the vertical axis. If the mentum rotates anteriorly under the symphysis pubis, vaginal delivery should be expected. Forceps, but not vacuum, can be applied to assist if prerequisites are met. However, **if the mentum rotates posteriorly, the fetal head will be unable to extend farther to complete the expulsive process.** Thus, mentum posterior cases and those with persistent mentum transverse must be delivered by cesarean birth. However, because final rotation from mentum transverse may occur only after a significant period of maternal pushing, patience is necessary. About half of the mentoposterior and mentotransverse presentations spontaneously rotate to a mentoanterior position. When delivered by spontaneous vaginal delivery (Figure 13-6) or low forceps (Figure 13-7), perinatal morbidity and mortality for face presentations are similar to those for vertex presentations.

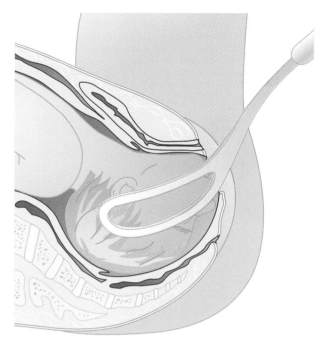

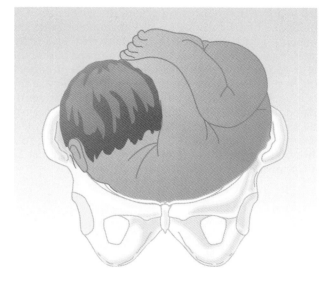

FIGURE 13-9   Shoulder presentation. Note the transverse lie of the fetus with the back down, which cannot be delivered vaginally.

FIGURE 13-7   Simpson forceps applied to a mentum anterior face presentation.

Other Presentations

Brow presentation occurs when the presenting part of the fetus is between the facial orbits and anterior fontanelle (Figure 13-8). This type of presentation arises as the result of extension of the fetal head such that it is midway between flexion (vertex presentation) and hyperextension (face presentation). **The incidence is about 1 in 1400 deliveries. With a brow presentation, the presenting diameter is the supraoccipitomental diameter,** which is much longer than the presenting diameter for a face or a vertex presentation.

The intrapartum management is expectant because the brow presentation is an unstable one. Fifty percent to 75% will convert to either a face presentation, through extension, or a vertex presentation, through flexion, and will subsequently deliver vaginally. **With a persistent brow presentation, the large presenting diameter makes vaginal delivery impossible, unless the fetus is very small or the maternal pelvis is very large, and delivery must be accomplished by cesarean birth.** There is an increased incidence of both prolonged labor (30% to 50%) and dysfunctional labor (30%). As with face presentations, midpelvic delivery and methods to convert the brow presentation to a vertex presentation are contraindicated. Perinatal morbidity and mortality are similar to those for vertex presentations.

A **compound presentation** occurs when a fetal extremity (usually the hand) prolapses alongside the presenting part (the head) and both parts enter the maternal pelvis at the same time. This presentation

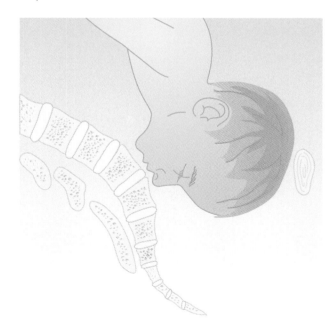

FIGURE 13-8   Brow presentation. Note the large presenting diameter (occipitomental).

occurs more frequently with premature gestations. The incidence of a hand or arm prolapsing alongside the presenting fetal head is 1 in 700 deliveries, and management is expectant. Usually, the prolapsed part of the fetus does not interfere with labor. If the arm prolapses, it is best to wait to see if it moves out of the way as the head descends. If it does not, the arm may be gently pushed upward while the head is simultaneously pushed downward by fundal pressure. If the complete extremity prolapses and the fetus then converts to a **shoulder presentation** (Figure 13-9), delivery must be accomplished by cesarean birth.

SUGGESTED READING

American College of Obstetricians and Gynecologists: Committee Opinion No. 265: Mode of term single breech delivery. Obstet Gynecol 98:1189-1190, 2001.

American College of Obstetricians and Gynecologists: Multiple gestation: Complicated twin, triplet, and high-order multifetal pregnancy. ACOG Practice Bulletin No. 56. Obstet Gynecol 104:869-883, 2004.

Cruikshank DP: Intrapartum management of twin gestations. Obstet Gynecol 109:1167-1176, 2007.

Schmitz T, Carnavalet C de C, Azria E, et al: Neonatal outcomes of twin pregnancy according to the planned mode of delivery. Obstet Gynecol 111:695-703, 2008.

Chapter 14

Hypertensive Disorders of Pregnancy

LONY C. CASTRO

The hypertensive disorders of pregnancy are major contributors to maternal and perinatal morbidity and mortality. **In the mother, they can cause multiorgan system dysfunction including renal failure, hepatic failure, central nervous system (CNS) hemorrhage and stroke, pulmonary edema, placental abruption and disseminated intravascular coagulation (DIC). Fetal and neonatal complications include growth restriction, prematurity, and perinatal death.** The Centers for Disease Control and Prevention (CDC) have reported that preeclampsia/eclampsia is the third leading cause of maternal mortality in the United States, primarily due to CNS hemorrhage. The combined incidence of hypertensive disorders in pregnancy varies depending on the population being studied and on the criteria used but is reported to range from 12% to 22%, whereas the preeclampsia/eclampsia syndrome occurs in about 5% to 8% of pregnancies.

■ Classification and Definitions

The general classification of hypertensive disorders recommended by the Working Group Report on High Blood Pressure in Pregnancy (2000) and adopted by the American College of Obstetricians and Gynecologists (ACOG) in 2002 is listed in Box 14-1. **Toxemia should not be used** because it represents the entire spectrum of hypertensive disorders of pregnancy and may also refer to isolated proteinuria.

Blood pressure readings vary depending on maternal position and the gestational age of the pregnancy. Maternal blood pressure tends to be lower in the left lateral decubitus position and higher in the sitting position. In the supine position, some pregnant women have elevated pressures, whereas others have supine hypotension due to compression of the vena cava by the uterus. In addition to positional variations, arterial blood pressure normally declines during the first and second trimesters of pregnancy and rises to prepregnant levels in the third trimester.

The diagnosis of hypertension should be reserved for patients with a systolic blood pressure of greater than or equal to 140 mm Hg or a diastolic pressure of greater than or equal to 90 mm Hg. Blood pressure measurements should be taken in the sitting position after the woman has rested at least 10 minutes. Arterial pressures may also be taken in the lateral decubitus position, but the measurements should be corrected to the level of the right atrium. In the hospitalized patient, either sitting or lateral decubitus measurements may be used, but consistency is advised. The length of the blood pressure cuff should be at least 1.5 times the circumference of the upper arm, and the fifth Korotkoff sound (disappearance) should be used for determining diastolic pressure.

PREECLAMPSIA/ECLAMPSIA

Preeclampsia is a syndrome unique to pregnancy, characterized by the new onset of hypertension and proteinuria in the latter half of gestation. Preeclampsia is classically considered to be a disease affecting the first pregnancy, but it also occurs in multiparas, especially if there are predisposing risk factors such as twins, diabetes mellitus, chronic hypertension, or a change in husband/partner. **When it arises in the early second trimester (14 to 20 weeks), a hydatidiform mole or choriocarcinoma should be considered.**

The following two criteria are essential for the diagnosis of preeclampsia: (1) the development of hypertension (systolic blood pressure ≥ 140 mm Hg or diastolic blood pressure ≥ 90 mm Hg), **in a woman whose blood pressures were previously normal, after the 20th week**

BOX 14-1 *General Classification of Hypertensive Disorders of Pregnancy*

- Preeclampsia or eclampsia (hypertension and proteinuria unique to pregnancy)
- Chronic hypertension
- Chronic hypertension with superimposed preeclampsia
- Gestational or transient hypertension

Based on the National Institutes of Health Working Group Report on High Blood Pressure in Pregnancy, 2000.

BOX 14-2 *Criteria for Severe Preeclampsia*

- Severe hypertension (systolic blood pressure ≥ 160 mm Hg, or diastolic blood pressure ≥ 110 mm Hg) at rest, on two occasions at least 6 hr apart
- Heavy proteinuria (at least 5 g in a 24-hr collection or a qualitative value of 3+ in urine samples collected 4 hr apart)
- Oliguria (<500 mL in 24 hr)
- Cerebral or visual disturbances
- Pulmonary edema or cyanosis
- Epigastric or right upper quadrant pain
- Impaired liver function (elevated liver enzymes)
- Thrombocytopenia
- Fetal growth restriction

Data from American College of Obstetricians and Gynecologists: Practice Bulletin No. 33. Washington, DC, ACOG, 2002.

of pregnancy; (2) **the development of new-onset proteinuria after the 20th week of gestation. Proteinuria is defined as more than or equal to 0.3 g protein in a timed 24-hour urine collection.** This usually correlates with a urinalysis report of 30 mg/dL (1+ on dipstick) or greater on a clean-catch urine sample.

In the past, a 30-mm Hg rise in systolic blood pressure or a 15-mm Hg rise in diastolic pressure was considered a sign of preeclampsia. Because of the previously described physiologic rise in blood pressure during the third trimester and the frequent lack of accurate prepregnant blood pressures for use as a baseline, this rise is no longer considered diagnostic if the blood pressure remains under 140/90 mm Hg. Despite this, **rising blood pressures should be of concern** because they may precede the development of the full preeclampsia syndrome. Similarly, **preeclampsia is often preceded by, or associated with, the development of generalized edema.** Dependent edema (edema of the lower extremities) is very common in normal pregnancies. Hand and facial edema are more likely to be associated with preeclampsia, but if unaccompanied by hypertension and proteinuria, they are not diagnostic of the preeclampsia syndrome.

Preeclampsia is divided into mild and severe forms, depending on the severity of the hypertension, the amount of proteinuria, and the degree to which other organ systems are affected. Box 14-2 lists specific criteria for the diagnosis of severe preeclampsia. If any of the symptoms, signs, or laboratory abnormalities listed in Box 14-2 is present in a woman with preeclampsia, it is very likely that she has severe disease, which is associated with much greater maternal and perinatal morbidity.

A variant of severe preeclampsia with particularly high morbidity is the HELLP syndrome. This syndrome occurs in preeclamptic women with evidence of *h*emolysis, *e*levated *l*iver enzymes, and *l*ow *p*latelets (thrombocytopenia). In contrast to more typical presentations of preeclampsia, the patient with HELLP syndrome is more likely to be multiparous, older than 25 years, and at less than 36 weeks' gestation.

Hypertension may be initially absent in 20% of the patients, whereas 30% will have mild elevations in blood pressure, and 50% will have severe elevations.

ECLAMPSIA

Eclampsia is the presence of tonic-clonic seizures in a woman with preeclampsia that cannot be attributed to other causes. Patients with severe preeclampsia are at the greatest risk for developing seizures, but the seizures can occur in so-called mild preeclamptic patients. Eclamptic seizures can also occur before the development of classic signs of preeclampsia. **There is a wide range in the reported frequency and timing of eclamptic seizures. Clinical practices,** including the use of magnesium sulfate intrapartum and postpartum for seizure prophylaxis in women with preeclampsia, as well as the timely recognition and delivery of women with severe preeclampsia, undoubtedly **influence these numbers. In a recent review of this subject, 38% to 53% of eclamptic seizures occurred before labor, 18% to 36% occurred during labor, and 11% to 44% occurred after delivery** (usually within the first 24 to 48 hours postpartum). When evaluating atypical cases of eclampsia (i.e., more than 48 hours postpartum or previous evidence of only mild disease) it is important to consider other causes of seizures such as underlying seizure disorder, hypertensive encephalopathy, metabolic abnormalities including hypoglycemia and hyponatremia, and CNS hemorrhage, thrombosis, mass, or infection.

CHRONIC HYPERTENSION

The diagnosis of chronic hypertension requires at least one of the following: known hypertension before pregnancy, development of hypertension before 20 weeks' gestation, or, in cases in which hypertension is first noted during pregnancy, persistence of elevated blood pressures greater than 12 weeks' postpartum.

Most pregnant women with chronic hypertension have essential hypertension, but **a small percentage have secondary hypertension** due to renal, vascular, endocrine, or behavioral causes (e.g., methamphetamine and cocaine use). Most of these conditions can be suspected on the basis of a thorough history and physical examination. Certain endocrine disorders, in particular hyperthyroidism, may present for the first time during pregnancy. Depending on the associated symptoms, signs, and response to medication, a workup to determine the etiology of the hypertension may be indicated. It is not uncommon for the physiologic stress of pregnancy to cause subclinical vascular or renal disease to become manifest. In these situations, it may be very difficult to differentiate between preeclampsia and an aggravated chronic hypertensive condition. Sometimes only careful follow-up postpartum will indicate the correct diagnosis.

CHRONIC HYPERTENSION WITH SUPERIMPOSED PREECLAMPSIA

Preeclampsia may become superimposed on chronic hypertensive disease. Superimposed preeclampsia can be very difficult to distinguish from poorly controlled chronic hypertension, especially if the woman is not seen until after the 20th week of gestation, but the two conditions are managed differently. In general, superimposed preeclampsia carries a worse prognosis than does either condition alone.

The diagnosis of superimposed preeclampsia should be reserved for those women with chronic hypertension who develop new-onset proteinuria (≥0.3 g in a 24-hour collection) after the 20th week of gestation. In pregnant women with preexisting hypertension and proteinuria, the diagnosis of superimposed preeclampsia should be considered if they experience sudden significant increases in blood pressure or proteinuria or any of the other signs and symptoms consistent with severe preeclampsia listed in Box 14-2, including thrombocytopenia or abnormally elevated liver enzymes.

GESTATIONAL HYPERTENSION

The diagnosis of gestational hypertension is made if hypertension without proteinuria first appears after 20 weeks' gestation or within 48 to 72 hours after delivery and resolves by 12 weeks postpartum. It is extremely difficult to differentiate this condition from the early stages of preeclampsia. A significant percentage of women with apparent gestational hypertension go on to develop proteinuria and the full preeclampsia syndrome at a later stage in pregnancy. Others have previously unrecognized chronic hypertension. **The diagnosis of gestational hypertension can only be made in retrospect, if the pregnancy has been completed without the development of proteinuria and if** the blood pressure has returned to normal before the 12th week postpartum.

Preeclampsia/Eclampsia

ETIOLOGY

Preeclampsia is called a "disease of theories," because genetic, immunologic, vascular, hormonal, nutritional, and behavioral factors have all been proposed as causes. No single, definitive "cause" has been identified, and the origins of the disease are considered to be multifactorial. **Because of the resolution of the preeclampsia after delivery, most attention has been focused on the placenta and the uterine-placental-fetal interface.**

Placental ischemia, or hypoxia, appears to be central to the development of the disease and has been attributed to failure of the cytotrophoblasts to adequately invade the uterine spiral arteries and establish the low-resistance uteroplacental circulation characteristic of normal pregnancy. Placental ischemia could also be due to underlying maternal vascular disease such as might occur in chronic hypertension, or to immunologically mediated placental vascular damage (see Chapter 6). Alternatively, ischemia could be caused by increased metabolic demand in the setting of a multiple gestation or a large singleton fetus.

It is postulated that uteroplacental ischemia results in oxidative stress leading to the production and release of toxins that enter the circulation and cause widespread inflammation, endothelial dysfunction, and activation of the coagulation system. The nature of these toxins has not yet been identified but may involve production of reactive oxygen and reactive nitrogen species. This is supported by the observation that preeclampsia is increased in pregnant women with underlying conditions such as obesity and diabetes that are associated with chronic inflammation and dyslipidemia. A hypoxic placenta may also shed microparticles derived from apoptosis of syncytiotrophoblasts, which can then lead to widespread endothelial injury. Antiangiogenic factors have also been shown to cause systemic hypertension, vascular injury, and activation of the coagulation system. Preeclamptic women have an imbalance in angiogenic and antiangiogenic proteins. **Circulating levels of the proangiogenic proteins** vascular endothelial growth factor (**VEGF**) and placental growth factor (**PlGF**) **are decreased,** whereas **levels of the antiangiogenic proteins** soluble fms-like tyrosine kinase 1 (**sFlt1**) **and soluble endoglin are markedly increased.** In animal models, overexpression of sFlt1 results in a preeclampsia-like syndrome.

Endothelial dysfunction leads to an imbalance between different classes of locally produced vasoconstrictors and vasodilators. Preeclampsia is associated with a disturbance in prostaglandin production, with a decrease in the ratio of the vasodilators prostaglandin E_2 (PGE_2) and prostacyclin to the vasoconstrictor PGF series and thromboxanes. **Endothelial changes also appear to involve a relative deficiency in the production of nitric oxide, a vasodilator and inhibitor of platelet aggregation, along with increased production of endothelin-I.** Endothelin-I is an extremely potent vasoconstrictor and activator of platelets. This shift in the production of locally acting vasoactive substances could enhance vasoconstriction in response to circulating pressor hormones.

The net effect of these processes would be widespread vasoconstriction leading to hypoxic and ischemic damage in different vascular beds, systemic hypertension, the HELLP syndrome (see later) or DIC, and worsening placental ischemia. The relative severity of the signs and symptoms of preeclampsia in any given individual would vary on the basis of which specific organ systems were most affected.

PATHOPHYSIOLOGY

Although the cause of preeclampsia is unknown, one of the primary underlying pathophysiologic abnormalities is generalized vasospasm. Cardiac output in untreated pregnant patients with preeclampsia is not significantly different from that of normal subjects in the last trimester of pregnancy, but systemic vascular resistance is significantly elevated.

Renal blood flow and glomerular filtration rate (GFR) are significantly lower than in patients with a normal pregnancy. The decrease in renal blood flow results from constriction of the afferent arteriolar system. **This afferent vasoconstriction may eventually lead to damage to the glomerular membranes, thereby increasing their permeability to proteins and leading to proteinuria.** The renal vasoconstriction and decrease in GFR also account for oliguria.

The cerebral vascular resistance is high in patients with preeclampsia and eclampsia. In hypertensive patients without convulsions, cerebral blood flow may remain within normal limits as a result of autoregulatory phenomena. In patients with convulsions, however, cerebral blood flow and oxygen consumption are significantly lower. Likewise, there is decreased blood flow and increased vascular resistance in the uteroplacental circulation, and color-flow Doppler studies suggest changes that are consistent with the development of increased vascular resistance.

Activation of the coagulation system (thought to be due at least in part to endothelial injury) is often clinically apparent with severe disease. The coagulation system abnormalities may be manifested by the HELLP syndrome (see later) or may accompany placental abruption. In addition, women with preexisting thrombophilias, either acquired or inherited, are at increased risk for developing preeclampsia.

PATHOLOGY

Three major pathologic lesions are classically associated with preeclampsia and eclampsia: (1) lack of decidualization of the myometrial segments of the spiral arteries; (2) glomerular capillary endotheliosis; and (3) ischemia, hemorrhage, and necrosis in many organs, presumably secondary to arteriolar constriction.

Under normal circumstances, the invasion of trophoblast results in the replacement of the muscular and elastic layers of the spiral arteries by fibrinoid and fibrous tissue, resulting in large, tortuous, low-resistance channels that extend through the myometrium. In preeclampsia, this change is mostly limited to the decidual segments of the vessels and may result in a 60% reduction in the diameter of the myometrial segment of a spiral artery. **The extent of placental infarction is increased in almost all preeclamptic pregnancies.**

The typical renal lesion of preeclampsia/eclampsia is *glomerular capillary endotheliosis,* **which is best seen by electron microscopy.** This disorder is manifested by marked swelling of the glomerular capillary endothelium and deposits of fibrinoid material in and beneath the endothelial cells. On light microscopy, the glomerular diameter is increased, with protrusion of the glomerular tufts into the neck of the proximal tubules and variable degrees of endothelial and mesangial cellular swelling.

Arteriolar vasospasm of relatively short duration (1 hour) can cause hypoxia and necrosis of sensitive parenchymal cells. Vasospasm of longer duration (3 hours) can lead to infarction of vital organs, such as the liver, placenta, and brain. In the liver, periportal necrosis and hemorrhage may occur, with subcapsular hematoma and hepatic rupture being rare complications. In the brain, focal areas of hemorrhage and necrosis may occur. In the retina, the clinical window to the arterial vasculature, vasospasm may be visualized on ophthalmoscopic examination. **Retinal hemorrhage is considered an extremely ominous sign** because it may signal similar phenomena in other vital organs.

CLINICAL AND LABORATORY MANIFESTATIONS

Many of the clinical and laboratory manifestations of preeclampsia and eclampsia can be explained on the basis of endothelial dysfunction, vasospasm, and activation of the coagulation system.

ANGIOTENSIN SENSITIVITY

One of the earliest signs of developing preeclampsia is a lowering of the effective pressor dose of infused angiotensin II. In normal pregnancy, the amount of angiotensin necessary to increase the diastolic pressure 20 mm Hg is increased, whereas in patients destined to develop preeclampsia, the effective pressor dose is lower.

WEIGHT GAIN AND EDEMA

Abnormal weight gain and edema occur early and reflect an expansion of the extravascular fluid compartment. This expansion is related to the endothelial injury and increased capillary permeability that allows fluid to diffuse from the intravascular to the extravascular space. Thus, many preeclamptic patients have an increase in total body fluid volume but are intravascularly volume depleted. **The hematocrit may also increase, reflecting the relative hypovolemia and hemoconcentration. For this reason, diuretic therapy is generally not advised unless there is evidence of pulmonary edema.**

ELEVATION OF BLOOD PRESSURE

The next sign usually detected is an elevation of blood pressure, particularly the diastolic pressure, which more closely mirrors changes in peripheral vascular resistance. In the antepartum period, the blood pressure changes may occur days to weeks after the onset of pathologic fluid retention.

PROTEINURIA

In the antepartum period, proteinuria may occur days or weeks after the onset of hypertension. If the disease first manifests during labor or in the immediate postpartum period, this progression of events is compressed into hours and sometimes minutes. The proteinuria of preeclampsia/eclampsia is likely due to afferent arteriolar constriction with increased glomerular permeability to proteins.

RENAL FUNCTION

The earliest change may be an increase in serum uric acid concentration. Creatinine clearance may decrease, and serum creatinine and blood urea nitrogen levels may rise. Renal involvement may progress to significant oliguria and frank renal failure.

COAGULATION SYSTEM

Thrombocytopenia is the most common abnormality. Although platelet counts tend to decline even in normal pregnancies, a value of less than 100,000 cells/mm^3 is clearly pathologic and, if accompanied by other signs of preeclampsia, is evidence of severe disease. **DIC may occur** especially if there is a placental abruption. **The specific combination of hemolysis (H), elevated liver function tests (EL), and low platelet levels (LP—the HELLP syndrome)** can occur without clinical manifestations of DIC and **is a sign of severe preeclampsia** even if blood pressures are normal or only minimally elevated.

LIVER FUNCTION

In the liver, vasospasm may result in focal hemorrhages and infarctions leading to right upper quadrant or epigastric pain and elevated serum enzyme levels (alanine aminotransferase and aspartate aminotransferase). Hepatic rupture is a rare, ominous complication of preeclampsia that is usually associated with the HELLP syndrome. When significant hemolysis is present, bilirubin levels are often elevated. Elevated alkaline phosphatase levels are frequently seen in pregnancy and are usually not of clinical significance because they are mostly due to placental production of this enzyme.

PLACENTAL FUNCTION

Vasospasm in the uteroplacental vascular bed may cause placental infarction and decreased uteroplacental perfusion. This ultimately leads to fetal compromise in the form of intrauterine growth restriction (IUGR), oligohydramnios, or fetal heart rate abnormalities. **Extensive placental infarctions can result in retroplacental hemorrhage or abruption,** which is an important cause of perinatal morbidity and mortality.

CENTRAL NERVOUS SYSTEM EFFECTS

Visual disturbances, such as blurred vision, spots, and scotomata, represent degrees of retinal vasospasm. Sudden loss of vision (cortical blindness) is due to occipital lobe ischemia. If the mother is expeditiously stabilized and delivered, full restoration of vision is likely to occur. A new-onset headache and **increased reflex irritability or hyperreflexia are extremely concerning signs** of CNS involvement and may connote imminent seizures.

◼ *Evaluation and Management of Preeclampsia*

There are three important questions the clinician must ask when managing a woman with preeclampsia. First, is the disease process mild or severe? Second, is there evidence of fetal compromise (i.e., growth restriction, oligohydramnios, or heart rate abnormalities)? Third, is the fetus mature enough for a reasonably uncomplicated course after delivery?

Delivery is the only definitive cure for preeclampsia, so it is always beneficial for the mother but may result in the delivery of a very preterm neonate. The goal of management is to decrease or prevent the maternal complications of severe preeclampsia, while minimizing the neonatal complications arising from prematurity. A woman with mild preeclampsia, without evidence of fetal compromise, whose disease does not appear to be progressing, will generally not be delivered unless the gestational age is 37 weeks or older, whereas **a woman with severe preeclampsia or eclampsia should usually be delivered after a period of stabilization, regardless of the gestational age of the fetus.**

The initial maternal assessment involves a complete medical history, physical examination, and laboratory evaluation. The history should focus on whether there is any past history of elevated blood pressures or renal disease, either before pregnancy or during previous pregnancies. The patient should be carefully questioned regarding symptoms of severe preeclampsia or its complications, including headache, visual changes, nausea, vomiting, abdominal or epigastric pain, and vaginal bleeding. Her medical record should be reviewed to determine when in the current pregnancy blood pressures started to rise and when proteinuria developed.

The physical examination should focus on the assessment of blood pressure, weight gain, edema, fundal height, and reflexes, and on a qualitative assessment of urinary protein excretion with a dipstick. In addition, findings consistent with severe preeclampsia such as epigastric or right upper quadrant tenderness, uterine tenderness, petechiae due to low platelets, and signs of pulmonary edema should be sought. If there is severe headache or visual symptoms, an ophthalmic examination may be indicated. The initial laboratory studies recommended are outlined in Box 14-3.

A careful fetal evaluation is also indicated. This should begin with an accurate determination of fetal gestational age based on clinical and sonographic data, if available. A fetal ultrasound should be performed to evaluate fetal growth, amniotic fluid index and the umbilical artery Doppler resistance index, or S/D ratio. **A nonstress test (NST) should also be done** to determine whether there is evidence of acute fetal compromise.

It is generally advisable to hospitalize patients with a presumed diagnosis of preeclampsia to determine the disease's severity and maternal and fetal stability. After the initial evaluation, **if the mother's disease is mild and if there is no evidence of fetal compromise, management consists of rest and observation.** There is no evidence that chronic antihypertensive therapy or diuretic therapy prevents the progression of mild preeclampsia to severe preeclampsia or improves maternal or fetal outcomes. Depending on the special circumstances surrounding each case, management can be carried out in the hospital or in some cases as an outpatient. The mother will require frequent reassessment of symptoms, blood pressure, and qualitative urine protein excretion along with weekly laboratory tests. The fetus needs to be followed with monitoring of fetal activity, heart rate reactivity, and amniotic fluid volume. **The patient should be delivered before she reaches 38 weeks, if she develops signs or symptoms of worsening disease, or if there is evidence of fetal compromise.**

If the initial evaluation is consistent with the diagnosis of severe preeclampsia, the patient should remain hospitalized for the remainder of the pregnancy. After 32 to 34 weeks' gestation, stabilization and delivery are appropriate for most patients. For those patients younger than 32 weeks with severe preeclampsia, the decision regarding delivery needs to be individualized after carefully weighing the risks to the neonate of prematurity vs. the potential maternal and fetal risks of continuing the pregnancy. Both the mother and fetus require very close monitoring with maternal laboratory parameters and fetal assessment testing repeated daily or more often if necessary. **In some instances, stabilization of the patient with bed rest, along with medical control of severe hypertension and corticosteroids for fetal lung maturity, will moderate the disease process and allow delivery to be delayed in the hope of advancing gestational age.** Deterioration in clinical status (e.g., uncontrollable hypertension, deteriorating renal function, pulmonary edema, evidence of HELLP or coagulopathy, CNS symptoms, abruption, or abnormal fetal testing) requires delivery.

INTRAPARTUM MANAGEMENT OF PREECLAMPSIA

Labor should be induced (or spontaneous labor allowed to continue) in the absence of obstetric indications for cesarean delivery such as failure to progress in labor, non-reassuring fetal status, or nonvertex presentation. The mother and fetus must be carefully monitored during labor and delivery. **Two of the most important maternal issues to be dealt with are seizure prophylaxis and control of hypertension.** Other potential maternal problems that may develop are oliguria, pulmonary edema, and thrombocytopenia or the HELLP syndrome.

If the fetus is growth restricted or if placental abruption occurs, the fetal heart rate tracing may show evidence of late decelerations, bradycardia, or other signs of fetal compromise necessitating cesarean delivery. In most instances, epidural anesthesia is the anesthetic of choice for operative delivery or pain relief during labor, unless there is evidence of coagulopathy.

SEIZURE PROPHYLAXIS

Because of the risk for seizures and their attendant morbidity and even mortality, a great deal of attention must be given to the level of CNS irritability. Peripheral

---

BOX 14-3   *Initial Laboratory Evaluation on a Patient with Preeclampsia*

- **Complete blood count, platelet count, lactate dehydrogenase:** If abnormal, order D-dimers, coagulation panel, and smear
- **Renal studies:** Serum blood urea nitrogen, creatinine, and uric acid; urinalysis; 24-hr urine for protein and creatinine
- **Liver function tests:** serum aspartate aminotransferase, alanine aminotransferase, and bilirubin

reflexes, particularly of the patella and ankle, are most extensively used as determinants of heightened instability. **In patients with preeclampsia, severe headaches and sustained clonus can be prodromal symptoms or signs of eclampsia.**

Seizure prophylaxis with magnesium sulfate should be instituted in most patients with preeclampsia during the intrapartum period and continued for about 24 hours after delivery, although the benefits in patients with mild preeclampsia are unproved. Patents with severe preeclampsia should have seizure prophylaxis instituted on admission and continued during the initial period of stabilization. If it is determined that they will not be delivered, the magnesium infusion can be stopped, restarted intrapartum, and continued for 24 hours postpartum or until there is evidence of resolution of the disease. **Randomized controlled trials have confirmed that magnesium sulfate is the agent of choice for the prevention and treatment of eclamptic seizures because it is efficacious and is associated with low neonatal morbidity.** Both intramuscular (IM) and intravenous (IV) routes are effective for prophylaxis, but the IM injections can be very painful.

Table 14-1 outlines the protocols for magnesium administration, and Table 14-2 reviews the relationship among serum magnesium concentrations, clinical response, and signs of toxicity. Therapeutic levels are generally accepted to be in the range of 4.8 to 9.6 mg/dL, but levels should not be allowed to rise above 7 to 8 mg/dL to avoid toxicity. **The magnesium ion is excreted exclusively through the kidneys, so careful monitoring of urine output is essential.** A magnesium overdose can have severe, even fatal, consequences. Magnesium should be given by a controlled infusion pump with a fail-safe mechanism to prevent errors in administration (i.e., inadvertent bolus infusion). **Serial assessments of urine output, deep tendon reflexes, and respirations are important for detecting signs of magnesium toxicity.** These clinical assessments should be supplemented with serial measurements of serum magnesium levels every 6 hours and arterial O_2 saturation through pulse oximetry. In a patient who has oliguria or a serum creatinine concentration of 1.1 or greater, maintenance infusion rates should be halved and serial magnesium levels measured every 2 hours. **Magnesium toxicity can occur even in a patient with apparently normal renal function.** Magnesium toxicity is treated by stopping infusion and administering calcium gluconate, 10 mL of a 10% solution, intravenously, and initiating resuscitative measures if necessary.

ANTIHYPERTENSIVE THERAPY

Arterial blood pressure greater than or equal to 160 mm Hg systolic or 105 mmHg diastolic must be treated promptly. In the setting of severe preeclampsia,

TABLE 14-1

ANTICONVULSIVE MAGNESIUM SULFATE THERAPY

Type of Treatment	Intravenous	Intramuscular
Prophylactic loading	4 g over 15-20 min	5 g in each buttock in 100 mL fluid
Maintenance	2 g/hr controlled IV infusion	5 g/4 hr infusion

TABLE 14-2

CLINICAL CORRELATES OF SERUM MAGNESIUM SULFATE LEVELS*

Clinical Response	Serum Levels (mg/dL)
Loss of patellar reflex	8-12
Warmth and flushing	9-12
Somnolence	10-12
Slurred speech	10-12
Paralysis and respiratory difficulty	15-17
Cardiac arrest	30-35

*Therapeutic range: 4.8-9.6.

blood pressures reaching these levels represent a hypertensive emergency. In some preeclamptic women, even elevations in the systolic blood pressure in the 150- to 159-mm Hg range require urgent treatment, especially those whose previous systolic blood pressures were in the 90- to 100-mm Hg range and who now have the HELLP syndrome or eclampsia. The goal of antihypertensive therapy in severe preeclampsia is to lower blood pressure carefully to prevent CNS hemorrhage. In general the blood pressure should not be lowered to "normal levels" or less than 130/80 mm Hg. **Caution must always be exercised to not lower the arterial pressure too much or too rapidly because either may result in decreased uteroplacental blood flow and fetal distress, which may necessitate emergent cesarean delivery in an unstable mother.**

The safest, most efficacious drugs for the acute control of severe hypertension complicating preeclampsia are **labetalol and hydralazine.** Although **hydralazine** has theoretical advantages over labetalol in that it is a direct vasodilator and does not induce bronchospasm, rapid bolus infusions are potentially more likely to induce precipitous hypotension. In general, either is acceptable, and their use will be determined by individual circumstances. Table 14-3 details the dosage, duration of action, and potential complications of these two drugs.

Oral **nifedipine** has been used successfully, starting at a dose of 10 mg orally and repeated in 20 to 30 minutes if necessary to a maximal dose of 30 mg. **Nifedipine should be used cautiously to avoid hypotension,** particularly when used in conjunction with magnesium

TABLE 14-3

EMERGENCY PARENTERAL THERAPY FOR SEVERE HYPERTENSION DURING PREGNANCY*

Agent	Action	Dose	Side Effects	Comment
Hydralazine	Direct vasodilator	5 mg IV over 1-2 min, then 5-10 mg IV every 20-30 min until blood pressure is 140-150/90-100 mm Hg. If no response after 25 mg, switch to another drug.	Headache, tachycardia, flushing, vomiting	Increases cardiac output and probably uterine and renal blood flow; has been drug of choice for short-term control historically.
Labetalol hydrochloride	Nonselective β_1- and α_1-blocker	Start with 20 mg IV bolus. If inadequate response after 10 min, give 40 mg IV followed by 80 mg IV every 10 min for two more doses if needed to lower blood pressure to 140-150/90-100 mm Hg. Total dose not to exceed 220 mg.	Nausea, vomiting, heart block, bronchoconstriction, dizziness	Increasing experience and efficacy reported; is current drug of choice in many centers. Avoid if evidence of asthma or acute heart failure occurs.

*Modification of Tables 21 and 23 from the Seventh Report of the Joint National Committee on Prevention, Detection, Evaluation, and Treatment of High Blood Pressure (JNC VII), 2004.

sulfate. Because of the potential for a precipitous drop in blood pressure, short-acting nifedipine is generally not advised in this setting. **Intravenous sodium nitroprusside has the advantage of providing minute-to-minute control of blood pressure** but may cause fetal cyanide toxicity with prolonged administration, so the use of this medication is generally limited to the postpartum period.

MANAGEMENT OF FLUID BALANCE

Accurately recorded intake and output data must be kept to calculate fluid requirements. **These patients experience vasoconstriction, have interstitial edema, and often demonstrate some degree of reduced intravascular volume, which may reduce urinary output.** In addition, they may be receiving several different therapeutic infusions, such as magnesium sulfate and oxytocin, which have a direct or indirect effect on urinary output.

The most common errors that occur in the management of these patients are fluid volume overload and excessive salt restriction. Water intoxication is rare with current management. The conservative approach is to replace documented output plus insensible loss with an appropriate electrolyte-containing fluid. Because of the multifaceted pathophysiology of this disease, central hemodynamic monitoring using a pulmonary artery catheter may aid in the management of refractory cases of oliguria or pulmonary edema.

MANAGEMENT OF ECLAMPSIA

Eclampsia is a true obstetric emergency, and all physicians involved in the care of pregnant women should be prepared to recognize the occurrence of an eclamptic seizure and begin initial resuscitative and stabilization efforts. The management of these patients should be carried out by a team of physicians and well-trained nurses in an isolated labor room, with minimal noise and not too much light. As with any seizure condition, the initial requirement is to protect the patient from injury, clear the airway, and give oxygen by face mask to relieve hypoxia. Blood pressure and pulse oximetry should be recorded every 10 minutes with the patient in the lateral position. A 16- to 18-gauge IV line should be placed for drawing blood and administering drugs and fluids. An indwelling catheter should be placed in the bladder and laboratory tests obtained as outlined in Box 14-3.

Pharmacologic stabilization consists of preventing recurrent convulsions and controlling hypertension. Randomized, controlled trials have confirmed that magnesium sulfate is the most efficacious drug for preventing recurrent eclamptic seizures and has the best safety profile for the mother and fetus. The administration of IV magnesium sulfate for the treatment of eclamptic seizures is similar to its prophylactic use as outlined in Table 14-1, except that the loading dose is generally increased from 4 to 6 g. The maintenance dose remains 2 g/hour if renal function appears normal. If diazepam (Valium) is used in addition to magnesium sulfate, personnel skilled in intubation should be readily available in case maternal respiratory depression occurs. In general, it is desirable to avoid polypharmacy.

Eclamptic seizures often induce a fetal bradycardia that usually resolves after maternal stabilization and correction of hypoxia. It is very important to stabilize the mother before any attempt is made to deliver the infant. Induction of labor or cesarean birth during the acute phase may aggravate the course of the disease. **Once hypoxia is corrected, convulsions controlled, and the diastolic blood pressures brought down to**

the 90- to 100-mm Hg range, delivery should be expedited, preferably by the vaginal route.

PROPHYLAXIS

At present there is no scientifically proven method for the prevention of preeclampsia. Although nutritional interventions have a sound theoretical and experimental basis, it is likely that dietary modifications and weight reduction will have to be implemented before conception in order to be successful. The current goal is to identify the disease early, monitor its effects on the mother and fetus, stabilize the patient if the disease is severe, and deliver the baby before there is evidence of major maternal or fetal morbidity.

MANAGEMENT OF CHRONIC HYPERTENSION

The major goals are to control hypertension and to detect the development of superimposed preeclampsia in the mother and IUGR in the fetus. In the patient with uncomplicated hypertension whose blood pressures are well controlled and who does not show signs of superimposed preeclampsia or fetal growth restriction, the outcome for both the mother and fetus should be good.

When a woman with chronic hypertension is first seen during the pregnancy, it is important to review previous records to determine whether she has essential hypertension or a secondary cause of high blood pressure. If no previous evaluations have been done, it may be appropriate to rule out some of the more common endocrine, renal, or cardiovascular causes of hypertension. Baseline laboratory tests similar to those outlined in Box 14-3, with the addition of an electrocardiogram (ECG), are useful. The purpose of these tests is to establish a baseline should the patient later develop superimposed preeclampsia as well as to look for evidence of end-organ dysfunction.

It is important to review the antihypertensive medications being taken and to discontinue any that are potentially teratogenic. **There is little evidence that lowering blood pressures below the 140/90 mm Hg range benefits the pregnancy.** In fact, lowering the blood pressure too much may result in decreased uterine perfusion pressure and iatrogenic fetal growth restriction. **In many women, blood pressures will decrease to normal in the second trimester, and no antihypertensive medication will be needed.**

As a general rule, the safest antihypertensive medication should be used at the lowest possible dose needed to keep blood pressures about 130/80 to 140/90 mm Hg. **Methyldopa** is considered to be the safest antihypertensive medication in pregnancy, and **calcium channel blockers** and **labetalol** are also considered to be safe. **Angiotensin-converting enzyme inhibitors and angiotensin II receptor blockers should be avoided at all stages of pregnancy because of** potential fetal toxicity. β-Blockers should be used with caution because they may cause fetal growth restriction and may affect the interpretation of the NST. In addition to pharmacologic control of blood pressure, the foundations of conservative management also include increased periods of rest in the lateral decubitus position. The risks and benefits of moderate exercise (i.e., walking) have not been well defined.

Because these pregnancies have a high incidence of IUGR, both early and serial sonographic examinations are indicated. The early ultrasound (before 12 weeks) is primarily for dating, and the 16- to 20-weeks ultrasound is for the assessment of fetal anomalies. Serial ultrasonic examinations (every 3 to 4 weeks after 24 to 28 weeks) are of great assistance in detecting growth restriction. Depending on the clinical circumstances, periodic fetal monitoring with NST and amniotic fluid assessment, supplemented by umbilical artery Doppler studies if there is evidence of IUGR or preeclampsia, may start as early as 26 to 28 weeks and should be commenced by 32 to 34 weeks in all hypertensive patients. **Maternal detection of daily fetal kick counts in the third trimester** or earlier are an important method of assessing fetal well-being.

A significant increase in hypertension or the development of proteinuria in a previously nonproteinuric patient with chronic hypertension are likely signs of superimposed preeclampsia. The incidence of superimposed preeclampsia varies from 15% to 25%. These patients should undergo repeat laboratory evaluation, as outlined in Box 14-3. Management should follow that outlined for severe preeclampsia.

The timing of delivery in the chronic hypertensive patient depends on the clinical circumstances. **For patients without evidence of fetal growth restriction in whom the blood pressure is well controlled and no signs of superimposed preeclampsia are present, a full-term gestation may be allowed, provided that fetal well-being is normal.** Any progression beyond the 40th week should be very carefully considered and probably avoided. The presence of growth restriction or blood pressure deterioration or the advent of proteinuria may dictate earlier delivery. If delivery is desirable but not imperative before 37 weeks, confirmation of fetal lung maturity should be obtained. **The route of delivery should be vaginal in the absence of obstetric reasons for cesarean delivery.**

Sequelae and Outcome

Uncomplicated mild preeclampsia at term in the primigravid patient carries essentially no long-term maternal sequelae. Such patients are at no greater risk for subsequent development of hypertensive cardiovascular disease than any other individual. However, patients with a pregnancy complicated by severe preterm preeclampsia are at higher risk for cardiovascular disease in later life and at very high risk for recurrent preeclampsia (up to 40%) in a subsequent pregnancy. Women with gestational hypertension also seem to have a higher incidence of developing chronic hypertension later in life. **The female offspring of preeclamptic women experience an increased risk for preeclampsia in their own pregnancies**, providing evidence of a genetic basis to the disease.

Pregnancy does not appear to affect the long-term prognosis in a patient with chronic hypertension. Some of the more serious complications of preeclampsia, such as cerebrovascular accidents and renal failure, may have long-term maternal sequelae. Overall, the mortality rate in women with hypertensive disease of pregnancy varies according to the severity of the disease, socioeconomic level, and quality of care received. Although at present there is no proven way of preventing preeclampsia, accessible, high-quality prenatal care should prevent most of the severe complications associated with the disease.

Fetal and neonatal sequelae are more difficult to determine because some of the morbidity and mortality associated with these hypertensive syndromes are related to IUGR, prematurity, and acute and chronic fetal distress. All of these may have long-term CNS effects.

SUGGESTED READING

American College of Obstetricians and Gynecologists: Chronic hypertension in pregnancy. ACOG Practice Bulletin No. 29. Clinical Management Guidelines for Obstetrician-Gynecologists, Washington, DC, ACOG, 2001.

American College of Obstetricians and Gynecologists: Diagnosis and management of pre-eclampsia and eclampsia. ACOG Practice Bulletin No. 33. Clinical Management Guidelines for Obstetrician-Gynecologists, Washington, DC, ACOG, 2002.

Berg CJ, Chang J, Callaghan WM, Whitehead SJ: Pregnancy-related mortality in the United States, 1991-1997. Obstet Gynecol 101:289-296, 2003.

Ilekis JV, Reddy UM, Roberts JM: Preeclampsia—a pressing problem: An executive summary of a National Institute of Child Health and Human Development workshop. Reprod Sci 14:508-523, 2007.

Joint National Committee: Seventh Report of the Joint National Committee on Prevention, Detection, Evaluation, and Treatment of High Blood Pressure (JNC VII), 2004.

Sibai BM: Diagnosis, prevention, and management of eclampsia. Obstet Gynecol 105:402-410, 2005.

Working Group Report on High Blood Pressure in Pregnancy: National High Blood Pressure Education Program. NIH Publication No. 00-3029, 2000.

Chapter 15

Rhesus Isoimmunization

LONY C. CASTRO

Rhesus (Rh) isoimmunization is an immunologic disorder that occurs in a pregnant, Rh-negative patient carrying an Rh-positive fetus. The immunologic system in the mother is stimulated to produce antibodies to the Rh antigen, which then cross the placenta and destroy fetal red blood cells.

◼ *Pathophysiology*

The Rh complex is made up of a number of antigens, **including C, D, E, c, e, and other variants, such as Dᵘ antigen.** More than 90% of cases of Rh isoimmunization are due to antibodies to D antigens. Therefore, this chapter is mainly limited to a discussion of the D antigen, although the same principles apply to any other antigen-antibody combination. A person who lacks the D antigen on the surface of the red blood cells is called "Rh negative," and an individual with the D antigen is considered "Rh positive."

Among African Americans, about 8% are Rh negative, whereas among white Americans, about 15% are Rh negative. **Only 1% to 2% of Asians and Native Americans are Rh negative. When Rh-negative patients are exposed to the Rh antigen, they may become sensitized.** Two mechanisms are proposed for this sensitization. The most likely mechanism is the occurrence of an undetected placental leak of fetal red blood cells into the maternal circulation during pregnancy. The other proposal is the "grandmother" theory. This theory suggests that an Rh-negative woman may have been sensitized from birth by receiving enough Rh-positive cells from her mother during her own delivery to produce an antibody response.

In general, two exposures to the Rh antigen are required to produce any significant sensitization, unless the first exposure is massive. The first exposure leads to primary sensitization, whereas the second causes an anamnestic response leading to the rapid production of immunoglobulins, which can cause a "transfusion reaction" or hemolytic disease of the fetus during pregnancy.

The initial response to exposure to Rh antigen is the production of immunoglobulin M (IgM) antibodies for a short period of time, followed by the production of IgG antibodies that are capable of crossing the placenta. If the fetus has the Rh antigen, these antibodies will coat the fetal red blood cells and cause hemolysis. If the hemolysis is mild, the fetus can compensate by increasing the rate of erythropoiesis. If the hemolysis is severe, it can lead to profound anemia, resulting in hydrops fetalis from congestive cardiac failure and intrauterine fetal death. High bilirubin levels can damage the central nervous system and lead to **neonatal kernicterus.** Before the widespread use of Rh immune globulin for prevention of Rhesus isoimmunization, neonatal kernicterus was one of the leading causes of cerebral palsy.

The fetal and maternal circulations are normally separated by the placental "barrier." Small hemorrhages occur in either direction across the intact placenta throughout pregnancy. With advancing gestational age, the incidence and size of these transplacental hemorrhages increase, with the largest hemorrhages usually occurring at delivery. **Most immunizations occur at the time of delivery, and antibodies appear either during the postpartum period or following exposure to the antigen in the next pregnancy.**

If a pattern of mild, moderate, or severe disease has been established with two or more previous pregnancies, the disease tends either to be of the same severity or to become progressively more severe with subsequent pregnancies. **If a woman has a history of fetal hydrops with a previous pregnancy, the risk for**

hydrops with a subsequent pregnancy is about 90%. Hydrops usually develops at the same time as, or earlier than, in the previous pregnancy.

Incidence

Although transplacental hemorrhage is very common, the incidence of Rh immunization within 6 months of the delivery of the first Rh-positive, ABO-compatible infant is only about 8%. In addition, the incidence of sensitization with the development of a secondary immune response before the next Rh-positive pregnancy is 8%. Therefore, the overall risk of immunization for the second full-term, Rh-positive, ABO-compatible pregnancy is about 1 in 6 pregnancies. The risk for Rh sensitization following an ABO-incompatible, Rh-positive pregnancy is only about 2%. The protection against immunization in ABO-incompatible pregnancies is due to the destruction of the ABO-incompatible cells in the maternal circulation and the removal of the red blood cell debris by the liver.

Transplacental hemorrhage may also occur before delivery. Establishment of the fetal circulation occurs at about 4 weeks' gestation, and the presence of the Rh D antigen has been demonstrated as early as 38 days after conception. Consequently, Rh isoimmunization can occur at any time during pregnancy, from the early first trimester on. In the first trimester, the most common causes of transplacental hemorrhage are spontaneous or induced abortions. **The incidence of immunization following spontaneous abortion is 3.5%, whereas that following induced abortion is 5.5%.** The risk is low in the first 8 weeks, but it rises to significant levels by 12 weeks' gestation. **The risk for immunization following ectopic pregnancy is about 1%. Transplacental hemorrhage can also occur in the setting of second- or third-trimester vaginal bleeding, after invasive procedures such as amniocentesis or chorionic villus sampling, after abdominal trauma, or after external cephalic version.** If necessary the amount of fetal blood entering the maternal circulation after an episode associated with transplacental hemorrhage can be estimated using the Kleihauer-Betke test (described later). **All pregnant Rh-negative women who are not sensitized to the D antigen should routinely receive prophylactic Rh immune globulin (Rh$_0$GAM) at 28 weeks of gestation, within 72 hours of delivery of an Rh-positive fetus, and at the time of recognition of any of the problems cited previously that are associated with transplacental hemorrhage.**

Detecting Fetomaternal or Transplacental Hemorrhage

The Kleihauer-Betke test is dependent on the fact that adult hemoglobin is more readily eluted through the cell membrane in the presence of acid than is fetal hemoglobin (HbF). The maternal blood is fixed on a slide with ethanol (80%) and treated with a citrate phosphate buffer to remove the adult hemoglobin. After staining with hematoxylin and eosin, the fetal cells can readily be distinguished from the empty maternal cells. All cells are then counted, and an estimate of the extent of the fetal to maternal hemorrhage (measured in milliliters) is made on the basis of the following equation:

$$\text{\# of fetal cells counted}/\text{\# of maternal cells counted} = \text{Estimated fetal blood volume (mL)}/$$

$$\text{Estimated maternal blood volume (mL)}$$

Recognition of the Pregnancy at Risk

A blood sample from every pregnant woman should be sent at the first prenatal visit for determination of the blood group and Rh type and for antibody screening. **In Rh-negative patients, whose anti-D antibody titers are positive (i.e., those who are Rh sensitized), the blood group and Rh status of the father of the baby should be determined. If the father is Rh negative, the fetus will be Rh negative, and hemolytic disease will not occur. If the father is Rh positive, his Rh genotype and ABO status should be determined.** This may be done by testing the father's red blood cells with the reagents available for the antigens D, E, C, e, and c. Newer molecular techniques are now available to assess fetal Rh genotype. If he is homozygous for the D antigen, every fetus he fathers will be Rh positive and could potentially be affected. If he is heterozygous, only half of his children will be affected. Information regarding the zygosity of the father is of value in absolutely predicting the presence or absence of the Rh antigen in the fetus if the father is homozygous and in signaling the potential need for fetal antigen testing if the father is heterozygous. About 56% of Rh-positive whites are heterozygous for the Rh D antigen. If it is not possible to test the antigen status and zygosity of the father, it must be assumed that he is antigen positive.

MATERNAL RH-ANTIBODY TITER

Anti-D antibody titers generally provide limited information regarding the severity of fetal hemolysis in Rh disease. However, many centers continue to use anti-D antibody titers to help guide their decision making regarding the initiation of testing procedures (e.g., amniocentesis, middle cerebral artery Doppler studies, and percutaneous umbilical blood sampling). The American College of Obstetricians and Gynecologists (ACOG) and other independent researchers have recommended that, **in an initially immunized pregnancy, the fetus is not in serious jeopardy if the titer remains below 1:16.** In patients with a positive titer less than 1:16, repeat titers should be obtained every 2 to 4 weeks.

If the titer rises to 1:16 or greater, a more detailed assessment and determination of fetal Rh status is indicated. The timing and methods of invasive testing will depend on the current clinical status of the fetus, the gestational age, and the patient's obstetric history. Titers are not generally useful for following a patient with a history of a previous fetus or neonate with hemolytic disease. In this setting, even if the titers are below the critical threshold, the patient should be followed and evaluated as if her titers were high.

TECHNIQUES FOR EVALUATING FETAL RH STATUS

In the United States, amniocentesis is the most commonly employed method to test fetal blood type in cases of a heterozygous paternal genotype. Most laboratories offering fetal red cell antigen typing on amniotic cells require an accompanying paternal blood sample, and with the discovery of an Rh D pseudogene in 21% of African Americans, a maternal blood sample should also be provided. Chorionic villus sampling has been used to determine fetal blood type but is discouraged because of the higher potential for transplacental hemorrhage and worsening fetal disease if the fetus is Rh D positive.

Flow cytometry has been successfully reported in sorting fetal cells from maternal blood. DNA amplification using a single fetal nucleated erythrocyte can be used to determine fetal Rh D blood type. Determination of free fetal DNA in maternal plasma or serum is another noninvasive test that is being increasingly used to detect fetal Rh D status.

ULTRASONIC DETECTION OF RH SENSITIZATION

Serial ultrasonic examinations of a woman with a fetus at risk for hemolytic disease can be a useful adjunct to amniocentesis in confirming fetal well-being and determining the advent of fetal hydrops. The examination should include a routine fetal assessment plus a determination of placental size and thickness and hepatic size. Both the placenta and the fetal liver are enlarged with hydrops. Fetal hydrops is easily diagnosed by the characteristic appearance of one or more of the following: ascites, pleural effusion, pericardial effusion, or skin edema. Appearance of any of these factors during an ultrasonic examination eliminates the need for diagnostic amniocentesis and necessitates therapeutic intervention based on fetal gestational age.

Doppler assessment of peak velocity in the fetal middle cerebral artery (MCA) in cm/sec has proved to be the most valuable tool for detecting fetal anemia. At-risk pregnancies should have this test performed every 1 to 2 weeks from 18 to 35 weeks of gestation. A fetal MCA peak systolic velocity (PSV) value above 1.5 multiples of the median for gestational age is predictive of moderate to severe fetal anemia and is an indication for percutaneous umbilical blood sampling for precise determination of fetal hemoglobin concentration. Intrauterine fetal transfusion should follow if indicated. After 35 weeks' gestation, this test may produce a higher false-positive rate (Figure 15-1), and amniotic fluid spectrophotometry may be indicated.

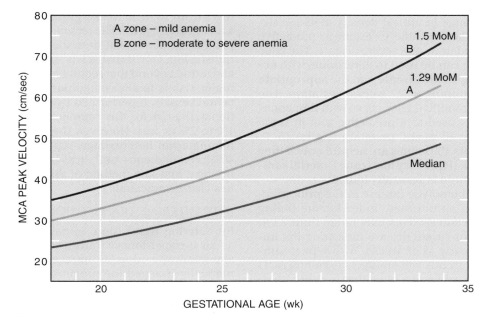

FIGURE 15-1   Middle cerebral artery (MCA) Doppler peak velocities based on gestational age. MoM, multiples of the median. *(Data from Moise KJ Jr: Management of rhesus alloisoimmunization. Obstet Gynecol 100:600-611, 2002.)*

AMNIOTIC FLUID SPECTROPHOTOMETRY

Before widespread use of MCA Doppler studies, analysis of amniotic fluid was the most frequently used method of gauging the severity of fetal hemolysis. It is still used in settings in which expertise in the performance of an MCA Doppler is not available, or occasionally, after 35 weeks of gestation. **There is an excellent correlation between the amount of biliary pigment in the amniotic fluid and the fetal hematocrit, beginning at 27 weeks' gestation.**

The most likely source of bilirubin in the amniotic fluid is tracheal and pulmonary efflux with some transudate from the umbilical and placental vessels. Because of the small concentrations found in the amniotic fluid, spectrophotometric analysis is the most widely used technique for estimating amniotic fluid bilirubin concentration.

The optical density deviation (ΔOD) at 450 μ from a baseline drawn between the optical density values at 365 and 550 μ forms a peak that can be used to calculate the change in ΔOD in nanomoles (nm) at 450 μ measuring the amniotic fluid unconjugated bilirubin, which correlates with the cord blood hemoglobin of the newborn at birth.

Bilirubin is oxidized to colorless pigments when it is exposed to light; therefore, the fluid should be protected from light. Heme pigments and meconium may cause falsely high spectrophotometric values.

Bilirubin is normally found in amniotic fluid in a concentration that gradually diminishes toward term. For predictive interpretation, Liley devised a spectrophotometric graph based on the correlation of cord blood hemoglobin concentrations at birth and the amniotic fluid change in optical density at 450 μ. Using this method, he was able to establish predictive zones for mild, moderate, and severe disease. **The Liley chart** (Figure 15-2) **can be used to determine, with accuracy, the severity of the disease and the appropriate management, beginning at 27 weeks' gestation.** The Queenan curve, a modified Liley curve with four zones instead of three, is used as a predictive tool in some centers from 14 to 40 weeks' gestation (Figure 15-3). **Because single ΔOD 450 values are helpful only if they are very high (zone III) or very low (zone I), serial sampling of amniotic fluid is generally indicated.**

The severity of hemolytic disease in the prior pregnancy provides an approximate index for the timing of the first amniocentesis. This may range from 22 to 30 weeks with prior severe disease indicating the initial procedure as early as 22 weeks. With repeat sampling one of three trends will emerge: (1) Falling ΔOD 450 values are indicative of a fetus that is either unaffected (e.g., Rh negative) or very mildly affected. No intervention is indicated in these patients (see Figures 15-1 and 15-2). (2) If the ΔOD 450 is either stable or rising, frequent ΔOD 450 determinations are necessary to determine the timing of delivery. (3) **If the ΔOD 450 enters zone III (refer to zone levels on the right side of** Figure 15-2) **before 34 weeks, percutaneous umbilical blood sampling is performed for determination of fetal hemoglobin followed by intrauterine transfusion if indicated.**

TECHNIQUE FOR AMNIOCENTESIS

An ultrasonic examination is performed to localize a pocket of amniotic fluid far enough away from the fetus and placenta to obtain a sample safely. A 22-gauge spinal needle is inserted, and 10 mL of fluid is aspirated using a sterile technique. The fluid is transferred to a dark or foil-wrapped tube to prevent deterioration due to light exposure and is sent for assessment of the ΔOD 450. **The incidence of fetal mortality from amniocentesis for hemolytic disease** is reported to be **less than 1 in 900** in experienced centers. Of potential concern is the procedure-related risk for fetomaternal hemorrhage, which may worsen the severity of the sensitization. **The incidence of fetomaternal hemorrhage is reported to be 8.4% to 11% per procedure.**

PERCUTANEOUS UMBILICAL BLOOD SAMPLING

Advances in fetal interventional techniques and high-resolution ultrasonography have made direct fetal blood sampling the most accurate method for the diagnosis of fetal hemolytic disease. **Percutaneous umbilical blood sampling (PUBS) can allow measurement of fetal hemoglobin, hematocrit, blood gases, pH, and bilirubin levels. The hemoglobin values for normal fetuses from 18 to 30 weeks' gestation range from about 11.5 to 13.4 $\pm$ 1 g/dL.** The technique for fetal blood sampling is similar to that described for fetal intravenous transfusion. One drawback is that it requires expertise above and beyond that required for amniocentesis. **The major risk is fetal exsanguination from tears in placental vessels.** If performed by an experienced practitioner, the risk for this complication and fetal death is 1% to 2% or less. **However, there is a greater risk for fetomaternal hemorrhage,** reported to be as high as 40%. Percutaneous umbilical blood sampling should not be a first-line method of assessing fetal status unless clearly indicated.

INTRAUTERINE TRANSFUSION

Intrauterine transfusion, initially introduced in 1963 as an intraperitoneal transfusion and presently usually administered as an intravascular transfusion has markedly changed the prognosis for severely affected fetuses. **The goal is to transfuse fresh group O, Rh-negative packed red blood cells.** In addition to routine blood screening, the blood for transfusion is irradiated, washed, processed through a leukocyte-poor filter,

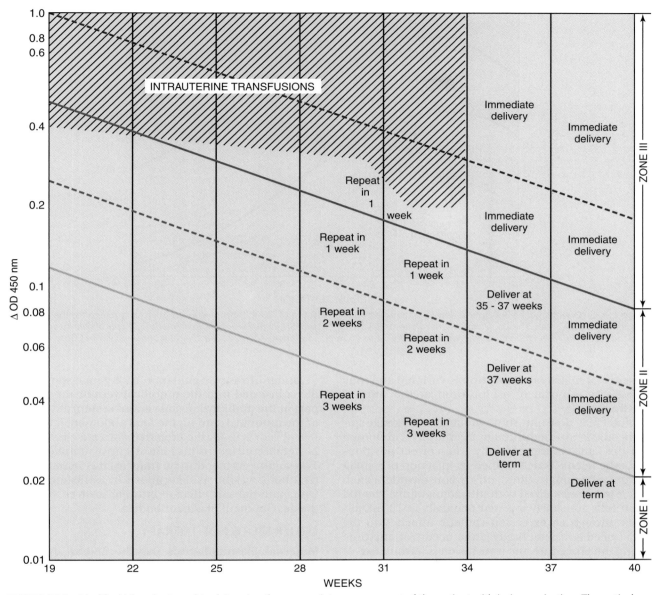

FIGURE 15-2   Modified Liley chart used to determine the appropriate management of the patient with isoimmunization. The optical density at a wavelength of 450-nm (ΔOD 450-nm) level in the amniotic fluid at a given weeks' gestation determines whether fetal transfusion or delivery is advisable.

and screened for cytomegalovirus. Curare is usually injected directly into the fetal thigh with a 22-gauge spinal needle before transfusion, regardless of method, to immobilize the fetus during the procedure. Repeat transfusions are generally scheduled at 1- to 3-week intervals. The final transfusion is typically performed at 32 to 34 weeks' gestation. In general, the fetus is delivered when the lungs are mature.

The overall survival rate following intrauterine transfusion is about 85%. In fetuses with no evidence of hydrops, the survival rate is about 90%, and for fetuses with hydrops before the transfusion, the survival rate is about 75%.

Fetal Intraperitoneal Transfusion

Red blood cells are absorbed through the subdiaphragmatic lymphatics and proceed through the right lymphatic duct into the fetal intravascular compartment. After transfusion, the absorption of blood may be monitored with serial transverse ultrasonic scans of the fetal abdomen. **In nonhydroptic fetuses, the blood should be absorbed within 7 to 9 days. In the**

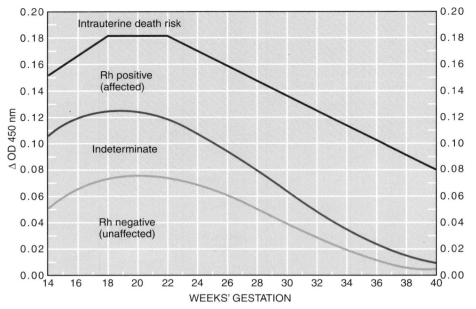

FIGURE 15-3   Queenan curve for optical density at a wavelength of 450-nm (ΔOD 450-nm) values for the management of the patient with isoimmunization. Rh, rhesus. *(Adapted from Queenan JT, Tomai TP, Ural SH, et al: Deviations in amniotic fluid optical density at a wavelength of 450-nm in Rh-immunized pregnancies from 14 to 40 weeks' gestation: A proposal for clinical management. Am J Obstet Gynecol 168:1370-1376, 1993.)*

presence of hydrops, absorption is variable and may necessitate removal of ascitic fluid at the time of transfusion.

Under real-time ultrasonic guidance, a 20-gauge spinal needle is inserted through the mother's abdomen into the fetal peritoneal cavity. The correct positioning of the needle is determined by injection of a small amount of normal saline and carbon dioxide, which can be easily visualized with ultrasonography. The red blood cells are slowly injected manually in 10-mL aliquots through an extension catheter attached to the spinal needle. If fetal bradycardia occurs at any time during the procedure, the transfusion is terminated.

For intraperitoneal transfusions, the volume to be infused is based on the following formula:

$$\text{Volume} = [\text{gestational age (weeks)} - 20] \times 10$$

For example, a 30-week fetus would require a 100-mL transfusion (30 weeks − 20 × 10 = 100 mL).

Intravascular Transfusion

Because many fetuses are not subjected to transfusion until ascites is present, intravascular fetal transfusion has become increasingly popular. In addition, transfusion into the peritoneal cavity can result in fetal bradycardia or a pseudosinusoidal fetal heart rate pattern following the procedure because of compression at the site of insertion of the umbilical cord.

Under ultrasonic guidance, a 22-gauge spinal needle is inserted into the umbilical vein or the hepatic part of the umbilical portal venous system at the level of the umbilical cord on the fetal abdomen. If the umbilical vein is used, the preferred sites are either at the placental cord insertion or into a loop of umbilical cord. The volume of blood to be transfused is based on the fetal body weight, as determined by ultrasonography. One maternal side effect of intrauterine transfusion is the development of alloantibodies.

OTHER MODES OF THERAPY

Maternal plasmapheresis may be helpful in severe erythroblastosis when intrauterine transfusions are not successful, but perinatal outcome with this technique has not been impressive. **Phenobarbital** has been used to induce fetal hepatic enzyme maturation, thereby increasing uptake and excretion of bilirubin by the liver. Treatment with phenobarbital is initiated 2 to 3 weeks before delivery.

Timing of Delivery in the Rh-Sensitized Fetus

In addition to serial ultrasounds for MCA Doppler studies and detection of hydrops, (or alternatively, serial amniocenteses for ΔOD 450 readings), these fetuses are evaluated at least twice weekly from 24 to 28 weeks for fetal well-being (NST, modified biophysical profile) and fetal growth. **While the goal is a term neonate,** the risks for intrauterine demise, including that from procedure-related losses, must be balanced against the risks for prematurity. There is no absolute gestational age cutoff for intrauterine transfusion, but after 34 weeks, the risk for an intrauterine loss in this setting may be greater than the risk for a neonatal death, and it may be prudent to deliver the fetus. If delivery is expected to occur before 34 weeks' gestation (or if amniocentesis suggests an immature lung profile), betamethasone should be given at least 48 hours before delivery to enhance fetal pulmonary maturation.

◼ Prevention of Rhesus Isoimmunization

Because Rh isoimmunization occurs in response to exposure of an Rh-negative mother to the Rh antigen, the mainstay for prevention is the avoidance of maternal exposure to the antigen. Rh immune globulin (Rh_O-GAM) diminishes the availability of the Rh antigen to the maternal immune system, although the exact mechanism by which it prevents Rh isoimmunization is not well understood.

Rh_O-GAM is prepared from fractionated human plasma obtained from hyperreactive sensitized donors. The plasma is screened for hepatitis B surface antigen and anti-HIV-1. The globulin is available in several dosages for intramuscular injection. Since the advent of its use in 1967, Rh immune globulin has dramatically reduced the incidence of Rh isoimmunization.

Because the greatest risk for fetal-to-maternal hemorrhage occurs during labor and delivery, Rh immune globulin was initially administered only during the immediate postpartum period. This resulted in a 1% to 2% failure rate, thought to be due to exposure of the mother to fetal red blood cells during the antepartum period. **The indications for the use of Rh immune globulin have therefore been broadened to include any antepartum event (such as amniocentesis) that may increase the risk for transplacental hemorrhage. The routine prophylactic administration of Rh immune globulin at 28 weeks' gestation is now the standard of care.** Despite adherence to this suggested Rh immune globulin protocol, 0.27% of primiparous Rh-negative patients still become sensitized.

INDICATIONS FOR ADMINISTRATION OF Rh_O-GAM

It is the responsibility of every health care practitioner who is involved in the care of pregnant women to prevent Rh isoimmunization. This is done by the timely administration of Rh_O-GAM to pregnant Rh-negative women, whose anti D titers are negative, at about the time of events associated with fetal-maternal hemorrhage. The following provides a practical approach to the administration of Rh immune globulin to an Rh-negative unsensitized patient.

All pregnant women should have a blood type and antibody screen on their first prenatal visit. **During an uncomplicated pregnancy, the Rh-negative woman whose initial antibody screen is negative should have a repeat antibody titer at 28 weeks' gestation. If the antibody screen is still negative, she should routinely receive an intramuscular injection of 300 μg of Rh_O-GAM prophylactically.** A positive antibody screen does not necessarily mean the woman is not a candidate for Rh_O-GAM. In this case, an antibody identification and titer must be requested. If the antibody is not an anti-D antibody, then she is still a candidate for Rh_O-GAM.

Rh_O-GAM should also be administered during the antepartum period at any gestational age to an Rh-negative unsensitized (anti-D–negative) woman at the time of spontaneous or induced abortion, treatment of an ectopic pregnancy, significant vaginal bleeding, performance of an amniocentesis, abdominal trauma, or external cephalic version. Before 12 weeks of gestation, 50 to 100 μg of Rh_O-GAM should be sufficient to prevent isoimmunization.

Because chorionic villi in gestational trophoblastic disease are avascular and are devoid of fetal erythrocytes, **Rh_O-GAM is probably not necessary following termination of a "complete" molar pregnancy. A "partial" molar pregnancy may have fetal tissue, and theoretically fetal cells could enter the maternal circulation.** At least one case of sensitization following a molar pregnancy has been reported.

The risk for transplacental hemorrhage increases at the time of delivery, especially with cesarean birth or manual removal of the placenta. At delivery, cord blood must be sent for determination of the fetal blood group, Rh type, and for a direct Coombs' test. **Rh_O-GAM (300 μg) is routinely given to all Rh-negative, anti-D–negative women who deliver an Rh-positive infant within 72 hours of delivery. If a transplacental hemorrhage of greater than 30 mL of fetal blood is suspected (as might occur in the setting of an abruption, manual removal of the placenta, or severe maternal abdominal trauma), a Kleihauer-Betke test is helpful in determining the volume of the hemorrhage. Additional Rh_O-GAM may then be given at a dose of 10 μg of Rh_O-GAM per 1 ml of fetal blood that entered the maternal circulation.**

Irregular Antibodies

Although Rh isoimmunization is the most common cause of hemolytic disease in the newborn, other blood group systems may be involved, such as **Kell, Duffy, or Kidd.** Kell antigen can elicit a strong IgG response similar to Rh isoimmunization. For this reason, any positive antibody screen in pregnancy, even in an Rh-positive woman, should be followed up with an antibody identification and titer. If the antibody screen is positive for one or more antibodies associated with hemolytic disease of the newborn, the pregnancy should be followed in a fashion similar to that advised for the Rh-sensitized pregnancy. A potential exception to this is Kell sensitization. Antibody titers and amniotic fluid spectrophotometry are not as reliable for detecting fetal anemia in this situation, probably because the anemia is due more to suppression of hematopoiesis than to hemolysis. The MCA PSV remains an excellent predictor of anemia in this setting. It is extremely important to test the Kell antigen status of the father of the fetus before any invasive testing because 90% of the population is Kell negative.

SUGGESTED READING

American College of Obstetricians and Gynecologists: Management of alloimmunization during pregnancy. ACOG Practice Bulletin No. 75. Washington DC, ACOG, 2006.

Brown S, Kellner LH, Munson M, et al: Non-invasive prenatal testing: Technical strategies to achieve testing of cell free fetal DNA (cffDNA) RHD genotype in a clinical lab. Am J Obstet Gynecol 197:S173, 2007.

Howe DT, Michailidis GD: Intraperitoneal transfusion in severe early-onset Rh isoimmunization. Obstet Gynecol 110:880-884, 2007.

Mari G, Deter RL, Carpenter RL, et al: Noninvasive diagnosis by Doppler ultrasonography of fetal anemia due to maternal red-cell alloimmunization. Collaborative Group for Doppler Assessment of the Blood Velocity of Anemic Fetuses. N Engl J Med 342:9-14, 2000.

Mari G, Deti L, Oz U, et al: Accurate prediction of fetal hemoglobin by Doppler ultrasonography: Obstet Gynecol 99:589-593, 2002.

Chapter 16

Common Medical and Surgical Conditions Complicating Pregnancy

LONY C. CASTRO • DOTUN OGUNYEMI

The more common medical, infectious, and surgical disorders that may complicate pregnancy are covered in this chapter. The pharmacologic agents recommended for these disorders have been classified by the Food and Drug Administration (FDA) for fetal risk (see Box 7-1 on page 73). Up to date information on these drugs can be found at *www.FDA.gov/* by selecting "Drugs" from the menu and searching for a specific agent.

◾ Endocrine Disorders

Diabetes mellitus and thyroid disease are the two most common endocrine disorders complicating pregnancy.

DIABETES MELLITUS

Incidence and Classification

The prevalence of diabetes mellitus has greatly increased in the last 20 years. Reports show a rate of 3% to 8% of gestational diabetes mellitus (GDM). Pregestational diabetes is present in about 1% of pregnancies. Overall, 90% of diabetes in pregnant women is gestational and about 10% pregestational.

GDM is defined as glucose intolerance with onset or first recognition during pregnancy. Pregnancy is associated with progressive insulin resistance. **Human placental lactogen, progesterone, prolactin, cortisol, and tumor necrosis factor are associated with increased insulin resistance during pregnancy.** Studies suggest that women who develop GDM have chronic insulin resistance and that GDM is a "stress test" for the development of diabetes in later life. Most obstetricians use **White's classification of diabetes during pregnancy.** This classification is helpful is assessing disease severity and the likelihood of complications (Table 16-1).

Complications

Maternal and fetal complications of diabetes are listed in Table 16-2. Diabetes often coexists with the metabolic syndrome. Most fetal and neonatal effects are attributed to the consequences of maternal hyperglycemia, or, in the more advanced classes, to maternal vascular disease. **Glucose crosses the placenta easily by facilitated diffusion, causing fetal hyperglycemia, which stimulates pancreatic β cells and results in fetal hyperinsulinism.** Fetal hyperglycemia during the period of embryogenesis is teratogenic. **There is a direct correlation between birth defects in diabetic pregnancies and increasing glycosylated hemoglobin levels (HbA$_{1C}$) in the first trimester. Fetal hyperglycemia and hyperinsulinemia cause fetal overgrowth and macrosomia, which predisposes to birth trauma, including shoulder dystocia and Erb's' palsy. Fetal demise is most likely due to acidosis, hypotension from osmotic dieresis, or hypoxia from increased metabolism coupled with inadequate placental oxygen transfer.**

In pregestational diabetes, maternal complications include worsening nephropathy and retinopathy, a greater incidence of preterm preeclampsia and a higher likelihood of diabetic ketoacidosis. **Hypoglycemia is much more common because of the tighter control attempted during pregnancy.** Fetal complications include an increased rate of abortions, anatomic birth defects, fetal growth restriction, and prematurity.

Diagnosis

Screening for gestational diabetes is generally performed between 24 and 28 weeks of gestation with a 50-g 1-hour oral glucose challenge test (GCT), given without regard to last oral intake. This timing will identify most gestational diabetic patients while providing several weeks of therapy to reduce potentially adverse consequences. **Screening is advised at the first**

TABLE 16-1

WHITE'S CLASSIFICATION OF DIABETES IN PREGNANCY

Class	Description	Therapy
A₁	Gestational diabetes; glucose intolerance developing during pregnancy; fasting blood glucose and postprandial plasma glucose normal	Diet alone
A₂	Gestational diabetes with fasting plasma glucose >105 mg/dL; or 2-hr postprandial plasma glucose >120 mg/dL, or 1-hr postprandial plasma glucose >140 mg/dL	Diet and insulin
B	Overt diabetes developing after age 20 yr and duration < 10 yr	Diet and insulin
C	Overt diabetes developing between ages 10 and 19 yr or duration 10-19 yr	Diet and insulin
D	Overt diabetes developing before age 10 yr or duration 20 yr or more or background retinopathy	Diet and insulin
F	Overt diabetes at any age or duration with nephropathy	Diet and insulin
R	Overt diabetes at any age or duration with proliferative retinopathy	Diet and insulin
H	Overt diabetes at any age or duration with arteriosclerotic heart disease	Diet and insulin

prenatal visit in pregnant women with risk factors such as maternal age greater than 25 years, previous macrosomic infant, previous unexplained fetal demise, previous pregnancy with GDM, family history of diabetes, history of polycystic ovarian disease, and obesity. If overt signs and symptoms of diabetes are present, a fetal scalp blood test should be undertaken first. **If the first-trimester screen is negative, it should be repeated at 24 to 28 weeks. Glucose values above 130 to 140 mg/dL on a GCT are considered abnormal** and have an 80% to 90% sensitivity in detecting GDM.

An abnormal screening GCT is followed with a diagnostic 3-hour 100-g oral glucose tolerance test. This involves checking the fasting blood glucose after an overnight fast, drinking a 100-g glucose drink, and checking glucose levels hourly for 3 hours. If there are two or more abnormal values on the 3-hour GTT, the patient is diagnosed with GDM (Table 16-3). **If the 1-hour screening (50-g oral glucose) plasma glucose exceeds 200 mg/dL, a glucose tolerance test is not required and may dangerously elevate blood glucose values.**

Management

THE DIABETIC TEAM. Management of gestational diabetes requires a team approach involving patient teaching and counseling, medical-nursing assessments and interventions, strategies to achieve maternal euglycemia, and avoidance of fetal-neonatal compromise. Ideally, this team should include the patient, obstetrician, maternal fetal medicine specialist, clinical nurse specialist, nutritionist, social worker, and neonatologist. **The patient is included as an active participant in formulating management strategies.**

ACHIEVING EUGLYCEMIA. The importance of strict metabolic control before and during pregnancy to decrease the incidence of congenital anomalies, perinatal morbidity, and perinatal mortality has been established. For optimal outcome, the fasting blood glucose should be less than 95 mg/dL, 1-hour postprandial glucose level less than 140 mg/dL, and 2-hour postprandial glucose level less than 120 mg/dL.

DIET. Caloric requirements are calculated on the basis of ideal body weight: 30 kcal/kg for those patients 80% to 120% of ideal body weight; 35 to 40 kcal/kg for those less than 80% of ideal body weight; and 24 kcal/kg for gravidas who are 120% to 150% of ideal body weight. The diet comprises about 50% carbohydrate, 20% protein, and 20% fat. The diet should also contain a generous amount of fiber. Caloric intake is divided into 25% at breakfast, 30% at lunch, 30% at dinner, and 15% at a bedtime snack.

THERAPY. Oral hypoglycemic agents have traditionally not been recommended for pregnant women because of the risks for teratogenesis and neonatal hypoglycemia. However, oral hypoglycemic agents (e.g., glyburide), which do not appear to enter the fetal circulation in appreciable quantities, have been used successfully to treat gestational diabetes after the first trimester.

Insulin use is the gold standard to maintain euglycemia in pregnancy. The peak action of lispro insulin is at 30 to 90 minutes, of regular insulin at 2 to 3 hours, and of NPH insulin at 6 to 10 hours. A combination of rapid-acting or short-acting (lispro or regular) and intermediate-acting (NPH) insulin is usually given in split morning and evening doses or more frequently to achieve euglycemia. A method for calculating insulin dosage is shown in Box 16-1.

EXERCISE. Diabetic patients should be encouraged to engage in mild to moderate aerobic exercise (e.g., brisk walking) for about half an hour after meals.

Antepartum Obstetric Management

Aside from achieving euglycemia, adequate surveillance should be maintained during pregnancy to detect and possibly mitigate maternal and fetal complications. In pregestational diabetic patients, or in those with GDMs diagnosed before 20 weeks, a first-trimester

TABLE 16-2

MATERNAL AND FETAL COMPLICATIONS OF DIABETES MELLITUS

Entity	Monitoring
MATERNAL COMPLICATIONS	
OBSTETRIC COMPLICATIONS	
Polyhydramnios	Close prenatal surveillance; blood glucose monitoring, ultrasonography
Preeclampsia	Evaluation for signs and symptoms
Infections, e.g., urinary tract infection and candidiasis	Urine culture, wet mount, appropriate therapy
Cesarean delivery	Blood glucose monitoring, insulin and dietary adjustment to prevent fetal overgrowth
Genital trauma	Ultrasonography to detect macrosomia, cesarean delivery for macrosomia
DIABETIC EMERGENCIES	
Hypoglycemia	Teach signs and symptoms; blood glucose monitoring; insulin and dietary adjustment; check for ketones, blood gases, and electrolytes if glucose > 300 mg/dL
Diabetic coma	
Ketoacidosis	
VASCULAR AND END-ORGAN INVOLVEMENT OR DETERIORATION (IN PATIENTS WITH PREGESTATIONAL DIABETES MELLITUS)	
Cardiac	Electrocardiogram first visit and as needed
Renal	Renal function studies, first visit and as needed
Ophthalmic	Funduscopic evaluation, first visit and as needed
Peripheral vascular	Check for ulcers, foot sores; noninvasive Doppler studies as needed
NEUROLOGIC	
Peripheral neuropathy	Neurologic and gastrointestinal consultations as needed
Gastrointestinal disturbance	
LONG-TERM OUTCOME	
Type 2 diabetes	Postpartum glucose testing, lifestyle changes (diet and exercise)
Metabolic syndrome	Lifestyle changes (diet and exercise)
Obesity	Lifestyle changes (diet and exercise)
Cardiovascular disease	Annual checkup by physician, lifestyle changes (diet and exercise)
FETAL AND NEONATAL COMPLICATIONS	
Maintenance of maternal euglycemia will decrease most of these complications.	
Macrosomia with traumatic delivery (shoulder dystocia, Erb's palsy)	Ultrasonography for estimated fetal weight before delivery; consider cesarean delivery if estimated fetal weight > 4250-4500 g
DELAYED ORGAN MATURITY	
Pulmonary, hepatic, neurologic, pituitary-thyroid axis; with respiratory distress syndrome, hypocalcemia	Avoid delivery before 39 weeks in the absence of maternal or fetal indications unless amniocentesis indicates lung maturity. Maintain euglycemia intrapartum.
CONGENITAL DEFECTS	
Cardiovascular anomalies	Preconception counseling and glucose control, HbA$_{1c}$ in the first trimester
Neural tube defects	Maternal serum alpha-fetoprotein screening; fetal ultrasonography and fetal echocardiogram; amniocentesis and genetic counseling
Caudal regression syndrome	
Other defects, e.g., renal	
FETAL COMPROMISE	
Intrauterine growth restriction	Serial ultrasonography for fetal growth and estimated fetal weight, serial fetal surveillance with nonstress test, amniotic fluid index, and fetal Doppler. Avoid postdates pregnancy.
Intrauterine fetal death	
Abnormal fetal heart rate patterns	

dating ultrasound followed by a detailed obstetric ultrasonic study, fetal echocardiogram, and maternal serum alpha-fetoprotein level should be obtained at 16 to 20 weeks to check for congenital malformations. Maternal renal, cardiac, and ophthalmic functions must be closely monitored. **The HbA$_{1C}$ should be obtained at the first prenatal visit, which is preferably scheduled early in the first trimester. Individuals with significantly elevated values (>8.5%) should be particularly targeted for careful ultrasonic assessment for congenital anomalies.** Regular electronic, biochemical, and ultrasonographic fetal monitoring should be performed. For

TABLE 16-3

THREE-HOUR ORAL GLUCOSE TOLERANCE TEST	
Test	Maximal Normal Blood Glucose (mg/dL)
Fasting	95
1 hr	180
2 hr	155
3 hr	140

From Carpenter and Coustan.

diabetic classes A, B, and C, fetal macrosomia is common and should be investigated, whereas for classes D, F and R, fetal growth restriction occurs more commonly.

Serial fetal testing should be performed in the third trimester. In patients with GDM on diet, fetal testing can be initiated at term; while in those on insulin, fetal testing should be initiated between 32 and 34 weeks of gestation or sooner if complications develop.

If the maternal state is stable, blood glucose is in the euglycemic range, and fetal studies indicate a healthy baby, spontaneous onset of labor at term may be awaited. Earlier intervention is indicated if these conditions are not met. For macrosomic babies, increased birth trauma to both mother and fetus should be kept in mind. **Cesarean delivery may be elected for large fetuses (>4250 to 4500 g).**

Intrapartum Management

Intrapartum management of a diabetic patient requires the establishment of maternal euglycemia during labor. This may be achieved by giving a continuous infusion of regular insulin. **Plasma glucose levels are measured frequently, and insulin dosage is adjusted accordingly to maintain a plasma glucose level between 80 and 120 mg/dL.** Not all insulin-dependent patients require exogenous insulin during labor. Continuous electronic **fetal heart rate monitoring is recommended for all diabetic patients.**

Postpartum Period

After delivery of the fetus and placenta, insulin requirements drop sharply because the placenta, which is the source of many insulin antagonists, has been removed.

BOX 16-1 *Method for Calculation of Starting Dose of Insulin*

Insulin units = body weight (kg)
×0.6 (First trimester)
×0.7 (Second trimester)
×0.8 (Third trimester)
Dosage schedule: give 2/3 in AM and 1/3 in PM
Before breakfast: 2/3 NPH, 1/3 regular or lispro
Before dinner: 1/2 NPH, 1/2 regular or lispro (if on lispro, administer additional dose before bedtime snack)

Many insulin-dependent diabetic patients may not require exogenous insulin for the first 48 to 72 hours after delivery. **Plasma glucose levels should be monitored and lispro or regular insulin given when plasma glucose levels are elevated.** Patients can be restarted on two thirds of the prepregnancy insulin dosage, with adjustments made as necessary. Gestational diabetic patients (with class A_1 and A_2 disease) frequently do not need insulin therapy postpartum. **A fasting blood glucose or a 75-g oral glucose tolerance test should be performed at 6 to 12 weeks postpartum.**

Patients should be counseled about changes in diet. The American Dietetic Association diet with the same distribution of carbohydrates, proteins, and fat should be maintained. If the mother is breastfeeding, 500 calories/day should be added to the prepregnant diet.

Sterilization should be discussed with patients who desire it and those with advanced vascular involvement.

THYROID DISEASES

Normal Thyroid Physiology during Pregnancy

With the increase in glomerular filtration rate that occurs during pregnancy, the renal excretion of iodine increases, and plasma inorganic iodine levels are nearly halved. Goiters due to iodine deficiency are not likely if plasma inorganic iodine levels are greater than 0.08 μg/dL. Inorganic iodine supplementation up to a total of 250 μg/day is sufficient to prevent goiter formation during pregnancy.

THYROID FUNCTION TESTS. The free thyroxine (free T_4) concentration is the only accurate method of estimating thyroid function that compensates for changes in thyroxine-binding globulin (TBG) capacity because serum levels of bound triiodothyronine (total T_3) and total T_4 are increased during pregnancy. Values of thyroid function tests during pregnancy are shown in Table 16-4.

FETAL THYROID FUNCTION. Before 10 weeks' gestation, no organic iodine is present in the fetal thyroid. By 11 to 12 weeks, the fetal thyroid is able to produce iodothyronines and T_4, and by 12 to 14 weeks, it is able to concentrate iodine. **Fetal thyroid-stimulating hormone (TSH), T_4, and free T_4 levels suggest that a mature, autonomous, thyroid-pituitary axis exists as early as 12 weeks' gestation.**

PLACENTAL TRANSFER OF THYROID HORMONE. Iodide freely crosses the placenta, but TSH does not. Limited transfer of T_4 occurs across the placenta and appears to be important for fetal neural development in the first trimester before fetal thyroid function begins. **Thyroid hormone analogues such as propylthiouracil and methimazole, with smaller molecular weights, cross the**

TABLE 16-4

THYROID FUNCTION TESTS IN NONPREGNANT WOMEN AND IN MATERNAL AND CORD BLOOD AT TERM

Test	Nonpregnant	Pregnant	Cord
Serum thyroxine (T_4) (µg/dL)	5-12	10-16	6-13
Free T_4 (ng/dL)	1.0-2.3	2.5-3.5	1.5-3.0
Serum triiodothyronine (T_3) (ng/dL)	110-230	150-250	40-60
Reverse T_3 (ng/dL)	15-30	35-65	80-360
Resin T_3 uptake (%)	20-30	10	10-15
Thyroxine-binding globulin (g/dL)	12-28	40-50	10-16
Serum thyroid-stimulating hormone (U/mL)	1.94	0-6	0-20

Note: Absolute values for these may vary according to the method used, but the ratio between maternal and cord values should remain constant.
Modified from Burrow GN, Ferris T (eds): Medical Complications during Pregnancy. Philadelphia, WB Saunders, 1972, p 194.

placental barrier and could potentially cause fetal hypothyroidism.

Thyroid-releasing hormone (TRH) can cross the placental barrier, but there is no significant placental transfer because of circulating low levels. Thyroid-stimulating antibodies also cross the placenta and can potentially cause fetal thyroid dysfunction.

Maternal Hyperthyroidism

The incidence of maternal thyrotoxicosis is about 1 per 500 pregnancies. It is accompanied by an increased incidence of prematurity, intrauterine growth restriction (IUGR), superimposed preeclampsia, stillbirth, and neonatal morbidity and mortality. Graves' disease is an autoimmune disorder caused by thyroid-stimulating antibodies and is the most common cause of hyperthyroidism. Other causes of hyperthyroidism in pregnancy include hydatidiform mole and toxic nodular goiter. Patients with Graves' disease tend to have a remission during pregnancy and an exacerbation during the postpartum period. The increased immunologic tolerance during pregnancy may lead to a decrease in thyroid antibodies to account for the remission.

CLINICAL FEATURES. The clinical diagnosis of hyperthyroidism in pregnancy is difficult because many of the signs and symptoms of the hyperdynamic circulation associated with hyperthyroidism are present in a normal euthyroid pregnant individual. A resting pulse rate greater than 100 beats/minute that fails to slow with a Valsalva maneuver, eye changes, loss of weight, failure to gain weight despite normal or increased food intake, and heat intolerance are all helpful in making the clinical diagnosis.

INVESTIGATIONS. An **elevated serum free T_4 level** and a **suppressed TSH level** establish the diagnosis of hyperthyroidism. Infrequently, a free T_3 determination might be needed to diagnose T_3 thyrotoxicosis.

THERAPY. Because radioactive iodine treatment is contraindicated during pregnancy, medical treatment is generally employed. Thioamides are the mainstay of antithyroid therapy. They block the synthesis but not the release of thyroid hormone. **Propylthiouracil (PTU) and methimazole (Tapazole)** have been used interchangeably, although PTU has the added advantage of blocking conversion of T_4 to T_3, and methimazole may cause fetal gastrointestinal defects. **Because these drugs readily cross the placenta, a concern during maternal treatment is the development of fetal goiter and hypothyroidism.** Although there is no conclusive evidence that PTU treatment leads to cretinism or abnormalities in physical or intellectual development, up to 1% to 5% of children exposed in utero will develop a goiter. **For this reason antithyroid drugs are reduced to the lowest dose that results in free T_4 levels within the upper range of normal.** Levels should be checked every 2 to 4 weeks. Antithyroid therapy can often be discontinued after 30 weeks of gestation.

Propylthiouracil excretion in breast milk is minimal, and no changes occur in the thyroid function tests of breastfed neonates.

Surgical management of the hyperthyroid pregnant patient during the second trimester is recommended only if medical treatment fails.

Thyroid Storm

The major risk in a pregnant patient with thyrotoxicosis is the development of a thyroid storm. Precipitating factors include infection, labor, cesarean delivery, or noncompliance with medication. It is not uncommon to mistakenly attribute the signs and symptoms of severe hyperthyroidism to preeclampsia. In the former, significant proteinuria is usually absent. The maternal mortality of thyroid storm exceeds 25% despite good medical management. **The signs and symptoms associated with a thyroid storm include hyperthermia,**

marked tachycardia, perspiration, and high output failure or severe dehydration.

Specific treatment is directed at (1) **blocking β-adrenergic activity with propranolol, 20 to 80 mg every 6 hours;** (2) **blocking secretion of thyroid hormone with sodium iodide, 1 g intravenously;** (3) **blocking synthesis of thyroid hormone and conversion of T_4 to T_3 with 1200 to 1800 mg of PTU** given in divided doses; (4) further blocking the deamination of T_4 to T_3 with 8 mg of **dexamethasone** per day; (5) **replacing fluid losses;** and (6) rapidly lowering the temperature with **hypothermic techniques.**

Neonatal Thyrotoxicosis

About 1% of pregnant women with a history of Graves' disease give birth to children with thyrotoxicosis due to transplacental transfer of thyroid-stimulating antibodies. It is transient and lasts less than 2 to 3 months but is associated with a neonatal mortality rate of about 16%. Fetal thyrotoxicosis can be suspected if the baseline fetal heart rate consistently exceeds 160 beats/minute. A fetal goiter can often be identified by ultrasonography in such cases. This situation is associated with an increase in perinatal morbidity and mortality and should be treated prenatally and postnatally.

Hypothyroidism

Pregnant women on appropriate thyroid replacement therapy can expect a normal pregnancy outcome, but **untreated maternal hypothyroidism has been associated with an increased risk for spontaneous abortion, preeclampsia, abruption, low-birth-weight or stillborn infants, and lower intelligence levels in the offspring.**

The most important laboratory finding to confirm the diagnosis of hypothyroidism is an elevated TSH level. Other findings include low levels of serum free T_3 and free T_4. Once diagnosed, therapy such as levothyroxine should be started and serum TSH levels performed monthly with appropriate adjustments in levothyroxine dosage.

NEONATAL HYPOTHYROIDISM. Thyroid hormone deficiency during the fetal and early neonatal periods leads to generalized developmental retardation. The severity of symptoms depends on the time of onset and the severity of the deprivation.

The incidence of congenital hypothyroidism (cretinism) is about 1 in 4000 births. The etiologic factors include thyroid dysgenesis, inborn errors of thyroid function, and drug-induced endemic hypothyroidism. **The most common cause of neonatal goiter is maternal ingestion of iodides present in cough syrup.** The goiters associated with maternal iodine ingestion are large and obstructive, unlike those associated with maternal PTU treatment.

Heart Disease

The categories of heart disease in pregnancy include **rheumatic and congenital cardiac disease** as well as **arrhythmias, cardiomyopathies** and other forms of acquired heart disease. Better treatment of rheumatic fever and improvements in medical and surgical management of congenital heart disease has meant that in a modern tertiary referral center, about 80% of patients with cardiac disease in pregnancy now have congenital heart disease.

RHEUMATIC HEART DISEASE

The most common lesion associated with rheumatic heart disease is mitral stenosis. Regardless of the specific valvular lesion, **patients are at higher risk for developing heart failure, subacute bacterial endocarditis, and thromboembolic disease.** They also have a higher rate of fetal wastage.

Pure mitral stenosis is found in about 90% of patients with rheumatic heart disease. During pregnancy, the mechanical obstruction worsens as cardiac output increases. **Asymptomatic patients may develop symptoms of cardiac decompensation or pulmonary edema as pregnancy progresses.** Atrial fibrillation is more common in patients with severe mitral stenosis, and **nearly all women who develop atrial fibrillation during pregnancy experience congestive heart failure.** However, pulmonary congestion and heart failure develop in only half of women in whom atrial fibrillation predates pregnancy. Tachycardia can result in decompensation because cardiac output in patients with mitral stenosis depends on an adequate diastolic filling time.

CONGENITAL HEART DISEASE

Congenital heart disease includes atrial or ventricular septal defects, primary pulmonary hypertension (Eisenmenger's syndrome), and cyanotic heart disease such as tetralogy of Fallot or transposition of the great arteries. If the anatomic defect has been corrected during childhood with no residual damage, the patient is expected go through pregnancy without complications. Patients with persistent atrial or ventricular septal defects and those with tetralogy of Fallot with complete surgical correction generally tolerate pregnancy well. However, **patients with primary pulmonary hypertension or cyanotic heart disease with residual pulmonary hypertension are in danger of undergoing decompensation during pregnancy.** Pulmonary hypertension from any cause is associated with an increased risk for maternal mortality during pregnancy or in the immediate postpartum period. In all these patients, care should be taken to avoid overloading the circulation and precipitating pulmonary congestion, heart failure, or hypotension with reversal of the left-right shunt, all of which may lead to hypoxia and sudden death. **In general, significant pulmonary hypertension with Eisenmenger's syndrome is a contraindication to pregnancy.**

CARDIAC ARRHYTHMIAS

Supraventricular tachycardia is the most common cardiac arrhythmia. It is usually benign and occurs secondary to structural changes in the heart that have presumably been present since birth. Atrial fibrillation and atrial flutter are more serious and are usually associated with underlying cardiac disease.

PERIPARTUM CARDIOMYOPATHY

This entity is rare but occurs exclusively during pregnancy. Patients have no underlying cardiac disease, and symptoms of cardiac decompensation appear during the last weeks of pregnancy or within 6 months postpartum. **Pregnant women particularly at risk for developing cardiomyopathy are those with a history of preeclampsia or hypertension and those who are poorly nourished.** It appears to be a dilational cardiomyopathy with decreased ejection fraction. Hypertensive cardiomyopathy, ischemic heart disease, viral myocarditis, and valvular heart disease must be excluded in patients with cardiac dysfunction before the diagnosis can be made. **The mortality rate is at least 20%.** About 30% to 50% of patients have persistent cardiac dysfunction, and recurrence occurs in about 20% to 50% of patients in a subsequent pregnancy.

MANAGEMENT OF CARDIAC DISEASE DURING PREGNANCY

The New York Heart Association's functional classification of heart disease is of value in assessing the risk for pregnancy in a patient with acquired cardiac disease and in determining the optimal management during pregnancy, labor, and delivery (Table 16-5). In general, the maternal and fetal risks for patients with class I and II disease are small, whereas **risks are greatly increased with class III and IV disease or if there is cyanosis.** However, the type of defect is important as well. Mitral stenosis and aortic stenosis carry a higher risk for decompensation than do regurgitant lesions. Other patients at high risk include those with significant pulmonary hypertension, a left ventricular ejection fraction less than 40%, Marfan syndrome, a mechanical valve, or a previous history of a cardiac event or arrhythmia.

Prenatal Management

As a general principle, **all pregnant cardiac patients should be managed with the help of a cardiologist.** A careful history and physical examination, along with an electrocardiogram and echocardiogram, should be performed. The patient should be counseled about

TABLE 16-5

NEW YORK HEART ASSOCIATION'S FUNCTIONAL CLASSIFICATION OF HEART DISEASE	
Class I	No signs or symptoms of cardiac decompensation
Class II	No symptoms at rest, but minor limitation of physical activity
Class III	No symptoms at rest, but marked limitation of physical activity
Class IV	Symptoms present at rest, discomfort increased with any kind of physical activity

risks associated with pregnancy and all options presented. Frequent prenatal visits are indicated, and frequent hospital admissions may be needed, especially for patients with class III and IV cardiac disease.

Avoidance of excessive weight gain and edema. Cardiac patients should be placed on a low-sodium diet (2 g/day) and encouraged to rest in the left lateral decubitus position for at least 1 hour every morning, afternoon, and evening to promote diuresis. Adequate sleep should be encouraged. If there is evidence of chronic left ventricular failure not adequately treated with sodium restriction, a loop diuretic and β blockers should be added. **Aldosterone antagonists should be avoided because of their potential antiandrogen effects on the fetus.**

AVOIDANCE OF STRENUOUS ACTIVITY. Individuals with significant heart disease are unable to increase their cardiac output to the same extent as healthy individuals to meet the increased metabolic demands associated with exercise.

AVOIDANCE OF ANEMIA. With anemia, the oxygen-carrying capacity of the blood decreases. Oxygen delivery to tissues is generally maintained by increased cardiac output. An increase in heart rate, especially with mitral stenosis, leads to a decrease in left ventricular filling time, resulting in pulmonary congestion and edema. Another factor that might lead to cardiac decompensation is the inability of the right ventricle to efficiently pump a percentage of the venous return.

ANTICOAGULATION. Women with mechanical valves require full anticoagulation with heparin in pregnancy. Warfarin may be restarted post partum.

Management of Delivery and the Immediate Postpartum Period

Cardiac patients should be delivered vaginally unless obstetric indications for cesarean are present. They should be allowed to **labor in the lateral decubitus position** with frequent assessment of vital signs, urine output, and pulse oximetry. Adequate pain relief is important.

Pushing should be avoided during the second stage of labor because the associated increase in intraabdominal pressure increases venous return and cardiac output and can lead to cardiac decompensation. The second stage of labor can be assisted by performing an **outlet forceps** delivery or by the use of a **vacuum extractor.**

The immediate postpartum period presents special risks to the cardiac patient. After delivery of the placenta, the uterus contracts, and about 500 mL of blood is added to the effective blood volume. **Cardiac output increases up to 80% above prelabor values in the first few hours after a vaginal delivery and up to 50% after cesarean delivery.** To minimize the risk for overloading the circulation, careful attention is paid to fluid balance and prevention of uterine atony. **Methergine should be avoided** owing to its vasoconstrictor effects.

Of particular concern is the risk for endocarditis. The 2007 guidelines from the American Heart Association state that delivery does not increase the risk for infectious endocarditis. **Antibiotic prophylaxis is only recommended for high-risk patients** (e.g., prosthetic valves, unrepaired or incompletely repaired congenital heart disease, congenital heart disease repaired with prosthetic material, previous history of bacterial endocarditis and valvulopathy in heart transplants) if bacteremia is suspected (such as in the setting of chorioamnionitis).

Acute cardiac decompensation with congestive heart failure should be managed as a medical emergency. Medical management may include administration of morphine sulfate, supplemental oxygen, and an intravenous loop diuretic (e.g., furosemide) to reduce fluid retention and preload. β Blockers should not be used in the setting of acute heart failure. Vasodilators such as hydralazine, nitroglycerin, and rarely nitroprusside are used to improve cardiac output by decreasing afterload. **Some patients may require inotropic support** with dobutamine or dopamine. The use of digitalis is controversial. **Angiotensin-converting enzyme inhibitors are contraindicated in pregnancy. Calcium channel blockers such as nifedipine may accelerate the progression of congestive heart failure and should be avoided.** Continuous pulse oximetry can be very helpful in managing these patients. Monitoring with a pulmonary artery catheter can provide a good index of left ventricular function but is discouraged in those with pulmonary hypertension.

Autoimmune Disease in Pregnancy

An autoimmune disease is one in which antibodies are developed against the host's own tissues. A summary of the interactions of primary immunologic disorders and pregnancy is shown in Table 16-6.

IMMUNE (IDIOPATHIC) THROMBOCYTOPENIA

In this condition thrombocytopenia occurs when peripheral platelet destruction exceeds bone marrow production. Idiopathic thrombocytopenia (ITP) is considered to be an autoantibody disorder in which immunoglobulins attach to maternal platelets leading to platelet sequestration in the reticuloendothelial system. ITP may be

TABLE 16-6

AUTOIMMUNE DISEASE IN PREGNANCY

Disease	Effect of Disease on Pregnancy		Effect of Pregnancy on Disease	Antibodies that Cross Placenta
	Mother	*Fetus*		
Rheumatoid arthritis	No significant effect	No significant effect Teratogenic effects of medication	Usually improved	None
Idiopathic thrombocytopenic purpura (ITP)	Antepartum, intrapartum, and postpartum hemorrhage	None (causes neonatal intracranial bleeding)	None	Platelet antibodies
Graves' disease	No significant effect (avoid magnesium sulfate)	Intrauterine growth restriction Neonatal thyrotoxicosis	Improved during pregnancy Exacerbation postpartum	Thyroid-stimulating immunoglobulins
Myasthenia gravis	No significant effect	Transient neonatal myasthenia	Variable during pregnancy Moderate exacerbation postpartum	Antiacetylcholinesterase
Systemic lupus erythematosus (SLE)	Increased incidence of uterine infection Increased incidence of preeclampsia	Abortion (spontaneous) Preterm preeclampsia Intrauterine growth restriction Stillbirth Congenital heart block Endomyocardial fibrosis	Exacerbation of disease Deterioration of renal condition Anemia, leukopenia, and thrombocytopenia	Anti-Ro (SS-A), anti-La (SS-B)

confused with gestational thrombocytopenia. The latter is unlikely to have a platelet count less than 70,000/µL, **is not associated with bleeding complications,** occurs late in pregnancy, and resolves after delivery.

Treatment

Therapy is usually not initiated unless platelet counts are less than 40,000/µL or petechial hemorrhages are present. **Prednisone** at a dose of 1 mg/kg per day is given initially, maintained for 2 to 3 weeks, then tapered slowly. Severe ITP can be treated with intravenous immunoglobulin (IVIG), or if the patient is Rh positive, anti-D antibody infusions, which can raise the platelet count within 12 to 48 hours. **In patients with life-threatening hemorrhage, platelet transfusions, combined with high-dose steroids and IVIG, may be required. Splenectomy is a last resort** for patients who fail to respond to medical therapy. Platelet transfusions are also indicated if the maternal platelet count is less than 20,000 before vaginal delivery, or less than 40,000 before cesarean delivery.

The neonate should be monitored for thrombocytopenia because placental transfer of maternal antiplatelet antibodies can occur. Rarely, neonatal intracranial hemorrhage occurs once the neonatal platelet count reaches its nadir after the first 2 to 3 days of life. There is no correlation between fetal platelet counts and neonatal outcome; thus, monitoring fetal platelet counts is not done in pregnancy. **Vaginal delivery is generally carried out** because there is no good evidence that the fetal outcome is improved by cesarean delivery, and surgery carries additional maternal risks.

SYSTEMIC LUPUS ERYTHEMATOSUS

Lupus occurs mainly in women. Associated antibodies include antinuclear, anti-RNP and anti-SM antibodies; anti-dsDNA is associated with nephritis and lupus activity; anti-Ro (SS-A) and anti-La (SS-B) are present in Sjögren's syndrome and neonatal lupus with heart block; while antihistone antibody is common in drug-induced lupus. The diagnosis of systemic lupus is made if 4 or more of the 11 revised criteria of the American Rheumatism Association are present, serially or simultaneously (Table 16-7).

During pregnancy, lupus improves in one third of women, remains unchanged in one third, and worsens in the remaining third. A lupus flare can be life threatening, but it is difficult to differentiate a lupus flare from superimposed preeclampsia (and both may coexist). Often only a trial of therapy will distinguish between the two. Flares and active disease can generally be managed with steroids, such as prednisone, 1 mg/kg per day.

Fetal and neonatal complications include an increased rate of preterm delivery, fetal growth restriction, and stillbirth, especially when associated with antiphospholipid antibodies. These pregnancies require close monitoring, often with weekly maternal and fetal assessments once they reach the third trimester. **There is about a 10% risk for neonatal lupus,** which is characterized by skin lesions, hematologic manifestations such as thrombocytopenia or hemolysis, systemic effects such as hepatic involvement, and occasionally congenital heart block.

ANTIPHOSPHOLIPID ANTIBODIES (LUPUS ANTICOAGULANT AND ANTICARDIOLIPIN)

Antiphospholipid antibodies are circulating antibodies to negatively charged phospholipids. They include lupus anticoagulant, anticardiolipin immunoglobulin G (IgG), or IgM antibodies and β_2-glycoprotein I antibodies. They may occur alone or in association with lupus. **Antiphospholipid antibody syndrome** is defined as the presence of at least one antibody in association with arterial or venous thrombosis with or without one or more obstetric complication (unexplained fetal demise after 10 weeks' gestation or severe preeclampsia or fetal growth restriction before 34 weeks' gestation). Lupus anticoagulant can be screened for with an activated partial prothrombin time or the dilute Russell

TABLE 16-7

AMERICAN RHEUMATISM ASSOCIATION 1997 REVISED CRITERIA FOR SYSTEMIC LUPUS ERYTHEMATOSUS	
Criteria*	**Comments**
Malar rash	Malar erythema
Discoid rash	Erythematous patches, scaling, follicular plugging
Photosensitivity	
Oral ulcers	Usually painless
Arthritis	Nonerosive involving two or more peripheral joints
Serositis	Pleuritis or pericarditis
Renal disorder	Proteinuria > 0.5 g/day or > 3+ dipstick, or cellular casts
Neurologic disorders	Seizures or psychosis without other cause
Hematologic disorders	Hemolytic anemia, leukopenia, lymphopenia, or thrombocytopenia
Immunologic disorders	Anti-dsDNA or anti-Sm antibodies, or false-positive VDRL, immunoglobulin M or G anticardiolipin antibodies, or lupus anticoagulant
Antinuclear antibodies	Abnormal titer of antinuclear antibodies

*If four criteria are present at any time during course of disease, systemic lupus can be diagnosed with 98% specificity and 97% sensitivity.

VDRL, Venereal Disease Research Laboratory.

From Hochberg MC: Updating the American College of Rheumatology revised criteria for the classification of systemic lupus erythematosus. Arthritis Rheum 40(9):1725, 1997. Copyright 1997 American College of Rheumatology. Reprinted with permission of John Wiley & Sons, Inc.

viper venom test (DRVVT); a sensitive and specific radioimmunoassay is available for the detection of anti-cardiolipin. In pregnancy, **a history of antiphospholipid antibody syndrome is treated with intermediate-dose heparin or low-molecular-weight heparin and baby aspirin,** unless there is a history of thrombosis, in which case full-dose anticoagulation is indicated.

▨ Renal Disorders

ACUTE RENAL FAILURE

Acute renal failure during pregnancy or in the postpartum period may be due to deterioration of renal function secondary to a preexisting renal disease or to a pregnancy-induced disorder. The underlying causative factors may be prerenal, renal, or postrenal. **With prerenal causes, a history of blood or fluid loss, such as occurs with obstetric hemorrhage, is usually apparent or can be elicited. Renal causes are usually suspected in a patient with a history of preexisting renal disease or with a hypercoagulable state,** such as thrombotic thrombocytopenic purpura or hemolytic-uremic syndrome **Prolonged hypotension can lead to acute cortical necrosis or acute tubular necrosis. Postrenal causes are less common but should be suspected in situations in which urologic obstructive lesions are present** or in which there is a history of kidney stones.

Laboratory Studies

Laboratory tests are directed at assessing renal function, cardiovascular status, and the patency of the urologic tract.

RENAL STUDIES. Renal studies include urine output, blood urea nitrogen (BUN)-to-creatinine ratio, fractional excretion of sodium, and urine osmolality. **Oliguria is defined as urine output of less than 25 mL/hour,** whereas anuria is the cessation of urine output. Not infrequently, a decrease in urine output alerts the physician to an impending crisis. **During pregnancy, the serum values of BUN and creatinine decrease, but the BUN-to-creatinine ratio remains about 20:1.** A ratio greater than 20:1 suggests tubular hypoperfusion (prerenal failure).

Urine osmolality greater than 500 mOsm/L or a urine-to-plasma osmolality ratio greater than 1.5:1 is highly suggestive of renal hypoperfusion. Urine specific gravity is of limited value, especially when the urine contains protein or hemolyzed blood.

CARDIOVASCULAR STUDIES. Acute blood and fluid losses are usually associated with orthostatic hypotension, tachycardia, decreased skin turgor, and reduced sweating. In a pregnant hypertensive or preeclamptic patient who is in labor, many of these signs are overlooked. If indicated, a Swan-Ganz catheter allows monitoring of right and left ventricular filling pressures, cardiac output, and pulmonary capillary wedge pressure. This can help to distinguish between congestive heart failure, cardiac tamponade, and volume depletion, any of which can lead to acute renal failure.

UROLOGIC TRACT STUDIES. A Foley catheter and renal sonogram are usually sufficient to diagnose obstructive lesions. Rarely, a one-shot intravenous pyelogram is needed. It is important not to mistake the **physiologic hydronephrosis of pregnancy** for true obstruction.

Treatment

PRERENAL CAUSES. Restoration of intravascular volume, cardiac output, and arterial pressure to normal values is sufficient to reverse oliguria. Careful attention should be given to electrolyte imbalance when large amounts of crystalloids are infused.

RENAL CAUSES. Acute tubular necrosis, acute cortical necrosis, or both, may be present. Because acute cortical necrosis is generally irreversible, treatment is directed toward preventing further damage. **A trial of diuretic therapy to increase urinary output appears to decrease the duration and severity of acute tubular necrosis and increase survival rates. Furosemide** (Lasix) is given initially and repeated every 4 to 6 hours for 48 hours in the presence of adequate urinary response. **If the diuretic therapy fails to increase the urine output, an oliguric fluid regimen (<500 mL/24 hr) is initiated.** Fluid intake should be limited to replacement of urine output and insensible water loss, and renal function studies should be monitored on a daily basis. For the first few days after the renal ischemic episode, renal function may worsen, but within 7 to 10 days, most patients with acute tubular necrosis show marked improvement. **If renal function deteriorates rapidly or fails to recover, hemodialysis is recommended.**

In some patients in whom acute renal failure is accompanied by oliguria, a diuretic phase coincides with the recovery period. The urine output may exceed 10 L/day, and if fluid and electrolyte losses are not replaced promptly, death ensues. **About 50% of obstetric patients who develop acute renal failure during pregnancy or the postpartum period recover enough renal function during the first year to survive without dialysis.**

POSTRENAL CAUSES. In many instances, simple measures, such as turning the patient on the left side to displace the gravid uterus away from the ureters, or inserting a Foley catheter into the bladder to overcome urethral obstruction, will resolve the problem. In situations in which a ureteral or renal pelvic obstruction is present (e.g., stones), surgical intervention is indicated to relieve the obstruction.

CHRONIC RENAL FAILURE

The outcome of pregnancies complicated by chronic renal disease is less favorable. Good pregnancy outcome may be expected in mild renal disease. There is increased risk for adverse fetal outcome and loss of maternal renal function with increasing renal insufficiency severity. **In general a serum creatinine greater than 1.5 to 2.0, especially if accompanied by hypertension or nephrotic syndrome, greatly worsens the prognosis for the mother and fetus.** Management principles include serial monitoring of renal function by 24-hour urinary creatinine clearance and protein excretion, and screening for asymptomatic bacteriuria. Diastolic pressure should be maintained at 90 mm Hg or less to prevent further renal damage. Superimposed preeclampsia is more difficult to diagnose because hypertension and proteinuria are already present. Fetal surveillance is important to assess fetal growth and well-being.

PREGNANCY FOLLOWING RENAL TRANSPLANTATION

Pregnancy after renal transplantation should not be considered before a thorough assessment of maternal, fetal, and neonatal risk factors is undertaken. Hypertension (up to 70%) and preeclampsia are common in women with renal transplantation, and up to 14% experience significant loss of graft function or graft rejection. **Fetal complications include steroid-induced adrenal and hepatic insufficiency, prematurity, and IUGR.** In addition, the infant may inherit the primary disease of the mother or other family members. The mother and neonate are at increased risk for infection because of immunosuppressive therapy.

Patients who are good candidates for pregnancy are those who are 1 to 2 years posttransplantation, have stable renal function (serum creatinine < 1.5 and proteinuria < 500 mg/day), are not significantly hypertensive, and are on low doses of prednisone and stable doses of azathioprine and cyclosporine. These medications do not appear to have significant teratogenic effects, but long-term consequences on growth, immune function, and neurocognitive development are unknown. Cyclosporine may have adverse maternal consequences, including a rise in blood pressure, a decline in renal function, hyperkalemia, hyperuricemia, and less frequently, hemolytic-uremic syndrome.

▨ *Gastrointestinal Disorders*

NAUSEA AND VOMITING DURING PREGNANCY

About 60% to 80% of pregnant women complain of nausea and vomiting during the first 8 to 12 weeks of gestation. The symptoms are usually mild and disappear during the early part of the second trimester. **The underlying causes of nausea and vomiting during pregnancy are not well understood.**

Treatment is usually symptomatic. Patients are instructed to refrain from eating large and late meals, to avoid the recumbent position, especially after meals, and to use an extra pillow to elevate the head when sleeping. Many patients respond to pyridoxine (vitamin B_6), whereas others may require antiemetics such as promethazine.

HYPEREMESIS GRAVIDARUM

Hyperemesis gravidarum is defined as persistent nausea and vomiting in pregnancy that is associated with ketosis and weight loss (>5% of prepregnancy weight). Even though the exact cause is unknown, proposed theories include psychological abnormalities, hormonal changes such as high human chorionic gonadotropin (hCG) and estradiol levels, gastric dysrhythmias, hyperacuity of the olfactory system, subclinical vestibular disorders, and impairment of mitochondrial fatty acid oxidation. **The overall incidence is about 1%. The disorder appears more frequently with first pregnancies, multiple pregnancies, and those with trophoblastic disease,** but tends to recur with subsequent pregnancies. **Pregnancy outcome is usually good.**

A history of intractable vomiting beginning in the first trimester and inability to retain food and fluid is usually elicited. Physical findings of weight loss, dry and coated tongue, and decreased skin turgor are very suggestive. **Significant abdominal pain and tenderness are generally absent.** Laboratory workup includes urine tests for ketonuria and blood tests for electrolytes and acetone. Electrolyte disturbances may include hypokalemia, hyponatremia, and hypochloremic alkalosis. Amylase and lipase levels may be elevated.

Treatment is symptomatic, but **if outpatient management fails, patients must be admitted for intravenous administration of fluids, electrolytes, glucose, vitamins, and medical therapy.** Vitamin B_6 (pyridoxine), doxylamine, antihistamines, antiemetics of the phenothiazine class, and promotility agents (e.g., metoclopramide), and droperidol are used. Acupressure and ginger have been shown to be beneficial. The few who do not respond to medical therapy may require nasogastric feeding or parenteral nutrition.

REFLUX ESOPHAGITIS

Reflux esophagitis or heartburn occurs in about 70% of pregnant women. The main symptoms include substernal discomfort aggravated by meals and the recumbent position and occasional hematemesis. An unusual symptom peculiar to reflux esophagitis is water brash, which is best described as the sudden filling of the mouth with clear, watery material that has a salty taste and produces a nauseous sensation.

Treatment

Treatment is usually symptomatic. Patients are instructed to refrain from eating large and late meals, to avoid the recumbent position, especially after meals, and to use an extra pillow to elevate the head when sleeping. Antacids can be helpful and should be taken 1 to 3 hours after meals and at bedtime. **A histamine-2 (H_2) blocker (cimetidine) or proton pump blocker (omeprazole) is indicated if there is no response to the above measures.**

PEPTIC ULCER

Pregnancy conveys relative protection against the development of peptic ulceration and may ameliorate an already present ulcer. Gastric acid secretion is probably not altered during pregnancy, although some studies suggest modest suppression. **The diagnosis of ulcer disease is mainly based on symptomatic improvement in response to conservative treatment. Endoscopy is reserved for patients who do not respond to treatment, have more severe gastrointestinal symptoms, or manifest significant gastrointestinal hemorrhage.** Treatment involves avoiding caffeine, alcohol, tobacco, and spicy foods and administering antacids, proton pump inhibitors, or H_2-receptor antagonists. Antibiotic therapy is indicated for patients with *Helicobacter pylori* infection.

ACID ASPIRATION SYNDROME (MENDELSON'S SYNDROME)

The pregnant patient in labor is at an increased risk for acid aspiration because of delayed gastric emptying. This is made worse when associated with increased anxiety or the use of sedatives, narcotics, and anticholinergic agents and **increased intraabdominal and intragastric pressure,** making regurgitation more likely. Damage to the pulmonary tissue is greatest when the pH of the aspirated fluid is less than 2.5 or the volume of the aspirate is greater than 25 mL. **Acute gastric aspiration is a cause of adult respiratory distress syndrome (ARDS).** Treatment consists of supplemental oxygen, measures to maintain the airway, and usual therapy for treatment of acute respiratory failure.

Preventive efforts are directed at decreasing the acid secretion by the stomach. Toward this end, women are usually not fed during labor. **Liquid magnesium and aluminum antacids may be given during labor to decrease the gastric acidity,** but they increase the volume of the gastric acid-antacid emulsion. If the patient is to undergo any surgical procedure that requires general anesthesia, a "full stomach" should be presumed and intubation performed.

CHRONIC INFLAMMATORY BOWEL DISEASE

The two entities described under this disorder are **Crohn disease (regional enteritis)** and **ulcerative colitis.** In about 25% of patients with inflammatory bowel disease, differentiation between these two disorders is difficult.

Patients with inflammatory bowel disease do well during pregnancy, provided there are no acute exacerbations. It seems unlikely that the natural history of the disease changes during pregnancy. **If inflammatory bowel disease is active at the time of conception, the spontaneous abortion rate is doubled.** If surgery is required for complications of inflammatory bowel disease, fetal survival is reduced.

Treatment

Treatment of an acute exacerbation is the same for pregnant and nonpregnant patients, although some of the more experimental drugs should not be used during pregnancy. **If diarrhea is the main complaint, dietary restriction of lactose, fruits, and vegetables is necessary.** If a lactose-free diet is used, calcium supplementation is needed. **Constipating agents, such as Pepto-Bismol and psyllium hydrophilic mucilloid (Metamucil), may be used daily and are quite effective.** The use of diphenoxylate-atropine (Lomotil) or loperamide (Imodium) should be restricted to patients in whom conservative management fails. **For those patients with mild to moderate symptoms, sulfasalazine may be beneficial.** Recently, several antibiotic regimens have been used to treat Crohn disease.

■ *Hepatic Disorders*

Liver disorders that are peculiar to pregnancy are discussed next.

INTRAHEPATIC CHOLESTASIS OF PREGNANCY

Although the pathogenesis of this syndrome is not known, some distinctive features are present: (1) **cholestasis and pruritus in the second half of pregnancy** without other major liver dysfunction, (2) **a tendency to recurrence** with each pregnancy, (3) **an association with oral contraceptives and multiple gestations,** (4) **a benign course** in that there are no maternal hepatic sequelae, and (5) an **increased rate of meconium-stained amniotic fluid and fetal demise.** There is a high prevalence in Latin America with rates of 4% to 22%. The highest rates occur in Chile in winter. The prevalence in the United States has been reported from between 0.001% and 0.32%, with a high prevalence of 5.6% reported in a Latina population in Los Angeles.

Most probably, genetic, geographic, or environmental factors are involved. A mutation in the *MDR3* gene may be associated with up to 15% of cases.

The main symptom is itching, without abdominal pain or a rash, which may occur as early as 20 weeks of gestation. Jaundice is rarely observed. **Laboratory tests show elevated levels of serum bile acids.** Serum levels of bilirubin and liver enzymes (e.g., aspartate and alanine transaminase) are usually normal but may be mildly elevated. If liver enzymes and bilirubin levels are significantly elevated, abdominal ultrasonography should be performed to exclude gallbladder obstruction, a hepatitis screen should be done to exclude viral hepatitis, and an autoantibody screen for primary biliary cirrhosis should also be undertaken.

Treatment

Local measures such as cold baths, bicarbonate washes, or phenol (0.5% to 1% in water-soluble creams) may be of some help. **The best results have been obtained with ursodeoxycholic acid.** It significantly ameliorates the pruritus and reduces serum levels of bile acids, aminotransferases, and bilirubin. **Serial fetal surveillance is performed in the third trimester, with delivery at term if testing remains reassuring.**

ACUTE FATTY LIVER OF PREGNANCY

Acute fatty liver of pregnancy is a serious complication that is peculiar to pregnancy. It is associated with diffuse microvesicular fatty infiltration of the liver resulting in hepatic failure. The incidence is about 1 per 10,000 pregnancies. It most commonly occurs in the third trimester of pregnancy or the early postpartum period. Although the cause is unknown, it may in some instances result from an inborn error of metabolism, possibly a deficiency of long-chain 3-hydroxyl coenzyme A dehydrogenase. **Presentation is variable, with abdominal pain, nausea and vomiting, jaundice, and increased irritability.** Extreme polydipsia or pseudodiabetes insipidus may be present. Hypoglycemia is infrequently present. **Hypertension and proteinuria are present in about half of patients, raising the issue of coexisting preeclampsia. Invariably, patients suffer hepatic coma and renal failure.**

Investigations

Laboratory findings include an increase in prothrombin time (PT) and partial thromboplastin time (PTT), hyperbilirubinemia, hyperammonemia, hyperuricemia, and a moderate elevation of the transaminase levels. Hematemesis and spontaneous bleeding become manifest as disseminated intravascular coagulation (DIC) develops. Liver failure is indicated by elevated blood ammonia levels.

Treatment

Termination of pregnancy and intensive supportive care are indicated on diagnosis. Treatment is mainly directed at supportive measures, such as administration of intravenous fluids with 10% glucose to prevent dehydration and severe hypoglycemia. For the coagulopathy of hepatic failure, vitamin K supplementation is not effective, and fresh-frozen plasma or cryoprecipitate should be given.

With early recognition, immediate delivery, and advances in critical care management, maternal mortality is about 7% to 18%, and fetal mortality about 9% to 23%. **In those who survive, recovery is complete, with no signs of chronic liver disease.**

Thromboembolic Disorders

Pregnancy is a hypercoagulable state and is associated with an increased risk for superficial thrombophlebitis, deep venous thrombosis (DVT), and pulmonary embolism. The risk increases postpartum and with cesarean delivery.

SUPERFICIAL THROMBOPHLEBITIS

This is more common in patients with varicose veins, obesity, or limited physical activity. **In most patients, superficial thrombophlebitis is limited to the calf area, and symptoms include swelling and tenderness of the involved extremity.** On physical examination, there is erythema, tenderness, warmth, and a palpable cord over the course of the involved superficial veins.

Superficial thrombophlebitis does not lead to pulmonary embolization. Bed rest, pain medications, and local application of heat are often sufficient treatment. **There is no need for anticoagulants, but antiinflammatory agents may be considered.** When symptoms disappear, patients may gradually begin to ambulate. **They should be instructed to wear support hose** to help avoid a repeat episode.

DEEP VENOUS THROMBOSIS

The incidence of DVT is 1 in 2000 patients antepartum and 1 in 700 patients postpartum. Virchow's triad of vascular injury, infection, and tissue trauma, coupled with the hypercoagulability and venous stasis of pregnancy, are the triggering factors for DVT.

CLINICAL FEATURES. The clinical diagnosis of DVT is difficult. Half of cases are asymptomatic. **DVT is much more common in the left than the right leg.** Pain in the calf in association with dorsiflexion of the foot **(positive Homans' sign)** is a clinical sign of DVT in the calf veins. Dull ache, tingling, tightness, or pain in the calf or leg, especially when walking, may be present. Acute swelling and pain in the thigh area and tenderness in the femoral triangle are suggestive of iliofemoral thrombosis.

INVESTIGATIONS. Compression ultrasonography with Doppler flow studies is a noninvasive technique that has high sensitivity and specificity and **is currently the primary mode of diagnosis** used for DVT. **Magnetic resonance imaging** (MRI) has been used to evaluate patients suspected of having pelvic thrombosis with a negative Doppler ultrasonic examination. **D-Dimers**

can be used in nonpregnant women to screen for DVT, but their use in pregnancy is unproved. The most reliable test for deep venous (noniliac) thrombosis is a well-performed **venogram,** but this is not generally performed because of the 2% risk for dye-induced phlebitis and radiation exposure, the latter dosage being between 0.05 and 0.628 Gy (see Table 16-8 on page 216).

Treatment

When a clinical diagnosis of DVT is made, anticoagulant therapy should be started pending the results of a diagnostic workup. If the workup fails to identify any iliofemoral or calf thrombosis, therapy may be discontinued.

Treatment of proven DVT during pregnancy is initiated with either intravenous unfractionated heparin or subcutaneous low-molecular-weight heparin (enoxaparin sodium) to achieve full anticoagulation. The unfractionated heparin dose is adjusted to 1.5 to 2.5 times the control activated PTT (aPTT). **Intravenous anticoagulation should be maintained for at least 5 to 7 days, after which treatment is converted to subcutaneous heparin, which must be continued for the duration of pregnancy and up to 6 weeks postpartum** with weekly monitoring of the aPTT. Alternatively, enoxaparin can be administered at a dose of 1 mg/kg subcutaneously every 12 hours. Although anti–factor Xa levels can be used to monitor enoxaparin's anticoagulant activity, they are not generally useful because of the long lag in receiving results. **Both forms of heparin may be associated with thrombocytopenia and osteoporosis.** Supplemental calcium and vitamin D are advised along with periodic platelet counts.

Warfarin is a vitamin K antagonist, which **crosses the placenta,** carries the risks for fetal hemorrhage and teratogenesis and, with few exceptions, **should only be used in the postpartum period.** The International Normalized Ratio (INR) is commonly used to measure the effects of warfarin, and the target INR is 2.5 (range, 2.0 to 3.0).

PULMONARY EMBOLISM

The incidence of pulmonary embolism during pregnancy is about 1 in 2500. **The maternal mortality rate is less than 1% if treated early and greater than 80% if left untreated.** It is one of the most common causes of pregnancy-related deaths in the United States. In about 70% of cases, DVT is the instigating factor.

CLINICAL FEATURES. Suggestive symptoms include pleuritic chest pain, shortness of breath, air hunger, palpitations, hemoptysis, and syncopal episodes. Suggestive signs include tachypnea, tachycardia, low-grade fever, a pleural friction rub, chest splinting, pulmonary rales, an accentuated pulmonic valve second heart sound, and even signs of right ventricular failure. In most obstetric patients, the signs and symptoms of a pulmonary embolus are subtle.

INVESTIGATIONS. An **electrocardiogram** can show sinus tachycardia with or without premature heartbeats or right ventricular axis deviation. On **chest film,** atelectasis, pleural effusion, obliteration of arterial shadows, and elevation of the diaphragm may be present. **Arterial blood gases obtained on room air may show an oxygen tension below 80 mm Hg. Pulmonary embolism is ultimately a radiologic diagnosis. Three algorithms may be used: (1) If bilateral compression ultrasonography of the lower extremities is positive for DVT, a pulmonary embolism may be assumed in a symptomatic patient. (2) A ventilation-perfusion scan** has minimal risk to the fetus, but it cannot be used in patients with an abnormal chest x-ray or in patients with asthma or chronic obstructive pulmonary disease. (3) **Helical computed tomography** has the advantage that the presence of a thrombus can be visualized by a noninvasive technique. It has comparative sensitivity to conventional pulmonary angiography and has been shown to be a cost-effective technique in pregnancy. **Pulmonary angiography is rarely required** because it is invasive, expensive, employs a higher radiation dose, and has a significant mortality.

Treatment of acute episodes and follow-up during pregnancy, labor, delivery, and the postpartum period are the same as for DVT.

THROMBOPHILIA EVALUATION. A thrombophilia workup should be considered in patients with a pulmonary embolus, especially those with recurrent thromboses or a positive family history. Tests to order include those for acquired (lupus anticoagulant, anticardiolipin antibody) and inherited thrombophilias (factor V Leiden mutation, protein C, protein S and antithrombin III deficiencies, and the prothrombin G20210A mutation).

PROPHYLACTIC ANTICOAGULANT THERAPY. In pregnant patients with a history of a pulmonary embolus or DVT during a previous pregnancy, prophylactic doses of heparin or low-molecular-weight heparin are given during pregnancy and the immediate postpartum period. **Minidose heparin (10,000 to 15,000 U/day) or enoxaparin sodium (40 mg once daily)** provides sufficient prophylaxis for most patients, although some pregnant women may require full anticoagulation.

Obstructive Lung Disease

BRONCHIAL ASTHMA

The incidence of bronchial asthma in pregnancy is about 5% to 9%. Status asthmaticus, the most severe form of asthma, complicates about 0.2% of pregnancies. Asthma is a chronic inflammatory airway disorder with a major hereditary component and usually an allergic stimulant. Asthma currently is classified according to severity as (1) mild intermittent, (2) mild persistent, (3) moderate persistent, and (4) severe persistent. The course during pregnancy is variable. About 33% of patients improve, and 33% deteriorate.

Pulmonary function studies done during an acute episode show (1) increased airway resistance; (2) increased residual volume, functional residual capacity, and total lung capacity; (3) decreased inspiratory and expiratory reserve volume; (4) decreased vital capacity; and (5) decreased 1-second forced expiratory volume (FEV_1), peak expiratory flow rate, and maximal mid-expiratory flow rate. **Severe asthma is associated with an increased rate of miscarriage, preeclampsia, intrauterine fetal death, fetal growth restriction, and preterm birth.** These complications may occur **as a result of intrauterine hypoxia.**

Obstetric Management

Pregnant asthmatic patients should be followed closely during pregnancy. The avoidance of dehydration, early and aggressive treatment of respiratory infections, and the avoidance of hyperventilation, excessive physical activity, and allergens are important. Serial measurements of peak expiratory flow rates can provide useful information on respiratory status. For those with mild intermittent asthma, **a short-acting inhaled β_2 agonist** can be used as needed. Patients with mild persistent asthma should be treated with **a low-dose inhaled corticosteroid.** The preferred treatment for moderate persistent asthma is a combination of a daily inhaled corticosteroid and a **long-acting β_2 agonist. Those with severe persistent asthma may require the addition of a systemic corticosteroid.** Alternative therapies include inhaled cromolyn sodium, leukotriene receptor antagonists, or sustained-release theophylline. Acute severe exacerbations must be treated aggressively with oxygen therapy, intravenous fluids, intravenous corticosteroids, and administration of β_2 agonists by nebulized aerosol and antibiotics if there is evidence of bacterial infection. A few patients may require endotracheal intubation and mechanical ventilation to maintain an adequate oxygen supply.

Serial fetal monitoring and ultrasonic assessment of fetal growth should be implemented. The timing of delivery is dependent on the status of both the mother and the fetus. If pregnancy is progressing well, there is no need for early intervention, and it is advisable to await the spontaneous onset of labor. **Early delivery can be considered for fetal growth restriction or maternal deterioration.**

Management of Labor and Delivery

Glucocorticoid therapy, including inhaled or high-potency topical use for more than 3 weeks, may suppress the hypothalamic-pituitary-adrenal axis. Delivery is probably associated with moderate surgical stress, and stress doses of steroids should be considered. A selective epidural block during labor reduces pain, anxiety, hyperventilation, and respiratory effort, all of which are known to aggravate the disease or precipitate an attack. **Vaginal delivery should be anticipated. Cesarean delivery is performed only for obstetric reasons.**

CYSTIC FIBROSIS

Because of improvements in diagnosis and treatment, most females with **cystic fibrosis** now survive to adulthood. Cystic fibrosis is due to mutations in cystic fibrosis conductance transmembrane regulator, or *CFTR*, which is the gene that regulates epithelial cell chloride channel function. **It is the most severe form of obstructive lung disease observed during pregnancy,** but **there is no evidence that pregnancy increases the maternal risk.** However, those with pulmonary hypertension should be counseled against pregnancy. There are risks for superimposed infections during pregnancy. Exocrine pancreatic insufficiency is present in about 90% of patients with cystic fibrosis. Women with malabsorption symptoms might become more emaciated during pregnancy. Preconception counseling is recommended. **The fetus is at increased risk for IUGR and premature delivery.**

For labor and delivery, epidural analgesia is recommended. Outlet forceps or vacuum-assisted delivery should also be considered. The Valsalva maneuver should be avoided because of the associated increase in maternal oxygen requirements. Breastfeeding is recommended unless the maternal condition does not allow it.

◼ *Seizures*

In most cases, seizure frequency does not change in pregnancy. Factors during pregnancy that may contribute to increased seizure frequency include nausea and vomiting leading to missed doses, decreased gastrointestinal motility, expanded intravascular volume lowering serum drug levels, induction of enzymes increasing drug metabolism, and increased glomerular filtration hastening drug clearance.

Treatment

If patients have no seizure activity for at least 2 years, antiepileptic drug (AED) therapy can be discontinued before conception. If patients are pregnant and their seizures are well controlled, no change in therapy should be attempted. The AED that is effective should be used. **Monotherapy should be attempted using the lowest drug dose that will control the seizures.** There is no ideal anticonvulsant in pregnancy, and all AEDs should be considered potential teratogens. **Valproate should probably not be used** because it is has been shown to be more teratogenic when compared with other AEDs.

Historically, the two most commonly used drugs for seizure treatment have been **phenytoin (Dilantin)** and **phenobarbital.** Phenobarbital at a dose of 100 to 250 mg/day may be given in divided doses. The serum levels are monitored, and the dose is increased gradually until a therapeutic level (10 to 40 μg/mL) is reached. **Phenytoin** may be given at 300 to 500 mg/day, in single or divided doses, to achieve serum levels of 10 to 20 μg/mL (1 to 2 μg/mL free level). Other first-generation AEDs include **trimethadione, clonazepam (Klonopin), and carbamazepine (Tegretol).** Second-generation AEDs **include** lamotrigine, topiramate, and gabapentin.

Women on AEDs should take 1 mg/day of folate supplementation. Those on carbamazepine or valproate should take 4 mg per day of folate supplementation. Oral vitamin K supplementation, 10 mg/day, should be considered in the last month of pregnancy for women taking enzyme-inducing AEDs (e.g., phenobarbital, carbamazepine, phenytoin, topiramate, oxcarbazepine). Phenytoin interferes with intestinal calcium absorption, leading to maternal and fetal hypocalcemia. In patients taking phenobarbital, primidone, or phenytoin, **vitamin D supplements** may be taken starting at about 34 weeks. Antacids and antihistamines should be avoided in patients receiving phenytoin because they lower plasma levels of phenytoin and may precipitate a seizure attack.

For the treatment of status epilepticus, immediate hospitalization is required. Management is similar to that in the nonpregnant adult. Patency of the airway and adequate oxygenation should be insured. After blood is drawn for plasma levels of anticonvulsants, **intravenous diazepam (or lorazepam) should be given slowly, followed by a loading dose of phenytoin (at a rate no faster than 25 to 50 mg/minute with continuous cardiac monitoring).** If seizure patterns continue, pentobarbital may be added, and the patient should be intubated and mechanically ventilated.

The management of labor and delivery follows obstetric indications. During labor and in the immediate postpartum period, anticonvulsant drugs must be continued. Postpartum, the dose of the anticonvulsant drug may be lowered, provided that a therapeutic level is maintained. **Although anticonvulsants are excreted in breast milk in small amounts, breastfeeding is not contraindicated.**

Complications

Pregnant patients with epilepsy have a twofold increase in such maternal complications as preeclampsia, abruption, hyperemesis, and premature labor. Fetal hypoxia is a potential consequence of maternal seizures, and there is a high incidence of intrauterine fetal demise. In the neonate, higher rates of coagulopathy, drug withdrawal symptoms, and neonatal morbidity and mortality are reported. **Congenital anomalies are more common in neonates exposed to AEDs in utero** compared with offspring of untreated women with epilepsy and women without epilepsy. **The overall risk for major malformations is 4% to 6%.** Small retrospective studies have raised the possibility of impaired cognitive and neurologic function in the offspring that may manifest later in life. The risk for a seizure disorder is greater among the children of mothers with epilepsy.

Human Immunodeficiency Virus and Other Infectious Diseases

Infections in pregnancy are a frequent cause of maternal and neonatal morbidity. In some cases (e.g., HIV and syphilis), treatment of the maternal infection will decrease the chance of fetal or neonatal infection.

HUMAN IMMUNODEFICIENCY VIRUS

About 16.4 million women have HIV worldwide; **mother-to-child transmission is the primary cause of the annual HIV infection rate of 600,000 in children.** Since 1994, significant progress has been made in reducing the vertical transmission rate.

The Virus

HIV is an RNA retrovirus that replicates in certain cell types, in particular in helper T4 lymphocytes in the hematopoietic system and in cells of the central nervous system. As with all retroviruses, HIV contains a reverse transcriptase in its core. HIV has specific surface proteins gp120 and gp41 and core proteins p18 and p24. HIV infects a cell by making contact with the gp120 protein. It then enters the cell, releases its core RNA, makes a DNA copy of itself with its reverse transcriptase, and inserts this DNA into the host genome. This viral gene then either enters into a latent state or begins making viral RNA and proteins with production of an infectious virus.

Laboratory Diagnosis

Indirect serologic methods that detect HIV antibody include the enzyme-linked immunosorbent assay (ELISA), Western blot, and immunofluorescence assay (IFA) tests. **The sensitivity of the ELISA is 93% to 99%, and the specificity is 99%.** Although rare, false-positive ELISA results can occur, so **a confirmatory test is always needed.** The Western blot test, which identifies the presence of HIV core and envelope antigens, is 99% sensitive and 98.5% specific. False-positive Western blot results are extremely uncommon. Indirect serology with the capture ELISA technique can also identify HIV antigen (e.g., p24 antigen test). **The virus** can also be identified by direct tissue culture or by HIV DNA polymerase chain reaction.

Disease Course

Infection with HIV results in a chronic progressive disease. **Seroconversion typically occurs 3 to 14 weeks after exposure but may take 6 months or more.** In 90% of cases, seroconversion is associated with a mononucleosis-like syndrome or aseptic meningitis. **Once the virus has been acquired, the patient enters an asymptomatic period,** but lifetime infection should be assumed. Because HIV has a predilection for helper (T4) cells, a gradual destruction of the patient's cell-mediated immunity occurs, rendering the host susceptible to opportunistic infections. Eventual reversal of the T4-to-T8 ratio to less than 1 is seen on laboratory analysis.

Typically, the patient develops asymptomatic lymphadenopathy, followed by the onset of constitutional symptoms (anorexia, fever, weight loss, diarrhea, nausea, and vomiting). **Eventually, opportunistic infections, secondary cancers** (Kaposi's sarcoma, non-Hodgkin's lymphoma), **or neurologic diseases** (dementia, neuropathy) **develop.** Opportunistic infections that may be seen include the following: *Pneumocystis carinii* pneumonia (PCP), tuberculosis, cryptococcal meningitis, cytomegalovirus (CMV) retinitis, atypical mycobacterial disease, cerebral toxoplasmosis, severe herpes, and cryptosporidiosis. **The average interval from initial infection to the onset of AIDS in adults not receiving potent antiviral therapy is 10 years.**

Pregnancy does not appear to accelerate the course of HIV infection. Pregnant women may be at increased risk for developing infectious complications during pregnancy. These infections include opportunistic infections, postpartum infections, antepartum urinary tract infections, and sexually transmitted diseases. **No direct detrimental effects on perinatal outcome have been documented.** Studies in the United States have not shown an increased risk for growth restriction, preterm labor, or premature rupture of the membranes. **In children, the disease progresses more rapidly.** Of infants infected with HIV, half develop AIDS in the first year of life, and 85% develop AIDS by age 3 years. Children have an extremely poor prognosis, the average survival time from diagnosis being 3 years.

Vertical Transmission

The risk for vertical transmission of HIV from an infected mother to her infant is between 20% and 30%. Such transmission accounts for 99% of cases of HIV infection in children. Vertical transmission may occur antepartum (transplacental), intrapartum, and postpartum. **It is suspected that more than 50% of transmissions occur near the time of or during labor and delivery.** Maternal-fetal transmission as a result of invasive procedures such as amniocentesis, chorionic villus sampling, umbilical blood sampling, or scalp electrode placement is theoretically possible, but the exact risk is unknown. **Breastfeeding may increase the risk for transmission by 10% to 20%.** There is no confirmed evidence that fetal HIV infection can result in structural anomalies. **It appears that women with advanced disease, recent HIV infection, or preterm delivery have an increased risk for vertical transmission to their infants.**

In 1994, Pediatric AIDs Clinical Trial 076 showed that the administration of the nucleoside reverse-transcriptase inhibitor **zidovudine** to the mother during pregnancy and labor and to the infant for 6 weeks postpartum reduced the maternal transmission to the newborn from 25.5% to 8.3%, with a 68% reduction in vertical transmission. More recently, **potent antiretroviral therapy,** which reduces the maternal plasma HIV RNA levels to less than 1000 copies per milliliter, has been shown to reduce the vertical transmission rate to only 1% to 2%.

The current management for pregnant women involves the use of multiple agents to minimize the development of drug resistance, and unless contraindicated, all drug regimens should include zidovudine. Antiretroviral drug classes currently used in pregnancy include nucleoside and nucleotide reverse transcriptase inhibitors (NRTIs); non-nucleoside reverse transcriptase inhibitors (NNRTIs), and protease inhibitors. A common regimen currently used is zidovudine plus lamivudine (Combivir) plus lopinavir and ritonavir (Kaletra). Pregnant women with HIV infection on nucleoside analogues should have liver enzymes and electrolytes monitored in the third trimester. Pregnant women on protease inhibitors should be screened for gestational diabetes at the initial visit in addition to the usual time at 24 to 28 weeks because these drugs can cause hyperglycemia. **For women who are immunocompromised,** with CD4 counts of $0.20 \times 10^9/L$ (200/μL) or below, **prophylaxis against PCP,** *Mycobacterium avium* **complex infection, and others should be offered.** Trimethoprim sulfamethoxazole is relatively safe for use in pregnancy and is the first choice for PCP prophylaxis.

Because the risk for vertical transmission increases with maternal plasma HIV RNA concentrations, the therapeutic goal is to keep the maternal viral load either undetectable or less than 1000 copies per milliliter. In general, pregnant women should be maintained on the same antiretroviral therapy they received in the nonpregnant state. Invasive fetal diagnostic procedures, such as amniocentesis and chorionic villus sampling, pose a theoretical risk for infecting the fetus and should probably be avoided.

Pregnant women should receive counseling on the risk for newborn infection and the delivery choices available. **Women who have viral loads greater than 1000 should be offered a cesarean delivery, which may reduce vertical transmission under these conditions.**

Such cesarean deliveries should be scheduled at about 38 weeks of gestation to reduce the chance of labor or rupture of membranes. **Women on antiretroviral therapy with viral loads less than 1000 HIV RNA copies per milliliter are at low risk (1% to 2%) of passing the virus on to the fetus or newborn.** Vaginal delivery should be offered to such patients. All procedures should be avoided that may increase the risk for fetal HIV infection, including artificial rupture of membranes, invasive fetal heart rate monitoring, fetal blood sampling, assisted delivery (forceps or vacuum), or episiotomy. **Once the membranes have ruptured, labor should be augmented with oxytocin to reduce the interval between membrane rupture and delivery.**

Regardless of the mode of delivery, all women should continue to receive antiretroviral medications as prescribed. **Zidovudine (2 mg/kg over 1 hour, followed by 1 mg/kg per hour) should be infused intravenously after the onset of labor or rupture of membranes until delivery or at least 3 hours before cesarean delivery.**

In the United States, **breastfeeding is not recommended** and should be discouraged.

Screening for HIV Infection in Pregnancy

All pregnant women should be tested for HIV unless they refuse. When counseling an HIV-positive pregnant woman, it is necessary to discuss the risk for perinatal transmission. Counseling on disease prevention, including a discussion of safe sexual practices, information on zidovudine therapy, and avoidance of breastfeeding, is imperative. Reproductive options with respect to the present pregnancy and future family planning need to be addressed. **Rapid HIV testing should be offered to pregnant women presenting intrapartum whose HIV status is unknown.** If the rapid test is positive, zidovudine prophylaxis should be administered and confirmatory testing sent.

RUBELLA (GERMAN MEASLES)

Rubella results from infection with a single-stranded RNA togavirus transmitted through the respiratory route, with highest attack rates occurring between March and May. It is highly contagious, with 75% of those infected becoming clinically ill. The incubation period is 14 to 21 days.

Diagnosis

The diagnosis of rubella is best made by serologic testing. **The IgM response is a rapid one** that begins at the onset of the rash and then declines and disappears by 4 to 8 weeks. **IgG response also begins at the onset of the rash and remains elevated for life.** The diagnosis can be made by the presence of a fourfold rise in the hemagglutination-inhibiting (HAI) antibody titer in paired sera obtained 2 weeks apart or by the presence of IgM. Rubella can also be diagnosed by culture and isolation

---

BOX 16-2   *Congenital Rubella Syndrome*

- Symmetrical IUGR
- Congenital deafness (detected after age 1 yr)
- Cardiac malformations
- Patent ductus arteriosus
- Pulmonary artery hypoplasia
- Eye lesions
- Cataracts
- Retinopathy
- Microphthalmia
- Hepatosplenomegaly
- Central nervous system involvement
- Microcephaly
- Panencephalitis
- Brain calcifications
- Psychomotor retardation
- Hepatitis
- Thrombocytopenic purpura

---

of the virus during the acute phase of infection, although this technique is slow. The presence of IgM in cord blood or IgG in an infant after 6 months of age supports the diagnosis of perinatal rubella infection.

Impact on Pregnancy

Between 10% and 15% of adult women are susceptible to rubella. In a review of all cases of infants with congenital rubella syndrome (CRS) in the United States reported to the National Congenital Rubella Syndrome Registry from 1997 to 1999, **83% were born to Hispanic mothers** and 91% were born to foreign-born mothers.

The disease course is unaltered by pregnancy, and the mother may or may not exhibit the full clinical disease. **The severity of the mother's illness does not have an impact on the risk for fetal infection.** Rather, it is the trimester in which infection occurs that has the greatest impact on fetal risk. **Infection in the first trimester carries up to 80% risk for development of CRS,** whereas the risk for CRS drops to 30% to 50% later in pregnancy. **CRS rarely occurs after 20 weeks of gestation.** Components of CRS are outlined in Box 16-2.

Routine rubella susceptibility testing should be performed in all pregnant women with a single IgG level. Those who are nonimmune should be vaccinated in the immediate postpartum period. It is recommended that women not become pregnant for at least 3 months after vaccination. Nonetheless, there are no reports of CRS after rubella immunization, and inadvertent immunization of a pregnant woman is not considered an indication for therapeutic abortion. Follow-up antibody titers should be obtained because up to 20% fail to develop an antibody response. **Women should be screened for rubella susceptibility at each pregnancy,** because immunity can wane.

Rubella is not a contraindication to breastfeeding. There is no specific treatment for rubella, and routine prophylaxis with γ-globulin after exposure is not recommended because it has not been shown to change the risk for fetal involvement.

CYTOMEGALOVIRUS

CMV is a DNA virus and a member of the herpesvirus family and thus has the ability to establish latency. The virus is transmitted in a number of ways, including blood transfusion, organ transplantation, sexual contact, breast milk, urine, or saliva. It may also be transmitted transplacentally, or at delivery by direct contact. **Between 30% and 60% of school-aged children are seropositive for CMV, as are 50% to 85% of all pregnant women.** Infection may be expressed as a mononucleosis-like illness, although subclinical infection is more common. Viral excretion may continue for months, and the virus may establish latency in lymphocytes, salivary glands, renal tubules, and the endometrium. Reactivation may occur years after primary infection, and reinfection with a different strain of the virus is also possible.

Diagnosis

The virus may be isolated on urine culture or by culture of other body secretions or tissues. Serologic testing is possible, with an elevation in IgM that peaks 3 to 6 months after infection and resolves by 1 to 2 years. IgG elevates rapidly and persists for life. **Problems with serologic testing include** (1) **the prolonged elevation in levels of IgM, making delineation of timing of infection difficult,** and (2) **a 20% false-negative rate in IgM testing.** In addition, the presence of IgG does not rule out the presence of persistent disease.

Impact on Pregnancy

CMV is the most common congenital viral infection in the United States, affecting 0.5% to 2.5% of all liveborn infants per year, and it is postulated that each year about 40,000 infants are born with congenital CMV infection. Fetal infection can occur when the mother does not exhibit symptoms. There is a 40% to 50% maternal-infant transmission rate.

About 10% to 15% of infected infants are symptomatic at birth, exhibiting nonimmune hydrops, symmetrical IUGR, chorioretinitis, microcephaly, cerebral calcifications, hepatosplenomegaly, and hydrocephaly. About 80% to 90% are asymptomatic at birth but may later exhibit mental retardation, visual impairment, progressive hearing loss, and delayed psychomotor development (Box 16-3). **Sensorineural hearing loss is the most frequent sequel of congenital CMV infection** and is observed in 40% to 50% of symptomatic children. Recurrent CMV infection is associated with a much lower fetal risk, with a 0.15% to 1% maternal-fetal transmission rate. Few cases of severely affected infants have been reported.

BOX 16-3   *Problems Associated with Congenital Cytomegalovirus Infection*

- Nonimmune hydrops
- Symmetrical growth restriction
- Chorioretinitis
- Microcephaly
- Cerebral calcifications
- Hepatosplenomegaly
- Hydrocephaly
- Later problems
- Visual impairment
- Hearing loss
- Delayed psychomotor development

Patients with a confirmed primary infection should have a detailed ultrasonic examination. Ultrasonic findings include fetal growth restriction, hydrocephaly, intracranial calcifications, microcephaly, echogenic bowel, hepatosplenomegaly, and nonimmune hydrops. **If the ultrasound is normal, an amniocentesis should be performed to test for CMV by polymerase chain reaction (PCR).** If the ultrasound shows signs of fetal anomalies, or the PCR test is positive, patients should be advised of options. Recently, **hyperimmune anti-CMV globulin** has been shown to be effective and can be offered. Ganciclovir has also been used in pregnancy with resolution of fetal CMV infection. The patient should also be advised of the option of termination.

VARICELLA-ZOSTER VIRUS

Acute varicella infection, or chickenpox, is caused by the varicella-zoster virus, which is a DNA herpesvirus transmitted by direct contact or through the respiratory route. The attack rate in susceptible individuals is more than 90%. The incubation period is 10 to 21 days. Infection is believed to be more severe in adults, and potential complications include encephalitis and pneumonia. **Because it is a herpesvirus, the varicella virus has the ability to establish latency in nerve ganglia. Reactivation of the virus results in herpes zoster (shingles).**

Diagnosis

The diagnosis of chickenpox is usually determined by the patient's clinical presentation, although the virus may be cultured from vesicles during the first 4 days of the rash. On serologic testing, varicella-zoster IgM will rise in 2 weeks on ELISA or complement fixation. Paired sera for IgG obtained 2 weeks apart may also detect infection.

Impact on Pregnancy

Between 5% and 10% of adult women are susceptible to the varicella virus. Acute varicella infection complicates 1 in 7500 pregnancies. **Potential maternal**

complications include preterm labor, encephalitis, and varicella pneumonia. Maternal management should be symptomatic, but a chest x-ray should be considered to rule out pneumonia. Varicella pneumonia complicates 16% of cases and carries a mortality rate of up to 40%. If pneumonia is confirmed or suspected, the patient requires immediate hospital admission and institution of antiviral therapy because rapid respiratory decompensation is not uncommon.

A congenital varicella syndrome has been described. Diagnosis of the syndrome is based on IgM-positive cord blood and clinical findings in the newborn, which include **limb hypoplasia, cutaneous scars, chorioretinitis, cataracts, cortical atrophy, microcephaly, and symmetrical IUGR.** The risk for this fetal syndrome is 2% if maternal infection occurred between 13 and 20 weeks and 0.4% if maternal infection occurred before 13 weeks of gestation. **Only rarely have cases been identified as a result of maternal infection past 20 weeks' gestation.** In the presence of fetal infection, ultrasound may reveal hydrops, organ calcifications, limb deformities, microcephaly, or growth restriction. However, **no reliable methods of definitive prenatal diagnosis are available.**

If maternal infection occurs 5 to 21 days before delivery and the infant develops infection, it is typically mild and self-limited. However, **if maternal infection occurs between 5 days before delivery and 2 days after delivery, transplacental transfer of maternal protective antibodies to the fetus has not occurred, and the infant is at great risk for developing a fulminant infection with a 30% mortality rate.** Varicella-zoster immune globulin (VZIG) should be given to these infants at birth, and they should be placed in contact isolation. The placenta and fetal membranes should be considered infectious.

For the exposed gravid woman who has no knowledge of a prior infection, a varicella IgG titer should be obtained immediately. **If the patient proves to be nonimmune, VZIG should be administered within 6 days of exposure,** although it is unclear whether this therapy modifies the disease course and risk to the fetus. **Administration of VZIG is also recommended after exposure to zoster.** Alternatively, VariZIG may be administered up to 96 hours after exposure. Varicella vaccine is composed of a live attenuated virus and, therefore, is contraindicated in pregnancy. **Herpes zoster does not occur more frequently in pregnancy. If it does occur, it poses no risk to the fetus.** If zoster develops close to delivery, varicella may be transmitted through contact with a lesion, so this should be avoided.

HEPATITIS B AND C VIRUSES

The hepatitis B virus is a DNA virus that is transmitted through blood, saliva, vaginal secretions, semen, and breast milk and across the placenta. The population at greatest risk includes intravenous drug users, homosexuals, individuals of Asian descent, and health care workers. Infection with the virus is either asymptomatic or expressed as acute hepatitis. Ten percent of individuals go on to develop chronic active or persistent hepatitis.

Impact on Pregnancy

The course of acute hepatitis is unaltered in pregnancy. Fetal infection may occur and is most likely if maternal infection occurs in the third trimester. **Chronic active hepatitis is associated with an increased risk for prematurity, low birth weight, and neonatal death.** Maternal prognosis is very poor if the disease is complicated by cirrhosis, varices, or liver failure.

The incidence of hepatitis B surface antigen (HBsAg) positivity (chronic carrier state) in pregnancy in the United States is 6 to 10 per 1000 pregnancies. Women who are asymptomatic HBsAg carriers are at no higher risk for antepartum complications than are the general population. However, **newborns delivered to mothers positive for HBsAg have a 10% risk for developing acute infection at birth. This is in contrast to those delivered to mothers positive for both HBsAg and hepatitis Be antigen (HBeAg), in which the infant's risk increases to 70% to 90%.** Infection in the infant may be fulminant and lethal. **If the infant survives, it has an 85% to 90% chance of becoming a chronic hepatitis carrier and a 25% chance of developing liver cirrhosis, hepatocellular carcinoma, or both.** Therefore, it is recommended that all pregnant women be screened for HBsAg carriage during pregnancy. Women in high-risk groups (Box 16-4) should be rescreened in the third trimester if the initial screen is negative.

If a pregnant woman is found on screening to be HBsAg positive, liver function tests and a complete hepatitis panel should be performed. Household members and sexual contacts should be tested and offered vaccination if they are susceptible. **Transmission to the infant is believed to occur by direct contact during delivery.** Therefore, the newborn is given hepatitis immune globulin and hepatitis vaccine soon after delivery, which reduces the risk for infection to less than 10%. **Pregnant women at high risk for becoming infected with hepatitis B who test negative for the HBsAg should be offered vaccination.** Available vaccines are produced by recombinant DNA technology and are therefore safe for use in pregnancy. The Centers for Disease Control and Prevention (CDC) have recommended that all children receive vaccination against hepatitis B as well.

Hepatitis C virus (HCV) is the most common chronic blood-borne infection in the United States. Vertical transmission in HCV RNA–negative pregnant women is about 1% to 3% vs. about 4% to 6% in HCV RNA–positive women. Coinfection with HIV has been shown to increase the risk for vertical transmission of HCV. In HIV-negative women, route of delivery does not influence vertical transmission. Amniocentesis is a potential risk for transmission. There is no clear evidence demonstrating an increased risk for HCV transmission in HIV-negative women who breastfeed.

There is currently no safe treatment for HCV infection during pregnancy. Given the lack of measures to prevent transmission and to treat the infection efficiently, **universal screening in pregnancy is currently not recommended.** Women with high risk factors (such as blood transfusion or organ donation before 1992, HIV or hepatitis B positive, intravenous drug use, high-risk sexual behavior) should be offered anti-HCV testing during pregnancy.

HERPES SIMPLEX VIRUS

Herpes simplex virus (HSV) is a member of the DNA herpes virus family and is transmitted by intimate mucocutaneous contact.

Impact on Pregnancy

PRIMARY GENITAL HERPES. Patients who acquire primary herpes in pregnancy have an increased risk for obstetric and neonatal complications. **Maternal infection has been associated with an increased risk for spontaneous abortion, IUGR, and preterm labor.** Fifty percent of infants born vaginally to mothers with a primary infection at delivery may develop HSV infection.

RECURRENT GENITAL HERPES. Complications from a recurrence in pregnancy are rare. However, 4% of infants born to mothers with recurrent infection at the time of delivery may have HSV infection.

NEONATAL HERPES. The reported incidence of neonatal herpes ranges from 4 to 31.2 per 100,000 life births. Neonatal infection is acquired in three ways: intrauterine (5%), peripartum (85%), or postnatal (10%) transmission. **Premature infants are at greatest risk for**

contracting infection, and they account for more than two thirds of reported cases. Symptoms typically present on day 2 to 3 of life, with rapid progression of disease thereafter. **Neonatal infection can be classified as (1) disseminated disease** with involvement of multiple major organs; **(2) central nervous system disease with encephalitis;** and **(3) skin, eye, or mouth infection** with localized involvement. Neonates with suspected neonatal herpes are treated with **intravenous acyclovir,** which has significantly reduced the mortality rate. Even with appropriate treatment, prognosis of **neonatal** encephalitis is still very poor. Between one third and one half of all treated neonates with disseminated disease die, and about two thirds of survivors have neurologic sequelae such as **microcephaly, mental retardation, seizures, and microphthalmos.**

Management in Pregnancy

Antenatal antiviral prophylaxis (valacyclovir and acyclovir) from 36 weeks until delivery is safe and has been shown to decrease asymptomatic viral shedding, decrease herpes outbreak at delivery, and reduce the need for cesarean delivery for genital herpes. Women with a prior history of herpes should be allowed to deliver vaginally if no genital lesions are present at the time of labor. **Patients with active lesions, either recurrent or primary, at the time of labor should be delivered by cesarean birth.** Those with active lesions at sites distant from the genital area may be delivered vaginally if the lesions are covered. Once delivered, isolation of the mother from her infant is not necessary as long as direct contact with lesions is avoided. **Mothers may breastfeed so long as no lesions are present on the breasts.**

Bacterial Infections

URINARY TRACT INFECTIONS

Urinary tract infections occur more frequently in pregnancy and the puerperium and are among the most common medical complications of pregnancy. This increased incidence appears to be a result of both hormonal (progesterone) and mechanical factors that increase urinary stasis.

Urinary tract infections in pregnancy may be either asymptomatic or symptomatic (e.g., cystitis, pyelonephritis). **By definition, asymptomatic bacteriuria is the presence of at least 100,000 organisms/mL in a clean urine specimen from an asymptomatic patient.** The incidence of asymptomatic bacteriuria in pregnancy is the same as in the nonpregnant sexually active population, ranging from 2% to 10%. Highest rates are found in inner city populations and in patients with sickle cell disease or trait. *Escherichia coli* **is the organism most frequently isolated (60%).** Other organisms encountered are *Proteus mirabilis,* enterococci, *Klebsiella* *pneumoniae,* and **group B streptococci. If the condition is left untreated, roughly 20% of pregnant women develop either acute cystitis or pyelonephritis later in pregnancy.** Initial therapy consists of either **nitrofurantoin, ampicillin** or a **cephalosporin.** After treatment, it is wise to follow with urine cultures because up to 25% of patients have a recurrence later in the pregnancy.

Acute cystitis complicates 1% to 2% of pregnancies and is characterized by dysuria, frequency, urgency, and hematuria. Systemic signs and symptoms, such as flank pain or fever, are absent. Urinalysis reveals bacteriuria, pyuria, and often hematuria. As in patients with asymptomatic bacteriuria, treatment is instituted on an outpatient basis while awaiting the results of sensitivity tests. Follow-up surveillance cultures are indicated.

Acute pyelonephritis occurs in about 2% to 4% of pregnancies, most frequently in the second trimester. It is characterized by flank pain, fever, rigors, and the urinary complaints of cystitis. It is a leading cause of septic shock and ARDS in pregnancy. Often, nausea and vomiting are present, and the patient may be markedly dehydrated. Physical examination reveals fever and costovertebral angle tenderness. **As a result of sepsis, premature uterine contractions are frequent.** Urinalysis reveals the same findings as are found with acute cystitis, and blood cultures are positive in 10% of cases. Organisms responsible are the same as those causing asymptomatic bacteriuria and cystitis.

Hospitalization, blood and urine cultures, intravenous antibiotic therapy, monitoring for preterm labor, and close observation of fluid status and pulse oximetry are indicated when a diagnosis of pyelonephritis is made. Usually, **ampicillin** or **cefazolin** therapy is initiated, with cefazolin or **gentamycin** gaining a great deal of popularity in areas in which resistance to ampicillin is prominent. Most patients (>80%) become asymptomatic and afebrile within 48 hours of initiation of antibiotic therapy and may be discharged at this point, continuing oral antibiotics for a 10-day course. **Serial urine cultures are indicated because 10% to 25% of patients have a recurrence later in the pregnancy.** Those with recurrent pyelonephritis should receive chronic antibiotic suppression and have an intravenous pyelogram performed 6 weeks postpartum to rule out urinary tract abnormalities.

GROUP B STREPTOCOCCI

Group B streptococci (GBS) are considered part of the normal flora of humans. The gastrointestinal tract is the major reservoir, although the organism has been isolated from the vagina, cervix, throat, skin, urethra, and urine of healthy individuals. **GBS may be transmitted to the genital tract by fecal contamination or sexual transmission from a colonized partner. Vaginal carriage rates vary from 15% to 40%,** but they are the same in pregnant women as in sexually active nonpregnant women. Two thirds of pregnant women who carry GBS do so intermittently or transiently, and only one third of all pregnant GBS carriers have the organism chronically.

Diagnosis

GBS grow readily on routine bacteriologic media and are easy to isolate from clinical specimens. A number of specific rapid assays for the detection of GBS have been developed, but none is sensitive enough for widespread use.

Impact on Pregnancy

GBS may be transferred from a colonized mother to her infant by vertical transmission at delivery. **Transmission rates of 35% to 70% have been reported, with the highest transmission rates occurring in women with heavy vaginal colonization. Other risk factors for transmission are preterm labor or delivery, preterm rupture of membranes, low birth weight, prolonged rupture of membranes (>12 to 18 hours before delivery), intrapartum fever, and a history of previously delivering an infected infant.**

GBS sepsis is the most common cause of neonatal sepsis in the United States, with 1 to 2 cases per 1000 live births per year reported. Neonatal infection with GBS is of two clinically distinct types: early-onset and late-onset disease. **Late-onset GBS infection** has been linked to a nosocomial source in the nursery, occurs after the first week of life (mean onset, 4 weeks), and usually **is exhibited as meningitis (80%) or another type of focal infection. Early-onset GBS infection is characterized by its rapid onset and fulminant course,** with presentation typically within the first 48 hours of life. Pathogenesis of this form of GBS sepsis is best explained by direct maternal-infant transmission at delivery. **The infant presents with respiratory distress and pneumonia, and 30% of infants develop meningitis. Septicemia, shock, and death may result even when antibiotics are begun expediently.** The overall infant mortality rate from early-onset disease is 50%. Preterm infants account for more than 90% of deaths. The risk for sepsis developing in a full-term infant with bacterial colonization is 1% to 2%, compared with 8% to 10% in the preterm infant.

GBS is the second most common cause of bacteriuria in pregnancy and is a major cause of puerperal infection. Infection with GBS accounts for 20% of cases of endomyometritis and is unique in its acute onset (within the first 48 hours postpartum) and typically fulminant course.

Treating carriers in labor will reduce the rate of transmission to the infant. Both the CDC and the Committee on Obstetric Practice of the American College of Obstetricians and Gynecologists support a screening program in which **vaginal and rectal group B streptococci cultures are obtained at 35 to 37 weeks for all**

gravidas except those who have GBS bacteriuria during the current pregnancy or a previous infant with invasive GBS disease. **Intrapartum antibiotic prophylaxis** would be indicated for pregnant women with (1) **a previous infant with invasive GBS disease,** (2) **GBS bacteriuria during the current pregnancy,** (3) **positive GBS screening culture during the current pregnancy,** or (4) **unknown GBS status with one of the high-risk factors** such as intrapartum fever (≥38°C), preterm delivery (<37 weeks of gestation), or prolonged membrane rupture (≥18 hours). Antibiotic prophylaxis is not indicated for those undergoing a scheduled cesarean delivery in the absence of labor or amniotic membrane rupture. Antibiotic prophylaxis is also not indicated for those who have risk factors but are GBS culture negative in the current pregnancy.

TUBERCULOSIS

Although the incidence of active tuberculosis (TB) in the United States is very low (0.6% to 1%), **about 10% of all women of childbearing age test positive on purified protein derivative (PPD) testing.** A positive PPD test indicates that the patient has been infected with tuberculosis in the past. Tuberculin skin testing is not a routine component of prenatal screening but should be performed in minority women of lower socioeconomic status and in women who live in areas in which large numbers of immigrants from Southeast Asia, Central America, or South America reside. HIV-positive patients should also have a PPD test.

Pregnancy does not alter the course of active tuberculosis, nor does it place the known PPD-positive woman at greater risk for disease reactivation. Tuberculosis can, however, **be passed to the fetus by a hematogenous route** across the placenta **or as a result of the fetus's swallowing infected amniotic fluid.** The risk for pregnancy wastage is increased, and **congenital tuberculosis may be evident at birth.** An affected infant exhibits low birth weight, failure to thrive, fever, respiratory distress, adenopathy, and hepatosplenomegaly and is at high risk for dying without rapid treatment. **Treatment of the mother with active disease during pregnancy eliminates the fetal risks.**

The pregnant patient who tests positive for tuberculosis should have a chest x-ray (with abdominal shielding) to rule out active disease. If the chest x-ray is suspicious for active disease, three sets of **sputum cultures** should be obtained. If the cultures are positive, therapy should be instituted without delay. If the chest x-ray is normal, no further treatment is required, but the patient should be followed with an annual chest x-ray. Prophylactic treatment with single-agent therapy is recommended for patients who are recent PPD converters, those who live with someone with active TB, and those who are immunosuppressed and PPD positive (e.g., AIDS sufferers).

Several drugs are available for therapy. All have potential risks, but untreated TB is believed to be of greater risk to both the mother and infant. **Isoniazid (INH) is the safest drug for use in pregnancy.** Fetal risks include potential central nervous system toxicity, but treating the mother with vitamin B_6 supplements eliminates this risk. The main risk to the mother is hepatitis, so monthly liver function tests should be performed. **Rifampin has been linked to limb reduction defects in the fetus and hepatitis in the mother. Ethambutol is safer than rifampin but is not as effective,** and it has been associated with a reversible maternal optic neuritis in 6% of patients. **Streptomycin is to be avoided in pregnancy** because of the risk for nephrotoxicity and permanent cranial nerve VIII damage in the fetus. **For women with active disease, current recommendations are for 9 months of therapy with INH and rifampin.** After delivery, newborns should be isolated from their mothers with active disease until the mothers are culture negative. **INH prophylaxis of the infant is recommended because 50% of infants develop active TB by 1 year of age without it.** Once the mother is culture-negative, she may breastfeed because only small concentrations of the drugs pass into the milk.

SYPHILIS

All pregnant women should be screened for syphilis at the first prenatal visit with either a Venereal Disease Research Laboratory (VDRL) test or a rapid plasma reagin (RPR) test. These tests carry a false-positive rate of between 0.5% and 14% because they are nonspecific for treponemes. Common causes of false-positive results are drug addiction, autoimmune disease, recent viral infection or immunization, and pregnancy. False-positive titers are usually 1:4 or less. **Specific treponemal tests, such as the fluorescent treponemal antibody absorption test (FTA-ABS), are performed to confirm the diagnosis.**

Impact on Pregnancy

Maternal infection can result in transplacental transmission to the fetus at any gestational age. **Mothers with primary and secondary syphilis are more likely to transmit the infection, with more severe manifestations occurring in the fetus.** Transmission rates for primary and secondary disease are between 50% and 80%. There is a wide range of fetal responses to infection.

Components of early congenital syphilitic infection include nonimmune hydrops, hepatosplenomegaly, profound anemia and thrombocytopenia, skin lesions, rash, osteitis and periostitis, pneumonia, and hepatitis. The perinatal mortality rate from congenital syphilis is roughly 50%.

Late congenital syphilis (diagnosed after 2 years of age) is a multisystem disease characterized by dental abnormalities (Hutchinson's teeth, mulberry molars); saber shins; saddle nose deformity; interstitial keratitis; eighth nerve deafness; and failure to thrive.

Treatment

Treatment of the condition in pregnancy is the same as that in the nonpregnant state. **Penicillin G is the therapy of choice.** Patients with primary, secondary, or latent syphilis of less than 12 months' duration are treated with a single dose of benzathine penicillin, 2.4 million U given intramuscularly. Those with syphilis of undetermined length or with latent infection for longer than 1 year receive this therapy weekly for 3 weeks. For patients with penicillin allergy, desensitization and use of penicillin is recommended. Patients with neurosyphilis require admission and prolonged intravenous penicillin therapy.

Women treated for syphilis during their pregnancy require careful follow-up with monthly VDRL or RPR titers to ensure that the treatment is successful. Patients with syphilis remain positive on FTA-ABS testing for the remainder of their lives. Sexual contacts should be referred for treatment and neonates evaluated and treated as indicated.

Parasitic Infections

TOXOPLASMOSIS

Toxoplasmosis is a systemic disease caused by the protozoan *Toxoplasma gondii.* Between 15% and 40% of women of reproductive age have antibodies (IgG) to toxoplasmosis and therefore are immune to future infection. The organism is acquired by ingesting undercooked meat or unpasteurized goat's milk, drinking contaminated water, exposure to feces from an infected cat, or rarely by tachyzoites from blood transfusion. In about 10% of maternal infections, **toxoplasmosis presents as a mononucleosis-like syndrome, but most infections are subclinical.**

Impact on Pregnancy

The incidence of primary infection in pregnancy is 1 in 1000. In immunocompromised women such as those with AIDS, a reactivation of toxoplasmosis could occur that would potentially be associated with a risk for fetal infection. **The risk for transmission to the fetus is 15% in the first trimester, 25% in the second trimester, and 65% in the third trimester.** However, the severity of fetal infection is greatest with first-trimester infection, and congenital defects are rarely seen if the infection occurs after 20 weeks of gestation. About 15% of infants with congenital infection are symptomatic at birth. A **classic triad of hydrocephalus, intracranial calcifications, and chorioretinitis is described.** Of the asymptomatic infants, 25% and 50% exhibit later sequelae (Box 16-5).

Diagnosis

Maternal infection is usually suspected if toxoplasmosis IgM antibodies are detected on routine screening. Occasionally pregnant women may be tested because of **mononucleosis-like symptoms.** A reference laboratory

---

BOX 16-5   *Manifestations of Congenital Toxoplasmosis Infection*

- Hydrocephalus
- Chorioretinitis
- Microcephaly
- Microphthalmia
- Hepatosplenomegaly
- Cerebral calcifications
- Adenopathy
- Convulsions
- Delayed mental development
- Rash
- Pneumonia
- Fever
- Anemia
- Later problems
- Visual impairment
- Hearing loss
- Delayed psychomotor development
- Seizure disorders
- Spasticity, palsies
- Mental retardation

---

is used to confirm primary toxoplasmosis infection. At about 18 to 20 weeks of gestation, amniocentesis for toxoplasmosis PCR should be offered to women with a confirmed diagnosis of primary toxoplasmosis to detect fetal infection.

Treatment

Toxoplasmosis is a self-limiting infection. Owing to the fetal risk, **spiramycin** is used for treatment of maternal primary infection, but it is obtainable in the United States only through special permission from the U.S. Food and Drug Administration. **If fetal infection is identified, therapy with pyrimethamine and sulfadiazine plus folinic acid should be given and has been shown to reduce the severity of fetal damage.** Most infected infants have no apparent physical abnormalities at birth, but without treatment, most of the infected infants develop morbidity related to chorioretinitis, hydrocephalus, or neurologic damage by the end of adolescence. Therefore **treatment of infected infants in the first year of life is recommended. To prevent infection, pregnant women should be advised to avoid contact with cat litter or feces, to wear gloves while gardening, and to avoid ingestion of undercooked meat or unpasteurized goat's milk and drink filtered water.**

Surgical Conditions during Pregnancy

Pregnancy substantially enhances the problems associated with surgery. Physiologic changes and the altered immunologic responses of pregnancy change the diagnostic parameters of surgical diseases. Surgery (especially abdominal surgery) can increase the rate of fetal loss. Reluctance to operate on a pregnant woman with an acute surgical condition may add to critical delays and increase the morbidity for both the fetus and the mother.

GENERAL PRINCIPLES

Elective surgery should be avoided in pregnancy. If surgery must be done, but not emergently (e.g., an ovarian neoplasm), **the second trimester is the safest time.** During this period, the risks for teratogenesis and miscarriage are much lower than in the first trimester, and the risk for preterm labor is lower than in the third trimester. Regional analgesia is preferred because it has lower mortality and morbidity than general anesthesia. There is little evidence of teratogenicity from commonly used anesthetics. **Pulmonary aspiration is more common.** All pregnant women should be treated as if they have a full stomach and premedicated with citrate and H_2-receptor blockers. **Precautions must be taken to avoid maternal hypotension and hypoxia, which have adverse effects on uteroplacental blood flow.** If possible, the patient should be in the left lateral decubitus position. Preoperative and postoperative fetal and uterine monitoring are indicated in the third trimester. If significant blood loss is anticipated and the patient is anemic, it is advisable to transfuse the patient preoperatively.

ACUTE CONDITIONS

The general approach to acute surgical emergencies during pregnancy is to manage the problem regardless of the pregnancy. Acute nonobstetric surgical emergencies occur in all three trimesters of pregnancy. The overall incidence is about 1 in 500 pregnancies. The more common acute conditions are discussed next.

Appendicitis

Appendectomy for presumed acute appendicitis is the most common surgical emergency during pregnancy. The incidence of acute appendicitis in pregnancy is about 0.05% to 0.1%, and it is constant throughout the three trimesters. The usual symptoms of acute appendicitis, such as epigastric pain, nausea, vomiting, and lower abdominal pain, may be less apparent during pregnancy, although **right lower quadrant pain is still the most common presentation. The differential diagnosis may be especially confusing** (Box 16-6). The enlarging uterus displaces the appendix superiorly and laterally as pregnancy progresses (Figure 16-1). **Tenderness and guarding are elicited more laterally than expected.** The increased white blood cell count seen in normal pregnancy further confuses the issue. Surgery may be delayed, resulting in an increased rate of rupture, premature labor, infant morbidity, and, rarely, maternal death.

BOX 16-6 *Differential Diagnosis of Acute Appendicitis in Pregnancy*

- Ruptured corpus luteum
- Torsion of an adnexal mass
- Pyelonephritis
- Nephrolithiasis
- Ectopic pregnancy
- Hyperemesis gravidarum
- Acute mesenteric lymphadenitis
- Inflammatory bowel disease
- Salpingo-ovarian abscess
- Acute mesenteric thrombosis
- Cholecystitis, cholelithiasis
- Concealed abruption

Imaging studies can increase the accuracy of the diagnosis of appendicitis. The American College of Radiology recommends nonionizing radiation techniques such as **ultrasonography** and **MRI** for imaging in pregnant women. On ultrasound, the abnormal appendix can be visualized as a noncompressible tubular structure measuring 6 mm or greater in the region of the patient's pain. Helical computed tomography has the disadvantage of radiation exposure, but appendicitis is suspected if right lower quadrant inflammation, an enlarged nonfilling tubular structure, or a fecalith is

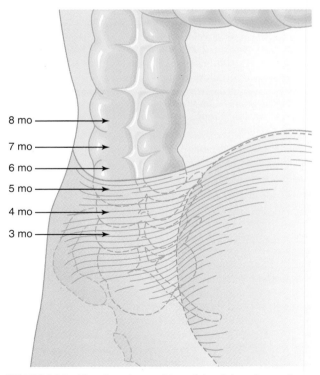

FIGURE 16-1 The changing position of the right colon and appendix as pregnancy progresses and the uterus enlarges.

noted. The estimated fetal radiation exposure is about 250 mrad. Exposure to less than 5 rad (0.05 Gy) has not been associated with an increase in fetal anomalies or pregnancy loss. Table 16-8 shows the dose of ionizing radiation to the fetus from common diagnostic radiologic procedures.

If acute appendicitis is diagnosed, laparotomy with appendectomy should be carried out. A McBurney, transverse, or Rockey-Davis incision can be employed.

Laparoscopic appendectomy may increase the risk for fetal loss. A potential concern is that carbon dioxide used for insufflation can be absorbed across the peritoneum into the maternal bloodstream and across the placenta, leading to fetal respiratory acidosis and hypercapnia. As gestation progresses, the likelihood increases that the pneumoperitoneum will decrease venous return, cardiac output, and uteroplacental blood flow. Laparoscopic appendectomy may be considered if specific recommendations are met (Table 16-9).

Acute Cholecystitis and Cholelithiasis

An increase in serum cholesterol and lipid levels in pregnancy, along with biliary stasis, leads to a higher incidence of cholelithiasis, biliary obstruction, and cholecystitis. High levels of estrogens in pregnancy increase the saturation of cholesterol in the bile. Virtually all of the gallstones associated with pregnancy are composed of crystallized cholesterol. Ultrasonography has revealed a fairly high incidence of cholelithiasis in pregnancy (4%). The incidence of hospitalization for cholecystitis in pregnancy is 1% to 2%, but only 1 in 2000 pregnant women require cholecystectomy.

Nausea and vomiting, along with right upper quadrant tenderness and guarding, generally suggest biliary tract disease. An increasing white blood cell count with elevated alkaline phosphatase and bilirubin levels, jaundice in the presence of stones, or increased thickness of the gallbladder wall on ultrasonography serves to authenticate the diagnosis. **Viral hepatitis must be considered in the differential diagnosis.** Markedly elevated aspartate transaminase and alanine

TABLE 16-8

ESTIMATED FETAL EXPOSURE FROM SOME COMMON RADIOLOGIC PROCEDURES

Procedure	Fetal Exposure*
Chest radiograph (two views)	0.02-0.07 mrad
Abdominal film (single view)	100 mrad
Intravenous pyelography	>1 rad†
Hip film (single view)	200 mrad
Mammography	7-20 mrad
Barium enema or small bowel series	2-4 rad
CT scan of head or chest	<1 rad
CT scan of abdomen and lumbar spine	3.5 rad
CT pelvimetry	250 mrad

*1 rad = 0.01 gray (Gy).
†Exposure depends on the number of films.
Data from American College of Obstetricians and Gynecologists: Guidelines for diagnostic imaging during pregnancy. ACOG Committee Opinion No. 299. Obstet Gynecol 104:649, 2004.

TABLE 16-9

SAGES GUIDELINES FOR LAPAROSCOPIC OPERATIONS DURING PREGNANCY AND PROPOSED GUIDELINES TO IMPROVE SAFETY OF THE PROCEDURE

SAGES Guidelines	Moreno-Sanz's Proposed Guidelines
Pneumatic compression devices	Same recommendation
Open abdominal access (Hasson)	Same recommendation
Pneumoperitoneum pressure ≤12 mm Hg*	Same recommendation
No routine prophylactic tocolytic therapy	Same recommendation
Obstetric consultation should be obtained preoperatively	Preoperative and postoperative obstetric consultation should be obtained*
Continuous intraoperative fetal monitoring	Preoperative and postoperative ultrasonographic examination and cardiotocography*
Maternal end-tidal CO_2 and/or arterial blood gases should be monitored	Maternal intraoperative end-tidal CO_2 monitoring (30-40 mm Hg)*
	Routine venous thrombosis prophylaxis with low-molecular-weight heparin†
	Use of harmonic scissors†

*Proposed guideline change.
†Proposed guideline.
SAGES, Society of American Gastrointestinal and Endoscopic Surgeons.
From Moreno-Sanz CJ: Laparoscopic appendectomy during pregnancy: Between personal experiences and scientific evidence. Am Coll Surg 205:37-42, 2007.

transaminase levels (>200 U/L), especially without leukocytosis, should suggest viral hepatitis.

Generally, cholecystitis can be managed medically in pregnancy. Parenteral fluids, gastric decompression, and dietary measures should be the primary approach. Endoscopic retrograde cholangiopancreatography (ERCP) can be safely performed in pregnancy with little ionizing radiation exposure to the fetus if the patient has cholangitis or pancreatitis due to a common bile duct stone. If symptoms and signs persist with progressive peritonitis despite medical management or ERCP, cholecystectomy is indicated. Laparoscopic cholecystectomy has been performed in pregnancy.

Acute Pancreatitis

Generally, pancreatitis is associated with cholecystitis, cholelithiasis, or alcoholism. It has also been associated with viral infections and drugs such as thiazide diuretics, furosemide, acetaminophen, clonidine, isoniazid, rifampin, tetracycline, propoxyphene, and steroids. It is less common in pregnancy, and the incidence in pregnancy varies from 1:1000 to 1:4000, increasing somewhat in the third trimester. However, **the mortality rate associated with pancreatitis is significantly higher when it does occur in pregnancy.**

The prime symptom of pancreatitis is severe, noncolicky epigastric pain radiating to the high back, which is relieved somewhat by leaning forward. Nausea and vomiting generally are present. Upper abdominal guarding may be difficult to assess in late pregnancy. **Elevated serum amylase** (>200 U/dL) and lipase levels **generally confirm the diagnosis,** although cholecystitis, peptic ulcer, diabetic ketoacidosis, and hyperemesis gravidarum may also be associated with elevations of serum amylase

Generally, the disease is self-limited and responds within 1 to 10 days to bed rest, parenteral fluids, pain relief, and nasogastric suction. Occasionally the disease becomes severe and protracted, with extensive pancreatic edema and autodigestion, massive ascites, hemoperitoneum, fever, and paralytic ileus. In such cases, maternal and fetal mortality is high, and peritoneal lavage, operative drainage, partial pancreatic resection, or some combination of these procedures may be required.

Bowel Obstruction

Bowel obstruction in pregnancy is usually associated with postoperative adhesions, although volvulus and intussusception are rare causes. It generally occurs in late pregnancy and is associated with traction on adhesions as the uterus enlarges. **An upright x-ray of the abdomen showing characteristic dilated loops of bowel and air-fluid levels serves to confirm the obstruction.**

Management does not differ from that in the nonpregnant patient. Nasogastric suction should be instituted and fluid and electrolyte balance carefully monitored. **If the obstruction does not resolve after 48 to 96 hours, an exploratory laparotomy should be carried out through an appropriate vertical incision.** If uterine contractions occur postoperatively, tocolytics may be employed.

Adnexal Torsion

Torsion of the uterine adnexa occurs somewhat more commonly in pregnancy, possibly because the supporting ligaments elongate as the gestation progresses. Ovarian tumors (e.g., cystic teratomas, corpus luteum cysts) may become ischemic if their vascular pedicles undergo torsion. Such ischemic events are usually heralded by the sudden onset of severe, intermittent abdominal pain, which may radiate to the flank and down the anterior thigh.

During the first and early second trimesters, a mass is usually felt on pelvic examination or is visualized by ultrasonography. Later in the pregnancy it may be impossible to palpate a mass clinically. Low-grade fever and leukocytosis may be present, and serum creatine phosphokinase levels may be elevated, depending on the extent of the infarction. In the first trimester, the differential diagnosis includes ectopic pregnancy and hemorrhagic corpus luteum; later in pregnancy, a degenerating myoma should be considered.

Although the pain may diminish somewhat after 24 hours, removal of the infarcted organ is indicated. If the excised ovary contains the corpus luteum, progesterone supplementation is generally necessary before 8 weeks' gestation.

Abdominal Trauma

By far, the most common abdominal trauma in pregnancy occurs in automobile accidents. Abruptio placentae, uterine contusions, and fetal skull fractures may result. Abruptio placentae is treated expectantly unless fetal monitoring indicates fetal distress, in which case immediate abdominal delivery is in order if the fetus is at a gestational age that is considered "viable" (23 to 24 weeks or greater). Abdominal exploration may be necessary to stop bleeding and repair uterine lacerations. Lap-shoulder harness seat belts, rather than lap belts, are advisable for pregnant women after 12 weeks' gestation.

Gunshot wounds of the abdomen are treated as in nonpregnant patients, with measures taken to stop bleeding and repair visceral or uterine injuries. So long as the pregnancy is intact, the uterus should not be disturbed. Careful monitoring of fetal well-being should be maintained before and after the operation.

Ovarian Tumors

Adnexal masses are not uncommon and are usually identified by pelvic examination or ultrasonography early in the pregnancy. Paraovarian cysts, corpus luteum cysts, and mature teratomas are the most common. About 50% to 70% are functional cysts (e.g., corpus luteum cysts) and spontaneously resolve as the gonadotropin levels fall during the second trimester. The risk for malignancy is about 3% to 7%, with germ cell and epithelial tumors both occurring. Abdominal and transvaginal ultrasonography should be used for initial diagnosis, and any complex mass that persists, or simple cyst that continues to enlarge, should be removed in the second trimester.

SUGGESTED READING

Abalovich M, Amino N, Barbour LA, et al: Management of thyroid dysfunction during pregnancy and postpartum: An Endocrine Society clinical practice guideline. J Clin Endocrinol Metab 92:s1-s47, 2007.

McKay DB, Josephson MA: Pregnancy in recipients of solid organs—effects on mother and child. N Engl J Med 354:1281-1293, 2006.

Perkins J, Dunn J, Jagasia S: Perspectives in gestational diabetes mellitus: A review of screening, diagnosis and treatment. Clin Diabetes 25:57-62, 2007.

Saleh MM, Abdo KR: Intrahepatic cholestasis of pregnancy: Review of the literature and evaluation of current evidence. J Womens Health 16:833-841, 2007.

Sulenik-Halevy R, Ellis M, Fejgin S: Management of immune thrombocytopenic purpura in pregnancy. Obstet Gynecol Surv 63:182-188, 2008.

Chapter 17

Obstetric Procedures

GLADYS A. RAMOS • THOMAS R. MOORE

As the fetus has become more accessible through technologic advances, the desire to intervene on behalf of the fetus has led to the development of a number of obstetric diagnostic and therapeutic procedures. Any procedure performed during pregnancy carries risk to both mother and fetus, so it is important to counsel the mother regarding the potential benefits and risks of all options before embarking on any intervention.

◼ Prenatal Diagnostic and Therapeutic Procedures

ULTRASOUND

Obstetric transvaginal and transabdominal sonography plays a pivotal role in contemporary obstetric care, with ultrasonic imaging being done in about 70% of pregnancies in the United States today. Human data have shown no adverse fetal effects of ultrasound. Box 17-1 lists common abnormalities that may be identified prenatally with ultrasound.

Transvaginal Ultrasound

Transvaginal ultrasound is useful in the first trimester of pregnancy because the close proximity of the intravaginal ultrasonic transducer allows for high-frequency scanning and thus better resolution of the pelvic organs and developing pregnancy than transabdominal imaging. Transvaginal ultrasound is commonly used in the first trimester to determine accurate **dating of the pregnancy** as well as **fetal location and number. The nuchal translucency measurement (first-trimester screening)**, a sonographically derived assessment of the subcutaneous fluid collection at the level of the fetal neck, is a screening test for chromosomal and structural abnormalities that is performed between 11 and 14 weeks' gestation, typically by a transabdominal but also a transvaginal approach (see Figure 7-2, pg 81). First-trimester vaginal ultrasound can also identify structural malformations. **Transvaginal sonographic measurement of cervical length in the mid-trimester can be used to identify patients at risk for preterm delivery.** The median length of the cervix at 24 to 28 weeks is 3.5 cm. Patients with a cervical length less than 2.0 cm are at significantly increased risk for preterm birth (threefold to fivefold). **Finally, transvaginal ultrasonic imaging of the lower uterine segment in the second or third trimester allows for very precise identification of placental location in relation to the internal cervical os.** In a patient with vaginal bleeding, excluding placenta previa is important in management.

Transabdominal Ultrasound

After 16 weeks' gestation, transabdominal ultrasound (second-trimester screening) is used to evaluate the fetus for structural abnormalities, provide a baseline assessment of fetal growth, and provide information regarding fetal well-being. The ability of a second-trimester scan to identify a fetus with an anomaly ranges from 17% to 74%. The reason various studies show such a wide range in sensitivity is probably due to variations in patient population and operator skill. The specificity, or the ability of ultrasound to correctly identify a normal fetus, approaches 100% in all studies. Thus **ultrasound is useful in ruling out fetal anomalies,** but it is not as reliable in detecting them.

In the third trimester, transabdominal ultrasound is useful in assessing fetal growth. Serial biometric measurements of the fetal head, abdomen, and limbs provide longitudinal information regarding the fetal growth trajectory. Software packages integral to the ultrasonic machines allow calculation of a fetal weight estimate from these measurements; this estimate is often used clinically. However, understanding that

BOX 17-1   *Examples of Fetal Abnormalities Detected by Prenatal Ultrasound*

Central Nervous System
- Hydrocephalus
- Anencephaly
- Spina bifida

Face
- Cleft lip and/or palate
- Hypoplasia of the nose

Neck
- Cystic hygroma
- Goiter
- Nuchal skin thickening

Heart
- Atrial septal defect
- Ventricular septal defect
- Tetralogy of Fallot
- Transposition of the great vessels
- Arrhythmias

Lungs
- Congenital cystic adenomatoid malformation (CCAM)
- Lung sequestration
- Diaphragmatic hernia

Abdominal Wall
- Gastroschisis
- Omphalocele

Gastrointestinal Tract
- Bowel atresia or obstruction
- Echogenic bowel

Urinary System
- Renal agenesis
- Polycystic kidney disease
- Hydronephrosis
- Posterior urethral valves

Skeletal Dysplasia

BOX 17-2   *Biophysical Profile**

Fetal breathing—30 seconds of rhythmic movement of the fetal thorax
Fetal movement—at least 3 movements of the fetal body or limb
Fetal tone—one extension and flexion of a limb joint
Amniotic fluid—single deepest vertical pocket of amniotic fluid > 2 cm
In conjunction with a 30-minute nonstress test (NST)

---

*Two points for each time these events are documented on real-time ultrasound and two points for a reactive NST. A score of 8-10 is considered normal.

these estimates may have an error of ±15% (a variation of ±1 lb or 450 g in a 7-lb or 3400-g fetus) limits the utility of ultrasonic fetal weight, especially in larger (>8 lb or 4000 g) fetuses.

Ultrasonic visualization of aspects of fetal behavior (body movement, breathing) provides highly predictive information regarding fetal oxygenation and well-being. These aspects are combined to determine the biophysical profile (Box 17-2). **The risk for fetal death within the week following a biophysical profile score of 8 or more is less than 1%.**

Doppler Sonography

Doppler sonography, which can precisely measure the velocity profile of blood flowing through fetal vessels, **allows for characterization of vascular impedance.** The umbilical artery, which normally has high-velocity flow during cardiac diastole, may have low, absent, or even reversed diastolic flow in a compromised fetus with high-resistance placental vasculature. Similarly, because the peak flow velocity through a blood vessel is inversely proportional to the viscosity of the liquid flowing through it, Doppler studies of the fetal middle cerebral artery are used as a noninvasive estimate of fetal hematocrit. This is useful in management of severe fetal anemia in pregnancies complicated by isoimmunization.

Finally, **ultrasound is used to assist in performing invasive obstetric procedures.** Amniocentesis, chorionic villus sampling (CVS), and percutaneous umbilical blood sampling (cordocentesis) are examples of procedures that require continuous ultrasonic guidance.

AMNIOCENTESIS

Amniocentesis, which involves removing a sample of fluid from the amniotic cavity, is the most common invasive prenatal diagnostic procedure. Using direct ultrasonic guidance, a 22-gauge needle is advanced into a clear pocket of amniotic fluid under sterile conditions, taking care to avoid maternal bowel and blood vessels, and the placenta if possible. About 20 mL of amniotic fluid is withdrawn for genetic studies. **Rh immune globulin (Rh_O-GAM) must be given to the Rh-negative gravida** because of the small risk for procedure-related isoimmunization.

Genetic Diagnosis

Amniocentesis for prenatal diagnosis of chromosomal anomalies is performed at **16 to 20 weeks of gestation**. The procedure-related **risks are an approximately 0.3% pregnancy loss rate and a 1% postprocedure measurable amniotic fluid leakage rate**. Early amniocentesis done before the 15th week of gestation is associated with a higher miscarriage rate (3% to 4%), a higher postprocedure leakage rate (3%), and an additional risk for limb deformities, including clubfoot (1%). Amniotic cells require 1 to 2 weeks of culture before final chromosomal analysis is possible, although fluorescent in situ hybridization (FISH) can be used with chromosome-specific probes (e.g., trisomy 21, 18, and 13) and gives preliminary results in 3 days.

Single gene defects that have been characterized at the molecular level are amenable to prenatal diagnosis through amniocentesis. **Using polymerase chain reaction (PCR), fetal DNA in the amniocytes can be amplified rapidly to allow for direct or indirect molecular analysis of genetic disorders.** Examples of common prenatally diagnosed genetic disorders include cystic fibrosis, Tay-Sachs disease, sickle cell disease, and fragile X syndrome.

Biochemical Testing

An example of biochemical testing that can be performed on amniotic fluid is **determination of the level of alpha-fetoprotein (AFP).** AFP is a fetal serum protein that should, under normal circumstances, be detectable in the amniotic fluid in only trace amounts. **In the event that the fetal dorsal or ventral wall is open (e.g., neural tube defect or gastroschisis), amniotic fluid AFP will be elevated,** allowing detection of these defects even if ultrasonic imaging is equivocal or nondiagnostic.

Diagnosis of Perinatal Infections

In the United States **the most commonly encountered prenatal infections with potential sequelae for the fetus include cytomegalovirus (CMV), parvovirus B19, varicella zoster virus (VZV), and toxoplasmosis.** Often these are accompanied by ultrasonographic findings on mid-trimester ultrasound, including abdominal, liver, and intracranial calcifications, fetal hydrops, echogenic bowel, ventriculomegaly, and intrauterine growth restriction. These findings can prompt amniotic fluid analysis by culture or PCR to identify the pathogen. **In addition, amniotic fluid Gram stain, white blood cell count, glucose level, and culture have been used to diagnose preterm chorioamnionitis, which is a major cause of premature labor.**

Other Diagnostic Testing

Amniocentesis is commonly used in the third trimester to determine the risk for neonatal lung immaturity in the case of impending premature birth or before elective delivery. This is performed by measuring the **pulmonary phospholipids or lamellar bodies,** which enter the amniotic fluid from the fetal lungs. **The presence of phosphatidylglycerol and a lecithin-to-sphingomyelin (L/S) ratio greater than 2 are associated with minimal risk for respiratory distress in the neonate.** In a case of suspected premature rupture of the membranes when the diagnosis is unclear using standard tests, infusion of 2 to 3 mL of indigo dye into the amniotic fluid may be performed. If the dye is then noted on a vaginally placed tampon, rupture of the membranes is confirmed.

Therapeutic Amniocentesis

The primary role of therapeutic amniocentesis has been in the management of polyhydramnios and twin-twin transfusion syndrome. Polyhydramnios, typically defined as a single deepest vertical pocket of amniotic fluid greater than 8 cm on ultrasound, can cause maternal respiratory embarrassment or premature labor. Excessive amniotic fluid volume may arise from lack of fetal swallowing or from excessive fetal urination. The latter condition occurs in the twin-twin transfusion syndrome (see Chapter 13). Serial amnioceteses to remove large volumes of excessive amniotic fluid from the sac of the recipient twin have been associated with improved perinatal outcome; however, recent data suggest that laser ablation of placental vascular connections between twin placentas with twin-twin transfusion syndrome is significantly better.

CHORIONIC VILLUS SAMPLING (CVS)

Another method to access fetal cells for prenatal genetic diagnosis is CVS of the placenta. The indications for CVS are similar to amniocentesis. **The advantage of CVS is that it is performed earlier than amniocentesis (typically between the 10th and 12th weeks of gestation), allowing for earlier prenatal diagnosis.** Although technically feasible, CVS is not performed before the 9th week because it has been associated with an increased risk for oromandibular and limb dystrophy, presumably from a vascular insult.

CVS may be performed under sterile conditions transcervically or transabdominally. In transcervical CVS, the distal 3 to 5 cm of a catheter is inserted through the cervix and into the placenta under sonographic guidance. A 20-mL syringe with nutrient medium is attached, and negative pressure is applied to obtain fragments of placental villi. Transabdominal CVS uses an 18- to 20-gauge needle inserted into the placenta transabdominally. With either approach, Rh_O-GAM should be administered to Rh-negative patients. **The procedure-related loss rate is less than 1%.**

Direct visual inspection of dividing villi cells obtained with CVS allows for detection of chromosomal abnormalities within 3 days, and tissue culture yields cytogenetic results in 6 to 8 days. **The diagnostic precision of CVS is somewhat less than the standard amniocentesis owing to a 1% risk for chromosomal mosaicism, which is often due to confined placental mosaicism.** A disadvantage of CVS is that amniotic fluid AFP levels cannot be assessed with this technique, and thus patients at risk for neural tube defects must be deferred to amniocentesis in the second trimester.

CORDOCENTESIS

Cordocentesis (percutaneous umbilical blood sampling) is a procedure in which fetal blood is obtained directly from the umbilical vein at the placental cord insertion site under direct ultrasonic guidance. Confirmation of the fetal origin of the blood specimen is obtained by measuring the fetal mean corpuscular

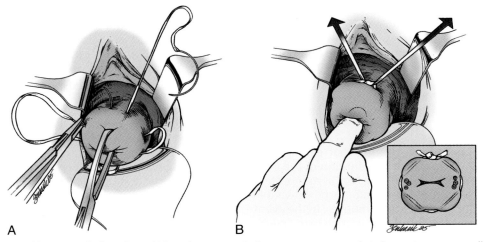

FIGURE 17-1 McDonald-type cervical cerclage. Although suture technique may vary somewhat, four sutures are usually placed high into the cervix using a nonabsorbable material such as Mersilene (**A**) and then tied, providing additional support at the level of the internal cervical os (**B**). This suture is cut for labor. *(From Gabbe SG, et al: Obstetrics, 5th ed. Philadelphia, Churchill Livingstone, 2007.)*

volume (MCV), which is typically greater than 120 fL (maternal MCV is usually less than 100 fL).

Historically, the most common indication for cordocentesis was to determine fetal hematocrit in the hemolytic disease, Rh isoimmunization. With the recent advent of fetal anemia assessment by Doppler of the fetal middle cerebral artery, cordocentesis for this indication is less frequent. **Today, cordocentesis is often performed for rapid fetal karyotype evaluation.** Unlike amniocytes, fetal leukocytes may be cultured rapidly, and results are typically available in 3 days.

The fetal loss rate is about 1% per procedure. In the case of a hydropic fetus, the risk for fetal loss may approach 7%. The cause of pregnancy loss may be due to chorioamnionitis, rupture of membranes, bleeding from the puncture site, bradycardia, or thrombosis of the umbilical vessel.

Cervical Cerclage

Cervical insufficiency or incompetence is defined as the inability of the uterine cervix to retain a pregnancy in the absence of contractions or labor (see Chapter 19). Cervical cerclage, a circumferential suture placed into the cervix, has been proposed as a surgical treatment for this condition. **The cerclage is usually placed at 13 to 16 weeks.**

The most common procedure, **McDonald's cerclage**, entails placement of a simple pursestring monofilament suture near the cervicovaginal junction (Figure 17-1). **Shirodkar's cerclage** differs in that the stitch is placed as close to the internal os as possible. The bladder and rectum are dissected off the cervix, the woven tape-like suture is tied, and the mucosa is replaced over the knot. Transabdominal cervicoisthmic cerclage is rarely indicated and is reserved for select patients with previously failed vaginal cerclage, cervical hypoplasia, or a cervix severely scarred from prior lacerations or prior surgery. This type of cerclage entails dissection of the bladder from lower uterine segment through an abdominal incision. **For transvaginal cerclage, the suture is typically removed before the onset of labor. For abdominal cerclage, cesarean delivery is performed.** Patients must be counseled thoroughly regarding the risks associated with cerclage, which include bleeding, infection, iatrogenic rupture of amniotic membranes, and damage to adjacent organs (bladder and bowel).

Operative Delivery

The incidence of an operative obstetric delivery in the United States today is about 35% to 40%, of which 10% to 15% are operative vaginal deliveries using either a forceps or vacuum device. **About 25% to 30% of all deliveries are cesarean births.** Each operative procedure has inherent benefits and risks.

OBSTETRIC FORCEPS

Forceps are instruments designed to provide traction and rotation of the fetal head when the expulsive efforts of the mother are insufficient to accomplish safe delivery of the fetus. Commonly used forceps are shown in Figure 17-2. There are two classes of obstetric forceps: classic forceps and specialized forceps. Forceps selection depends on the obstetric indication.

Classic or standard forceps are used to effect delivery by applying traction to the fetal skull. The components of each blade are illustrated in Figure 17-3. The blades have a **cephalic curve** designed to conform to the curvature of the fetal head. Simpson forceps (an

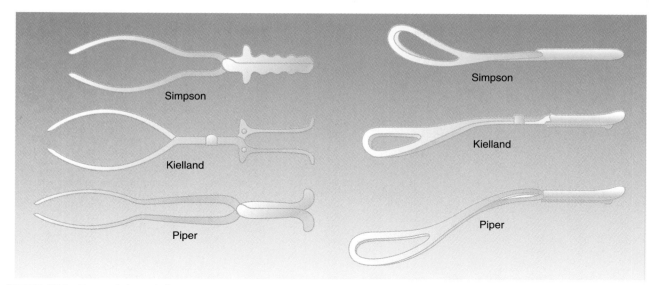

FIGURE 17-2 Types of obstetric forceps in use. Simpson forceps are an example of classic or standard forceps. Kielland forceps (for midforceps rotation) are an example of specialized forceps and are used infrequently. Piper forceps are used for breech delivery of the aftercoming head (see Figure 17-4).

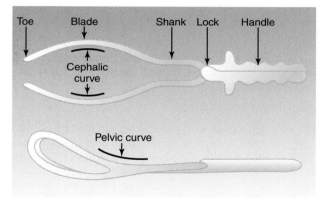

FIGURE 17-3 Components of classic forceps.

example of classic or standard forceps) have a tapered cephalic curve that is designed to fit on a molded fetal head. The **pelvic curve** of classic forceps approximates the shape of the birth canal.

Indications

In general, there are four indications for an operative vaginal delivery:
1. **Prolonged second stage of labor.** In nulliparous women, this is defined as lack of continuing progress for 2 hours without regional anesthesia or 3 hours with regional anesthesia. In multiparous women, it is defined as lack of continuing progress for 1 hour without regional anesthesia or 2 hours with regional anesthesia.
2. **Suspicion of immediate or impending fetal compromise**

3. **To stabilize the aftercoming head during a breech delivery** (Figure 17-4)
4. **To shorten the second stage of labor for maternal benefit.** Maternal conditions such as hypertension, cardiac disorders, or pulmonary disease, in which strenuous pushing in the second stage of labor is considered hazardous, may be indications for forceps delivery. Epidural analgesia, which also decreases strenuous pushing during the second stage of labor, may also be recommended for this purpose.

Types of Forceps Operations

Forceps application is classified according to the station and position of the presenting part at the time the forceps are applied. The American College of Obstetricians and Gynecologists (ACOG) has proposed the following classification:
1. **Outlet forceps:** Scalp is visible at the introitus without separating the labia, fetal head is at perineum, fetal skull is at pelvic floor, sagittal suture is in anteroposterior or right/left occiput anterior or posterior position, and rotation of the fetal head does not exceed 45 degrees.
2. **Low forceps:** Leading part of the fetal skull is at station +2 cm or more. Low forceps have two subdivisions: rotation of 45 degrees or less and rotation of more than 45 degrees.
3. **Mid forceps:** Fetal head is engaged, but the leading point of the skull is above station +2 cm.

Before performing a forceps-assisted vaginal delivery, appropriate consent from the patient regarding potential risks and benefits should be obtained. The

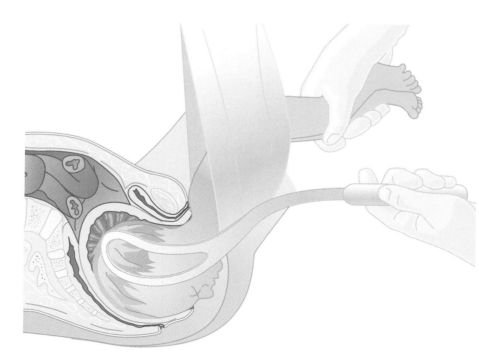

FIGURE 17-4   Delivery of the after-coming head, using Piper forceps.

indication for the procedure should be clearly outlined to the patient and in the medical record. **The cervix must be fully dilated, membranes ruptured, and the fetal head engaged into the pelvis.** Clinical assessment to determine the level of the presenting part, estimation of the fetal size, and adequacy of the maternal pelvis is mandatory. **There must be no doubt regarding the position of the fetal head.** This evaluation is performed by palpation of the sutures and fontanelles in comparison to the maternal pelvis. **Anesthesia must be adequate** by either pudendal nerve block with local infiltration (for outlet forceps only) or regional anesthesia. **The bladder should be emptied** to prevent damage to that structure and to provide more room to effect delivery.

Forceps Technique

The forceps blades are inserted sequentially into the vagina such that the sagittal suture of the fetal head is directly between and perpendicular to the shanks. Damage to maternal tissues may be avoided by placing one operator hand into the vagina to guide the toe of the blade along the natural pelvic curve of the birth canal. With the next maternal pushing effort, the forceps are locked, and traction is applied. The direction of pull should be parallel to the axis of the birth canal at that level, such that typically there is downward traction initially, followed by ever-increasing upward traction as delivery of the fetal head occurs. With complete delivery of the head, the shanks are nearly perpendicular to the floor. **If progress of the fetal head is**

not obtained with appropriate traction, the procedure should be abandoned (failed forceps) in favor of a cesarean delivery.

VACUUM EXTRACTION

The vacuum extractor is an instrument that uses a suction cup that is applied to the fetal head. Because of relative ease of use compared with forceps, vacuum delivery has become more prevalent in the United States. After confirming that no maternal tissue is trapped between the cup and the fetal head, the vacuum seal is obtained using a suction pump. Traction is then applied using similar principles described previously for a forceps delivery. **Flexion of the fetal head must be maintained to provide the smallest diameter to the maternal pelvis by placing the posterior edge of the suction cup 3 cm from the anterior fontanelle squarely over the sagittal suture.** This is illustrated in Figure 17-5. With the aid of maternal pushing efforts, traction is applied parallel to the axis of the birth canal. Detachment of the suction cup from the fetal head during traction is termed a *pop-off.* If progress down the birth canal is not obtained with appropriate traction, or if two pop-offs occur, the procedure should be discontinued in favor of a cesarean delivery. **The indications for vacuum delivery are the same as for forceps delivery.**

The prerequisites for use of the vacuum extractor are also the same as for forceps, with a few exceptions. **The vacuum extractor is contraindicated in preterm**

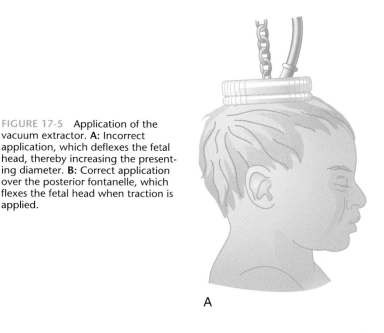

FIGURE 17-5 Application of the vacuum extractor. **A:** Incorrect application, which deflexes the fetal head, thereby increasing the presenting diameter. **B:** Correct application over the posterior fontanelle, which flexes the fetal head when traction is applied.

A

B

delivery because the preterm fetal head and scalp are more prone to injury from the suction cup. The vacuum extractor is suitable for all vertex presentations, but unlike forceps, **it must never be used for delivery of fetuses presenting by the face or breech**.

COMPARISON OF FORCEPS AND VACUUM DELIVERY

Understanding the potential advantages and disadvantages of each operative vaginal delivery instrument allows the operator to counsel the mother appropriately and choose the device that is best suited for the particular clinical situation.

Forceps have a higher overall success rate for vaginal delivery. **The failure rate for forceps is 7%, whereas the failure rate for vacuum extraction is 12%. In general, forceps deliveries cause higher rates of maternal injury**, and **vacuum extraction causes higher rates of fetal morbidity**. Forceps have an increased risk for trauma to vaginal and perineal tissues and damage to the maternal anal sphincter. In contrast, neonates delivered by vacuum have more **cephalohematomas** (accumulation of blood beneath the periosteum) and exclusively have **subgaleal hematomas** (blood in the space above the periosteum that has a large potential space and can allow significant blood loss). **Sequential use of one instrument followed by the other has been associated with a disproportionately high fetal morbidity rate** and should be avoided or approached with extreme caution. Long-term retrospective studies of adolescents delivered by normal vaginal delivery, forceps, vacuums, and cesarean delivery have shown little difference in physical and cognitive impairment.

CESAREAN DELIVERY

Cesarean delivery is delivery of the fetus through an incision in the maternal abdomen and uterus. Hospitals offering obstetric services must have the personnel and equipment to perform an emergent cesarean delivery within 30 minutes.

Cesarean delivery is the most common major operation performed in the United States today. **The rate of cesarean deliveries has increased more than fivefold, from 5% of births in 1970 to nearly 30% of births currently**. The dramatic increase in the cesarean delivery rate has been attributed to many factors, including assumed benefit for the fetus, relatively low maternal risk, societal preference, and fear of litigation.

The perinatal benefits of cesarean section are largely based on unquantified and scanty evidence. There has been more than a 10-fold decrease in perinatal mortality in the United States over the past 40 years concurrent with advances in prenatal, intrapartum, and neonatal care. How much of this improvement is due to the increased use of cesarean delivery is debatable, with the exception of management of the term breech delivery. **Perinatal and neonatal mortality and significant neonatal morbidity have been shown to improve from 5.0% for those breeches delivered vaginally to 1.6% for those delivered by cesarean.**

The overall mortality rate from cesarean delivery is currently less than 1 in 1000, but this is about 5 times greater than that from vaginal delivery. However, **recent**

studies have shown that the maternal mortality rate for an elective cesarean delivery approximates that of vaginal delivery. This is due to advances in surgical techniques, anesthetic care, blood transfusions, and antibiotics.

The maternal morbidity with cesarean delivery is increased compared with vaginal delivery, owing to increased postpartum infections, hemorrhage, and thromboembolism.

Indications

Four indications account for 90% of the marked increase in cesarean delivery over the past 40 years: dystocia (30%), repeat cesarean delivery (25% to 30%), breech presentation (10% to 15%), and fetal distress (10% to 15%). An absolute indication for a cesarean delivery is a previous full-thickness, nontransverse incision through the myometrium. This occurs in all classic cesarean deliveries and some myomectomy surgeries. All pregnancies complicated by placenta previa should also be delivered by cesarean birth.

Types of Cesarean Deliveries

Cesarean deliveries are classified by the uterine incision (Figure 17-6), not the skin incision. In the low transverse cesarean delivery (LTCD), the uterine incision is made transversely in the lower uterine segment after establishing a bladder flap. The advantages of this approach include decreased rate of rupture of the scar in a subsequent pregnancy and a reduced risk for bleeding, peritonitis, paralytic ileus, and bowel adhesions.

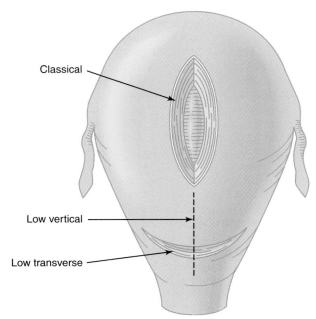

Classical

Low vertical

Low transverse

FIGURE 17-6 Types of cesarean delivery incisions.

In the classic cesarean delivery, a vertical incision is made in the upper segment of the uterus through the myometrium of the uterus. A vertical incision may also be made in the lower segment, in which case the procedure is referred to as a low vertical cesarean delivery, although the incision invariably extends into the upper segment of the uterus. The common indications for a classic cesarean delivery include the preterm breech with an undeveloped lower uterine segment, transverse back-down fetal position, poor access to the lower segment due to myomas or adhesions, or a planned cesarean hysterectomy.

The type of uterine incision has important implications regarding risk for uterine rupture in future pregnancies. Uterine rupture, defined as separation of the uterine incision, may cause significant maternal complications due to massive hemorrhage and fetal damage or death. An LTCD incision is associated with less than a 1% risk for symptomatic uterine rupture in the subsequent pregnancy, although this risk may be higher if labor induction or augmentation is carried out. A classic cesarean delivery carries a 4% to 7% risk for uterine rupture. Patients with a classic uterine incision are thus destined to have repeat cesarean deliveries for all subsequent pregnancies.

Prevention

Two clinical interventions have been shown to reduce cesarean delivery rates: external cephalic version (ECV) and vaginal birth after cesarean delivery (VBAC).

ECV converts a malpresenting fetus to the vertex position to avoid a cesarean delivery for breech presentation. This procedure is performed in labor and delivery, after the 36th or 37th week of gestation, under ultrasonic guidance. A tocolytic may be given to decrease uterine tone. Using external manipulation, the fetus is gently guided to the vertex presentation. Fetal risks due to umbilical cord entanglement and placenta abruption are low (<1%).

The success rate of ECV is about 60%. Parity, gestational age, placental location, and dilation or station affect this success rate. An ECV program can decrease the rate of cesarean delivery in this group of patients by more than half and an obstetric service's overall cesarean birth rate by about 2%.

Women with a prior cesarean delivery represent the second most common overall cause of cesarean delivery, VBAC (25% to 30%). In fact, about 10% to 15% of pregnant women have had a previous cesarean delivery.

A trial of labor may be offered if one or two previous LTCDs were performed, the uterine incision did not extend into the cervix or uterine upper segment, and there is no history of prior uterine rupture. Adequate maternal pelvic dimensions should be noted by clinical examination. Personnel and equipment should be immediately available in case emergent cesarean delivery is required.

The overall success rate of VBAC is about 70%, although this ranges from 60% (dystocia) to 90% (malpresentation), depending on the indication for the previous cesarean delivery. Compared with repeat cesarean delivery, a successful vaginal delivery is associated with less maternal morbidity without an increase in perinatal morbidity. However, if uterine rupture does occur, there may be a 10-fold increase in perinatal mortality as well as substantial maternal morbidity.

SUGGESTED READING

American College of Obstetricians and Gynecologists: Cervical insufficiency. ACOG Practice Bulletin No. 48. Washington, DC, ACOG, 2003.

American College of Obstetricians and Gynecologists: Vaginal birth after previous cesarean delivery. ACOG Practice Bulletin No. 54. Obstet Gynecol 104:203–212, 2004.

American College of Obstetricians and Gynecologists: Screening for fetal chromosomal abnormalities. ACOG Practice Bulletin No. 77. Obstet Gynecol 109:217–227, 2007.

Fox NS, Chervenak FA: Cervical cerclage: A review of the evidence. Obstet Gynecol Surv 63:58-65, 2008.

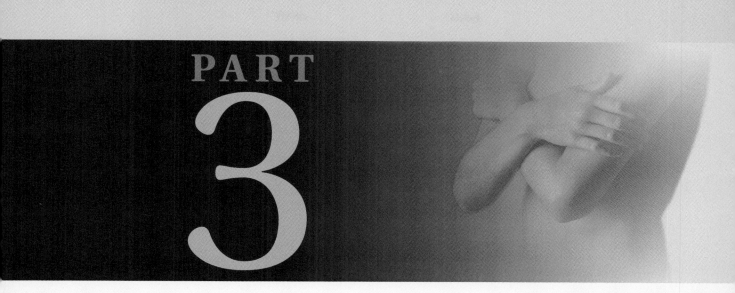

PART
3

GYNECOLOGY

Chapter 18

Congenital Anomalies and Benign Conditions of the Vulva and Vagina

ANITA L. NELSON • JOSEPH C. GAMBONE

Vulvovaginal problems are among the 10 leading disorders encountered by primary care clinicians. Definitive diagnosis may be delayed even though the woman may complain of pruritus and irritation because these problems are nonspecific and can be caused by a wide range of conditions. **It is important to establish an accurate diagnosis before initiating therapy.**

In this chapter, benign lesions of the vulva and vagina are described in the broad categories of congenital anomalies, benign neoplastic conditions, dermatologic changes, trauma, and functional disorders. Infectious conditions of the vulva and vagina are covered in Chapter 22.

◼ *Vulva*

CONGENITAL ANOMALIES OF THE VULVA

Congenital anomalies of the external genitalia are quite variable. Ambiguous genitalia can present with **clitoromegaly, bifid clitoris,** or **midline fusion of the labioscrotal folds. Clitoral agenesis** is also possible as a result of failure of the genital tubercle to develop. Many of these defects are associated with other problems such as bladder extrophy. Incomplete development of the genitalia can result in a **cloaca** with no definite separation of the bladder and vagina. **Hernial sacs** may present in the newborn as vulvar masses. Similarly, any of the cell types normally found in the vulva can present at birth with overexuberant tissue development, such as a **hemangioma** or **neuroma.**

The **problems of sexual identification posed by ambiguous genitalia are particularly important at birth. Caution, sensitivity, and the avoidance of hasty decisions and confusing terminology should be the rule when dealing with anxious parents and relatives.** Careful physical examination, pelvic ultrasonography, hormonal studies, examination of a buccal smear for sex chromatin, karyotyping, and consultation with specialists may be necessary before the sex of rearing

is assigned. In general, when there is any suboptimal development of penile or scrotal structures, the infant will be assigned a female gender because it is easier to reconstruct ambiguous genitalia to female structures than it is to build functional male genitalia. The assignment of sex will determine the need for any corrective surgery or hormonal manipulation and the manner in which the parents rear the child. These factors are all critical to the child's proper gender identification.

Female pseudohermaphroditism is caused by masculinization occurring in utero, the infant presenting with ambiguous genitalia. Masculinization of the genetically female fetus occurs secondary to the endogenous hormonal milieu, **as in congenital adrenal hyperplasia, or as a result of exogenous hormonal ingestion by the mother.** Androgen-producing tumors of the ovary or adrenal gland, although rare, also cause this problem. **Enlargement of the clitoris is the most conspicuous abnormality.** Fusion of the labioscrotal folds also occurs in various degrees, producing a hypospadiac urethral meatus and a malpositioned vaginal orifice. Internal genital development is normal.

However, **when the genetic sex is male (46 XY), there may be external phenotypic development along female lines. This occurs in the complete androgen insensitivity syndrome (testicular feminization),** a genetic abnormality most commonly inherited as an X-linked recessive disorder. Because of a genetic deficiency of androgen receptors, the external genital development occurs along female lines. Testes are usually undescended and are located in the inguinal canals or the labial areas. After puberty, external genitalia are generally normal for females on examination, with the exception that the public hair is scanty or absent. In many cases, there is sufficient vaginal development to allow adequate coital activity. In utero, müllerian inhibiting substance is produced by the 46 XY fetus, which results in a lack of müllerian duct

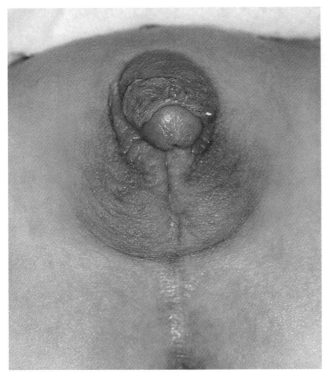

FIGURE 18-1 Ambiguous genitalia in a child with an XY karyotype and partial androgen insensitivity. *(From McKay M: Vulvar manifestations of skin disorders. In Black M, McKay M, Braude P, et al [eds]: Obstetric and Gynecologic Dermatology, 2nd ed. Edinburgh, Mosby, 2003, p 121.)*

development and explains the absence of uterus or fallopian tubes. After puberty, the testes must be removed because malignant neoplastic transformation is possible. Ambiguous genitalia in an XY child can occur with *partial* androgen insensitivity (Figure 18-1).

Male pseudohermaphroditism may occur with varying degrees of virilization and müllerian development. This is most commonly the result of genetic mosaicism, such as 45 XO/46 XY. Many factors must be taken into account in the determination of gender role in these cases, and a full discussion of this problem is beyond the scope of this book. In a phenotypic female with a Y chromosome, localization and removal of the gonadal tissue and subsequent hormonal management are necessary (as with androgen insensitivity syndrome) because malignant neoplastic transformation may occur in these gonads.

In true hermaphroditism, which is rare, dual gonadal development occurs, either in the form of an ovotestis or as a separate ovary and testis. Although some of these cases represent mosaicism of the normal female and male chromosomal complement, the usual chromosomal pattern is 46 XX. Most true hermaphrodites have some degree of both female and male development internally and externally. The extent to which masculinization

occurs depends on the relative amount of testicular tissue and its relative contribution of testosterone. Confirmation of the diagnosis requires laparotomy.

BENIGN CONDITIONS OF THE VULVA

Significant noninfectious conditions that may affect the vulva are covered in this section. Infectious conditions are covered in Chapter 22.

Structural and Benign Neoplastic Conditions

Young girls can develop **labial agglutination,** which is easily treated by estrogen cream and massage to separate the labia majora. **Fox-Fordyce disease** is characterized by a series of pruritic, raised, yellowish retention cysts (often inflamed) in the axilla, mons, or labia, which result from keratin-plugged apocrine glands.

Other cysts can also develop in the vulva, reflecting the variety of dermoid structures present. The most common are **epidermal inclusion cysts** and **sebaceous cysts** located below the epidermis, which are mobile, nontender, spherical, and slow growing. Sebaceous cysts are slightly firmer than other inclusion cysts; they are filled with dry caseous material. Most such inclusion cysts require no treatment if they are asymptomatic. The mucous glands of the vestibule and periurethral areas can become obstructed and form cystic structures. The milk line extends from the axilla to the vulva, and postpartum women can form **galactoceles** in the labia. **Vulvar varicosities** can enlarge, especially in pregnancy, to cause discomfort and pose possible risks for rupture or thrombosis.

Urethral caruncles appear as small, fleshy outgrowths of the distal edge of the urethra (Figure 18-2). In children, this results from spontaneous prolapse of the urethral epithelium. On the other hand, in postmenopausal women, the caruncle occurs when the hypoestrogenic vaginal epithelium contracts and everts the urethral epithelium.

Vulvar vestibulitis (vestibular adenitis) is a relatively rare condition in which one or more of the minor vestibular glands becomes inflamed. This condition is characterized by severe introital dyspareunia and, occasionally, vulvar pain. On examination, the lesions may be visualized as 1- to 4-mm erythematous dots that are exceedingly tender when gently touched with a cotton-tipped swab. Although described as an "itis," vestibulitis is not an infectious process and does not respond to antibiotic therapy. Topical estrogen creams or hydrocortisone may be tried, but surgical therapy to remove the glandular area may ultimately be required. Other interventions may be necessary to deal with the associated sexual dysfunction. Women with psoriasis may complain of vulvar pruritus and burning with minimal or no apparent lesions in the vulvar area. Box 18-1 lists other chronic, noninfectious vulvar conditions commonly associated with pruritus.

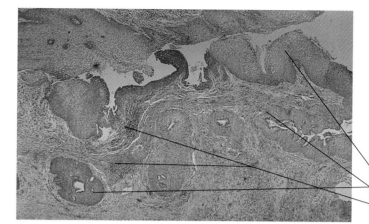

Squamous epithelium
Transitional epithelium
Chronic inflammation

FIGURE 18-2 Urethral caruncle. This lesion usually presents as a small, painful, red lump at the urethral meatus. In this example, transitional epithelium can be recognized, and there is a papillomatous pattern involving small, neighboring glands. A little chronic inflammation is seen.

BOX 18-1 *Chronic, Noninfectious Conditions Commonly Associated with Vulvar Pruritus*

Dermatoses
Atopic and contact dermatitis
Lichen sclerosus, lichen planus, lichen simplex chronicus
Psoriasis
Genital atrophy

Neoplasia*
Vulvar intraepithelial neoplasia, vulvar cancer
Paget's disease

Vulvar Manifestations of Systemic Disease
Crohn disease

---
*See Chapter 40.
Data from American College of Obstetricians and Gynecologists (ACOG): ACOG Practice Bulletin, No. 93, May 2008. Diagnosis and management of vulvar skin disorders. Obstet Gynecol 111:1243-1253, 2008.

The external genitalia can also be the site of benign growths. Both **lentigo** (freckles) and **nevi** (moles) can be found on the labia and must be clearly distinguished from melanomas. Often excisional biopsy is needed. **Fibromas** are the most common benign solid tumors that form in the deeper connective tissue of the vulva. Although fibromas are slow growing and most are 1 to 10 cm in diameter, they can become gigantic (>250 lb). **Lipomas** are also slow-growing tumors of the vulva, composed of adipose cells. Other tumors derive from tissue found in the external genitalia, such as **hidradenoma** (the apocrine gland tumor), **syringoma** (eccrine gland tumor), **granular cell myoblastoma** (neural sheath Schwann cell tumor), and **neurofibroma** (from von Recklinghausen's disease). These lesions should be removed surgically if they cause any problems. Small cherry **angiomas** can develop in the fourth and fifth decade and appear as multiple red lesions 2 to 3 mm in diameter.

Clitoromegaly may develop after birth in response to excessive androgen exposure. In the nonerect state, the clitoris usually is 0.5 cm wide and 1 to 1.5 cm long. **Clitoromegaly is a sign of virilization** and is diagnosed when the product of the external clitoral length times the width at the base of the clitoris exceeds 35 mm^2 (in a nonerect state) in an adult woman, or the width at the base is more than 1 cm.

TRAUMATIC LESIONS

Blunt trauma to the female genitalia from falls, motor vehicle crashes, or sexual assault (see Chapter 28) most commonly results in **vulvar bruising, lacerations**, and **hematomas**. Close observation and occasionally surgical exploration may be necessary to determine the full extent of the injuries and to repair them appropriately.

Genital body piercing and tattoos can cause infection or skin irritation. The area around the piercing can develop localized skin thickening and even trauma after sexual activity.

Female genital mutilation (**often termed** *female circumcision*) has been performed on more than 150 million women worldwide and continues to be a common practice, especially in some African and Eastern Asian countries where the roles of women are tightly restricted. Box 18-2 contains the World Health Organization (WHO) classification of the four types of female genital mutilation, updated in 2008. The degree of anatomic change has a profound effect on infection risk, sexual function, and vaginal delivery.

Women who have suffered **obstetric lacerations** or **episiotomies** posteriorly into the rectum, anteriorly into the urethra, or laterally into the labia have scarring that reflects these injuries or their repairs.

EPITHELIAL CONDITIONS

In postmenopausal women, estrogen deficiency generally produces significant signs of genital atrophy. The labia minora regress. The subcutaneous fat

BOX 18-2   *World Health Organization (WHO) Classification of Female Genital Mutilation*

Type I—Partial or total removal of the clitoris and/or prepuce (clitoridectomy)

Type II—Partial or total removal of the clitoris and labia minor, with or without the excision of the labia majora (excision)

Type III—Narrowing of the vaginal orifice with creation of a covering seal by cutting and appositioning the labia minora and/or the labia majora, with or without excision of the clitoris (infibulation)

Type IV—All other harmful procedures to the female genitalia for nonmedical purposes, for example, pricking, piercing, incising, scraping, and cauterizing

in the labia majora shrinks, reducing the size of those structures. The most prominent change is the vaginal introitus, which can assume a prepubertal appearance and caliber, making coitus uncomfortable.

Lichen simplex chronicus (squamous cell hyperplasia) is a local thickening of the epithelium that may result from a prolonged itch-scratch cycle. Women may note pruritus and pain. Examination reveals a white or reddish, thickened, leathery, raised surface. The effects of scratching may be evident as linear excoriations. The lesions tend to be discrete but may be multiple and coexist with other vulvar pathology. Histologically, the rete ridges deepen, and there is hyperkeratosis of the superficial layer of the epidermis (Figure 18-3). Treatment includes moderate-strength steroid ointments with antipruritic agents.

Lichen sclerosis often causes intense pruritus, dyspareunia, and burning pain. Although it can develop in any body area in any aged person, it is most frequently found on the vulva of menopausal women. On examination, the skin is thin, inelastic, and white, with a crinkled, tissue paper appearance. Ultimately, lichen sclerosis can involve all the genital area from the mons to the anal area in a keyhole pattern. **Biopsy reveals a thin epithelium with loss of rete ridges and inflammatory cells lining the basement membrane** (Figure 18-4). Diagnosis is important because this is a chronic, progressive disease with the potential to constrict and destroy the normal genital architecture. When untreated, there is the possibility of progression to vulvar intraepithelial neoplasia (VIN), differential type. In the long term, the labia minora are lost, the labia majora flatten, the introitus becomes severely constricted, and the clitoris becomes inverted and trapped (Figure 18-5). Combinations of lichen sclerosis and dysplasia, hyperplasia, or carcinoma are possible. Multiple biopsies may be necessary to characterize completely all the pathologies present in one woman. Treatment of lichen sclerosis involves the use of potent topical steroids such as 0.05% clobetasol. Eighty percent of lesions respond. Long-term therapy with lower-potency steroids or topical emollients may be necessary.

Lichen planus presents as purplish, polygonal papules that may appear in their erosive form. Lichen planus may involve the vagina and the mouth as well as the vulva (vulvar-vaginal-gingival syndrome). The patient generally complains of vulvar burning or severe dyspareunia, especially in advanced stages when

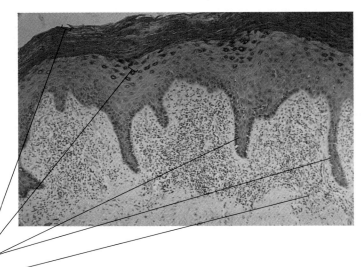

Thick keratin layer (hyperkeratosis and parakeratosis)
Granular layer
Elongated rete ridges
Chronic inflammatory infiltrate

FIGURE 18-3   Squamous cell hyperplasia. Microscopy shows marked hyperkeratosis and parakeratosis with a prominent granular layer. Acanthosis, with prolongation of rete ridges, is also seen, and there is a dense infiltrate of chronic inflammatory cells, mainly lymphocytes, in the superficial dermis.

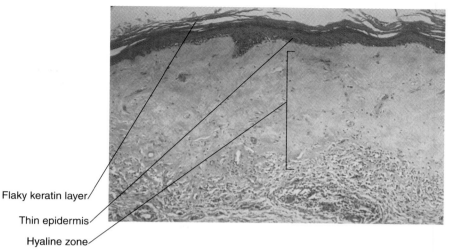

FIGURE 18-4 Lichen sclerosis. Histology shows hyperkeratosis, but the epidermis is thinner than normal. The most striking feature of lichen sclerosis is the presence of a hyaline zone in the superficial dermis. This is the result of edema and degeneration of the collagen and elastic fibers of the dermis.

Flaky keratin layer

Thin epidermis

Hyaline zone

vaginal stenosis may develop. Topical and systemic steroids are recommended for treatment.

The epithelium of the vulva is susceptible to dermatologic disorders found elsewhere on the body surface, although the clinical manifestations of those disorders may be slightly different because of the vulva's moist environment. A correct diagnosis is critical, and tissue punch biopsy may be required (Figure 18-6). **Psoriasis** generally appears velvety but may lack the characteristic scaly patches found on the flexor surfaces (e.g., knees and elbows). **Eczema** has a more erythematous presentation and may be difficult to diagnose unless lesions that are more characteristic can be found on the scalp, umbilicus, or extremities. Even in these circumstances, diagnostic biopsy may be needed to rule out conditions that are more serious. **Pemphigus** is an autoimmune blistering disease involving the vulvovaginal and conjunctival areas. **Behçet's syndrome** classically involves ulcerations in the genital and oral areas, as well as superficial ocular lesions. The genital lesions are distinctive and can result over time in a scarred, fenestrated vulva. The etiology is unknown, as is an effective treatment. Diagnosis is based on the concurrence of vulvar, oral, and ocular involvement, the recurrent nature of the disease, and the exclusion of other conditions, such as syphilis and Crohn disease.

Crohn disease is primarily a gastrointestinal (GI) disorder, but vulvar ulcers can precede the development of GI ulcerations. The vulvar ulcers are slit-like or "knife-cut" ulcers with prominent edema. Draining sinuses and fistulas to the rectum may occur. **Aphthous ulcers,** which are superficial and painful, can be found not only on the labia but also in the mouth. **Decubitus ulcers** can develop in frail women over the bony prominences of their ischial tuberosities or sacrococcygeal region or in areas susceptible to friction from indwelling catheters.

Acanthosis nigricans is most commonly found in the intertriginous area, in the axilla or on the nape of

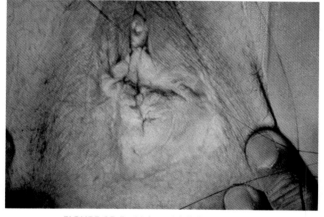

FIGURE 18-5 Vulva with lichen sclerosis.

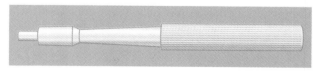

FIGURE 18-6 A disposable cutaneous punch biopsy instrument.

the neck (see Chapter 32, Figure 32-4). It is recognizable by its darkly pigmented velvety or warty surface. **Acanthosis nigricans** is related most closely to insulin resistance but can be linked less commonly to other benign conditions and malignancy.

The labia are exposed to a wide range of chemicals and other foreign materials that can induce **contact dermatitis** (erythema and burning) or irritative changes. A careful history may identify the use of a specific irritant, such as harsh soaps, perfumed toilet paper, deodorant spray, panty liners, or latex condoms. Physical examination may reveal erythema, edema, and occasionally excoriation or ulceration. In the more chronic state, the epidermis can thicken (see discussion of squamous cell hyperplasia, earlier). **Biopsy of any thickened or suspicious area is imperative at the initial examination.** Later biopsy of areas unresponsive to therapy may be necessary. In the acute phase, management involves stopping all exposure to potential irritants and keeping the area dry. The use of topical mild to moderate potency corticosteroids for 1 to 4 weeks may calm the inflammatory response. Antihistamines, cold packs, and bland emollients may provide relief from the pruritus.

Vulvar intraepithelial neoplasia, Paget's disease of the vulva, and invasive tumors of the vulva are discussed in Chapter 40.

FUNCTIONAL

Vulvodynia is a term used to describe chronic vulvar discomfort or pain with no obvious pathology. This condition, along with a similar condition called *vulvar vestibulitis* (see earlier), may be responsible for dyspareunia and has been associated with a visible lesion of the vulva called *vestibular papillomatosis*. Vulvodynia can be localized but generally is described as a burning, aching, stinging sensation involving isolated areas or the entire external genital area. Other pathology must be ruled out before the diagnosis can be applied. Many women who suffer vulvodynia share a history of prior vulvar treatments with laser, loop electrosurgical excisional procedures, or multiple topical medications. Others have a history of herpes simplex virus infection or fibromyalgia. It is thought that many of the women with vulvodynia may be suffering from peripheral neuropathy. Treatment is challenging but starts by removing all irritants. If this fails, providing a trial of low-dose tricyclic antidepressants, gabapentin-carbamazepine, or pregabalin to treat peripheral neuropathy may be effective. Pruritus may be addressed with a variety of agents, including doxepin given orally or topically. Newer treatments with estrogen, capsaicin ointments, and even botulinum toxin type A (by injection) are showing promise.

◼ *Vagina*

CONGENITAL ABNORMALITIES

Many variations and combinations of anomalies of the vagina occur. The more common anomalies of the vagina include canalization defects such as imperforate hymen, longitudinal and transverse vaginal septa, partial development (vaginal atresia), and double vagina. Congenital absence of the vagina (agenesis) is less common.

Imperforate hymen represents the mildest form of these canalization abnormalities. It occurs at the site where the vaginal plate contacts the urogenital sinus. After birth, a bulging, membrane-like structure may be noticed in the vestibule, usually blocking egress of mucus. If not detected until after menarche, an imperforate hymen may be seen as a thin, dark bluish or

thicker, clear membrane blocking menstrual flow at the introitus (Figure 18-7). A similar anomaly, the **transverse vaginal septum,** is most commonly found at the junction of the upper and middle thirds of the vagina (Figure 18-8). At times, a transverse vaginal septum will have a sinus tract or small perforation that allows menstruation. Thus, the septum may become apparent only after intercourse is impeded. Patients with an imperforate hymen or transverse vaginal septum usually have normal development of the upper reproductive tract.

Atresia of the vagina generally represents a more substantial lack of canalization at the caudal or cranial end of the vaginal plate. If cranially placed, the upper vagina and cervix may be absent, whereas the uterine fundus and fallopian tubes remain unaffected.

A midline longitudinal septum may be present, creating a double vagina. The longitudinal septum may be only partially present at various levels in the upper and middle vagina, either in the midline or deviated to one side. In addition, a longitudinal septum may attach to the lateral vaginal wall, creating a blind vaginal pouch, with or without a communicating sinus tract. These septa are usually associated with a double cervix and one of the various duplication anomalies of the uterine fundus, although the upper tract is often entirely normal.

Vaginal agenesis represents the most extreme instance of a vaginal anomaly, with total absence of the vagina except for the most distal portion that is derived from the urogenital sinus. If the uterus is absent but the fallopian tubes are spared, the defect is **müllerian agenesis or Rokitansky-Küster-Hauser syndrome.** Isolated vaginal agenesis with normal uterine and fallopian tube development is rare and is thought to be the end result of isolated vaginal plate malformation.

Adenosis of the vaginal wall consists of islands of columnar epithelium in the normal squamous epithelium. It is often located in the upper third of the vagina. The incidence of this finding is much higher in women exposed in utero to diethylstilbestrol (Figure 18-9).

Dysontogenic cysts of the vagina are generally thickwalled, soft cysts resulting from embryonic remnants. **Gartner's duct cysts** are the most common of these. They arise from the remnant of the wolffian duct (mesonephros). They vary in size from 1 to 5 cm and are found on the anterolateral walls in the upper half of the vagina and more laterally in the lower vagina. Most are asymptomatic and require no intervention.

BENIGN CONDITIONS OF THE VAGINA

Structural and Benign Neoplastic Conditions

Urethral diverticula are small (0.3 to 3 cm), sac-like projections that can be found in the anterior vagina along the posterior urethra. As obstructed periurethral glands, they may or may not communicate with the urethra. Urethral diverticula can cause recurrent urinary tract infections,

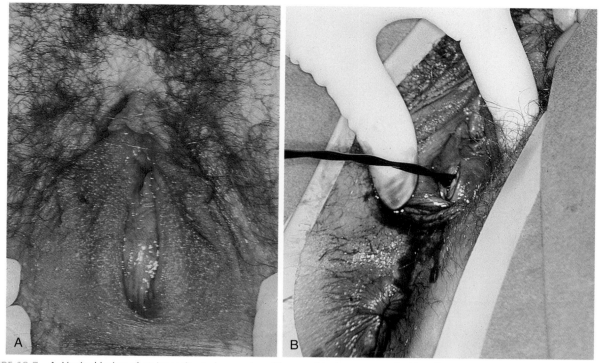

FIGURE 18-7 **A:** Vaginal bulge of an imperforate hymen in a 13-year-old who presented with pelvic pain, now constant but cyclical in the past. **B:** Old blood (hematocolpos) and some mucus (mucocolpos) are released after a stab incision is made through the hymen. *(From McKay M: Vulvar manifestations of skin disorders. In Black M, McKay M, Braude P, et al [eds]: Obstetric and Gynecologic Dermatology, 2nd ed. Edinburgh, Mosby, 2003, p 122.)*

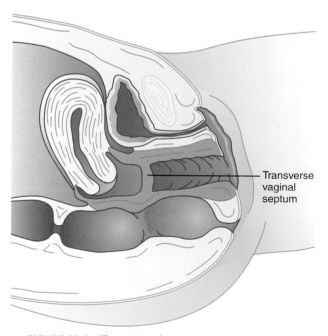

Transverse vaginal septum

FIGURE 18-8 Illustration of a transverse vaginal septum.

dysuria, dyspareunia, and occasionally, urinary dribbling. **Most women with urethral diverticula have symptoms of chronic urinary tract infection.** Urethral dilation or surgical excision of a diverticulum may be necessary.

Inclusion cysts are common lesions that result from an infolding of the vaginal epithelium. They are usually located in the posterior or lateral wall of the lower third of the vagina. They are most frequently associated with lacerations from childbirth or gynecologic surgery.

Bartholin's cyst is the most common vulvovaginal tumor. It presents as a swelling posterolaterally in the introitus, usually unilaterally. The cyst is usually less than 3 cm in diameter and is frequently asymptomatic. Careful examination of the base of the cyst is necessary (especially in a woman older than 40 years) to rule out an underlying Bartholin's carcinoma (see Chapter 40). Infection of the gland may result from blockage and accumulation of purulent material. When infected, a large, painful inflammatory mass can develop, and an inflatable bulb-tipped tube (Word catheter) can be inserted through a small stab incision into the mass and left in place for 4 to 6 weeks. This allows for an epithelialized tract to form that will remain open for drainage. When Bartholin's cysts are large, symptomatic, and not infected, a marsupialization procedure can be performed (Figure 18-10).

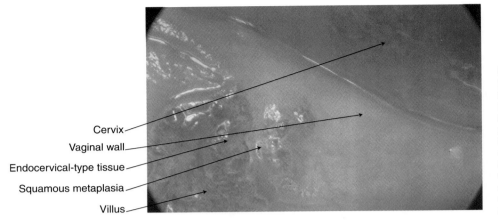

Cervix

Vaginal wall

Endocervical-type tissue

Squamous metaplasia

Villus

FIGURE 18-9   Vaginal adenosis photographed at the time of colposcopy. Glands are not normally present in the vagina, and columnar epithelium should not be seen. In vaginal adenosis, endocervical-type glands with columnar epithelium on the surface are seen in the vaginal wall. This condition is more common in women who were exposed to diethylstilbestrol (DES).

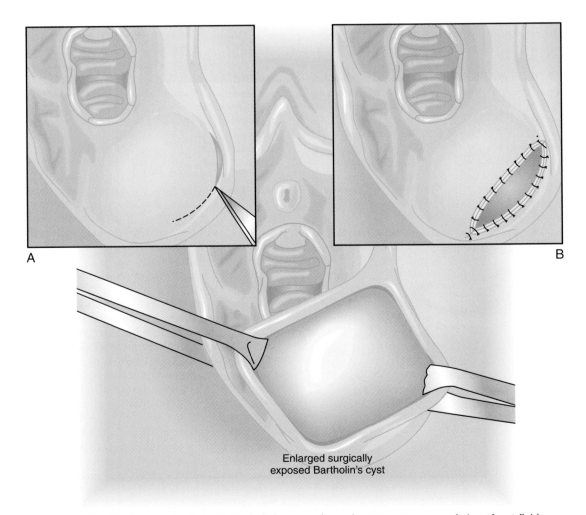

A

B

Enlarged surgically
exposed Bartholin's cyst

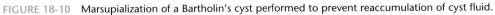

FIGURE 18-10   Marsupialization of a Bartholin's cyst performed to prevent reaccumulation of cyst fluid.

Another cystic structure that may be found in the upper third of the vagina is an implantation of endometriosis. **Endometriosis** presents as steel-gray or black cysts that may bleed slightly at the time of menstruation.

Structural changes that develop over time generally result from the loss of pelvic support. **Cystoceles,** now referred to as anterior vaginal prolapse, **rectoceles** or posterior vaginal prolapse, and **enteroceles** are more thoroughly discussed in Chapter 23. **Ureterovaginal, vesicovaginal, and rectovaginal fistulas** may result from infection, complications of surgery or radiation therapy, obstetric injury, or invasive cancer. They cause chronic vaginal discharge and considerable vulvovaginal irritation.

TRAUMA

The most common cause of vaginal trauma is sexual assault, although some superficial vaginal abrasions can occur with consensual intercourse. Focal abrasions may result from tampons (especially when used on low-flow days), a poorly fitted diaphragm, or prolonged pessary use. A lost or forgotten tampon or retained vaginal packing material most often presents with a foul-smelling vaginal discharge. Vaginal trauma can also result from other foreign objects, straddle injuries, and childbirth. Lacerations and hematomas from vaginal trauma pose significant and immediate challenges, but potential damage to surrounding bladder and bowel structures must also be evaluated.

DERMATOLOGIC

An unavoidable consequence of estrogen deficiency after menopause or with breastfeeding is vaginal atrophy. The vaginal rugations flatten, and the vaginal epithelium becomes thin, pale, and inelastic. Secretions from the Bartholin's glands and the vaginal vault in response to sexual arousal diminish. The vaginal pH rises. This combination of atrophy at the introitus and dry, inelastic vaginal walls leads to dyspareunia and even traumatic injury with attempted coitus.

Erosive lichen planus, with its characteristic erythematous papules, can involve the vagina as well as the vulvar vestibule. Condylomata acuminata and flat warts from human papillomavirus can be found in the vaginal vault, as can herpes simplex infections.

FUNCTIONAL

Vaginismus is an involuntary contraction of the vaginal introital and levator ani muscles. Vaginismus may preclude, or render very painful, vaginal penetration during coitus, pelvic examination, or tampon use. Often a history of sexual abuse or phobias about vaginal trauma is associated with vaginismus; these misconceptions and phobias may respond to education and desensitization (see Chapter 27).

SUGGESTED READING

American College of Obstetricians and Gynecologists (ACOG): ACOG Practice Bulletin, No. 93, May 2008. Diagnosis and management of vulvar skin disorders. Obstet Gynecol 111: 1243-1253, 2008.

Bikoo M: Female genital mutilation: Classification and management. Nurs Stand 22:43-49, 2007.

Guntner J: Vulvodynia: New thoughts on a devastating condition. Obstet Gynecol Surv 62:812-819, 2007.

Kaufman RH, Faro S, Brown D (eds): Benign Diseases of the Vulva and Vagina, 5th ed. Philadelphia, Elsevier Mosby, 2005.

Kondi-Pafiti A, Graspa D, Papakonstantinou K, et al: Vaginal cysts: A common pathologic entity revisited. Clin Exp Obstet Gynecol 3591:41-44, 2008.

Zamirska A, Reich A, Berny-Moreno J, et al: Vulvar pruritus and burning sensation in women with psoriasis. Acta Derm Venereol 88:132-135, 2008.

Chapter 19

Congenital Anomalies and Benign Conditions of the Uterine Corpus and Cervix

ANITA L. NELSON • JOSEPH C. GAMBONE

Benign conditions of the uterine corpus and cervix are commonly encountered in gynecologic practice because they affect a woman's fertility and can cause abnormal uterine bleeding or pelvic pain. In this chapter, congenital anomalies, benign neoplasms, epithelial changes, and functional disorders of the uterus (corpus and cervix) are discussed along with conventional and emerging therapies.

Congenital Anomalies of the Uterine Corpus and Cervix

The upper vagina, cervix, uterine corpus, and fallopian tubes are formed from the paramesonephric (müllerian) ducts. **The absence of a Y chromosome and the resultant absence of müllerian inhibiting substance lead to the development of the paramesonephric system, with the regression of the mesonephric system.** The paramesonephric ducts first arise at 6 weeks' gestation lateral to the cranial pole of the mesonephric duct and expand caudally. By 9 to 10 weeks, they fuse in the midline at the urogenital septum to form the uterovaginal primordium. Later, dissolution of the septum between the fused paramesonephric ducts leads to the development of a single uterus and cervix.

The most common anomalies of the uterus result from either incomplete fusion of the paramesonephric ducts, incomplete dissolution of the midline fusion of those ducts, or formation failures. Figure 19-1 shows variations of uterine and cervical development and demonstrates that communication between the dual systems can exist at several levels. Failure of fusion is most evident in **uterus didelphys,** which presents with two separate uterine bodies, each with its own cervix and attached fallopian tube and vagina. A **bicornuate uterus with a rudimentary horn** also represents a fusion failure. Less complete fusion failure is seen in the **bicornuate uterus with or without double cervices.** Incomplete dissolution of the midline fusion of the paramesonephrica explains the **septate uterus.** Failure of formation can be seen in the **unicornuate uterus. In müllerian agenesis, there is complete lack of development of the paramesonephric system.** The affected woman generally has incomplete development of the fallopian tubes associated with the absence of the uterus and most of the vagina. All these conditions occur in normal karyotypic and phenotypic females but can be associated with important anomalies of the urinary system such as a horseshoe or pelvic kidney.

The most common congenital cervical anomalies are the result of malfusion of the paramesonephric (müllerian) ducts with varying degrees of separation, as seen in the didelphys cervix or septate cervix.

These different anatomies may have a significant effect on a woman's risk for infertility and early pregnancy loss and may also cause dysmenorrhea and dyspareunia. Women with fusion anomalies may present with menstrual blood trapped in a noncommunicating uterine horn or vagina.

In addition to these macroscopic differences, subtle anomalies may exist within the uterine vascular system, such as an **arteriovenous malformation,** rupture of which may cause life-threatening hemorrhage.

Although all these anomalies can occur spontaneously, they may also be caused by early maternal exposure to certain drugs. The most notable of these drugs is diethylstilbestrol (DES). A **DES-exposed female infant has an increased risk for a small, T-shaped endometrial cavity** (Figure 19-2A) **or cervical collar deformity** (Figure 19-2B). DES exposure in utero can also produce fallopian tube abnormalities, although it does not appear to cause abnormalities of the urinary tract.

240

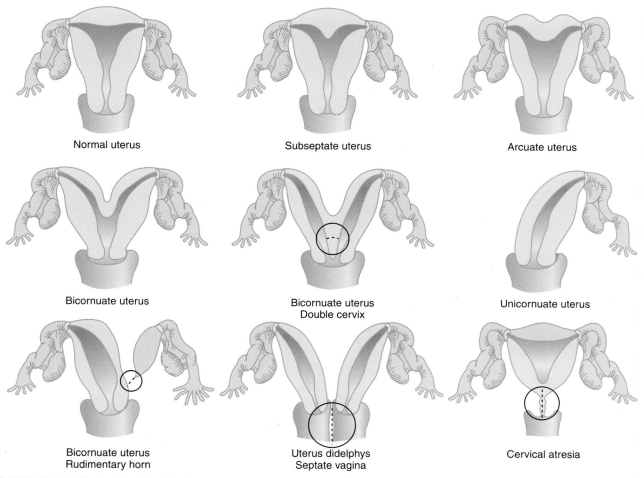

Normal uterus

Subseptate uterus

Arcuate uterus

Bicornuate uterus

Bicornuate uterus
Double cervix

Unicornuate uterus

Bicornuate uterus
Rudimentary horn

Uterus didelphys
Septate vagina

Cervical atresia

FIGURE 19-1   Variations in uterine development. The *dotted lines within circles* represent potential sites of communication or obstruction.

■ *Benign Neoplastic Conditions*

UTERINE LEIOMYOMAS

Uterine leiomyomas ("fibroids") are benign tumors derived from the smooth muscle cells of the myometrium. They are the most common neoplasm of the uterus. Estimates are that more than 45% of women have leiomyomas by the fifth decade of life, but most are asymptomatic. However, **leiomyomas can cause excessive uterine bleeding, pelvic pressure and pain, and infertility.** They are the primary indication for about 200,000 hysterectomies in the United States each year. Although leiomyomas have the potential to grow to impressive sizes, **their malignant potential is minimal.** Sarcomatous changes occur in less than 1 per 1000 uteri with fibroids.

Risk factors for developing leiomyomas include increasing age during the reproductive years, ethnicity (African American women have at least a twofold to threefold increased risk compared with white women),

nulliparity, and family history. The data are suggestive that higher body mass index is associated with a greater risk for leiomyomas. Oral contraceptive pills and depot medroxyprogesterone acetate (DMPA) injections may be associated with reduced risk.

Pathogenesis of Leiomyomas

Factors that initiate leiomyomas are not known, but ovarian sex steroids are important for their growth. Leiomyomas rarely develop before menarche and seldom develop or enlarge after menopause, unless stimulated by exogenous hormones. **Leiomyomas can also enlarge dramatically during pregnancy.** Leiomyomas have increased levels of estrogen and progesterone receptors compared with other smooth muscle cells. Estrogen stimulates the proliferation of smooth muscle cells, whereas progesterone increases the production of proteins that interfere with programmed cell death (or apoptosis). Leiomyomas also have higher levels of growth factors that stimulate the

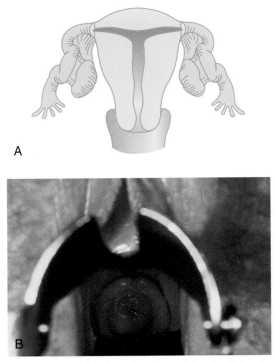

A

B

FIGURE 19-2   Typical T-shaped endometrial cavity (**A**) and cervical collar deformity (**B**) more commonly seen in women exposed to diethylstilbestrol in utero. *(Courtesy of Dr. William Growdon, UCLA-Santa Monica Medical Center.)*

production of fibronectin and collagen, major components of the extracellular matrix that characterizes these lesions.

Characteristics of Leiomyomas

Leiomyomas are usually spherical, well-circumscribed, white, firm lesions with a whorled appearance on cut section. Although the leiomyoma appears discrete, it does not have a true cellular capsule. Compressed smooth muscle cells on the tumor's periphery provide the false impression of such a capsule. **Few blood vessels and lymphatics traverse the pseudocapsule,** leading to degenerative changes as the tumors enlarge. **The most commonly observed degenerative change is that of hyaline acellularity,** in which the fibrous and muscle tissues are replaced with hyaline tissue. If the hyaline substance breaks down from a further reduction in blood supply, **cystic degeneration may occur. Calcification may occur in degenerated fibroids,** particularly after the menopause. **Fatty degeneration may also occur** but is rare. **During pregnancy, 5% to 10% of women with fibroids undergo a painful red or carneous degeneration** caused by hemorrhage into the tumor.

Leiomyomas always arise within the myometrium **(intramural),** but some migrate toward the serosal

surface **(subserosal)** or toward the endometrium **(submucosal),** as depicted in Figure 19-3. Individual tumors may migrate further when they develop large pedicles. The submucosal leiomyomas can extend through the endometrial canal and abort from the cervical os. An aborting leiomyoma causes significant bleeding and cramping pain. A subserosal leiomyoma on a long pedicle can present as a mass that feels separate from the uterus. Rarely, pedunculated subserosal myomas attach to the blood supply of the omentum or bowel mesentery and lose their uterine connections to become **parasitic leiomyomas.** Leiomyomas can also arise in the cervix, between the leaves of the broad ligament (intraligamentous), and in the various supporting ligaments (round or uterosacral) of the uterus. Leiomyomas can invade and fill the vena cava retrograde up to the level of the atrium (intravenous leiomyomatosis).

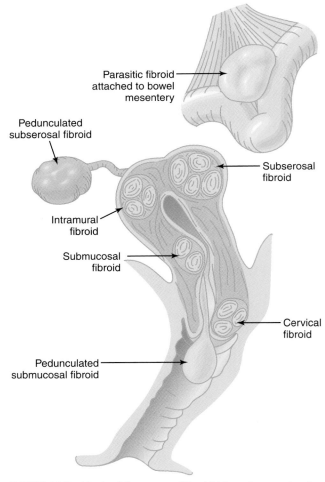

Parasitic fibroid attached to bowel mesentery

Pedunculated subserosal fibroid

Subserosal fibroid

Intramural fibroid

Submucosal fibroid

Cervical fibroid

Pedunculated submucosal fibroid

FIGURE 19-3   Uterine leiomyomas (fibroids) in various anatomic locations.

Symptoms of Leiomyomas

Most uterine leiomyomas cause no symptoms. On occasion, the patient may complain of a lower abdominal mass if the fibroid protrudes above the pelvis. Symptomatic women **may complain of pelvic pressure, congestion, bloating, a feeling of heaviness in the lower abdomen, or lower back pain.** If the fibroid presses on the bladder, there may be a problem with frequency of urination. Urinary retention and hydronephrosis are rare but result from the fact that the bladder and large leiomyomas compete for space within the pelvis.

Prolonged or heavy menstrual bleeding may be associated with intramural or submucosal myoma. Intermenstrual bleeding is not characteristic of these tumors but may occasionally occur with submucous myomas ulcerating through the endometrial lining. Excessive bleeding may result in anemia, weakness, dyspnea, and even congestive heart failure.

Fibroids are not generally painful, but **severe pain may be associated with red degeneration (acute infarction) within a fibroid,** which occurs most commonly during pregnancy. In addition, pressure pains may occur in the lower abdomen and pelvis if a myomatous uterus becomes incarcerated within the pelvis. Dyspareunia is also common with incarceration. There is an increased incidence of secondary dysmenorrhea in women with uterine myomas, generally caused by more frequent episodes of uterine bleeding. Although many women with uterine myomas become pregnant and carry their pregnancies to term, submucosal leiomyomas **may be associated with an increased incidence of infertility** because of placentation challenges.

Signs of Leiomyomas

Very large fibroids can be palpated abdominally. Those smaller than 12- to 14-week gestational size are usually confined to the pelvis. The bladder should be emptied before examination to avoid confusion with urinary retention. Although submucous fibroids may not be palpable, **on bimanual pelvic examination, a firm, irregularly enlarged uterus with smoothly rounded or bosselated protrusions may be felt if the tumors are subserosal or intramural.** The tumors are usually nontender. Their consistency may vary from rock hard, as in the case of a calcified postmenopausal leiomyoma, to soft or even cystic, as in the case of cystic degeneration of the tumor. In general, the myomatous masses are in the midline, but sometimes a large portion of the tumor lies in the lateral aspect of the pelvis and may be indistinguishable from an adnexal mass. **If the mass moves with the cervix, it is suggestive of a leiomyoma.** Often the presence of a leiomyoma precludes a proper evaluation of the adnexa, but ultrasound imaging (Figure 19-4) can help to distinguish adnexal masses from laterally placed myomas.

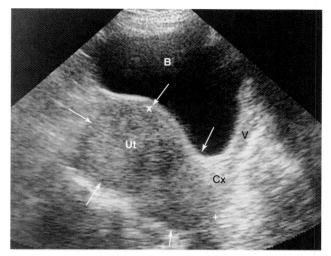

FIGURE 19-4   Ultrasound image of a uterus (Ut) enlarged and irregularly distorted by multiple leiomyomas (*arrows*). Such studies are useful to exclude ovarian enlargement. B, bladder; Cx, cervix; V, vagina. *(From Mettler FA: Essentials of Radiology, 2nd ed. Philadelphia, Saunders, 2005.)*

Differential Diagnosis for Leiomyomas

The differential diagnosis of a leiomyoma is extensive and includes other uterine pathology, such as uterine sarcoma, and other processes, such as inflammation, that can cause pelvic masses. **The most common differential diagnoses are an ovarian neoplasm, a tubo-ovarian inflammatory mass, a pelvic kidney, a diverticular or inflammatory bowel mass, or cancer of the colon.** Ultrasonography may visualize the fibroids and identify normal ovaries apart from the leiomyomas. Adenomyosis usually results in a uniformly enlarged uterus (see Chapter 25, Figure 25-5) but may on occasion be diagnosed as a leiomyoma. Figure 19-5 shows the gross appearance of an irregularly enlarged uterus with multiple fibroids.

Management of Leiomyomas

In general, if a small, asymptomatic fibroid is detected, treatment is not necessary. Unless the fibroid uterus is excessively large (>12-week gestational size) or is implicated as a cause of infertility in a woman seeking pregnancy, the first line of treatment is targeted to her symptoms.

Medical Management

Heavy or prolonged menstruation caused by fibroids may be managed hormonally in many cases. **Progestin-only therapies** (oral or injected medroxyprogesterone acetate, progestin-only oral contraceptive pills, or levonorgestrel-releasing intrauterine devices) **or combination hormonal contraceptive methods** (oral contraceptive pills, vaginal rings, or patches) **are usually the first therapeutic option.** The goal is to reduce

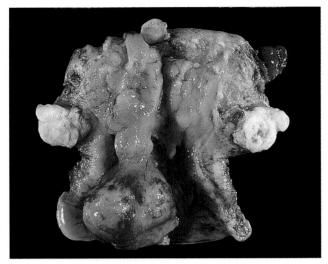

FIGURE 19-5 Gross appearance of an irregularly enlarged uterus with multiple leiomyomas. *(From Voet RL: Color Atlas of Obstetric and Gynecologic Pathology. St. Louis, Mosby, 1997.)*

monthly menstrual blood loss with cyclic hormonal methods or to eliminate menses with extended or continuous use of these methods. Dysmenorrhea is also markedly reduced by these measures.

Gonadotropin-releasing hormone (GnRH) agonists block ovarian steroidogenesis, which halts endometrial proliferation and reduces the volume of the myometrium and sometimes the volume of the leiomyomas. However, because of the intense vasomotor symptoms and the deleterious effect the GnRH agonists may have on bone mineral density, only short courses of these agonists can be administered. Usually their use is confined to women preparing for surgical treatments, such as endometrial ablation, myomectomy, or hysterectomy. Intermittent GnRH agonist administration has been shown to reduce side effects while achieving therapeutic goals longer term. **Combining GnRH agonists with hormonal agents, such as low-dose progesterone or estrogen-progestin combinations, may minimize some adverse effects of hypoestrogenism (such as osteoporosis), but long-term data are not available. GnRH agonists are very expensive, even in the short term.**

Clinical trials using the selective antiprogesterone receptor antagonist, mifepristone (RU 486), to reduce the size of uterine myomas have shown a reduction of 50% by volume over a 3-month period. Doses of 5, 25, or 50 mg/day for up to 6 months have been used to reduce the size of uterine myomas without producing the changes in bone density noted with GnRH agonists and without untoward glucocorticoid effects. However, this drug is not routinely available for this treatment.

Surgical Management Options

For women desiring to preserve their fertility, myomectomy may be an option if the number and size of the fibroids is limited. The surgical approach depends on the location of the myoma. Magnetic resonance imaging (MRI) can localize and estimate the volume of each myoma. Submucosal myomas may be resected hysteroscopically. Pedunculated, subserosal, and some intramural myomas may be removed laparoscopically. Laparotomy is generally reserved for larger myomas. If the endometrial cavity is entered during myomectomy, future delivery must be by cesarean birth. Myomectomy may not be successful in avoiding hysterectomy. At the time of myomectomy, if an inadequate amount of uterine tissue remains, a hysterectomy may be needed. New fibroids may form in the future, and about 25% of women treated with myomectomy require a subsequent operation.

For women desiring uterine preservation but not future fertility, surgical management of excessive bleeding is possible using procedures that ablate the endometrium. With endometrial ablation, more than 70% of women have a significant and satisfactory decrease in menstrual blood loss after one treatment, whereas others require repeat ablation or undergo hysterectomy. For women who desire uterine preservation and possible future fertility, uterine artery embolization (UAE) may be an option when a few small to moderate-sized tumors are present. UAE is a procedure performed under conscious sedation in which microspheres or small coils are introduced into the uterine artery by a transcutaneous femoral approach. These coils and particles occlude the artery feeding the fibroid, leading to necrosis of the fibroid. Fibroids often shrink 40% to 60% in size, and bleeding is reduced. After UAE is performed, pregnancy is still possible but is higher risk.

Hysterectomy provides definitive therapy. About 200,000 hysterectomies are done annually in the United States to treat fibroids. If the uterus is large or bulky, laparotomy is generally the preferred approach. Vaginal hysterectomy and total laparoscopic hysterectomy are both excellent options for women with smaller myometrial uteri. If a woman desires a supracervical hysterectomy, the vaginal approach is not possible. Usually ovarian preservation is encouraged unless the woman is older than 60 years or has risk factors for ovarian carcinoma. Table 19-1 summarizes the more common nonmedical options for patients with leiomyomas.

Other technologies have been developed to offer new treatment options. Cryomyolysis is a technique for destroying the myoma by the insertion of probes under laparoscopic guidance. These probes are cooled using liquid nitrogen or differential gas exchange. MRI-guided focused ultrasonography produces energy that penetrates through soft tissue to produce regions of protein

TABLE 19-1

INTERVENTION FOR PATIENTS WITH LEIOMYOMAS NOT AMENABLE TO MEDICAL THERAPY*

Clinical Presentation	Nonmedical Options	Comments
Desired fertility	Myomectomy or uterine artery embolization (UAE)†	Usually used for a limited number of leiomyomas
Desired uterine preservation or poor surgical risk	Endometrial ablation or UAE	UAE only for a limited number of leiomyomas
No desired fertility or uterine preservation	Endometrial ablation or hysterectomy	Hysterectomy is definitive therapy
Rapidly growing uterus (double in size in 6 months)	Exploratory laparotomy, abdominal hysterectomy	More extensive surgery if malignancy discovered

*Generally, failed medical therapy or large (>12-14 weeks' gestational size) uterus.
†Pregnancies after UAE are at higher risk.

denaturation and necrosis, reducing the volume of myomas. Radiofrequency ablation through a laparoscope can also be used to treat individual myomas. Each of these newer technologies lacks long-term follow-up data.

ENDOMETRIAL POLYPS

Endometrial polyps form from the endometrium to create abnormal protrusions of friable tissue into the endometrial cavity. They can cause menorrhagia and spontaneous bleeding during the reproductive years and postmenopausal bleeding after menopause. On ultrasound, endometrial polyps may appear as a focal thickening of the endometrial stripe. **They can be more clearly recognized on saline infusion sonography or visualized directly by hysteroscopy** (see Chapter 34, Figure 34-1). Endometrial polyps may evade detection by endometrial aspiration or dilation and curettage (D&C) because they are too large to be aspirated through the sampling orifice and are very flexible and can fold out of the path of the sharp curette. Histologic evaluation of the polyp is imperative because although most are benign, endometrial hyperplasia, endometrial carcinoma, and carcinosarcomas may also present as polyps.

NORMAL CERVIX

At birth, a pale pink squamous epithelium covers the outer rim of the cervix. The inner region of the ectocervix is covered with the taller columnar cells. The junction between the two is called the *original squamocolumnar junction* (Figure 19-6). The columnar epithelium appears redder because of the closer proximity of its underlying blood vessels to the surface. **With acidification of the vagina at menarche, the ectocervix undergoes an accelerated rate of squamous metaplasia in a radial pattern, from the squamocolumnar junction inward, which produces the transformation zone.** A new squamocolumnar junction is formed that moves progressively up the endocervical canal (see Chapter 38, Figure 38-1). Younger women are often found to have a reddish ring of tissue surrounding the os, which is sometimes called a ***cervical ectropion,*** but in reality, this is an area of columnar epithelium that has not yet undergone squamous metaplasia.

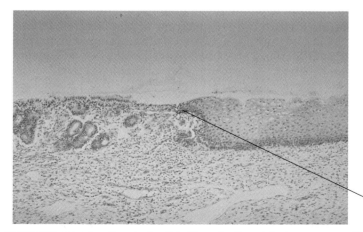

Squamocolumnar junction

FIGURE 19-6   Squamocolumnar junction. In the "ideal" cervix, the original squamous epithelium abuts the columnar epithelium. The squamocolumnar junction thus formed may be situated at the external cervical os, but in most women of childbearing age, the original squamocolumnar junction is located on the vaginal portion of the cervix.

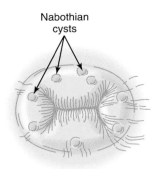

FIGURE 19-7   Cervix of a multiparous woman with nabothian cysts.

Under the influence of estrogen (birth control pills, pregnancy), the columnar epithelium of more mature women may evert and present a similar-appearing ectropion. The columnar cells produce mucus and are more vulnerable to trauma and infection with chlamydia. Therefore **women with a cervical ectropion may notice more vaginal secretions and, occasionally, postcoital spotting.** Once other etiologies have been ruled out, no treatment is needed for the friable tissue.

Nabothian cysts on the cervix are so common that they are considered a normal variant. They result from the process of squamous metaplasia. A layer of superficial squamous epithelium entraps an invagination of columnar cells beneath its surface. The underlying columnar cells continue to secrete mucus, and a mucous retention cyst is created. Nabothian cysts are opaque, with a yellowish or bluish hue. They vary generally in size from 0.3 to 3 cm (Figure 19-7), although larger nabothian cysts have been reported.

CERVICAL POLYPS

Ectocervical and endocervical polyps are the most common benign neoplastic growths of the cervix. A polyp is a localized proliferation of cells (usually columnar) located in the endocervix. Endocervical polyps tend to be more beefy red in color and arise from the endocervical canal on a long, pedunculated stalk. Ectocervical polyps are less common, are generally pale, and arise from the ectocervix to create a broad-based protrusion. Cervical polyps may be isolated or multiple and vary in diameter from a few millimeters to several centimeters. **If symptomatic, they most commonly cause coital bleeding or menorrhagia.** Narrow-based polyps are removed by twisting the polyp off at its base. Broader-based polyps may be better removed with cautery or other modalities that can control bleeding after removal. **Although the incidence of malignancy is low (1% or less), both squamous cell carcinomas and adenocarcinomas can present as polyps.** All specimens must be sent for pathologic examination.

▨ Trauma of the Uterine Corpus and Cervix

Most trauma to the uterus has an obstetric basis, such as uterine rupture from prolonged labor, caused by a Bandl's ring, or along a previous uterine scar. However, uterine perforation is also possible with operative procedures such as D&C, endometrial aspiration, or intrauterine contraceptive placement. Similarly, most traumatic injuries to the cervix occur during vaginal delivery. The cervix can tear if the infant is delivered through an incompletely dilated cervical os. Lacerations can also occur when instruments such as forceps are used for delivery or during gynecologic operations, such as cervical conization, hysteroscopy, or abortion. Trauma to the cervix can occur with sexual assault.

▨ Epithelial Conditions of the Uterine Corpus and Cervix

ENDOMETRIAL HYPERPLASIA

Endometrial hyperplasia represents an overabundant growth of the endometrium generally caused by persistent levels of estrogen unopposed by progesterone. **Hyperplasia is most frequently seen at the extremes of a woman's reproductive years when ovulation is infrequent.** It also occurs in association with unopposed estrogenic stimulation, such as the following:
1. **Polycystic ovary syndrome**
2. Estrogen-producing tumors such as **granulosa–theca cell tumors**
3. **Obesity** because of peripheral conversion of androgens to estrogen in adipose cells
4. Prolonged use of **exogenous estrogens** without progestins
5. Use of **tamoxifen**

A spectrum of histologic variations exists. **There are two categories (simple hyperplasia and complex hyperplasia) and two subcategories (with and without atypia).** Complex atypical hyperplasia has the greatest malignant potential; about 20% to 30% of cases progress to endometrial carcinoma, if untreated. Figure 19-8 shows photomicrographs of normal proliferative endometrium, simple hyperplasia (without atypia), and complex hyperplasia (with atypia).

Diagnosis

Endometrial hyperplasia should be suspected especially when a woman develops intermenstrual bleeding or when a high-risk woman develops unexplained heavy or prolonged bleeding. Endometrial sampling is necessary to obtain a histologic diagnosis. Other

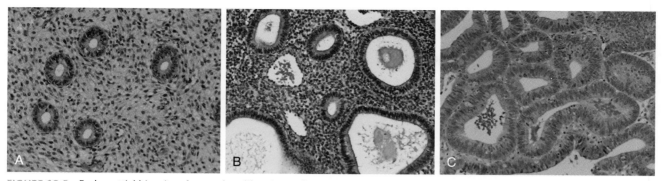

FIGURE 19-8   Endometrial biopsies of normal proliferative endometrium (**A**), simple endometrial hyperplasia without atypia (**B**), and complex endometrial hyperplasia with cellular atypia (**C**). *(From Espindola D, Kennedy KA, Fischer EG: Management of abnormal uterine bleeding and the pathology of endometrial hyperplasia. Obstet Gynecol Clin North Am 34:717-737, 2007.)*

procedures, such as fractional D&C or hysteroscopically directed biopsy, may be needed to rule out carcinoma or other pathology. **In postmenopausal women, a thin (<4 mm) endometrial stripe on transvaginal ultrasound is reassuring.**

Treatment

Treatment of hyperplasia in reproductive-aged women without atypia generally consists of a thorough, coordinated sloughing of the hyperplastic endometrium and therapies directed at preventing recurrence. **Simple hyperplasia without atypia should be treated initially with a progestin, such as 10 days each month for 3 months,** then biopsy should be repeated to confirm normalization of the endometrium. **Complex hyperplasia must be evaluated with a fractional D&C and should be initially treated with daily progestin therapy for 3 to 6 months. Test of cure with another biopsy is then needed.** In the long run, a source of progestin must be supplied. **Complex hyperplasia with atypia is best treated by hysterectomy** after carcinoma has been excluded. **Endometrial ablation is absolutely contraindicated in any of these situations until the endometrium normalizes.**

ASHERMAN'S SYNDROME

The endometrium is denuded and the endometrial cavity filled with adhesions in patients with Asherman's syndrome. Bleeding disorders can range from irregular bleeding to amenorrhea depending on the amount of intrauterine scarring. Most commonly, the scarring results from curettage in high-risk settings, such as postpartum hemorrhage or septic abortion, although vigorous scraping under any circumstances can result in the loss of the endometrium and consequent adhesion of opposing myometrial surfaces. Endometrial ablation procedures are designed to deliberately destroy the endometrium and create such scarring.

▮ *Functional Conditions of the Uterine Corpus and Cervix*

Noncongenital cervical stenosis usually arises after trauma (endocervical curettage, conization) or **hypoestrogenism** (menopause, prolonged DMPA use). Problems arise if blood from the endometrium cannot escape into the vagina, in which case the uterus becomes grossly distended (**hematometra**). Similarly, sperm may be unable to enter the upper genital tract. Cervical stenosis may also cause cervical sampling for microscopic evaluation to be incomplete.

Cervical incompetence is a condition in which the cervix is unable to maintain closure under the pressure of a progressively enlarging pregnant uterus and painlessly dilates, resulting in pregnancy loss, most commonly in the second trimester (see Chapter 12). **Cervical incompetence may be intrinsic** (caused by poor ground substance in the cervix), **the result of cervical surgery** (especially loop electrosurgical excision procedure and cold-knife conization) for cervical dysplasia, **or the result of DES exposure in utero.**

SUGGESTED READING

American College of Obstetricians and Gynecologists (ACOG): Surgical alternative to hysterectomy in the management of leiomyomas. Practice Bulletin No.16. Washington, DC, ACOG, May 2000.

Cheng MH, Wang PH: Uterine myoma: A condition amenable to medical therapy. Emerg Drugs 13:119-133, 2008.

Espindola D, Kennedy KA, Fischer EG: Management of abnormal uterine bleeding and the pathology of endometrial hyperplasia. Obstet Gynecol Clin N Am 34:717-737, 2007.

Marshburn PB, Matthews ML, Hurst BS: Uterine artery embolization as a treatment option for uterine myomas. Obstet Gynecol Clin North Am 33:125-144, 2006.

Viswanathan M, Hartman K, McDoy N, et al: Management of uterine fibroids: An update of the evidence. Evid Rep Technol Assess 154:1-122, 2007.

Chapter 20

Congenital Anomalies and Benign Conditions of the Ovaries and Fallopian Tubes

ANITA L. NELSON • JOSEPH C. GAMBONE

The ovaries and fallopian tubes, along with the blood vessels, ligaments, and connective tissues located along both sides of the uterus, are referred to as the *adnexa*. In this chapter, the normal development of the ovaries and fallopian tubes is discussed to facilitate a better understanding of the workup and management of benign adnexal masses.

Congenital Anomalies of the Ovaries and Fallopian Tubes

Abnormal embryologic development of the ovaries is uncommon. Congenital duplication or absence of ovarian tissue may occur, as may ectopic ovarian tissue and supernumerary ovaries. Although rare, the sexual bipotentiality noted in embryologic development can progress without the usual regression of one system, producing an ovotestis and subsequent intersex problems.

Genetic chromosomal disorders, such as **Turner syndrome (45 XO),** are associated with a lack of normal gonadal development, as evidenced by the rudimentary streaked ovaries that are a hallmark of the disorder. **Women with Turner syndrome usually progress through puberty and develop secondary sexual characteristics but enter menopause shortly thereafter.** This provides evidence that two X chromosomes are required for normal ovarian development. Testicular predominance occurs with the addition of a single Y chromosome, even in the face of multiple X chromosomes. Such predominance is seen in **Klinefelter syndrome (47 XXY),** in which testicular development occurs embryologically. In **complete androgen insensitivity syndrome (46 XY), which is also known as testicular feminization,** the lack of androgen receptors produces a phenotypic female in the face of

a Y chromosome. The gonads in these women (functioning testes) should be removed (usually after puberty) because of their significant malignant potential.

Isolated anomalies of the fallopian tubes, the end result of abnormal development of the proximal unfused portions of the paramesonephric ducts, are rare. **Aplasia or atresia,** usually of the distal ampullary segment of the fallopian tube, is most commonly unilateral in the presence of otherwise normal development. Bilateral aplasia is noted in some cases of uterine and vaginal agenesis. **Complete duplication** of the fallopian tubes is rarely seen, but distal duplication and accessory ostia are relatively common.

In addition, women exposed in utero to certain drugs, such as diethylstilbestrol (DES), may have abnormalities in the architecture of the fallopian tubes; **with DES exposure, the tubes may be shortened, distorted, or clubbed.**

Benign Conditions of the Ovaries

FUNCTIONAL AND BENIGN OVARIAN TUMORS

The human ovary has a striking propensity to develop a wide variety of tumors, most of which are benign. As indicated in Table 20-1, ovarian masses may be functional, inflammatory, metaplastic, or neoplastic. During the childbearing years, 70% of noninflammatory benign ovarian tumors are functional. The remainder are either neoplasms (20%) or endometriomas (10%). The management of ovarian tumors, whether functional, benign, or malignant, involves difficult decisions that may affect a woman's hormonal status or her future fertility. Although only functional cysts and benign ovarian neoplasms are considered in detail in this chapter, diagnostic methods to differentiate benign masses from malignant ones are discussed.

TABLE 20-1

DIFFERENTIAL DIAGNOSIS OF OVARIAN MASSES	
Pathogenesis	**Specific Type**
Functional	Follicular cysts Lutein cysts Polycystic ovaries
Inflammatory	Salpingo-oophoritis Pyogenic oophoritis—puerperal, abortal, or related to an intrauterine device Granulomatous oophoritis
Metaplastic	Endometriomas
Neoplastic	Premenarchal years—10% are malignant Menstruating years—15% are malignant Postmenopausal years—50% are malignant

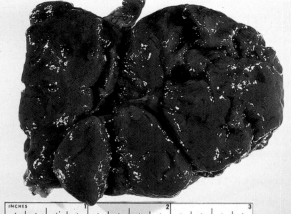

FIGURE 20-1   Gross appearance of a luteoma of pregnancy. Note the multiple brown nodules. *(From Voet RL: Color Atlas of Obstetric and Gynecologic Pathology. St. Louis, Mosby, 1997.)*

Functional Ovarian Cysts and Tumors

Dozens of ovarian follicles form the "cohort of follicles" of each menstrual cycle. **To be classified a *functional cyst*, the follicle must reach a diameter of at least 3 cm.** Functional cysts may cause pelvic pain, a dull sensation, or heaviness in the pelvis.

A **follicular cyst,** lined by one or more layers of granulosa cells, develops when an ovarian follicle fails to rupture. Similarly, a **lutein cyst** may develop if the corpus luteum becomes cystic, grows to larger than 3 cm, and fails to regress normally after 14 days. **Hemorrhagic cysts,** especially hemorrhagic corpus luteum cysts, are more likely to cause symptoms and are more vulnerable to rupture toward the end of the menstrual cycle. The hemorrhage within the cyst results from invasion of the ovarian vessels into the corpus luteum cyst 2 to 3 days after ovulation.

Other specific types of lutein cysts may occur with abnormally high serum levels of human chorionic gonadotropin (hCG) or increased ovarian sensitivity to gonadotropins. **Theca-lutein cysts** may develop in association with the high levels of hCG present **in patients with a hydatidiform mole or choriocarcinoma. Patients undergoing ovulation induction with gonadotropins or clomiphene may also develop theca-lutein cysts.** Theca-lutein cysts are usually bilateral, may become quite large (>30 cm), and characteristically regress slowly after the gonadotropin level falls. Rarely, when follicles are stimulated with gonadotropins, theca-lutein cysts can become so extensive as to cause massive ascites and dangerous problems with systemic fluid imbalance.

A **luteoma of pregnancy** is a related condition in which there is a hyperplasic reaction of ovarian theca cells, presumably from prolonged hCG stimulation during pregnancy. The luteomas characteristically appear as brown to reddish-brown nodules that may be cystic or solid. A luteoma of pregnancy (Figure 20-1)

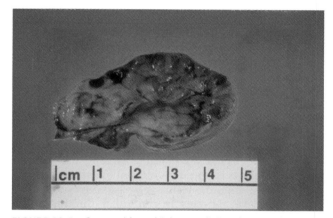

FIGURE 20-2   Ovary with multiple cysts lining the capsule consistent with polycystic ovary syndrome. *(Courtesy of Dr. Sathima Natarajan, Ronald Reagan–UCLA Medical Center.)*

may be associated with multifetal pregnancies or hydramnios. They can cause maternal virilization in 30% of women and, less often, ambiguous genitalia in a female fetus. Although ovarian enlargement may be impressive, surgical resection is not indicated because luteomas regress spontaneously postpartum.

Polycystic ovary syndrome, a functional disorder generally associated with chronic anovulation and hyperandrogenism, can also produce enlarged ovaries with multiple simple follicles (Figure 20-2). The hormonal aspects of this syndrome are discussed further in Chapter 32.

CLINICAL FEATURES. An ovarian follicular cyst is usually asymptomatic and unilocular (simple) and can reach 15 cm in diameter. It usually regresses during the subsequent menstrual cycles. In general, a lutein cyst is apt

TABLE 20-2

CALCULATION OF THE RISK OF MALIGNANCY INDEX* FOR AN OVARIAN MASS

Criteria	Scoring System
A. Menopausal Status	
Premenopausal	1
Postmenopausal	3
B. Ultrasonic Features	
Multiloculated	1 feature = 1
Solid areas	≥2 features = 3
Bilaterality	
Ascites	
C. Serum CA-125 Titer	Absolute value

*Risk of Malignancy Index = A × B × C. A cut-off value of 200 discriminates a benign from a malignant mass with a sensitivity of 87% and a specificity of 97%.

Data from Jacobs I, Oram D, Fairbanks J, et al: A risk of malignancy index incorporating CA 125, ultrasound and menopausal status for the accurate preoperative diagnosis of ovarian cancer. Br J Obstet Gynaecol 97:922, 1990.

TABLE 20-3

MODALITIES FOR THE EVALUATION OF ADNEXAL MASSES

Modality	Sensitivity (%)	Specificity (%)
Gray-scale transvaginal ultrasonography	0.82-0.91	0.68-0.81
Doppler ultrasonography	0.86	0.91
Computed tomography	0.90	0.75
Magnetic resonance imaging	0.91	0.88
Positron emission tomography	0.67	0.79
CA-125 level measurement	0.78	0.78

Data from Agency for Healthcare Research and Quality (AHRQ): Management of adnexal mass. AHRQ Publication No. 06-E004. Rockville, MD, AHRQ, 2006.

to be smaller but more firm or even solid in consistency and is more likely to cause pain or signs of peritoneal irritation. Because it may continue to produce progesterone, it is also more likely to cause delayed menses. On occasion, a functional ovarian cyst may undergo **torsion** (see later) or may **rupture,** which may produce acute lower abdominal pain and tenderness and significant hemoperitoneum.

DIAGNOSIS. The presumptive diagnosis of a functional ovarian tumor is usually made when a 5- to 8-cm cystic adnexal mass is noted on bimanual examination; it is confirmed when the lesion regresses over the course of the next several cycles. **In general, a functional cyst is mobile, unilateral, and not associated with ascites**. On rare occasions, the mass may exceed 8 cm and be quite tender to palpation. On occasion, hemorrhagic lutein cysts may have a solid rather than a cystic consistency. A pelvic ultrasound will confirm the cystic nature of the mass, but it cannot differentiate with certainty between a functional and a neoplastic tumor.

All suspicious adnexal masses in premenopausal and postmenopausal women must be carefully evaluated. Table 20-2 contains a useful risk assessment tool, the **risk for malignancy index** (RMI), which can be used to help identify those ovarian masses that could be malignant. The RMI has high sensitivity (87%) and specificity (97%).

When a patient has delayed menses, abnormal uterine bleeding, or severe pelvic pain, the differential diagnosis must include ectopic pregnancy, pelvic abscess, or adnexal torsion of a neoplastic cyst. A pregnancy test (hCG), diagnostic laparoscopy, or rarely, laparotomy may be needed. Table 20-3 lists the current modalities that are available to evaluate adnexal masses along with the sensitivity and specificity as calculated by the U.S. Agency for Healthcare Research and Quality. None of these modalities is accurate enough to be used alone for diagnosis.

MANAGEMENT. When a reproductive-aged patient who is asymptomatic or experiencing only mild symptoms presents with an adnexal cyst, a pelvic ultrasound and serum CA-125 titer should be obtained and the RMI determined. If the RMI is low and the cyst is considered to be functional, it is appropriate to wait and reexamine the patient after her next menses. Low-dose contraceptive agents may be given to suppress gonadotropin levels and prevent development of another cyst.

If the lesion does not fulfill the requirements for observation because it is solid, painful, or fixed or has an elevated RMI, surgical exploration or referral to a gynecologic oncologist is indicated. Laparoscopic cystectomy to allow histologic evaluation may be needed to differentiate between a functional and a neoplastic ovarian cyst. Aspiration of the fluid as a diagnostic tool is inappropriate because the false-negative rate for the cytologic examination is high and slow leakage of the fluid disseminates cancer if the cyst is malignant.

When the patient is in her late 40s, the chances of an ovarian neoplasm are increased, and observational delays should be undertaken with caution.

Benign Neoplastic Ovarian Tumors

Ovarian neoplasms may be divided generally by cell type of origin into three main groups: epithelial, stromal, and germ cell. Taken as a group, the epithelial tumors are by far the most common, although **the single most common benign ovarian neoplasm is the benign cystic teratoma (dermoid cyst)**, which is a germ cell tumor.

EPITHELIAL OVARIAN NEOPLASMS. These tumors are believed to be derived from the mesothelial cells lining the peritoneal cavity and also lining the surface of the

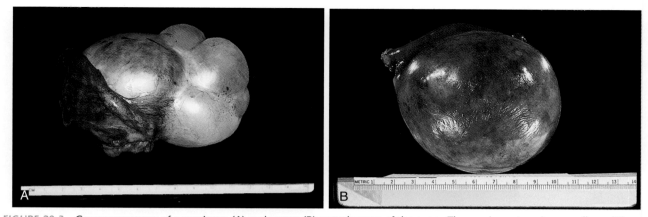

FIGURE 20-3   Gross appearance of a mucinous (**A**) and serous (**B**) cystadenoma of the ovary. The mucinous type is generally multilocu-lated and can be quite large. (**A**, *From Voet RL: Color Atlas of Obstetric and Gynecologic Pathology. St. Louis, Mosby, 1997, Fig. 6.31;* **B**, *from Voet RL: Color Atlas of Obstetric and Gynecologic Pathology. St. Louis, Mosby, 1997, Fig. 6.20.)*

ovary. The mucinous ovarian neoplasm cytologically resembles the endocervical epithelium, the endome-trioid neoplasm resembles the endometrium, and se-rous tumors resemble the lining of the fallopian tubes. The most common epithelial ovarian tumors are serous cystadenomas. Figure 20-3 shows the gross appearance of a mucinous and serous cystadenoma.

Each of the epithelial ovarian neoplasms has char-acteristic clinical and histologic features. The serous tumors are bilateral in about 10% of cases. **Of all se-rous tumors, about 70% are benign, 5% to 10% have borderline malignant potential, and 20% to 25% are malignant,** depending largely on the patient's age. Larger serous cystadenomas tend to be multilocular, although small unilocular serous cystomas also occur. Histologically, serous tumors characteristically form **psammoma bodies** (from the Greek *psammos,* mean-ing sand), which are calcific, concentric concretions. Psammoma bodies occur occasionally in benign serous neoplasms and frequently in serous cystadenocarcino-mas. Papillary patterns are also common.

The mucinous neoplasms of the ovary can attain a huge size, often filling the entire pelvis and abdomen. They are often multilocular, and benign mucinous tu-mors are bilateral in less than 10% of cases. **About 85% of mucinous tumors are benign.** Mucinous tumors are often associated with a mucocele of the appendix. **Rarely, a benign mucinous tumor may be complicated by pseudomyxoma peritonei,** a condition in which a great many benign implants are seeded onto the sur-face of the bowel and other peritoneal surfaces and produce large quantities of mucus.

The **Brenner tumor** is a small, smooth solid ovarian neoplasm, usually benign, with a large fibrotic compo-nent that encases epithelioid cells that resemble tran-sitional cells of the bladder (Figure 20-4). In about 33%

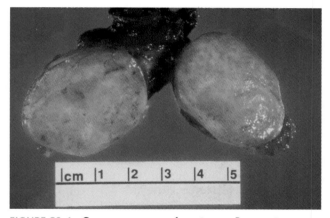

FIGURE 20-4   Gross appearance of a cut-open Brenner tumor. *(Courtesy of Dr. Sathima Natarajan, Ronald Reagan–UCLA Medical Center.)*

of cases, Brenner tumors are associated with mucinous epithelial elements.

SEX CORD–STROMAL OVARIAN NEOPLASMS. These tumors include fibromas, granulosa-theca cell tumors, and Sertoli-Leydig cell tumors. Combinations of the latter two types are termed *gynandroblastomas.*

The tumors in this category derive from the sex cords and specialized stroma of the developing gonad. The embryologic origins of granulosa and theca cells, as well as their counterparts in the testes, the Sertoli and Leydig cells, arise from cells that make up this spe-cialized gonadal stroma. If the ultimate differentiation of cell types occurring in the tumor is feminine, the neoplasm becomes a **granulosa cell tumor,** a **theca cell tumor,** or in many instances, a **mixed granulosa-theca cell tumor.** Neoplasms containing cells that take on a masculine differentiation become **Sertoli-Leydig cell**

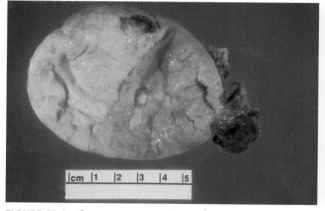

FIGURE 20-5   Gross appearance of an ovarian fibroma. *(Courtesy of Dr. Sathima Natarajan, Ronald Reagan–UCLA Medical Center.)*

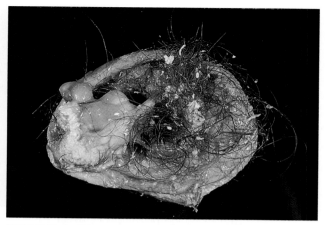

FIGURE 20-6   Gross appearance of a cut-open dermoid cyst. Note the presence of hair-bearing skin. *(From Voet RL: Color Atlas of Obstetric and Gynecologic Pathology. St. Louis, Mosby, 1997.)*

tumors. This is far less common. The **fibroma** represents a stromal cell neoplasm developing from mature fibroblasts in the ovarian stroma.

The granulosa-theca cell neoplasms, as well as their androgenic counterparts, are generally referred to as *functioning* **(not functional) ovarian tumors.** They occur in any age group, from birth on, but more commonly in the postmenopausal years. Their functioning characteristics are responsible for a variety of associated presenting signs and symptoms. **The granulosa-theca cell tumors promote feminizing signs and symptoms,** such as precocious menarche, precocious thelarche, or premenarchal uterine bleeding during infancy and childhood. In the reproductive years, menorrhagia (with alternating amenorrhea), endometrial hyperplasia, and not infrequently, endometrial cancer, breast tenderness, and fluid retention occur. Postmenopausal bleeding may occur in older women with granulosa-theca cell tumors. In contrast, **the less frequent Sertoli-Leydig cell tumors are responsible for virilizing effects,** such as hirsutism, temporal baldness, deepening of the voice, clitoromegaly, and a defeminizing change in body habitus to a muscular build. Fifteen percent of these tumors produce no obvious endocrinologic effects. **Except for the pure thecoma, all these tumors have low malignant potential** and are discussed further in Chapter 39.

The **ovarian fibroma,** another ovarian stromal tumor, forms a solid, encapsulated, smooth-surfaced tumor made up of interlacing bundles of fibrocytes. It is not hormonally active. It is glistening white on its cut surface (Figure 20-5), as opposed to the soft yellow appearance of the granulosa-theca cell or the smaller hilus cell tumor. On occasion, this tumor is associated with ascites caused by the transudation of fluid from the ovarian fibroid. The flow of this ascitic fluid through the transdiaphragmatic lymphatics into the right pleural cavity may result in **Meigs' syndrome** (ascites and

hydrothorax in association with an ovarian fibroma). The ovarian fibroma may be associated with theca cell elements called a *fibrothecoma.*

GERM CELL TUMORS. Germ cell neoplasms can occur at any age. They make up about 60% of ovarian neoplasms occurring in infants and children.

The most common ovarian neoplasm is the benign cystic teratoma, a germ cell tumor that can take on a great variety of forms, with virtually all adult tissues being represented within the mass. Ten percent to 15% of teratomas are bilateral. The benign cystic teratoma, commonly referred to as a *dermoid cyst,* is composed primarily of ectodermal tissue (such as sweat and sebaceous glands, hair follicles, and teeth), with some mesodermal and rarely endodermal elements. These are slow-growing tumors. Half are diagnosed in women between 25 and 50 years of age. Most are less than 10 cm in diameter. Because of the oily secretion of the sebaceous glands, the desquamated squamous cells, the presence of hair, and the presence of a dermoid tubercle (of Rokitansky), which often contains a hard, well-formed tooth, the dermoid cyst has a characteristic gross and histologic appearance (Figure 20-6). Other tissue components commonly found in benign cystic teratomas include mature brain, bronchus, thyroid, cartilage, intestine, bone, and carcinoid cells. As opposed to similar tissues found in a malignant immature teratoma, the tissues making up the benign (mature) teratoma are all of an adult, well-differentiated form.

MIXED OVARIAN NEOPLASMS. The most common ovarian tumor in which the neoplastic elements are composed of more than one cell type is the **cystadenofibroma,**

or the fibrocystadenoma. These tumors generally take their characteristics from the epithelial component, although they tend to be more solid than the epithelial ovarian neoplasms.

The **gonadoblastoma** is a tumor composed of cells resembling those of a dysgerminoma and others resembling granulosa and Sertoli cells. Characteristically, calcific concretions are a prominent feature of this neoplasm. **Almost all patients with a gonadoblastoma have dysgenetic gonads, and a Y chromosome has been detected in more than 90% of cases.** Although the gonadoblastoma is initially benign, about half of these tumors may predispose to the development of dysgerminomas or other malignant germ cell tumors.

DIAGNOSIS OF BENIGN OVARIAN TUMORS. The clinical features of benign ovarian tumors are often nonspecific. Except for the functioning ovarian neoplasms, **most benign ovarian tumors are asymptomatic unless they undergo torsion or rupture**. They usually enlarge very slowly, so that an increase in abdominal girth or pressure on surrounding organs is not perceived until the later stages of growth. Any pelvic pain is generally mild and intermittent, unless the tumor twists on its pedicle (torsion), when infarction may induce severe pain and tenderness. On rare occasions, an ovarian cyst may rupture spontaneously from internal hemorrhage or intracystic pressure, resulting in pain and peritoneal irritation. A cyst may also rupture occasionally during or after a bimanual pelvic examination or with intercourse. Depending on the cystic contents, pain of varying degrees of severity can result. The escape of thin serous fluid without hemorrhage may evoke little pain or tenderness, but the oily contents of a dermoid cyst or the thick mucinous fluid of a mucinous cystadenoma may be irritating to both the parietal and the visceral peritoneum, with the development of chemical peritonitis and possibly the subsequent formation of troublesome intraabdominal adhesions.

Bimanual pelvic examination generally indicates the presence of the tumor in the pelvis, but the tumor may be too small to be palpated. On the other hand, if the tumor is large enough, it may be detected by abdominal palpation. Examination may suggest a cystic mass or a solid tumor. Movement of the mass separate from the uterus supports the suspicion of an adnexal mass instead of a uterine leiomyoma. Percussion of the abdomen in a patient with a large ovarian cyst reveals dullness anteriorly with tympany in the flanks as the bowel is displaced laterally by the tumor.

If the tumor undergoes torsion and infarction or rupture, signs of peritoneal irritation may be present. If complete infarction has occurred, there may be abdominal rigidity. Paralytic ileus may also be present.

Pelvic ultrasonography, particularly **transvaginal ultrasonography,** with or without color Doppler, may be helpful. A pelvic ultrasound will be highly suggestive of a dermoid cyst, especially if it is found to include a tooth-like calcification.

Tumor markers, such as **serum CA 125,** as part of the RMI (see Table 20-2) may help to distinguish between benign and malignant masses, particularly in a postmenopausal patient. When clinical evaluation, pelvic ultrasonography, and tumor markers all indicate malignancy, the positive predictive value of the combination is high in postmenopausal women. Such patients should be referred to a gynecologic oncologist for surgical evaluation.

Laparoscopy is helpful in distinguishing between a uterine myoma, a quiescent hydrosalpinx, and an ovarian tumor, but it will not distinguish between a functional cyst, a benign neoplasm, and an encapsulated malignant ovarian neoplasm. On occasion, laparoscopy may identify endometriosis on the surface of the ovary. An ovarian endometrioma cannot be distinguished unequivocally from an ovarian neoplasm by visualization alone. In general, laparotomy is preferable to laparoscopy in the ultimate evaluation of a suspicious adnexal mass unless the entire mass can be removed laparoscopically without rupture for histologic examination.

Management of Ovarian Neoplasms

No persistent ovarian neoplasm should be assumed to be benign until proved so by surgical exploration and pathologic examination. The indications for exploratory laparotomy in a patient with a pelvic mass have been discussed under functional tumors. If laparotomy is indicated, any ascitic fluid should be collected on opening the peritoneal cavity and sent for cytologic examination. A frozen-section histologic diagnosis should be obtained intraoperatively to exclude malignancy. The definitive treatment will depend on the type of neoplasm, the patient's age, and her desire for future childbearing.

Benign epithelial ovarian neoplasms are generally treated by unilateral salpingo-oophorectomy. The contralateral ovary must be carefully inspected to exclude a bilateral lesion. Because of the possible coexistence of an appendiceal mucocele with a mucinous cystadenoma, appendectomy should also be performed in such patients. If the patient is young and nulliparous, the ovarian neoplasm is unilocular, and there are no excrescences within the cyst, an ovarian cystectomy with preservation of the ovary may be performed. **In an older woman, a total abdominal hysterectomy and bilateral salpingo-oophorectomy may be appropriate,** particularly if there is any suspicion of malignancy.

Stromal cell neoplasms of the ovary are generally treated by unilateral salpingo-oophorectomy when future pregnancies are a consideration. Ovarian fibromas, even when associated with ascites and a right hydrothorax (Meigs' syndrome), are almost always benign and might even be treated by resection from the ovary in a young woman.

Cystic teratomas ("dermoids") can be treated by ovarian cystectomy. Because 15% to 20% are bilateral, the contralateral ovary should be carefully evaluated and any cysts resected.

In a patient with a gonadoblastoma, dysgenetic ovaries are usually present, necessitating bilateral salpingo-oophorectomy, particularly in the presence of a Y chromosome. With embryo transfer now available to these patients, the uterus should be left in situ if future fertility is desired.

Benign Conditions of the Fallopian Tubes

Most benign "tumors" of the fallopian tubes are infectious or inflammatory (e.g., hydrosalpinx and pyosalpinx [Figure 20-7]). Benign neoplasms of the oviducts are rare. Although the tubes, uterine corpus, and uterine cervix are from the same müllerian anlage (primordial tissue), the tubes have less of a tendency toward neoplastic transformation.

Tubal neoplasms that do occur are **epithelial adenomas and polyps, myomas** from the tubal musculature, **inclusion cysts** from the mesothelium, or **angiomas** from the tubal vasculature.

It is quite difficult to differentiate a tubal neoplasm from other adnexal masses on examination, and operative exploration is generally necessary to confirm the diagnosis. Salpingectomy represents the definitive treatment, although if pathologic evaluation confirms the benign nature of the neoplasm, normal portions of the tube may be preserved for fertility reasons in selected cases.

As the name parovarian (beside the ovary) implies, **parovarian neoplasms are generally located within the broad ligament** between the tube and

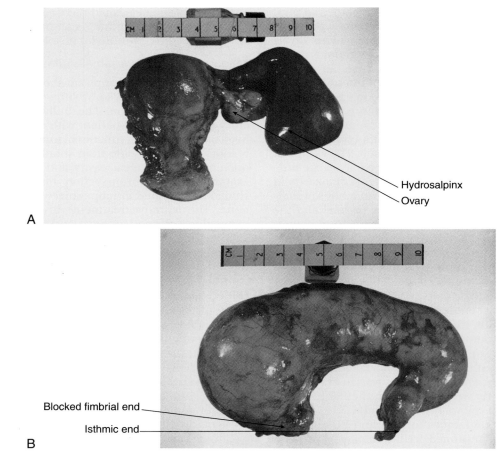

Hydrosalpinx
Ovary

A

Blocked fimbrial end
Isthmic end

B

FIGURE 20-7 **A:** Hydrosalpinx. A gross photograph of a hydrosalpinx of the right fallopian tube. In this example, the ovary is not involved in the inflammatory process. Sometimes the acute inflammation may spread to the ovary from the tube, giving rise to a tubo-ovarian abscess. **B:** Pyosalpinx. In this gross photograph, the isthmic end of the tube is at the right, and the blocked fimbrial end is on the left.

the ovary. These tumors are generally small compared with ovarian cysts, measuring less than 8 cm in diameter. Histologically, most appear to be derived from paramesonephric (müllerian) structures or occasionally from mesonephric (wolffian) remnants. Although the malignancy rate is less than 10%, it is necessary to resect the cystic mass to obtain a pathologic assessment.

Torsion either of the ovary alone or of both the ovary and fallopian tube (adnexal torsion) represents an acute surgical emergency. Torsion is a complication of benign ovarian tumors, parovarian cysts, and tubal ligation remnants. Adnexal torsion causes severe acute, unilateral lower abdominal pain, which starts often as less severe pain alternating with a dull soreness. This pattern results from intermittent twisting and untwisting of the mass. With torsion, the venous blood supply is occluded, which increases pressure in the mass and can cause hemorrhage into the mass. With more prolonged and extensive torsion, the arterial supply is occluded, and the mass undergoes necrosis.

The diagnosis may be confusing because the patient may also have fever, nausea, vomiting, and leukocytosis suggestive of appendicitis. Ultrasonic studies, including Doppler color-flow studies, can help pinpoint the diagnosis preoperatively, but prompt surgical intervention is required. If the mass has not necrosed, it may be untwisted. Cystectomy or other procedures to remove the underlying pathology will be necessary. In some cases, the ovary may be sutured to the pelvic side wall to prevent recurrence. If the tube has undergone necrosis, a unilateral salpingectomy or salpingo-oophorectomy may be necessary.

Ovarian remnant syndrome may be the cause of cyclic pelvic pain and deep dyspareunia in women who have previously undergone hysterectomy with salpingo-oophorectomy. A residual part of the ovary may be left inadvertently and adhere to the vaginal cuff or the retroperitoneal space near a ureter. Surgical excision of the small mass is required to relieve the pain.

The ovarian remnant syndrome must be distinguished from the **residual ovary syndrome.** In the latter, an ovary is intentionally left at the time of hysterectomy but subsequently causes deep dyspareunia if it becomes adherent to the vaginal cuff.

SUGGESTED READING

Agency for Healthcare Research and Quality (AHRQ): Management of adnexal mass. Evidence Based Report/Technology Assessment No. 130. AHRQ Publication No. 06-E004. Rockville, MD, AHRQ, 2006.

American College of Obstetricians and Gynecologists (ACOG): ACOG Practice Bulletin, Number 83, July 2007. Management of adnexal masses. *In* Compendium of Selected Publications (ACOG), Washington, DC, 2007, pp 1372–1383.

Boyle KJ, Torrealday S: Benign gynecologic conditions. Surg Clin North Am 88:245-264, 2008.

Grimes DA, Jones LB, Lopez LM, Schulz KF. Oral contraceptives for functional ovarian cysts. Cochrane Database Syst Rev CD006134, 2006.

Trimbos B, Hacker NF: The case against aspirating ovarian cysts. Cancer 72:828, 1993.

Chapter 21

Pelvic Pain

ANDREA J. RAPKIN • JOSEPH C. GAMBONE

Pelvic pain is a frequent complaint in gynecology. It may be cyclic and associated with menstruation, sudden in onset (acute), or chronic, lasting for more than 6 months. **Half of all menstruating women are affected by** painful menstruation or **dysmenorrhea,** making it the most common type of pelvic pain. Ten percent of these women have severe symptoms necessitating time off from work or school.

◼ Dysmenorrhea

Dysmenorrhea may be **primary,** when there is no readily identifiable cause, or **secondary** to organic pelvic disease. The typical age range of occurrence for primary dysmenorrhea is between 17 and 22 years, whereas secondary dysmenorrhea is more common in older women.

PRIMARY DYSMENORRHEA

Pathophysiology

Primary dysmenorrhea occurs during ovulatory cycles and usually appears within 6 to 12 months of the menarche. The etiology of primary dysmenorrhea has been attributed to uterine contractions with ischemia and production of prostaglandins. Women with dysmenorrhea have increased uterine activity, which results in increased resting tone, increased contractility, and increased frequency of contractions. During menstruation, prostaglandins are released as a consequence of endometrial cell lysis, with instability of lysosomes and release of enzymes that break down cell membranes.

The evidence that prostaglandins are involved in primary dysmenorrhea is convincing. Menstrual fluid from women with this disorder have higher than normal levels of prostaglandins (especially prostaglandin $F_{2\alpha}$ [$PGF_{2\alpha}$] and PGE_2), and these levels can be reduced to below normal with nonsteroidal antiinflammatory drugs (NSAIDs), which are effective treatments. Infusions of $PGF_{2\alpha}$ or PGE_2 reproduce the discomfort and many of the associated symptoms such as nausea, vomiting, and headache. Secretory endometrium contains much more prostaglandin than proliferative endometrium. Women with primary dysmenorrhea have upregulated cyclooxygenase (COX) enzyme activity as a major cause of their pain. **Anovulatory endometrium (without progesterone) contains little prostaglandin, and these menses are usually painless.**

Figure 21-1 summarizes the relationships among endometrial cell wall breakdown, prostaglandin synthesis, uterine contractions, ischemia, and pain.

Clinical Features

The clinical features of primary dysmenorrhea are summarized in Box 21-1. Cramping usually begins a few hours before the onset of bleeding and may persist for hours or days. It is localized to the lower abdomen and may radiate to the thighs and lower back. The pain may be associated with altered bowel habits, nausea, fatigue, dizziness, and headache.

Treatment

Box 21-2 lists the treatment options for primary dysmenorrhea. **NSAIDs, which act as COX inhibitors, are highly effective in the treatment of primary dysmenorrhea.** Typical examples include **ibuprofen** (400 mg every 6 hours), **naproxen sodium** (250 mg every 6 hours), and **mefenamic acid** (500 mg every 8 hours). Decreasing prostaglandin production by enzyme inhibition is the basis of all NSAIDs. Hormonal contraceptives such as **oral contraceptive pills (OCs), patches, or transvaginal rings reduce menstrual flow**

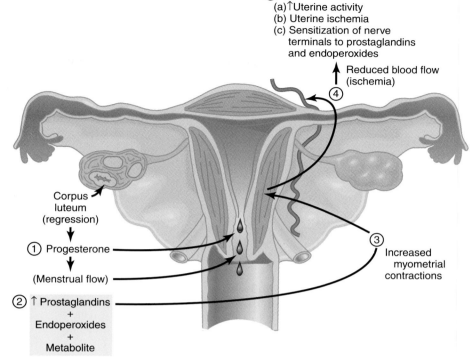

⑤ **PAIN**
(a)↑Uterine activity
(b) Uterine ischemia
(c) Sensitization of nerve
    terminals to prostaglandins
    and endoperoxides

↑ Reduced blood flow
(ischemia)

④

③

Increased
myometrial
contractions

Corpus
luteum
(regression)

① Progesterone

(Menstrual flow)

② ↑ Prostaglandins
+
Endoperoxides
+
Metabolite

FIGURE 21-1   Postulated mechanism of pain generation in primary dysmenorrhea. Nonsteroidal anti-inflammatory drugs inhibit cyclooxygenase, the enzyme that catalyzes the formation of prostaglandins from arachidonic acid. Hormonal contraceptives that block ovulation significantly reduce the formation of prostaglandins. Both drugs mitigate this mechanism of pain and are effective treatment for primary dysmenorrhea. *(Modified from Dawood MY: Hormones, prostaglandins and dysmenorrhea.* In *Dawood MY [ed]: Dysmenorrhea. Baltimore, Williams & Wilkins, 1981.)*

BOX 21-1   *Features of Primary Dysmenorrhea*

Initial Onset

About 90% experience symptoms within 2 years
of menarche (i.e., when ovulation begins).

Duration and Type of Pain

Dysmenorrhea begins a few hours before or just after
the onset of menstruation and usually lasts 48 to 72
hours.
Pain is described as cramp-like and is usually strongest
over the lower abdomen and may radiate to the back
or inner thighs.

Associated Symptoms

Nausea and vomiting
Fatigue
Diarrhea
Lower backache
Headache

Pelvic Examination Findings

Normal

BOX 21-2   *Treatment of Primary Dysmenorrhea*

General Measures

Reassurance and explanation

Medical Measures

Nonsteroidal antiinflammatory drugs
Hormonal contraceptives (including hormone-releasing
    intrauterine devices and vaginal rings)
Progestins
Tocolytics
Analgesics

Other Measures

Transcutaneous nerve stimulation
Acupuncture
Psychotherapy
Hypnotherapy

---

and inhibit ovulation and are also effective therapy for primary dysmenorrhea. Extended cycle use of OCs or the use of long-acting injectable or implantable hormonal contraceptives or progestin-containing intrauterine devices minimizes the number of withdrawal bleeding episodes that users have. Some patients may

benefit from using both hormonal contraception and NSAIDs.

Resistant cases may respond to tocolytic agents (e.g., **salbutamol**), a calcium blocker (e.g., **nifedipine**), or high-dose continuous daily progestogens (especially **medroxyprogesterone acetate** or **dydrogesterone**). Nonpharmacologic pain management, particularly acupuncture or **transcutaneous electrical stimulation,** may be useful, as are **psychotherapy, hypnotherapy, and heat patches**. Surgical procedures such as presacral neurectomy and uterosacral ligament section have been largely abandoned.

If a patient fails to respond to hormonal contraception and NSAID therapy, the diagnosis of primary dysmenorrhea should be questioned and consideration given to a secondary cause. Ultrasonic imaging, laparoscopy, and hysteroscopy with directed biopsy should be performed to exclude pelvic disease.

SECONDARY DYSMENORRHEA

Pathophysiology

The mechanism of pain in secondary dysmenorrhea depends on the underlying (secondary) cause and in most cases is not well understood. Prostaglandins may also be involved in this type of dysmenorrhea, although NSAIDs and hormonal contraceptives that do not suppress menses altogether are less likely to provide satisfactory pain relief.

Clinical Features

The clinical features of some of the underlying causes of secondary dysmenorrhea are summarized in Box 21-3. In general, secondary dysmenorrhea is not limited to the menses and can occur before as well as after the menses. In addition, secondary dysmenorrhea is less related to the first day of flow, develops in older women (in their 30s or 40s), and is usually associated with other symptoms such as dyspareunia, infertility, or abnormal uterine bleeding.

Treatment

Management consists of the treatment of the underlying disease. The treatments used for primary dysmenorrhea (Box 21-2) are often helpful. Other specific treatments are discussed in the chapters dealing with the underlying causes.

◼ *Acute Pelvic Pain*

Acute pain is sudden in onset and is usually associated with significant neuroautonomic reflexes such as nausea and vomiting, diaphoresis, and apprehension. It is important for the gynecologist to be aware of both the gynecologic and nongynecologic causes of acute pelvic pain (Box 21-4). Delay of diagnosis and treatment of acute pelvic pain increase the morbidity and even mortality.

Adnexal accidents, including **torsion or rupture of an ovarian** (Figure 21-2) **or fallopian tube cyst,** can cause severe lower abdominal pain. Normal ovaries and fallopian tubes rarely undergo torsion, but cystic or inflammatory enlargement predisposes to these adnexal accidents. The pain of adnexal torsion can be intermittent or constant, is often associated with nausea, and has been described as reverse renal colic because

BOX 21-3 *Characteristics of Some Causes of Secondary Dysmenorrhea*

Endometriosis

Pain extends to premenstrual or postmenstrual phase or may be continuous; may also have deep dyspareunia, premenstrual spotting, and tender pelvic nodules (especially on the uterosacral ligaments); onset is usually in the 20s and 30s but may start in teens.

Pelvic Inflammation

Initially pain may be menstrual, but often with each cycle it extends into the premenstrual phase; may have intermenstrual bleeding, dyspareunia, and pelvic tenderness.

Adenomyosis, Fibroid Tumors

Uterus is generally clinically and symmetrically enlarged and may be mildly tender; dysmenorrhea is associated with a dull pelvic dragging sensation.

Ovarian Cysts (Especially Endometriosis and Luteal Cysts)

Should be clinically evident

Pelvic Congestion

A dull, ill-defined pelvic ache, usually worse premenstrually, relieved by menses; often a history of sexual problems

BOX 21-4 *Causes of Acute Pelvic Pain*

Gynecologic

Adnexal accidents (e.g., ovarian cyst torsion, rupture, hemorrhage)
Acute infections (e.g., endometritis, pelvic inflammatory disease)
Pregnancy complications (e.g., ectopic gestation, abortion)

Nongynecologic

Gastrointestinal (e.g., appendicitis, enteritis, or intestinal obstruction)
Genitourinary (e.g., cystitis, ureteral stones, urethral syndrome)
Other (e.g., pelvic thrombophlebitis, vascular aneurysm, porphyria)

it originates in the pelvis and radiates to the loin. An enlarging pelvic mass is found on examination and ultrasound with decreased or absent blood flow to the adnexa on Doppler ultrasound studies. The need for surgical intervention is common and urgent.

Functional ovarian cysts (e.g., corpus luteum or follicular cysts) **may rupture,** causing leakage of fluid or blood that causes acute pain from peritoneal irritation. When there is significant associated bleeding, the pain may be followed by a hemoperitoneum and hypovolemia. Surgical intervention is mandatory in this setting, after adequate resuscitation with packed red cells and intravenous fluids.

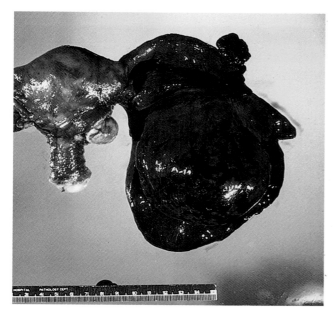

FIGURE 21-2   Torsion of an ovarian cyst. *(From Clement PB, Young RH: Atlas of Gynecologic Surgical Pathology. Philadelphia, WB Saunders, 2000.)*

Acute reproductive organ infections such as **endometritis** or **salpingo-oophoritis** (commonly referred to as pelvic inflammatory disease [PID]) can present acutely. Rupture of a tubo-ovarian abscess is a surgical emergency that can progress to hypotension and oliguria after initially presenting with diffuse lower abdominal pain. Pelvic infection is covered in greater detail in Chapter 22.

Several complications of early pregnancy, such as **ectopic gestation** (see Chapter 24) and **threatened or incomplete abortion** can cause acute pelvic pain and are generally associated with abnormal bleeding. Ectopic tubal pregnancies produce pain as the fallopian tube dilates and ruptures into the abdominal cavity and can be life-threatening when not diagnosed expeditiously.

Nongynecologic causes of acute lower abdominal pain (see Box 21-4) are frequently seen in the differential diagnosis when a woman presents with pelvic pain. **Appendicitis** is a common gastrointestinal cause of acute lower abdominal pain that eventually localizes to the right lower quadrant of the abdomen (McBurney's point). The unilateral intensity of the pain usually differentiates it from salpingo-oophoritis. Rupture of an infected appendix into the pelvic cavity can have a significant adverse effect on female fertility. Diverticular abscess is also not uncommon but usually occurs in postmenopausal women.

Acute cystitis and **ureteral stone formation** (lithiasis) and passage are both frequently painful. **Urethral syndrome** can present acutely and become chronic over time when not recognized and treated. Urinary tract disorders are covered in more detail in Chapter 23.

Chronic Pelvic Pain

Chronic pelvic pain (CPP) refers to pelvic pain of more than 6 months' duration that has a significant effect on daily function and quality of life. CPP includes reproductive and nonreproductive organ–related pelvic pain that is primarily acyclic. Although CPP is an enigmatic entity, it is one of the most common presenting complaints in a gynecologic practice. As a health problem, it results in great cost to society in terms of hospital services, loss of productivity, and human misery.

Obviously, not all lower abdominal and low back pain is of gynecologic origin. **Careful evaluation is needed to distinguish gynecologic pain from that of orthopedic, gastrointestinal, urologic, neurologic, and psychosomatic origin.** The relationship between pelvic pain and the underlying gynecologic pathology is often inexplicable and frequently thought to be psychosomatic. The discovery of the role of prostaglandins in primary dysmenorrhea, however, formerly believed to be a neurotic affectation, calls for caution when making a diagnosis of psychosomatic pelvic pain. There is still much to be learned about the mechanisms involved in the production and perception of pelvic pain.

Anatomy and Physiology

The pain fibers to pelvic organs are shown in Table 21-1. Painful impulses that originate in the skin, muscles, bones, joints, and parietal peritoneum travel in somatic nerve fibers, whereas those originating in the internal organs travel in visceral nerves.

Visceral pain is more diffusely spread than somatic pain because of a phenomenon called *viscerosomatic convergence* and the lack of a well-defined projection area in the sensory cortex for its identification. Viscerosomatic convergence occurs in all second-order neurons in the dorsal horn of the spinal cord that receive visceral input. No second-order neurons in the dorsal horn receive only visceral input. The viscerosomatic neurons have larger receptive fields than do the somatic second-order neurons, and the number of somatic second-order neurons vastly exceeds the number of viscerosomatic neurons. Visceral pain is therefore usually referred to the skin, which is supplied by the corresponding spinal cord segment (**referred pain**). For example, the initial pain of appendicitis is referred to the epigastric area, as both structures are innervated by the thoracic cord segments T8, T9, and T10.

The structures of the female genital tract vary in their sensitivity to pain. The skin of the external genitalia is exquisitely sensitive. Pain sensation is variable in the

TABLE 21-1

NERVES CARRYING PAINFUL IMPULSES FROM THE PELVIC ORGANS

Organ	Spinal Segments	Nerves
Perineum, vulva, lower vagina	S2-4	Pudendal, inguinal, genitofemoral, posterofemoral cutaneous
Upper vagina, cervix, lower uterine segment, posterior urethra, bladder trigone, uterosacral and cardinal ligaments, rectosigmoid, lower ureters	S2-4	Pelvic parasympathetics
Uterine fundus, proximal fallopian tubes, broad ligament, upper bladder, cecum, appendix, terminal large bowel	T11-12, L1	Sympathetics through hypogastric plexus
Outer two thirds of fallopian tubes, upper ureter	T9-10	Sympathetics through aortic and superior mesenteric plexus
Ovaries	T9-10	Sympathetics through renal and aortic plexus and celiac and mesenteric ganglia
Abdominal wall	T12-L1 T12-L1 L1-2	Iliohypogastric Ilioinguinal Genitofemoral

vagina; the upper segment is somewhat less sensitive than the lower. **The cervix is relatively insensitive to small biopsies but is sensitive to deep incision or to dilation.** The uterus is quite sensitive. The ovaries are insensitive to many stimuli, but they are sensitive to rapid distention of the ovarian capsule or compression during physical examination.

■ Patient Evaluation

HISTORY

A pain history should be obtained during the first visit. Characteristics of the pain, including its location, radiation, severity, and alleviating and aggravating factors as well as effects on menstruation, level of stress, work, exercise, and intercourse should be determined. Symptoms related to the gastrointestinal, genitourinary, and musculoskeletal and neurologic systems should be elicited. This process can be guided by the Pain History Mnemonic outlined in Box 21-5.

PHYSICAL EXAMINATION

The examination of the abdomen should be performed gently to prevent involuntary guarding, which may obstruct the findings. The patient should be asked to point to the exact location of the pain and its radiation, and an attempt should be made to duplicate the pain by palpation of each abdominal quadrant. The severity of the pain should be quantified on a 0 to 10 scale (0 = no pain, 10 = hitting thumb with a hammer).

A gentle but thorough pelvic examination should be performed with an attempt to reproduce and localize the patient's pain. The examination may be suggestive of specific pelvic pathology. For example, patients with endometriosis may have a fixed retroverted uterus with

BOX 21-5 *Pain History Mnemonic (OLD CAARTS)*

Onset: When and how did the pain start? Does it change over time?
Location: Localize specifically—Can you put a finger on it?
Duration: How long does it last?
Characteristics: Cramping, aching, stabbing, itching
Alleviating/aggravating factors: What makes it better (e.g., position change, medication, stress reduction) or worse (e.g., menstrual cycle, stress, specific activity)?
Associated symptoms:
  Gynecologic (e.g., dyspareunia, dysmenorrhea, abnormal bleeding, discharge)
  Gastrointestinal (e.g., constipation, diarrhea, bloating, gas, rectal bleeding)
  Genitourinary (e.g., urinary frequency, dysuria, urgency, incontinence)
  Neurologic: specific nerve distribution of the pain
Radiation: Does the pain move to other areas of the body?
Temporal: What time of day? —relationship to daily activities
Severity: Scale of 0 to 10 (from no pain to the most severe imaginable)

From Rapkin AJ, Howe CN: Chronic pelvic pain: A review. *In* Family Practice Recertification. Monroe Township, NJ, Medical World Communications, 2006, pp 59-67.

tender uterosacral nodularity. Chronic salpingitis may be suggested by bilateral, tender, irregularly enlarged adnexal structures. A prolapsed uterus may account for pelvic pressure, pain, or low backache.

The abdominal wall should be examined for evidence of myofascial trigger points and for iliohypo

gastric (T12, L1), ilioinguinal (T12, L1), or genito-femoral (L1, L2) nerve entrapment. Each dermatome of the abdominal wall and back is palpated with a fingertip, and points of motion tenderness or "jump signs" are marked with a pen. The patient is asked to tense the abdominal muscles by performing a straight-leg raising maneuver (both legs raised at least 6 inches with both knees straight) or a partial sit-up. Points that are still tender or more tender or that reproduce the patient's pain suggest that the etiology of the pain is in the abdominal wall, generally nerve entrapment, impingement, or trigger point pain, and should be injected with 2 to 3 mL of 0.25% bupivacaine. Chronic abdominal wall pain is confirmed if the pain level is reduced by at least 50% and outlasts the duration of the local anesthetic.

FURTHER INVESTIGATIONS

Psychological evaluation should be requested if an obviously traumatic event has occurred with the onset of pain; if there is obvious depression, neurosis, psychosis, or secondary gain; or to aid in the planning of pain management sessions. The latter may involve cognitive behavioral and stress reduction therapy.

Laboratory studies are of limited utility in the diagnosis of CPP, although a complete blood cell count, erythrocyte sedimentation rate (ESR), and urinalysis are indicated. The ESR is nonspecific and will be increased in any type of inflammatory condition, such as subacute salpingo-oophoritis, tuberculosis, or inflammatory bowel disease. Patients who are engaging in sexual intercourse should have a pregnancy test if they have a uterus and are not postmenopausal. Pelvic ultrasonography should be performed because the pelvic examination may miss an adnexal mass, particularly in obese patients and those who are unable to relax for the complete examination. If bowel or urinary signs and symptoms are present, an abdominal and pelvic computed tomography (CT) scan, endoscopy, cystoscopy, or CT urogram may be useful. Similarly, if there is clinical evidence of musculoskeletal disease, a lumbosacral x-ray, CT, magnetic resonance imaging, or orthopedic consultation may be in order.

Diagnostic laparoscopy is the ultimate method of diagnosis for patients with CPP of undetermined etiology. Laparoscopic examination and bimanual examination may differ in 20% to 30% of cases. Laparoscopy should only be performed if no etiology for the pain can be identified.

■ Differential Diagnosis

ORGANIC CAUSES OF CHRONIC PELVIC PAIN

Of women with CPP who are subjected to diagnostic laparoscopy, about one third have no apparent pathology, one third have endometriosis, one fourth have

---

BOX 21-6 *Gynecologic Causes of Chronic Pelvic Pain*

> Endometriosis
> Salpingo-oophoritis (pelvic inflammatory disease)
> Ovarian remnant syndrome
> Pelvic congestion syndrome
> Cyclic pelvic (uterine) pain
> Myomata uteri (degenerating)
> Adenomyosis
> Adhesions

---

adhesions or stigmata of chronic PID, and the remainder have other causes (Box 21-6).

Endometriosis

Endometriosis may be missed visually at the time of diagnostic laparoscopy in as many as 20% to 30% of women who have the disease proven histologically, so it is justifiable to initiate treatment based on a presumptive diagnosis of the disease once other etiologies have been ruled out.

The size and location of the endometriotic implants do not appear to correlate with the presence of pain, and the reasons for the pain are not fully understood.

Chronic Pelvic Inflammatory Disease (PID)

Chronic PID may cause pain because of recurrent exacerbations that require active antibiotic therapy or because of hydrosalpinges and adhesions between the tubes, ovaries, and intestinal structures. **Before ascribing symptoms to adhesions, one must have specifically noted adhesions in the area of pain localization** because some patients with extensive pelvic adhesions discovered incidentally during surgery for other reasons are asymptomatic.

Ovarian Pain

Ovarian cysts are usually asymptomatic, but episodic pain may occur secondary to rapid distention of the ovarian capsule. **An ovary or ovarian remnant may occasionally become retroperitoneal secondary to inflammation or previous surgery, and cyst formation in these circumstances may be painful.** Some women, for unknown reasons, may develop multiple recurrent hemorrhagic ovarian cysts that appear to cause pelvic pain and dyspareunia on an intermittent basis.

UTERINE PAIN

Adenomyosis (or endometriosis interna) may cause dysmenorrhea, dyspareunia, and menorrhagia, but rarely does it cause chronic daily intermenstrual pain. **Uterine myomas usually do not cause pelvic pain unless they are degenerating, undergoing torsion (twisting on their pedicles), or compressing pelvic nerves. On occasion, a submucous leiomyoma may attempt** to deliver through the cervix, which may cause considerable pelvic pain akin to childbirth. Uterine myomas may cause pain from rapid growth or infarction during pregnancy.

Pelvic pain is not likely to be caused by variations in uterine position, but **deep dyspareunia may occasionally be associated with uterine retroversion,** especially when the uterus is fixed in place by scarring or adenomyosis. The pain has been ascribed to irritation of pelvic nerves by the stretching of the uterosacral ligaments as well as to congestion of pelvic veins secondary to retroversion. The dyspareunia is typically worse during intercourse in the missionary position and is improved in the female superior position. A tender uterus that is in a fixed retroverted position usually signifies other intraperitoneal pathology, such as endometriosis or PID, and diagnosis rests on laparoscopic findings.

Pelvic Congestion Syndrome

The concept of a pelvic congestion syndrome still has many proponents. **This entity has been described in multiparous women who have pelvic vein varicosities and congested pelvic organs.** The pelvic pain is worse premenstrually and is increased by fatigue, standing, and sexual intercourse. Many women with this condition are noted to have a uterus that is mobile, retroverted, soft, boggy, and slightly enlarged. **There may be associated menorrhagia and urinary frequency.** Dilated veins may be seen on venographic studies. Factors other than venous congestion may be involved, however, because most women with pelvic varicosities have no pain. Surgery for this condition, consisting of hysterectomy and oophorectomy, may be beneficial for women who have completed their families, as are ovarian hormone suppression (decreased blood flow to the pelvic organs) and cognitive behavioral therapy.

Genitourinary Pelvic Pain

A variety of genitourinary problems result in pelvic pain. **Urinary retention, urethral syndrome, trigonitis, and interstitial cystitis are prime examples. Urinary urgency, frequency, nocturia, and pelvic pain may suggest early interstitial cystitis.** A thorough genitourinary evaluation is an important part of the workup for CPP. As many as one in five women have interstitial cystitis.

Gastrointestinal Pain

Gastrointestinal sources of CPP include penetrating neoplasms of the gastrointestinal tract, irritable bowel syndrome, partial bowel obstruction, inflammatory bowel disease, diverticulitis, and hernia formation. Because the innervation of the lower intestinal tract is the same as that of the uterus and fallopian tubes, the patient's complaint of pelvic pain may be confused with pain of gynecologic origin. Irritable bowel syndrome is the most common gastrointestinal cause of pelvic pain.

Neuromuscular Pain

Pain of neuromuscular origin, which is experienced as low back pain, usually increases with activity and stress. Trigger points and myalgia of the pelvic floor muscles can cause pelvic pain, vulvodynia, and dyspareunia. **Chronic low back pain without lower abdominal pain is seldom of gynecologic etiology.** Fibromyalgia, or generalized myofascial pain syndrome, can also cause pelvic pain. On occasion, neuromuscular symptoms are accompanied by a pelvic mass, and surgical exploration may reveal a neuroma or bony tumor. Entrapped or compromised nerves in the abdominal wall (iliohypogastric and ilioinguinal nerve most commonly) or pelvic floor (pudendal nerve) are often unrecognized sources of pain. The nerves may become entrapped after surgery or physical trauma, pregnancy and delivery, or occupational injury.

PSYCHOLOGICAL FACTORS

A pathologic diagnosis may not be made in about one third of patients with CPP, even after laparoscopy, which has led to the postulation that **psychological factors** may be etiologic. The patients have been assumed to be anxious, neurotic, anorgasmic, and insecure in their roles as women or as mothers. **When subjected to the Minnesota Multiphasic Personality Inventory (MMPI), these patients have shown a greater degree of anxiety, hypochondriasis, and hysteria than control subjects. The profiles are similar, however, in patients who have chronic pain with organic pathology, indicating that chronic pain per se engenders a complex, debilitating, psychological response.** Chronic pain patients with and without pathology tend to feel depressed, helpless, and passive. They withdraw from social and sexual activity and are preoccupied with pain and suffering. Many have posttraumatic stress disorder from emotional, physical, or sexual trauma. Women with CPP are also at risk for chronic fatigue syndrome.

Pain Perception Factors

Chronic pain is characterized by physiologic, emotional, and behavioral responses that are different from those of acute pain. Although both acute and chronic pain consists of a stimulus and a psychic response, for acute pain these may be adaptive and appropriate, whereas for chronic pain this may not be the case. In fact, **the response to chronic pain may be greatly affected by learning. The patient's reaction to pain and the reaction of significant others to the patient and her pain may be so reinforcing that the behavior may persist even after the painful stimulus has resolved.** In acute pain, the pain perception, suffering, and behavior are *usually* commensurate with the degree of sensory input. **In chronic pain, the suffering and behavioral responses to a given sensory input may be quite exaggerated and may persist even after the stimulus has remitted.**

Modulation of Sensation

Pain impulses are subjected to a large amount of modulation en route to and within the central nervous system. **The first synapse in the dorsal horn is an important focus of enhancement, inhibition, or facilitation. Modulation of sensations may also occur within the spinothalamic system, the descending inhibitory neurosystems, and the frontal cortex.** Various neurotransmitters and neuromodulators are present in the dorsal horn and at other higher levels of the neuraxis. Excitatory modulators include substance P, glutamate, aspartate, calcitonin gene-related peptide, and vasoactive intestinal peptide. Inhibitory neuromediators include endogenous opioid peptides, norepinephrine, serotonin, and γ-aminobutyric acid (GABA). Nerve axons that have been compromised after inflammation as well as stretch or crush injury also develop abnormal sodium channels. These changes play an important role in the development of allodynia (pain with gentle touch) and hyperalgesia (pain with stimuli that are not normally painful) in many women with CPP.

Within this context, anxiety and other psychological states are also considered to be facilitators or inhibitors of neurologic transmission. It is possible that many forms of CPP, in particular those without sufficient pathology, may result from modulation of afferent impulses or abnormality of descending inhibition in the dorsal horn, spinal cord, or brain.

■ *Management*

When treating patients with CPP, a therapeutic, supportive, and sympathetic (but structured) physician-patient relationship should be established. The patient should be given regular follow-up appointments and should not be told to call only if the pain persists. This reinforces pain behavior as a means of procuring sympathy and medical attention.

A negative evaluation or the finding of pathology not amenable to therapy (e.g., dense pelvic adhesions) does not mean that the patient should be discharged from care without therapy directed toward her symptoms. **After initial reassurance that there is no serious underlying pathology, and education as to the likely mechanisms of pain production, including central nervous system factors, symptomatic therapy should be undertaken. The symptoms of pain should be approached with the seriousness and direction afforded to any other condition.**

TEAM MANAGEMENT

The most productive strategy for the management of patients with CPP is referral to a multidisciplinary pain clinic or creation of a multidisciplinary team within a specific practice setting. The personnel at such a facility should include a gynecologist, a psychologist who also has expertise in chronic pain and sexual and marital counseling, a physical therapist with pelvic floor muscle expertise, and for more complex cases, an anesthesiologist. An acupuncturist is often helpful for referrals. It is the role of the psychologist to provide cognitive behavioral pain management and stress reduction, assertiveness training, and adaptive coping strategies. Marital and sexual counseling or psychiatric referral for psychopharmacology may be needed as well. This aspect of therapy is crucial because many of these patients have become severely depressed and often are interpersonally, sexually, and sometimes even occupationally withdrawn. Depression may be secondary to pain, but without treatment of the depression, the pain may persist. **Relaxation, cognitive, and behavioral therapies are employed to replace the pain behavior and its secondary gain with effective behavioral responses. Multidisciplinary management has been shown to be more effective than traditional gynecologic management.** When a designated multidisciplinary pain clinic is not available, it is important to involve other specialists by referral.

MEDICAL AND SURGICAL MANAGEMENT

The gynecologist continues to assess progress, coordinate care, and provide periodic gynecologic examinations. **In the initial stages of therapy, a trial of ovulation with or without menstrual suppression with combined hormonal contraception (pills, patches, rings; cyclic or continuous), high-dose or intrauterine progestins or a gonadotropin-releasing hormone agonist may be helpful.** Ovulation with or without menstrual suppression is especially helpful in patients who have midcycle, premenstrual, or menstrual exacerbation of pain and in those who have ovarian pathology, such as parovarian adhesions or recurrent functional cyst formation. **NSAIDs are also useful.** Pharmacologic approaches to increase inhibitory neuromodulators such as norepinephrine, serotonin (5-HT), and GABA or sodium channel blockers are frequently used in the form of tricyclic antidepressants, serotonin norepinephrine reuptake inhibitors, anticonvulsants, or other GABAergic agents and local anesthetics.

Surgical procedures that have not proved effective for CPP without pathology include unilateral adnexectomy for unilateral pain or total abdominal hysterectomy, presacral neurectomy, and uterine suspension for generalized pelvic pain. Lysis of adhesions is also usually nonproductive, with the possible exception

4-QUADRANT INJECTION TECHNIQUE

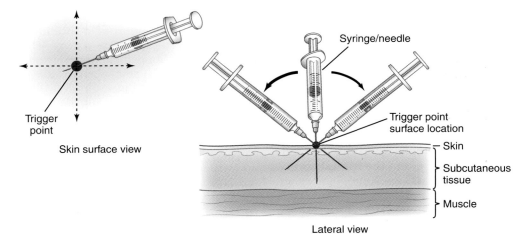

FIGURE 21-3   Trigger point injection technique for the abdominal wall in a patient with chronic pelvic pain. *(From Auerbach PS: Wilderness Medicine, 5th ed. Philadelphia, Mosby, 2007.)*

of the situation in which the site of adhesions, visualized by the laparoscope, specifically coincides with the localization of pain. However, pelvic adhesions often recur after surgical lysis. **Without proof of organic pathology or a reasonable functional explanation for the pelvic pain, a thorough psychosomatic evaluation should be carried out before a surgical corrective procedure is considered.**

ANESTHESIA

Acupuncture, nerve blocks, and trigger-point injections of local anesthetics may provide prolonged pain relief. Acupuncture has been used successfully for dysmenorrhea, and trigger-point injections and nerve blocks with local anesthetics have been used successfully for pelvic pain. Acupuncture probably increases spinal cord endorphins. In patients who complain of pelvic pain, trigger points are usually found on either the lower abdominal wall, lower back, or vaginal and vulvar areas. **A significant percentage of patients with pelvic pain have abdominal wall trigger points or nerve entrapments that respond to biweekly injections of a local anesthetic (usually up to five injections is sufficient).** Anesthesia of trigger points (Figure 21-3) may abolish pain by lowering the impulses from the area of referred pain, thereby diminishing the afferent impulses

reaching the dorsal horn to a level below the threshold for pain transmission. Local anesthetic nerve blocks on a repeated basis for areas of nerve impingement combined with instructions to patients about alteration in physical activity can be helpful. When needed, a prescription for nerve threshold–altering medications, as mentioned previously, can be given. These interventions can downregulate neural hypersensitivity and permanently decrease or eliminate pain.

SUGGESTED READING

American College of Obstetricians and Gynecologists (ACOG) Committee on Practice Bulletins: ACOG Practice Bulletin No. 51. Chronic pelvic pain. Obstet Gynecol 103:589-605, 2004.

Gambone JC, Mittman BS, Munro MG, et al: Consensus statement for the management of chronic pelvic pain and endometriosis: Proceedings of an expert panel consensus process. Fertil Steril 78:961-972, 2002.

Peng PW, Tumber PS: Ultrasound-guided interventional procedures for patients with chronic pelvic pain: A description of techniques and review of the literature. Pain Physician 11(2):215-224, 2008.

Rapkin AJ, Howe CN: Chronic pelvic pain: A review. Parts 1 and 2. *In* Family Practice Recertification. Monroe Township, NJ, Ascend Media 2006, 49-56, 59-67.

Tu FF, Holt J, Gonzales J, Fitzgerald CM: Physical therapy evaluation of patients with chronic pelvic pain: A controlled study. Am J Obstet Gynecol 198:272-277, 2008.

Chapter 22

Vulvovaginitis, Sexually Transmitted Infections, and Pelvic Inflammatory Disease

JAMES A. MCGREGOR • JOEL B. LENCH

Infectious diseases are interesting and challenging disorders in gynecology. Some are difficult to treat and have frequent recurrences. Antibiotic resistance has recently changed the recommended treatment for one of the original "venereal diseases," and vaccination has been introduced as a preventive tool for one of the more prevalent pelvic infections. The diagnosis and management of common reproductive tract infections in nonpregnant women are covered in this chapter.

Reproductive Tract Infections

Infections of the vulva, vagina, and cervix (lower reproductive tract) and the uterine corpus, fallopian tubes, and ovaries (upper reproductive tract) are common gynecologic problems. Many of these infections are sexually transmitted and require partner treatment for effective care. The term **sexually transmitted infection (STI)** is replacing sexually transmitted disease (STD) as a more accurate and appropriate term for these frequently asymptomatic disorders, emphasizing their infectious nature and the need for screening, early recognition, and treatment. **A person with an STI may be infected and infect others without actually "having a disease."** The most common STIs are **chlamydia, genital herpes, human papillomavirus** (HPV), and **gonorrhea.**

Vulvovaginitis is a common pelvic infection caused by yeast, bacteria, or trichomonads, and **pelvic inflammatory disease** (PID) is the most serious form of upper reproductive tract infection. PID is frequently a consequence of an unrecognized or inadequately treated lower tract STI. PID is a common cause of infertility and is the reproductive tract infection that is most likely to require hospitalization and even surgery for adequate treatment.

Maintaining and restoring normal vaginal physiology and microbiology is an important measure for preventing pelvic infections.

Normal Physiology and Microecology of the Vagina

The vagina is lined by nonkeratinized stratified squamous epithelium, which is powerfully influenced by estrogen and progesterone. **The vagina of the newborn is colonized by aerobic and anaerobic bacteria acquired while passing through the birth canal.** The newborn's vaginal epithelium is strongly estrogenized and rich in glycogen, which supports growth of lactic acid–producing lactobacilli. This results in a low pH (<4.7), which promotes further growth of acidophilic-protective microflora. **Within days of birth, estrogen decreases,** and the vaginal epithelium becomes thin, atrophic, and largely devoid of glycogen. In this environment, **the pH rises,** and acidophilic organisms no longer have a selective advantage. **As a consequence, the predominant vaginal microflora becomes diverse gram-positive cocci and bacilli.**

With the onset of puberty and ovarian steroidogenesis, the vagina again becomes estrogenized, and the glycogen content increases. **Lactic acid– and hydrogen peroxide (H_2O_2)–producing lactobacilli again predominate,** resulting in a self-sustaining vaginal pH of between 3.5 and 4.5. Even so, a wide variety of aerobic and anaerobic bacteria can be cultured from the normal vagina. Most women harbor at least three to eight types of bacteria at any given time. Lactic acid, H_2O_2, and other substances produced by "healthy" lactobacilli provide some protection in the lower reproductive tract from STIs, including human immunodeficiency virus (HIV).

Multiple factors may alter this protective microflora. **Antibiotics** suppress growth of commensal organisms, which can allow pathogenic strains (e.g., yeasts) to predominate. **Douching with water or nonbuffered solutions** may transiently alter the pH or selectively suppress endogenous bacteria. **Sexual intercourse with introduction of semen** raises the pH to as high as 7.2 for 6 to 8 hours, making the vaginal milieu receptive to STI pathogens. During coitus, vaginal transudate increases vaginal fluid and serves as lubrication. Vaginal transudate has the same pH as blood (7.4), which also favors attachment of abnormal microflora. **The presence of a foreign body** (e.g., forgotten diaphragm or tampon in adults or various small objects in children) dramatically disrupts normal vaginal cleansing mechanisms and may lead to secondary infection.

PHYSIOLOGIC VAGINAL FLUIDS

Vaginal fluid is a mixture consisting of cervical mucus (the major component), endometrial and oviductal fluid, exudates from the Bartholin's and Skene's glands, transudate from the vaginal squamous epithelium together with exfoliated squamous cells, and metabolic products of the microflora. Vaginal fluid is composed of proteins, polysaccharides, amino acids, enzymes, and immunoglobulins. Physiologic increases in vaginal and endocervical fluid occur during pregnancy, at mid menstrual cycle, and during intercourse. **In postmenopausal women (not using estrogens), vaginal fluid may become markedly decreased, which predisposes to infection** with various exogenous microflora (e.g., *Escherichia coli* and staphylococcal, and streptococcal species).

INVESTIGATION OF VAGINAL DISCHARGE

Patients with a vaginal infection frequently complain of a nonbloody vaginal discharge. The characteristics of the discharge (e.g., color, texture, viscosity, and odor) are helpful in making the correct diagnosis. Normal vaginal fluid has a pH of less than 4.7 in ovulatory women. Vaginal pH can be easily determined by using pH paper with an appropriate pH range (3.5 to 7.0). Self-care over-the-counter (OTC) tests, such as "pH on a stick" and "pH glove," are available to test vaginal pH.

Testing for the presence of an amine odor (referred to as a *positive whiff test*) **is performed by putting a few drops of 10% potassium hydroxide (KOH) in the spoon of a vaginal speculum** after it is removed from the vagina. With healthy vaginal fluid, no odor is noted. **An "amine" or "fishy" odor suggests trichomoniasis or bacterial vaginosis (BV).**

A wet-mount preparation of the discharge should be evaluated. Using a cotton-tipped applicator, a sample of vaginal discharge from the posterior fornix is suspended in 2 mL of normal saline. A drop of this solution is placed on a glass slide, covered with a coverslip, and examined under the microscope. **Motile trichomonads may be seen on this type of wet mount** (Figure 22-1). Also, epithelial cells with irregular, granular edges (**clue cells**) are indicative of clumped bacteria on the cell wall and are **highly suggestive of BV if present in more than 20% of epithelial cells** (Figure 22-2). If the cells are not sufficiently separated, **an aliquot of fluid is placed in a drop of saline or 10% to 20% KOH** (to eliminate cellular and other debris while leaving mycelia) and examined microscopically, to visualize the pseudohyphae or spores of *Candida* infection. In complicated or atypical cases, bacterial and yeast cultures are required.

■ *Vaginal Discharge Etiology*

Vaginitis and complaints referable to the vagina (e.g., discharge, pruritus, burning, and "late" dysuria) are common. A correct diagnosis can be difficult because symptoms and signs may be nonspecific, patients frequently self-medicate with OTC products, multiple

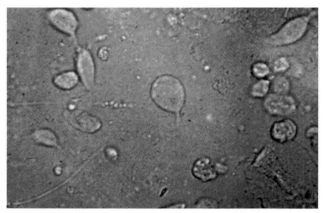

FIGURE 22-1 Microscopic view (high power) of a trichomonad in a saline wet-mount preparation. The organisms are usually motile in this type of preparation.

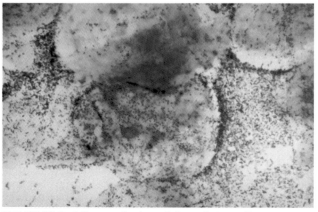

FIGURE 22-2 Microscopic view of clue cells in a saline wet-mount preparation. Note the irregular or serrated cell walls.

causes may be present, and accurate diagnostic tools are either not available or not properly employed.

Up to 90% of cases of vaginitis appear to be caused by three conditions. **Bacterial vaginosis accounts for 40% to 50%, vulvovaginal candidiasis (VVC) for 20% to 25%, and trichomoniasis for 15% or less of cases. Mucopurulent cervicitis ("mucopus") caused by chlamydia, _Neisseria gonorrhoeae_, mycoplasma, or BV-associated bacteria (see Figure 22-6) may also cause vaginal irritation and discharge.** Less common types include **atrophic vaginitis** (overgrowth with aerobic or anaerobic microflora in the absence of lactobacilli and with hypoestrogenized tissues), **foreign-body vaginitis, genital ulcer diseases** such as herpes and syphilis, **desquamative vaginitis** (most commonly group B streptococcal overgrowth), and **lichen planus. Irritation from sexual activity and allergen-containing substances can also mimic infectious vaginitis.**

Standard clinic or office diagnosis of vaginitis requires a working microscope, pH paper, KOH, saline solution, slides, coverslips, and the ability to recognize an amine odor (whiff test). In many settings, these rudimentary tools are not available. Newer, inexpensive "point of care" products can detect vaginal sialidase, amines, and proline aminopeptidase and other biomarker substances or nucleic acid–based tests. In difficult or refractory cases, additional tests for vaginal agents may be used such as culture for _Trichomonas vaginalis_, _Candida_, mycoplasmas, or predominant vaginal aerobic bacterial. Table 22-1 lists the common causes, characteristics, and treatments for vulvar and vaginal infections.

BACTERIAL VAGINOSIS

BV is the most common cause of vaginal discharge but is often without other symptoms. BV occurs subsequent to a significant disruption of "healthy" vaginal microflora, (typically _Lactobacillus jensenii_ and _Lactobacillus crispatus_) by a characteristic set of BV-complex microorganisms: _Gardnerella vaginalis_, genital mycoplasmas _(Mycoplasma hominis, Ureaplasma urealyticum)_ and vaginal anaerobic bacteria, including _Prevotella_, _Bacteroides_, and _Mobiluncus_ species. Risk factors for acquisition of BV include a new sexual partner, smoking, intrauterine device (IUD) use, and frequent douching.

Classic features of BV discharge include a profuse, milky, nonadherent discharge that demonstrates an amine or fishy odor after alkalization with a drop of KOH (positive whiff test).

The presence of BV heightens a nonpregnant woman's risk for PID, postoperative infections (e.g., after hysterectomy or pregnancy termination), and HIV transmission. **Partner treatment is generally not recommended.**

VULVOVAGINAL CANDIDIASIS

VVC is the second most common cause of vulvovaginal-related symptoms. Wide use of OTC antifungal products for self-diagnosed candidiasis has resulted in a decreased frequency of doctor visits, but women who do present are less likely to present with textbook findings. _Candida albicans_ formerly caused more than 90% of cases of VVC, but **now less azole-susceptible species, such as _Candida glabrata_, are recognized as causative agents in 15% of cases.** These less susceptible yeasts necessitate prolonged or alternative treatments. Because of _Candida's_ requirement for estrogenated tissues, VVC becomes more common after menarche and less common after menopause. An estimated 75% of women acquire VVC at some time in their life, and 5% suffer frequent symptomatic recurrences. VVC is considered recurrent when at least four episodes occur

TABLE 22-1			
COMMON CAUSES OF VULVOVAGINITIS			
Infection	**Symptoms/Findings**	**Diagnosis**	**Treatment**
Yeast	Vaginal burning, itching, irritation; curdy white discharge	Wet prep and/or KOH microscopic examination shows pseudohyphae, or budding yeast	Butoconazole 2% cream*, 5 g intravaginally for 3 days, or fluconazole, 150 mg orally in a single dose†
Bacterial vaginosis	Asymptomatic, or vaginal odor; odor after intercourse, or increased discharge	Wet prep "clue cells"; release of amine odor; positive whiff test with KOH; vaginal fluid pH > 4.5	Metronidazole, 500 mg orally twice a day for 7 days or clindamycin cream 2%, one applicator (5 g) intravaginally at bedtime for 7 days†
Trichomoniasis	Asymptomatic, or increased thin or thick, green or yellow foul-smelling discharge; frothy in 2% to 3% of cases; strawberry cervix in 2% to 3% of cases	Motile trichomonads on microscopic examination of wet mount	Metronidazole, 2 g orally in a single dose or tinidazole, 2 g orally in a single dose (for resistant cases)†

*Over-the-counter preparation.
†See Centers for Disease Control and Prevention website for a more complete list and identification of the latest recommended and alternative treatments at http://www.cdc.gov.

within 1 year. **Risk factors for recurrent VVC include high-dose oral contraceptives, diaphragm use with a spermicide, diabetes mellitus, antibiotic use, pregnancy, immunosuppression from any cause** (HIV/AIDS, transplantation, steroid use), and possibly **tight occlusive clothing.**

The classic presentation of VVC includes vaginal itching, burning, irritation, and possibly postvoiding dysuria. The discharge is usually odorless, has a pH of less than 4.7, and is thick or curdy with the appearance of cottage cheese (Figure 22-3). Examination often shows vulvovaginal erythema, with evidence of acute or chronic excoriation.

Microscopic examination of a wet-mount preparation is positive for budding yeast cells, pseudohyphae, or mycelial tangles (Figure 22-4) in 50% to 70% of cases. **Women with suggestive clinical findings but absent wet preparation evidence may benefit from fungal culture.**

First-line treatments include topical or oral antifungal (imidazole) agents. Documented cases of recurrences can be effectively treated by confirming the diagnosis and treating with weekly suppressive doses of topical imidazoles. Boric acid (600 mg vaginal gelatin capsules) 3 times daily for 1 week is an effective treatment for imidazole-resistant species. Although VVC is not thought to be sexually transmitted in most cases, male partners sometimes reinfect their partners and are routinely treated by some practitioners.

TRICHOMONIASIS

Trichomoniasis (cervicitis, vaginitis, and urethritis) is caused by the protozoan *T. vaginalis*. **About 50% of cases in women and men are asymptomatic.** Symptomatic infection is classically manifested by a green-yellow, frothy vaginal discharge (Figure 22-5), with a "musty" odor. Dyspareunia, vulvovaginal irritation, and occasionally dysuria may be present. **Male partners are often asymptomatic even though they demonstrate nongonococcal urethritis on direct examination.**

The diagnosis of trichomoniasis in patients and their sexual partners should be followed by screening for other prevalent STIs and empiric treatment of partners. Diagnosis is usually made on clinical grounds and can be confirmed by seeing the characteristic motility of trichomonads on a saline wet mount. Much more sensitive techniques, including culture, polymerase chain reaction (PCR), and antigen testing, are becoming available.

In addition to vulvovaginitis and urethritis, trichomoniasis is associated with upper reproductive tract symptoms, an increased risk for adverse pregnancy outcomes (prematurity, low birth weight), and increased transmission of HIV infection.

Metronidazole (2 g single oral dose) **is the recommended treatment** (see Table 22-1). Patients should

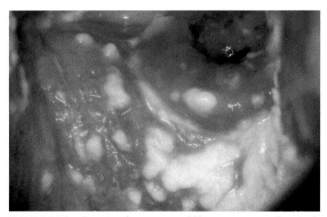

FIGURE 22-3　Cottage cheese or curd-like appearance of vaginal discharge is typical of vulvovaginitis due to yeast.

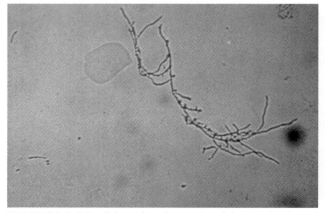

FIGURE 22-4　Mycelial tangles of yeast pseudohyphae in KOH wet-mount preparation.

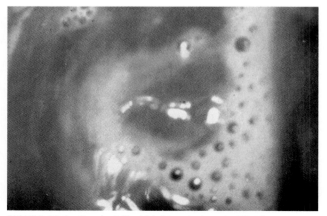

FIGURE 22-5　Purulent "bubbly" cervical-vaginal fluid characteristic of trichomoniasis.

not consume alcohol for 2 days after treatment. Although metronidazole is not known to be teratogenic in recommended dosages, it has been traditionally avoided during the first 12 weeks of pregnancy. Prompt early treatment during pregnancy relieves symptoms, reduces the risk for HIV transmission, and may improve pregnancy outcomes. Trichomoniasis should be treated before vaginal surgical procedures.

Metronidazole resistance is increasing and may be overcome by using tinidazole (now available in the United States; see Table 22-1) **or using higher doses of metronidazole** (2 g daily for 7 days). Reversible side effects of metronidazole include an "Antabuse-like reaction" with alcohol exposure, neutropenia, and peripheral neuropathy. Higher-dose treatment for resistant trichomoniasis in pregnancy should be prescribed with caution in consultation with experts.

ATROPHIC VAGINITIS

Atrophic vaginitis is the most common cause of vaginal irritation among climacteric patients. As the term indicates, **the atrophy of the vaginal epithelium results in secondary infection.** The vulva and introitus quickly become involved because of the associated discharge, and the situation may be exacerbated by a foreign body (such as a pessary). Patients complain of vulvar irritation and discharge, which may be clear or purulent and yellow but occasionally will be blood tinged. Associated symptoms of frequency, urgency, and stress incontinence may occur.

Examination of the external genitalia may reveal a watery discharge with generalized vulvar erythema, often with excoriation. Speculum examination reveals a pale epithelium with patches of erythema. Superficial blood vessels are visible and may bleed easily on contact. If bleeding is present, the examiner must consider the possibility of a coexistent neoplasm. The discharge has a pH of 4.7 or higher. **A simple evaluation of the epithelial cells using a saline wet-mount preparation or Papanicolaou (Pap) smear confirms the diagnosis, with immature basal cells and parabasal cells replacing superficial vaginal epithelial cells.**

The treatment of choice is topical estrogen available in vaginal creams, suppositories, or rings. If systemic hormonal treatment is desirable, oral tablets, transdermal patches, sprays, and gels are available. Aerobic cultures for predominant microorganisms should be obtained in refractory cases and when infection is suspected.

FOREIGN-BODY VAGINITIS

When a mother states there is discharge on the baby's diaper or the child has vulvar itching, infection, or a bloody vaginal discharge, a foreign body should be suspected in addition to sexual abuse. In adults, forgotten or lost tampons, diaphragms, or condoms may be the cause of vaginitis. With removal of the foreign body and vaginal application of some form of sulfa cream (or estrogen cream in children), rapid improvement usually occurs.

Other Common Sexually Transmitted Infections

GENITAL HERPES

Genital herpes is the most prevalent STI in the United States, with an estimated 50 million adults infected (active or latent) with herpes simplex virus (HSV) and about 1.5 million new cases occurring every year. It is a chronic lifelong viral infection with the potential for rare to frequent recurrences. This infection may have devastating emotional and social consequences. Unfortunately, **only 10% to 20% of infected persons know that they are infected, and 70% of transmissions are from asymptomatic viral shedding from infected partners with no visible lesions.** Individuals who are infected with HSV are at increased risk for acquiring and transmitting HIV.

HSV has two serotypes, HSV-1 and HSV-2. HSV-1 is most commonly associated with oral lesions (cold sores), but about 30% of primary genital herpes is due to HSV-1. HSV-2 is the cause of 70% of primary genital herpes and 95% of recurrent genital herpes. The frequency of recurrences is much higher after a primary infection with HSV-2 than HSV-1. The virus enters the body through mucosa or microabrasions in the skin and follows the sensory nerves to the dorsal spinal ganglion, where it remains dormant until reactivated. Transmission occurs through intimate genital, oral, or anal contact. **An infected mother can transmit the virus to her infant during delivery resulting in significant fetal mortality and morbidity.** Regular condom use decreases transmission by about 50%, especially from men to women.

Primary genital herpes infection occurs when the infected person has no HSV-2 or HSV-1 antibodies. **The usual clinical presentation is multiple, bilateral, and painful anogenital vesicles or ulcers with an erythematous base.** Systemic symptoms may also be present, such as fever, headache, malaise, and lymphadenopathy. Acute cervicitis may be present. The lesions heal without scarring in 14 to 21 days.

Recurrent genital herpes infection occurs when the infected person has HSV antibodies to the same serotype. The lesions are fewer, unilateral, and less painful. Systemic symptoms and lymphadenopathy are rare. The lesions heal without scarring in 5 to 7 days in immunocompetent individuals.

Laboratory tests that are used to confirm the diagnosis include (1) **viral culture** that requires live cells from a lesion, which is expensive, time-consuming, and has a relatively low sensitivity (50% to 80%); (2) **PCR**, which is expensive and very accurate, is very useful for testing cerebrospinal fluid, but is not used routinely on genital lesions; and (3) **type-specific serologic tests** for HSV-1 and HSV-2 antibodies. These are highly sensitive and specific tests that can identify infected individuals who are asymptomatic.

The goals of treatment for genital herpes are symptom relief, acceleration of lesion healing, and a decrease in frequency of recurrences. Education and supportive counseling are also important. The antiviral agents (**acyclovir, famciclovir**, and **valacyclovir**) are safe and effective for treating primary and episodic outbreaks and for providing suppressive therapy for patients with chronic disease. No treatment can eradicate the latent virus from the dorsal ganglia of the spinal cord. Work is underway to develop an HSV vaccine.

HUMAN PAPILLOMAVIRUS (HPV)

Genital **HPV** is a common viral STI with an estimated 20 million infected persons in the United States and 5 million new cases every year. It is believed that about 75% of sexually active adults will be infected sometime in their life. **Most HPV cases are latent infections with no visible lesions and are only diagnosed by DNA hybridization testing performed in the evaluation of an abnormal Pap smear.** Subclinical infections have lesions that are only visible during colposcopy. Clinical infections are characterized by readily visible "warty" growths called *condylomata acuminata* on the vulva, vagina, cervix, urethra, and perianal area.

There are about 1 million new cases of these external genital (venereal) warts every year in the United States. HPV infection usually clears spontaneously within 2 years, but recurrences are common. **There are about 200 HPV subtypes. Some have been strongly associated with genital neoplasia and cancers, especially cervical** (see Chapter 38). Biopsies of atypical or persistent lesions are needed to rule out neoplastic disease. Because these growths may also mimic condylomata lata, syphilis must be excluded if the lesions are atypical or do not respond to treatment. Transmission of HPV can occur even when there are no visible lesions. Regular condom use may provide some degree of protection. During pregnancy, condylomata may increase in number and size, but **transmission from mother to infant is rare.**

An HPV-like particle vaccine (Gardasil) is now available that protects against four HPV serotypes (6, 8, 16, and 18), which together are responsible for 70% of cervical cancers and 90% of genital warts. This vaccine was licensed in 2006 for use in females aged 9 to 26 years. Another vaccine against HPV types 16 and 18 only (Cervarix) may be available soon (from 2008). These vaccines are highly effective (>95%) in women who have not been exposed to these HPV types.

The reasons for treating genital warts are to relieve symptoms (pain and bleeding) and to ameliorate psychological and cosmetic concerns of the patient. Multiple therapeutic modalities are available, and all are comparable. Provider-applied topical therapies include (1) **podophyllin resin** 10% to 25% in tincture of benzoin and (2) **trichloroacetic acid** (TCA) or **bichloracetic acid** (BCA) 80% to 90%. Patient-applied topical therapies include (1) **podofilox** 0.5% solution or gel and (2) **imiquimod** 5% cream. Surgical therapies include (1) **cryotherapy**, (2) **surgical excision**, (3) **electrocautery**, (4) **laser vaporization**, and (5) **intralesional interferon. Podophyllin, podofilox, and imiquimod should not be used during pregnancy.**

CHLAMYDIA

Chlamydia **has the highest incidence of any bacterial STI in the United States**, with 3 million new cases every year. Most cases (75%) are found in individuals who are younger than 25 years, and about half of cases are in adolescents.

Chlamydia trachomatis is an obligate intracellular bacteria that grows in vitro only in tissue culture. It can infect the columnar epithelium of the endocervix, urethra, endometrium, fallopian tubes, and rectum. This organism can persist for long periods in an asymptomatic carrier state. There is no vaccine available, and even though chlamydia antibodies are produced, they do not protect against reinfection. Because **about 70% of infected females and 50% of infected males have no symptoms,** it is very difficult to diagnose and treat this "hidden" infection. In those cases in which symptoms are present, the clinical manifestations of lower genital tract chlamydia infection are (1) mucopurulent cervicitis or mucopus, which is a yellow discharge coming from a swollen, red, friable cervix that bleeds easily (see Figure 22-3), and (2) acute urethritis with dysuria but minimal frequency and urgency and a negative urine culture.

Various **laboratory tests** are used to confirm the diagnosis of chlamydia: (1) **tissue culture**, which requires live cells and is expensive; (2) **antigen tests,** which are inexpensive and rapid with a high sensitivity and specificity; and (3) **DNA hybridization tests** and **nucleic acid amplification tests** (PCR and ligase chain reaction), which are rapid and very accurate. **These newer DNA amplification tests can be done on urine specimens as well as cervical swabs and therefore they are very convenient for screening purposes.** Selective screening should be performed at least annually on all sexually active females younger than 26 years and all women with risk factors (e.g., unmarried, multiple partners, inconsistent use of barrier contraception, previous history of any STI, and all pregnant women). **It is estimated that 30% of untreated chlamydial cervicitis will progress to PID. Aggressive screening** and appropriate early treatment have been shown to decrease the incidence of PID. Screening may also be performed after partner change or for any concern.

General treatment guidelines for lower genital tract chlamydial infection include the following: (1) **presumptive treatment with appropriate antibiotics** (e.g., azithromycin, 1 g orally in a single dose, or doxycycline, 100 mg twice a day for 7 days); (2) **treatment of all sexual contacts within the past 60 days before diagnosis**; (3) **testing for other STIs**, including gonorrhea, syphilis, hepatitis B, and HIV; and (4) **abstinence from sexual contact for 7 days** after last partner has started antibiotic therapy. Test of cure is not necessary; however, rescreening in 3 to 4 months to check for reinfection is recommended.

Chlamydial infection during pregnancy can cause adverse outcomes for both mother and infant. These include **preterm labor, chorioamnionitis,** and **postpartum endometritis.** Intrapartum transmission to the infant can cause **neonatal conjunctivitis and pneumonia.**

GONORRHEA

N. gonorrhoeae is the second most common bacterial STI in the United States, with 600,000 new cases annually. The organism is a gram-negative diplococcus, and it infects the same columnar epithelium as chlamydia. Additionally, it can infect the pharynx in about 10% of the cases. It can also survive in the host as an asymptomatic carrier. **There is no vaccine available, and no immunity is conferred even though antibodies are produced.**

Most infected women, but as few as 5% of infected men, have no symptoms. If symptoms are present, the clinical manifestations of lower genital tract gonococcal infections are the same as for chlamydia and include mucopurulent cervicitis, which involves a swollen, red, friable cervix; contact bleeding; and acute urethritis, producing dysuria with minimal frequency and urgency and usually a negative urine culture.

Laboratory tests that can be used to confirm the diagnosis include **Gram stain of the discharge** or cervix, which is rapid and inexpensive. The presence of **gram-negative diplococci in the leukocytes** is very sensitive in men; however, in women, the sensitivity is only 50%. **Thayer-Martin or Transgrow media culture** is inexpensive but takes longer with a sensitivity of 90% and a specificity of 97%. **DNA hybridization test** is inexpensive and rapid, with a high sensitivity and specificity, and **nucleic acid amplification tests** (PCR and ligase chain reaction [LCR]) are more expensive and rapid with high sensitivity and specificity. These tests can be done on urine or cervical swabs. **Because most women with gonococcal cervical infection are asymptomatic, selective screening of high-risk persons is essential in attempting to control the progression and spread of** this disease. About 15% of untreated gonococcal cervical infections progress to PID.

Resistant strains of gonorrhea include penicillinase-producing *N. gonorrhoeae*, chromosomal mediated–resistant *N. gonorrhoeae*, tetracycline-resistant *N. gonorrhoeae*, and quinolone-resistant *N. gonorrhoeae*. **A Centers for Disease Control and Prevention (CDC) update (April 2007) recommends that quinolones no longer be used for the treatment of gonococcal infections due to significant resistance.**

General treatment guidelines for lower genital tract gonococcal infection include (1) **treatment with appropriate antibiotics** (e.g., cefixime, 400 mg orally in a single dose, or ceftriaxone 125 mg intramuscularly in a single dose); (2) **simultaneous treatment for** *chlamydia* (i.e., 1 g of azithromycin orally in a single dose is indicated because 20% to 40% of gonococcal cervical infections also have chlamydia); (3) **treatment of all sexual contacts within the 60 days** before diagnosis; (4) **abstinence from sexual activity for 7 days** after the start of antibiotic therapy; (5) **testing for other STIs**, including chlamydia, syphilis, hepatitis B, and HIV. Test of cure is not necessary; however, rescreening in 3 to 4 months to check for reinfection may be helpful.

Gonococcal infection during pregnancy can cause adverse outcomes for both the mother and infant. These include **preterm labor and delivery, chorioamnionitis,** and **postpartum endometritis.** Intrapartum transmission to the infant can cause **neonatal conjunctivitis** *(ophthalmia neonatorum).*

Pelvic Inflammatory Disease

PID is a morbid and costly sexually transmitted bacterial upper reproductive tract infection affecting nonpregnant and occasionally pregnant women. Studies demonstrate the importance of pathogenic lower reproductive tract microorganisms ascending from the endocervix to mediate endometritis, salpingitis, and sometimes peritonitis.

EPIDEMIOLOGY AND PATHOGENESIS

More than 10% of reproductive-aged women report a history of PID. PID is an expensive public health problem. It has been estimated that the direct costs of treating PID in the United States exceed $6 billion annually. These costs do not include the indirect costs of treating sequelae such as infertility, ectopic pregnancy, and preterm birth.

The most important single-agent causes of PID include *C. trachomatis, N. gonorrhoeae,* **and genital mycoplasmas** *(M. hominis, U. urealyticum,* and *Mycoplasma genitalium).* Each of these is an STI with inoculation occurring most commonly during intercourse. *M. hominis, U. urealyticum,* and *M. genitalium* are widely recognized causes of nongonococcal urethritis in males and females. Both *C. trachomatis* and *N. gonor-rhoeae* have well-defined molecular virulence factors that mediate genital attachment and cell damage. Unlike gonorrhea, which occurs more frequently within inner-city and minority populations, chlamydial infections are broadly distributed among most racial, ethnic, and economic groups.

PID develops in 15% to 30% of women with inadequately treated gonococcal or chlamydial cervicitis. There are an estimated 3 million chlamydial genital infections yearly in the United States. The highest rates of chlamydial cervicitis occur in sexually active adolescents and young adults between the ages of 20 and 25 years. The largely asymptomatic nature of chlamydial cervicitis in women and urethritis in men makes routine screening and treatment for chlamydia necessary for the prevention of PID.

The most common microbial isolates recovered from patients at laparoscopy or at drainage of pelvic abscesses are endogenous lower reproductive tract or gastrointestinal microflora, including *E. coli, Bacteroides* and *Prevotella* species, *G. vaginalis,* and anaerobic streptococci. These common sexually transmitted and endogenous agents should be covered during antibiotic treatment for PID.

COMPLICATIONS

The sequelae of PID are much more common, morbid, and costly than previously recognized. A seminal study of PID was performed in Lund, Sweden, where 2500 women with PID were followed from 1960 to 1984. **Women with clinical PID were 6 times more likely to have an ectopic pregnancy and 14 times more likely to have tubal factor infertility than women without PID.** Women with a history of PID were 6 to 10 times more likely than healthy controls to have the diagnosis of **endometritis,** suffer from **chronic pelvic pain**, or **require a hysterectomy. Women with prior salpingitis are at increased risk for premature labor.**

SYMPTOMS

Women with symptomatic PID commonly have lower abdominal pain and tenderness (especially when walking or during coitus), abnormal vaginal discharge, chills, and fever. Less common symptoms include irregular vaginal bleeding, dysuria, nausea, and vomiting. **No specific combination of symptoms is consistently associated with PID.** Some women are asymptomatic.

SIGNS

Clinical signs in women with laparoscopically confirmed PID most frequently include **lower abdominal tenderness,** with or without rebound tenderness; **uterine and adnexal tenderness** to palpation and motion; and findings of **mucopurulent cervicitis** (Figure 22-6). Fever is the least common finding. A pregnancy test

should be performed when symptoms or signs of pregnancy are present.

INVESTIGATIONS

Nucleic acid, antigenic, or culture tests should be done to detect chlamydial and gonococcal infections. Confirmatory laboratory evidence includes **leukocytosis, increased erythrocyte sedimentation rate, or C-reactive protein level,** and microscopic or leukocyte esterase test evidence of purulent cervical discharge (mucopus). **Pelvic ultrasonic studies** may show enlarged, tender fallopian tubes as well as cul-de-sac fluid.

Laparoscopy is no longer considered clinically necessary for diagnosis of PID or tubo-ovarian abscess (TOA) because it is invasive and costly, and safer, effective antimicrobial regimens are now available for empiric use. Laparoscopy is generally not performed unless differentiation from other processes (e.g., appendicitis) is required.

DIAGNOSIS

PID should be diagnosed and treated empirically in sexually active young women and women with risk factors who have uterine and adnexal or cervical motion tenderness. The CDC cautions that PID is unlikely if the patient does not have a mucopurulent cervical discharge (see Figure 22-6) or white blood cells on vaginal wet mount. Abnormal findings that make the diagnosis more secure include fever, elevated erythrocyte sedimentation rate, elevated C-reactive protein, and documented cervical infection with gonorrhea or chlamydia.

TREATMENT

Therapeutic goals for treating PID are elimination of reproductive tract infection and inflammation, improvement of symptoms and physical findings, prevention or minimization of long-term sequelae, and eradication of causal agents from the patient and her sexual partner.

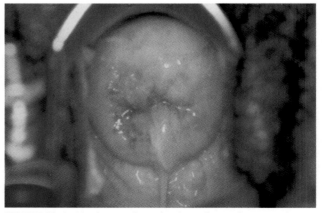

FIGURE 22-6   Uterine cervix at the time of speculum examination with mucopus protruding from the os.

Empiric antibiotic regimens should be aimed at treating likely causative agents, that is, *N. gonorrhoeae,* *C. trachomatis,* genital mycoplasmas, and BV-associated endogenous microflora. The latter include anaerobic (*Bacteroides* and *Prevotella* species and anaerobic streptococci) as well as aerobic organisms (*G. vaginalis,* *E. coli,* and facultative streptococci). Except for *N. gonorrhoeae* and some anaerobes, resistance is not yet a clinical problem.

The need for hospitalization is an important treatment decision (Box 22-1). **Women with severe infections or an inability to take and absorb oral antibiotics** (nausea, vomiting, possible peritonitis, and ileus) **should be hospitalized** and treated until clinical improvement is evident. Similarly, women with **a questionable diagnosis, pregnancy,** or unreliability, should be admitted initially and treated with parenteral agents to ensure compliance and treatment efficacy, as should **those who fail to respond to outpatient therapy.**

Table 22-2 lists antibiotic regimens for inpatient and outpatient management, as recommended by the CDC. Other recommended and alternative treatments are listed on their website, http://www.cdc.gov.

Outpatient treatments may be selected for most women, who will return promptly if no improvement is seen within 24 to 48 hours and who are likely to be compliant. Direct observation of initial oral treatment is preferred.

Patients should be reevaluated 3 to 4 weeks after treatment. Pelvic examination should be done at that time to ensure adequacy of treatment. Counseling regarding preventative strategies for STIs and HIV infection, as well as contraceptive advice, should be repeated at the follow-up visit.

PREVENTION

Developments in diagnostic testing and the use of single-dose antibiotic treatments for gonococcal and chlamydial infections, trichomoniasis, and BV have led to new opportunities to prevent PID. The practice of routine screening for and treatment and prevention of chlamydial infections has dramatically reduced rates of PID in the United States.

Use of sensitive and specific nucleic acid diagnostic techniques such as PCR and LCR for common STIs allows for relatively inexpensive screening and diagnosis in both high- and low-prevalence populations. Although direct cervical or urethral sampling is preferable, both females and males may now submit either urine samples or self-collected swabs for accurate and inexpensive nucleic acid–based testing. **Use of urine-based testing greatly facilitates identification of infected asymptomatic carriers.**

Single-dose regimens, such as azithromycin, 1 g orally (for chlamydial infections), and cefixime, 400 mg, or intramuscular ceftriaxone, 125 mg, **simplify**

BOX 22-1 *Pelvic Inflammatory Disease: Clinical Criteria for Hospitalization and Parenteral Treatment*

1. Surgical emergencies (e.g., appendicitis) not ruled out
2. Pregnancy (decrease fetal wastage from preterm birth)
3. Failed oral treatment (no improvement with short-term treatment)
4. Compliance questionable (i.e., patient unable to follow or tolerate outpatient regimen)
5. Severe illness (toxicity: nausea, vomiting, high fever)
6. Tubo-ovarian abscess shown or suspected

TABLE 22-2

CENTERS FOR DISEASE CONTROL AND PREVENTION RECOMMENDED TREATMENTS FOR PELVIC INFLAMMATORY DISEASE, 2006*

Regimen A	Regimen B
INPATIENT TREATMENT	
Cefoxitin, 2 g IV q6hr *or* Cefotetan, 2 g IV q12hr *plus* Doxycycline, 100 mg IV q12hr until improved, followed by doxycycline, 100 mg orally twice daily, to complete 14 days	Clindamycin, 900 mg IV q8hr *plus* Gentamicin, 2 mg/kg IV once, followed by 1.5 mg/kg IV q8hr until improved, followed by doxycycline, 100 mg orally bid, to complete 14 days
OUTPATIENT TREATMENT	
Ceftriaxone, 250 mg IM in a single dose, plus doxycycline, 100 mg twice daily, to complete 14 days *with or without* Metronidazole, 500 mg orally twice daily for 14 days	Cefoxitin, 2 g IM single dose, and probenecid, 1 g orally, *plus* Doxycycline, 100 mg twice daily, to complete 14 days *with or without* Metronidazole, 500 mg orally twice daily for 14 days

IM, intramuscularly; IV, intravenously.

*See Centers for Disease Control and Prevention website for verification of latest recommended dose and a more complete list of alternative treatments at http://www.cdc.gov.

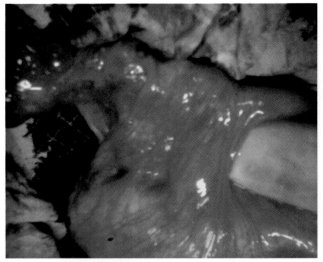

FIGURE 22-7   View of agglutinated adhesions of the female reproductive organs at the time of laparotomy typical of recurrent episodes of pelvic inflammatory disease.

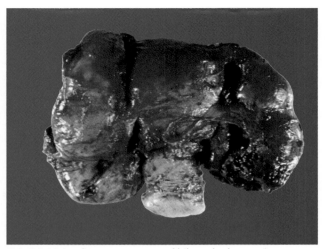

FIGURE 22-8   Gross appearance of bilateral tubo-ovarian abscesses. *(From Kumar V, et al: Robbins and Cotran Pathologic Basis of Disease, 7th ed. Philadelphia, Saunders, 2005.)*

treatment and ensure greater compliance. Directly observed therapy also ensures compliance.

To minimize the risk for reinfection, partners for the past 60 days should be identified, diagnosed, and given specific treatment or treated empirically for both chlamydial infection and gonorrhea. Most infected male partners are asymptomatic. This practice should minimize recurrence and reinfection that can lead to permanent adhesions (Figure 22-7).

■ Other Clinical Issues Related to STIs

INTRAUTERINE DEVICE USE

Studies are reassuring with respect to a lack of an association between PID and IUD use. However, these devices are intended only for couples who are in stable, mutually monogamous relationships. It is prudent, however, to screen patients for common STIs and to treat for BV before insertion to minimize the risk for endometrial contamination.

TUBO-OVARIAN ABSCESS (TOA)

TOA involving fallopian tubes, ovaries, bowel, and possibly other pelvic structures is a potentially lethal complication of PID. Inflammatory complexes also represent severe infection but do not contain significant amounts of pus and are more easily treated with antibiotics.

TOAs occur in about 10% of women hospitalized for PID. A TOA in the course of the initial episode of PID represents severe infection in which the host is unable to localize tissue damage. Some TOAs are caused by reactivation of past infection or repeated infections, whereas others may occur as a result of postpartum or postoperative infections.

Rupture of a TOA causes spreading peritonitis, which can be rapidly lethal in the absence of expeditious surgical drainage, antimicrobial treatment, and systemic vital organ support. TOAs may cause considerable long-term morbidity from irreversible tubal and ovarian damage, with subsequent infertility, chronic pain, and gonadal failure. Rarely, death results from uncontrolled sepsis. Figure 22-8 shows a gross postoperative specimen of a uterus with bilateral TOAs.

A TOA is distinguished from uncomplicated endometritis or salpingitis by the presence of a tender inflammatory adnexal mass. Confirmation of the diagnosis may require the use of imaging techniques such as ultrasonography, computed tomography, or magnetic resonance imaging, as depicted in Figure 22-9. Drainage of a TOA under ultrasonic guidance can be both diagnostic and therapeutic. Laparotomy or laparoscopy may be required to distinguish TOAs from inflammatory complexes, twisted or infected adnexal structures, or pelvic abscesses from other sources (e.g., appendicitis or diverticulitis). **If there is doubt regarding the diagnosis, laparoscopy should be performed promptly.** If laparoscopy or laparotomy is performed, the TOA or pyosalpinx should be drained (extraperitoneally if possible), followed by copious irrigation.

Broad-spectrum intravenous antibiotic treatment, including coverage for endogenous pelvic microorganisms (*E. coli, B. fragilis,* and aerobic and anaerobic cocci) and *N. gonorrhoeae,* **should be started promptly after obtaining microbiologic tests from the cervix.** Intensive antibiotic treatment for TOAs should consist of **broad coverage, multiagent regimens.**

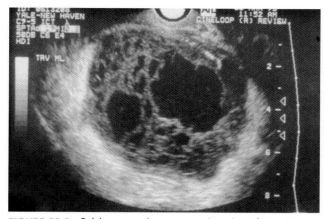

FIGURE 22-9 Pelvic magnetic resonance imaging of a patient with tubo-ovarian abscesses.

Such regimens are associated with curative response rates of about 85%. Some meta-analyses have found improved results if clindamycin is included in a multiagent regimen. **Empiric oral antibiotic treatment** such as oral doxycycline (100 mg twice daily), amoxicillin-clavulanic acid (250 mg 3 times a day), or metronidazole (500 mg twice a day) **is traditionally given for at least 7 days after response to parenteral treatment.**

In the face of clinical deterioration or the absence of obvious clinical improvement after 24 to 48 hours of antibiotic treatment, other modalities should be used. Aspiration using vaginal, abdominal, or rectal ultrasonic guidance should be considered initially. When uterine and ovarian preservation is a goal, drainage of the abscess, possibly combined with salpingectomy, may be required. Total abdominal hysterectomy and bilateral salpingo-oophorectomy may be necessary in refractory cases, usually by a laparotomy.

LESS COMMON SEXUALLY TRANSMITTED INFECTIONS AND INFESTATION

Chancroid is caused by *Haemophilus ducreyi*. The lesions, called *soft chancres*, are painful and are usually accompanied by pelvic adenopathy. Diagnosis is made clinically and confirmed with cultures. Treatment is with azithromycin, 1 g orally in a single dose, or ceftriaxone, 250 mg intramuscularly in a single dose.

Granuloma inguinale (donovanosis) is caused by *Calymmatobacterium granulomatis*. The lesions are red and raised. Treatment is with doxycycline, 100 mg twice a day for a minimum of 3 weeks.

Lymphogranuloma venereum is caused by *C. trachomatis*. Vesicles progress to bubo formation. A complement fixation test is available for diagnosis. Treatment is with doxycycline, 100 mg twice a day for at least 3 weeks.

Molluscum contagiosum is caused by **Poxviridae**. The raised papules with waxy cores are desiccated or treated with cryotherapy or topical imiquimod.

Syphilis is relatively uncommon in the United States. It is particularly important, however, for the obstetrician to recognize this infection in the pregnant patient (see Chapter 16) or in the patient who may become pregnant. Syphilis is caused by *Treponema pallidum*. Treatment is with parenteral (intramuscular) benzathine penicillin G.

Pediculosis pubis is caused by the crab louse *Phthirus pediculosis*, a millimeter-sized insect that infests the pubic area. Treatment is with permethrin 1% crème rinse.

Scabies is caused by a microscopic mite, *Sarcoptes scabiei*. Infestation is common and found worldwide. Treatment is with permethrin 5% crème or ivermectin.

HIV/AIDS AND REPRODUCTIVE-TRACT INFECTIONS IN WOMEN

Lower and upper reproductive tract infections may increase HIV risk in multiple ways. The presence of vaginal, cervical, and endometrial infection may amplify both the susceptibility to HIV infection and its transmission to sexual partners. Both ulcer- and non–ulcer-causing STIs appear to increase the susceptibility to HIV by damaging host defenses or increasing the number and efficiency of HIV viral receptors. Conversely, genital tract inflammation increases local release of HIV virus, which potentiates transmission to sexual partners and vaginally delivered babies. Screening for and treatment of STIs provides an opportunity to reduce the risks for HIV acquisition and transmission.

SUGGESTED READING

Centers for Disease Control and Prevention: Sexually transmitted diseases: Treatment guidelines. MMWR Morb Mortal Wkly Rep 55:1-92, 2006. Updates and ordering available online at: http://www2.cdc.gov/nchstp_od/piweb/stdorderform.asp or by telephone at 404-639-3311.

McClelland RS: Trichomonas vaginalis infection: Can we afford to do nothing? J Infect Dis 197:487-489, 2008.

Paavonen J, Lehtinen M: Introducing human papillomavirus vaccines: Questions remain. Ann Med 40:162-166, 2008.

U.S. Preventive Services Task Force (USPSTF): Recommendations for human immunodeficiency virus (HIV) of adults and adolescents in healthcare settings. Am Fam Physician 77: 819-824, 2008.

Vanvranken M: Prevention and treatment of sexually transmitted diseases. Am Fam Physician 76:1827-1832, 2007.

Chapter 23

Genitourinary Dysfunction
PELVIC ORGAN PROLAPSE, URINARY INCONTINENCE, AND INFECTIONS

CHRISTOPHER M. TARNAY • NARENDER N. BHATIA

A better understanding of the anatomic basis of pelvic relaxation defects has led to less invasive techniques and better outcomes for the treatment of female genitourinary dysfunction.

Normal Pelvic Anatomy and Supports

Anatomically, the pelvic organs, including the vagina, uterus, bladder, and rectum, are maintained within the pelvis by the bilaterally paired and posteriorly fused levator ani muscles. **The anterior separation between the levator ani is called the _levator hiatus._ Inferiorly, the levator hiatus is covered by the urogenital diaphragm. The urethra, vagina, and rectum pass through the levator hiatus and urogenital diaphragm as they exit the pelvis. The endopelvic fascia is a visceral pelvic fascia that invests the pelvic organs and forms bilateral condensations referred to as _ligaments_ (i.e., pubourethral, cardinal, and uterosacral ligaments).** These ligaments attach the organs to the fascia of the pelvic side walls and bony pelvis. Damage to the vagina and its support system allows the urethra, bladder, rectum, and small bowel to herniate and protrude into the vaginal canal.

The **perineal body** is a central point for the attachment of the perineal musculature. **Although the contents of the abdominal cavity bear down on the pelvic organs, they remain suspended in their relation to each other and to the underlying levator sling and perineal body.**

Pelvic Organ Prolapse

Pelvic organ prolapse (POP) refers to protrusion of the pelvic organs into the vaginal canal or beyond the vaginal opening. It results from a weakness in the endopelvic fascia investing the vagina, along with its ligamentous supports. Defects in vaginal support may occur in isolation (e.g., anterior vaginal wall only) but are more commonly combined. The nomenclature of POP has evolved such that cystocele, rectocele, and enterocele have been replaced by more anatomically precise terms (Figure 23-1).

ANTERIOR VAGINAL PROLAPSE (CYSTOCELE)

The anterior vagina is the most common site of vaginal prolapse. Women with this type of defect describe symptoms of vaginal fullness, heaviness, pressure, and discomfort that often progress over the course of the day and are most noticeable after prolonged standing or straining. Women may have to apply manual pressure to empty their bladder completely. Other symptoms include stress urinary incontinence (SUI), urinary urgency, frequency, and nocturia. Significant anterior vaginal wall prolapse that protrudes beyond the vaginal opening (hymen) can cause urethral obstruction due to kinking, resulting in urinary retention.

POSTERIOR VAGINAL PROLAPSE (RECTOCELE AND ENTEROCELE)

Posterior vaginal defects occur when there is weakness in the rectovaginal septum. Symptoms can be indistinguishable from other types of prolapse because the discomfort, pressure, and sense of a vaginal bulge are nonspecific. However, when difficulties with bowel function and defecation occur, lower posterior vaginal prolapse is likely. Straining or the need to manually splint for complete bowel elimination may occur. Upper posterior vaginal wall prolapse is nearly always associated with herniation of the pouch of Douglas, and because this is likely to contain loops of bowel, it is called an **enterocele.**

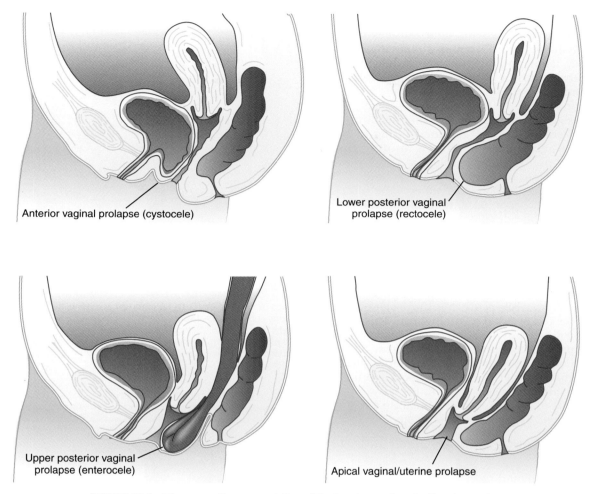

Anterior vaginal prolapse (cystocele)

Lower posterior vaginal prolapse (rectocele)

Upper posterior vaginal prolapse (enterocele)

Apical vaginal/uterine prolapse

FIGURE 23-1   Diagrammatic representation of the four types of vaginal/uterine prolapse.

APICAL VAGINAL AND UTERINE PROLAPSE

Although vaginal prolapse can occur without uterine prolapse, the uterus cannot descend without carrying the upper or apical portion of the vagina with it.

Complete procidentia (uterine prolapse through the vaginal hymen) represents failure of all the vaginal supports (Figure 23-2). Hypertrophy, elongation, congestion, and edema of the cervix may sometimes cause a large protrusion of tissue beyond the hymen, which may be mistaken for a complete procidentia. **Vaginal vault prolapse or eversion of the vagina may be seen after vaginal or abdominal hysterectomy** and represents failure of the supports around the upper vagina.

Symptoms of POP mainly affect quality of life. However, significant sequelae of POP can occur in neglected cases of procidentia, which may be complicated by **excessive purulent discharge, decubitus ulceration, bleeding, and rarely, carcinoma of the cervix.**

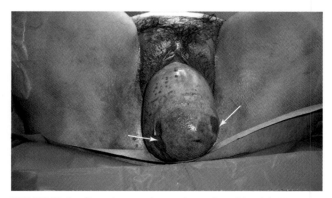

FIGURE 23-2   Complete uterine prolapse (procidentia). Note the lesions on either side of cervical dimple (*arrows*) representing pressure ulcerations from clothing/undergarments. *(Courtesy of CM Tarnay, MD, Ronald Reagan–UCLA Medical Center.)*

ETIOLOGY OF PROLAPSE

The pelvic fascia, ligaments, and muscles may become attenuated from excessive stretching during pregnancy, labor, and difficult vaginal delivery, especially with forceps or vacuum assistance. Asian and black women appear less likely than white women to develop prolapse.

Increased intraabdominal pressure resulting from a chronic cough, ascites, repeated lifting of heavy weights, or habitual straining as a result of constipation may predispose to prolapse. Atrophy of the supporting tissues with aging, especially after menopause, also plays an important role in the initiation or worsening of pelvic relaxation. **Iatrogenic factors include failure to adequately correct all pelvic support defects at the time of pelvic surgery, such as hysterectomy.**

DIAGNOSIS

Vaginal examination is facilitated by using a single-blade speculum. While depressing the posterior vaginal wall, the patient is asked to strain down. This demonstrates the descent of the anterior vaginal wall consistent with prolapse and urethral displacement. Similarly, retraction of the anterior vaginal wall during straining will accentuate posterior vaginal defects and uncover enterocele and rectocele if present. **Rectal-vaginal examination is often useful to demonstrate a rectocele and to distinguish it from an enterocele.**

QUANTIFYING AND STAGING PELVIC ORGAN PROLAPSE

The preferred method to describe and document the severity of POP is the **Pelvic Organ Prolapse Quantification (POP-Q) system.** The extent of prolapse is evaluated and measured relative to the hymen, which is a fixed anatomic landmark. The anatomic position of the six defined points for measurement is denoted in centimeters above the hymen (negative number) or centimeters below the hymen (positive number). The plane at the level of the hymen is defined as zero (Figure 23-3).

Stages of POP can be assigned according to the most severe portion of the prolapse after the full extent of the protrusion has been determined. An ordinal system is used for measurements of different points along the vaginal canal and allows for better communication among clinicians. This staging system enables more objective tracking of surgical outcomes (Table 23-1).

MANAGEMENT

Prophylactic measures to mitigate the symptoms of POP include identifying and treating chronic respiratory and metabolic disorders, correction of constipation and intraabdominal disorders that may cause repetitive increases in intraabdominal pressure, and

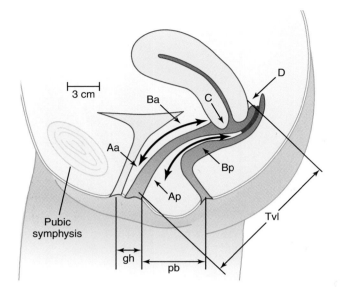

FIGURE 23-3 Illustration showing a side view of female pelvis. Six sites (points Aa, Ba, C, D, Bp, and Ap), genital hiatus (gh), perineal body (pb), and total vaginal length (tvl) used for pelvic organ support quantitation. *(Reproduced with permission from Bump RC, et al: The standardization of terminology of female pelvic organ prolapse and pelvic floor dysfunction. Am J Obstet Gynecol 175:10, 1996.)*

TABLE 23-1

PELVIC ORGAN PROLAPSE STAGING SYSTEM

Stage	Characteristics
0	No prolapse Aa, Ba, Ap, Bp are −3 cm and C or D ≤ −(tvl −2) cm
1	Most distal portion of the prolapse −1 cm (above the level of hymen)
2	Most distal portion of the prolapse ≥ −1 cm but ≤ +1 cm (≤1 cm above or below the hymen)
3	Most distal portion of the prolapse > +1 cm but < +(tvl − 2) cm (beyond the hymen; protrudes no farther than 2 cm less than the total vaginal length)
4	Complete eversion; most distal portion of the prolapse ≥ +(tvl − 2) cm

Aa, point A of anterior wall; Ba, point B of anterior wall; Ap, point A of posterior wall; Bp, point B of posterior wall; −, above the hymen; +, beyond the hymen; tvl, total vaginal length.

Reproduced with permission from Harvey MA, Versi E: Urogynecology and pelvic floor dysfunction. *In* Ryan KJ, Berkowitz RS, Barbieri RL, Dunaif A (eds): Kistner's Gynecology and Women's Health, 7th ed. St. Louis, Mosby, 1999. Copyright © 1999 Elsevier.

administration of estrogen to menopausal women. **Failure to recognize and treat significant support defects at the time of concomitant gynecologic surgery may lead to progression of existing prolapse** and the development of urinary incontinence or retention and urinary tract infections (UTIs).

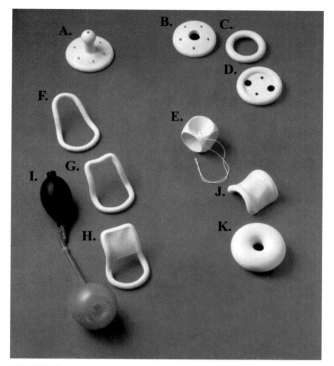

FIGURE 23-4 Some types of vaginal pessaries used for prolapse: Gellhorn (**A**), Shaatz (**B**), ring (**C**), ring with support (**D**), cube (**E**), Smith (**F**), Hodge (**G**), Hodge with support for cystocele (**H**), Inflatoball (**I**), Gehrung (**J**), and doughnut (**K**).

Nonsurgical Treatment

When only a mild degree of pelvic relaxation is present, pelvic floor muscle exercises may improve the tone of the pelvic floor musculature. Pessaries, which provide intravaginal support (Figure 23-4), may be used to correct prolapse by "propping up" the vagina. They can be considered when the patient is medically unfit or refuses surgery or during pregnancy and the postpartum period. They are also useful to promote healing of a decubitus ulcer before surgery for prolapse.

Pessaries require proper fitting and selection of the appropriate type and size. They should be removed, cleaned, and reinserted every 6 to 12 weeks. They may cause vaginal irritation and ulceration. **Neglect may result in serious consequences,** including fistula formation, impaction, bleeding, and infection.

Surgical Treatment

The main objectives of surgery are to relieve symptoms and restore normal anatomic relationships and visceral function. Preservation or restoration of satisfactory coital function when desired and a lasting operative result are also important goals.

REPAIR OF VAGINAL PROLAPSE. Anterior colporrhaphy corrects anterior vaginal wall prolapse and helps support the urethra. It involves **plication of the pubocervical fascia** to support the bladder and urethra.

When the anterior prolapse involves a direct detachment of lateral vaginal support, it is considered a **paravaginal defect.** Paravaginal defect repairs involve exposure of the retropubic space. **Interrupted permanent sutures are used to reattach bilaterally the anterosuperior vaginal sulci to the arcus tendineus fasciae ("white line")** extending from the ischial spine to the lower edge of the pubic ramus. In the presence of SUI, additional supportive measures are taken to achieve suspension of the bladder neck and proximal urethra.

Posterior colporrhaphy corrects a posterior vaginal wall prolapse and is similar in principle to anterior colporrhaphy. Site-specific posterior vaginal repairs can be performed after identification of the discrete endopelvic fascial breaks and reapproximating this thicker tissue identified during rectal examination. Perineorrhaphy repairs a deficient perineal body.

Recent modifications of these procedures involve the use of permanent suture or the addition of graft materials to augment the durability of the repair. These modifications can be accomplished using minimally invasive techniques.

REPAIR OF APICAL PROLAPSE. When the uterus is present, hysterectomy may be performed to facilitate exposure of the apical support structures. Hysterectomy, however, is not a requirement in settings in which uterine removal is not desired. The repair of apical defects may require peritoneal entry for the **repair of an enterocele.** After identification of the enterocele, the contents are reduced, the neck of the peritoneal sac is ligated, and the defect is repaired by approximating the uterosacral ligaments and levator ani muscles to restore continuity in the endopelvic fascia.

Vaginal vault suspension (colpopexy) for apical prolapse is performed to secure a durable fixation point for the top of the vagina. This can be accomplished vaginally or abdominally by suspending the vaginal vault to the sacrum, sacrospinous ligaments, uterosacral ligaments, or other firm points of fixation.

VAGINAL CLOSURE PROCEDURES. For women with advanced vaginal prolapse who no longer desire coital function, there are less invasive surgical options. A LeFort colpocleisis involves suturing the partially denuded anterior and posterior vaginal walls together in such a way that the uterus remains in situ and is supported above the partially occluded vagina. **In women with posthysterectomy prolapse, a complete colpocleisis** involves total obliteration of the vagina. These "obliterative" procedures are traditionally reserved for elderly women who are not likely to tolerate more invasive reparative surgery.

■ Urinary Incontinence

Urinary incontinence is defined as the involuntary loss of urine that is objectively demonstrable and is a social or hygienic problem. Urinary incontinence has been reported to affect 15% to 50% of women. The problem increases in prevalence with age, reaching more than 50% in elderly persons in nursing homes. **It is estimated that the direct financial cost of urinary incontinence in the United States is between $10 and $15 billion per year.**

ANATOMY AND PHYSIOLOGY OF THE LOWER URINARY TRACT

In the adult female, the urethra is a muscular tube, 3 to 4 cm in length, lined proximally with transitional epithelium and distally with stratified squamous epithelium. It is surrounded mainly by smooth muscle. **The striated muscular urethral sphincter, which surrounds the distal two thirds of the urethra, contributes about 50% of the total urethral resistance and serves as a secondary defense against incontinence.** It is also responsible for the interruption of urinary flow at the end of micturition.

The two posterior pubourethral ligaments provide a strong suspensory mechanism for the urethra and serve to hold it forward and in close proximity to the pubis under conditions of stress. They extend from the lower part of the pubic bone to the urethra at the junction of its middle and distal third.

INNERVATION

The lower urinary tract is under the control of both parasympathetic and sympathetic nerves. **The parasympathetic fibers originate in the sacral spinal cord segments S2 through S4.** Stimulation of the pelvic parasympathetic nerves and administration of cholinergic drugs cause the detrusor muscle to contract. Anticholinergic drugs reduce the vesicle pressure and increase the bladder capacity.

The sympathetic fibers originate from thoracolumbar segments (T10 through L2) of the spinal cord. The sympathetic system has α- and β-adrenergic components. The β-fibers terminate primarily in the detrusor muscle, whereas the α-fibers terminate primarily in the urethra. α-Adrenergic stimulation contracts the bladder neck and urethra and relaxes the detrusor. β-Adrenergic stimulation relaxes the urethra and detrusor muscle. **The pudendal nerve (S2 to S4) provides motor innervation to the striated urethral sphincter.**

FACTORS INFLUENCING BLADDER BEHAVIOR

Sensory Innervation

Afferent impulses from the bladder, trigone, and proximal urethra pass to S2 through S4 levels of the spinal cord by means of the pelvic hypogastric nerves. The sensitivity of these nerve endings may be enhanced by acute infection, interstitial cystitis, radiation cystitis, and increased intravesical pressure. The latter may occur in the standing or bending-forward position or in association with obesity, pregnancy, or pelvic tumors.

Inhibitory impulses, probably relayed by the pudendal nerve, also pass to S2 through S4 after mechanical stimulation of the perineum and anal canal. Their passage may explain why pain in this region can cause urinary retention.

Central Nervous System

In infancy, the storage and expulsion of urine are automatic and controlled at the level of the sacral reflex arc. Later, connections to the higher centers become established, and by training and conditioning, this spinal reflex becomes socially influenced so that voiding can be voluntarily accomplished. Although organic neurologic diseases may interrupt the influence of the higher centers on the spinal reflex arc, patterns of micturition may also be profoundly altered by mental, environmental, and sociologic disturbances.

CONTINENCE CONTROL

The bladder must store and hold urine painlessly and then, at the appropriate social setting, empty urine effectively. The normal bladder holds urine because the intraurethral pressure exceeds the intravesical pressure. The pubourethral ligaments and surrounding endopelvic fascia support the urethra so that abrupt increases in intraabdominal pressure are transmitted equally to the bladder and proximal third of the urethra, thus maintaining a pressure gradient between the two structures. In addition, a reflex contraction of the levator ani compresses the mid-urethra, decreasing the likelihood of urine loss.

■ Stress Urinary Incontinence

SUI is involuntary leakage of urine in response to physical exertion, sneezing, or coughing.

ETIOLOGY

The most commonly accepted theory for the pathogenesis of SUI is urethral hypermobility due to vaginal wall relaxation, displacing the bladder neck and proximal urethra downward. When this occurs, increased intraabdominal pressure from coughing, sneezing, or physical exertion is no longer transmitted *equally* to the bladder and proximal urethra. The normal urethral resistance is overcome by this increased bladder pressure, and leakage of urine results.

The second possible mechanism is intrinsic sphincter deficiency, where the urethra fails to close in response to increases in intraabdominal pressure. This cause of SUI is analogous to having a leaky "valve" in the urethra.

Factors that contribute to SUI include childbearing, previous urogenital surgery, pelvic radiation, estrogen deficiency (menopause), and medications such as diuretics and α-adrenergic blockers.

PELVIC EXAMINATION

Inspection of the vaginal walls should be performed with a single-blade speculum, which allows optimal visualization of the anterior vaginal wall and urethrovesical junction. Scarring, tenderness, and rigidity of the urethra from previous vaginal surgeries or pelvic trauma may be indicated by a scarred anterior vaginal wall. Because the distal urethra is estrogen dependent, the patient with urogenital atrophy also has atrophic urethritis.

DIAGNOSTIC TESTS

Stress Test

The patient is examined with a full bladder in the lithotomy position. While the physician observes the urethral meatus, the patient is asked to cough. SUI is present if short spurts of urine escape simultaneously with each cough. A delayed leakage, or loss of large volumes of urine, suggests uninhibited bladder contractions. If loss of urine is not demonstrated in the lithotomy position, the test should be repeated with the patient in a standing position.

Cotton Swab (Q-Tip) Test

This test determines the mobility and descent of the urethrovesical junction on straining and allows differentiation from anterior vaginal laxity alone. With the patient in the lithotomy position, the examiner inserts a lubricated cotton swab into the urethra to the level of the urethrovesical junction and measures the angle between the cotton swab and the horizontal. The patient then strains maximally, which produces descent of the urethrovesical junction. Along with the descent, the cotton swab moves, producing a new angle with the horizontal. **The normal change in angle is up to 30 degrees. In patients with pelvic relaxation and SUI, the change in cotton swab angle ranges from 30 to 60 degrees or more** (Figure 23-5).

Urethrocystoscopy

Urethrocystoscopy allows the physician to examine inside the urethra, urethrovesical junction, bladder walls, and ureteral orifices. This procedure is useful to detect bladder stones, tumors, diverticula, or sutures from prior surgeries.

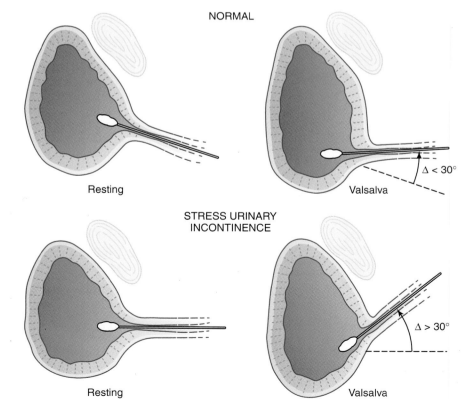

FIGURE 23-5 Diagrammatic representation of the Q-tip (cotton swab) test, showing mobility of the urethrovesical junction in a continent patient and a patient with stress urinary incontinence.

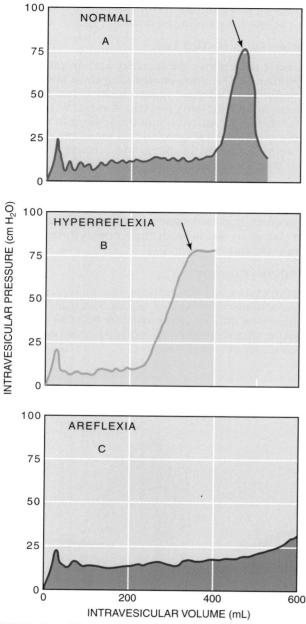

FIGURE 23-6   Water cystometrogram in a normal patient (**A**), a patient with detrusor hyperreflexia (**B**), and a patient with detrusor areflexia (hypotonic bladder) (**C**). *Arrows* in **A** and **B** indicate peak of bladder contraction.

Cystometrogram

Cystometry consists of distending the bladder with known volumes of water and observing pressure changes in bladder function during filling. **The most important observation is the presence of a detrusor reflex and the patient's ability to control or inhibit this reflex.**

The first sensation of bladder filling should occur at volumes of 150 to 200 mL. The critical volume (400 to 500 mL) is the capacity that the bladder musculature tolerates before the patient experiences a strong desire to urinate. At this point, if the patient is asked to void, a terminal contraction may appear and is seen as a sudden rise in intravesical pressure. At the peak of the contraction, the patient is instructed to inhibit this reflex (indicated by *arrows* in Figure 23-6). A normal person should be able to inhibit this detrusor reflex and thereby bring down intravesical pressure (see Figure 23-6A). In a urologically or neurologically abnormal patient, the detrusor reflex may appear without the specific instruction to void, and the patient cannot inhibit it (see Figure 23-6B); this observation is referred to as an **uninhibited detrusor contraction.** Other terms for this disorder include overactive bladder, detrusor dyssynergia, detrusor hyperreflexia, irritable bladder, hypertonic bladder, unstable bladder, and uninhibited neurogenic bladder.

These cystometric procedures allow differentiation between patients who are incontinent as a result of uninhibited detrusor contraction and those who have SUI. Conversely, the hypotonic bladder accommodates excessive amounts of gas or water with little increase in intravesical pressure, and the terminal detrusor contraction is absent when the patient is asked to void (see Figure 23-6C).

Urethral Pressure Measurements

A low urethral pressure may be found in patients with SUI, whereas an abnormally high urethral closing pressure may be associated with voiding difficulties, hesitancy, and urinary retention.

Urethral function can be evaluated with cystometric testing. The urethral closing pressure profile (UCPP) is a graphic record of pressure along the length of the urethra. The urethral closing pressure normally varies between 50 and 100 cm H_2O. A Valsalva maneuver or abdominal leak point pressure of less than 60 cm H_2O or urethral closure pressure of less than 20 cm H_2O are suggestive of the diagnosis of **intrinsic sphincteric deficiency (ISD).**

Uroflowmetry

Uroflowmetry records rates of urine flow through the urethra when the patient is asked to void spontaneously.

Voiding Cystourethrogram

In this radiologic investigation, fluoroscopy is used to observe bladder filling, the mobility of the urethra and bladder base, and the anatomic changes during voiding. The procedure provides valuable information regarding bladder size and the competence of the bladder neck during coughing. It may detect any bladder trabeculation; vesicoureteral reflux during voiding;

funneling of the bladder neck, bladder, and urethral diverticula; and outflow obstruction.

Ultrasonography

Employing real-time or sector ultrasonography, information can be obtained about the inclination of the urethra, flatness of the bladder base, and mobility and funneling of the urethrovesical junction, both at rest and with a Valsalva maneuver. In addition, bladder or urethral diverticula may be identified.

Video urodynamics incorporates fluoroscopy with concurrent measurement of bladder and urethral pressures. Dynamic **magnetic resonance imaging** studies are employed to detect pelvic floor and relaxation defects in incontinent patients.

SUMMARY

For a significant percentage of patients with SUI, a good history and physical examination, the cotton swab test, and the cough stress test are adequate investigations. The addition of uroflowmetry, cystourethroscopy, and the cystometrogram are appropriate when more detailed information is needed for diagnosis and treatment. Additional urodynamic, electromyographic, electrophysiologic, and radiologic studies may be necessary in patients with a history of multiple previous surgeries for urinary incontinence and for patients with associated neurologic disease.

TREATMENT

Medical Therapy

In postmenopausal incontinent women, **estrogens improve urethral closing pressure, vaginal epithelial thickness and vascularity, and reflex urethral function.** α-Adrenergic stimulants, such as phenylpropanolamine and pseudoephedrine, may enhance urethral closure and improve continence but are unproved in placebo controlled trials. The search for an effective medication to treat SUI is still ongoing.

Physical Therapy

Pelvic floor muscle exercises (PFMEs) also known as Kegel exercises, are proven first-line therapy to improve or cure mild to moderate forms of SUI. PFMEs require diligence and willingness to practice at home and at work. Many women find them difficult, fatiguing, or time-consuming. Kegel exercises before and after delivery may help patients with postpartum urinary incontinence.

Intravaginal Devices

Larger sizes of pessaries (see Figure 23-4) have been used to elevate and support the bladder neck and urethra. They have been shown to be effective for SUI.

Surgical Therapy

Surgery is the most commonly employed treatment for SUI. The aim of all surgical procedures is to correct the pelvic relaxation defect and to stabilize and restore the normal supports of the urethra. The approach may be vaginal, abdominal, or combined abdominovaginal.

ABDOMINAL APPROACH. **Abdominal retropubic urethropexy has a long-term success rate of 85% to 95%. The retropubic urethropexy is performed extraperitoneally (in the space of Retzius) by placing sutures in the fascia lateral to and on each side of the bladder neck and proximal urethra and elevating the vesicourethral junction by attaching the sutures to the symphysis pubis (Marshall-Marchetti-Krantz procedure) or to Cooper's ligament (Burch procedure).**

Postoperatively, a transurethral or suprapubic catheter is left in the bladder for continuous bladder drainage for 48 to 72 hours before instituting spontaneous voiding. Some patients (20% to 30%) may need prolonged postoperative bladder drainage (more than 7 days). An occasional patient may develop osteitis pubis after the Marshall-Marchetti-Krantz procedure.

The recent popularity of operative laparoscopy for many gynecologic procedures has resulted in the **use of the laparoscope for bladder neck suspension procedures. Their long-term success rates, however, have been disappointing.**

VAGINAL APPROACH. **Suburethral sling procedures have long been used to treat refractive patients or patients with severe SUI.** Conventional slings often required harvesting a patient's own fascial tissue to be placed under the bladder neck but were plagued by high rates of urinary retention.

The latest modification of the sling procedure is the use of tension-free synthetic (polypropylene) mesh made of polypropylene **placed at the level of the mid-urethra.** This pioneering technique, developed in Sweden, was introduced in the United States in the late 1990s. **The tension-free vaginal tape** was developed as a minimally invasive technique for the surgical correction of genuine SUI and has a high success rate. **Traditionally, a mid-urethral sling is placed retropubically.** A variation in placement for the mid-urethral sling is the transobturator approach. Rather than retropubic passage, the sling is passed through the obturator foramen laterally. The potential advantage of this approach, which avoids the space of Retzius, is reduction in bladder, bowel, or vascular injury.

SPECIAL PROCEDURES

Conventional surgical procedures for incontinence sometimes fail in patients with a diagnosis of ISD. ISD is a subtype of SUI marked by a very poorly functioning urethral sphincter. These patients are treated with a suburethral sling procedure or **periurethral bulking injections** to improve urethral function. A commonly used bulking material is **bovine collagen (Contigen).** This collagen gel causes periurethral compression after injection and becomes a fibrous network that serves as a matrix for host connective tissue. Collagen, however, is ultimately degraded by the body, and this type of therapy usually requires reinjection at frequent intervals, usually several months. **A nonabsorbable bulking agent is calcium hydroxylapatite,** which is nontoxic and nonantigenic and is less likely to degrade.

Urge Urinary Incontinence and Overactive Bladder

The two terms are often used interchangeably to describe a problem with bladder control that is associated with a strong desire to pass urine with a decreased ability to control it. Urge urinary incontinence (UUI) is defined as the involuntary leakage of urine accompanied by or immediately preceded by urgency. UUI can be associated with small losses of urine between normal micturitions or large volume losses with complete bladder emptying. **Overactive bladder (OAB),** previously described as UUI associated with detrusor muscle instability, is a more descriptive symptom-based term and more accurately encompasses the common clinical presentation. **OAB is defined as "urgency, with or without urge incontinence, usually with frequency and nocturia."** OAB has become the preferred term because it comprises symptoms of urgency, urge urinary incontinence, frequency, and nocturia.

The incidence of overactive bladder increases with age, approximating 30% in the geriatric patient population. **In most patients, the exact etiology of bladder instability remains unknown,** but a number of risk factors are associated with its development (Box 23-1).

Classically, women with OAB describe a sudden strong urge to urinate with an inability to suppress the feeling, rushing to the bathroom, and leaking before making it to the toilet. Awakening several times a night to urinate is also a prominent feature.

TREATMENT

The optimal treatment of OAB starts with behavioral modification, adding pharmacologic and physical interventions, such as electrical stimulation, as needed. Identification of any dietary triggers, like caffeine, alcohol, or carbonated beverages, is important. The use of a self-reported bladder diary can be helpful for obtaining this information.

BOX 23-1 *Risk Factors Associated with Overactive Bladder*

- Older age
- Chronic disorders (e.g., multiple sclerosis, dementia, Alzheimer's disease, spinal cord injury, stroke, diabetes mellitus)
- Pregnancy (may contribute to neural injury or development of pelvic organ prolapse)
- Menopause (estrogen deficiency causes urogenital atrophy and impaired bladder capacity)
- Pelvic surgery (scarring or operative trauma may injure nerves and supportive structures)
- Obesity (increases bladder pressure)
- Immobility (impairs ability to toilet, particularly in older patients)
- Medications (e.g., diuretics, calcium channel blockers, and psychotropic agents)
- Smoking (increases risk for chronic coughing)

Behavioral Modification

Reducing fluid intake and avoiding liquids during the evening hours are good initial behavioral changes. Gradually **increasing the intervals between voidings** and doing pelvic floor muscle strengthening exercises, such as **Kegel exercises**, are effective for attaining better bladder control.

Pharmacologic Treatment

Antimuscarinics, or anticholinergics, have become the mainstays of drug treatment for OAB.

The mainstays of drug therapy include **oxybutynin chloride (Ditropan)** and **tolterodine (Detrol).** Oxybutynin chloride has been shown to improve symptoms of urinary urgency in about 70% of patients. **Tolterodine also** has anticholinergic activity. Because of its bladder specificity, tolterodine has a more favorable side-effect profile than oxybutynin. It is also dosed less frequently, which improves patient compliance. Both are available in immediate release and long-acting formulations. Oxybutynin is also available for delivery in a transdermal patch.

Trospium chloride, solifenacin, and **darifenacin** are newer agents used in the treatment of OAB. All significantly improve OAB symptoms compared with placebo. Evidence suggests that side-effect profiles will be similar or lower than the less specific antimuscarinics.

Imipramine hydrochloride is a tricyclic antidepressant that acts through its anticholinergic properties to increase bladder storage. The drug improves bladder compliance rather than counteracting uninhibited detrusor contractions. It is given in doses greatly reduced from those recommended for use as an antidepressant. It also blocks postsynaptic noradrenaline uptake and thereby increases bladder outlet resistance. With its dual action, imipramine may be effective in patients with both stress incontinence and OAB (mixed incontinence). It should be dosed in the evening because it may be sedating, and should be used with caution in elderly patients owing to potential orthostatic hypotension.

Functional Electrical Stimulation

Functional electrical stimulation offers an alternative for treating stress or urge incontinence when other treatments fail. A vaginal or rectal probe is inserted, usually twice daily for 15 to 30 minutes, to provide electrical stimulation to the pelvic floor muscles or to the nerves to these structures. Stimulation of the afferent fibers of the pudendal nerve can produce contractions of the pelvic floor and periurethral skeletal muscles, improving their tone and function in women with SUI.

◼ Overflow Incontinence

Urinary retention and overflow incontinence may result from detrusor areflexia or a hypotonic bladder, as is seen with lower motor neuron disease, spinal cord injuries, or autonomic neuropathy (diabetes mellitus). These patients are best managed by intermittent self-catheterization.

Overflow incontinence may also occur when there is an outflow obstruction. Straining to void, poor stream, retention of urine, and incomplete emptying may indicate an obstructive disorder. Overdistention of the bladder because of unrecognized urinary retention may occur in the postoperative period. This is a temporary problem related to postoperative pain and may be managed by continuous bladder drainage for 24 to 48 hours.

◼ Urinary Fistula

Fistulas are an uncommon cause of urinary incontinence in the United States. Obstetric fistulas, however, are a tremendous source of social and physical distress in developing countries. Obstetric injuries, once the leading cause of urinary fistulas, have almost disappeared in developed countries. They usually result from operative deliveries (e.g., forceps) rather than from neglected labor and pressure necrosis.

Pelvic surgery, irradiation, or both now account for 95% of the vesicovaginal fistulas in the United States. More than 50% occur after simple abdominal or vaginal hysterectomy. About 1% to 2% of radical hysterectomies are followed in 10 to 21 days by a urinary fistula, usually **ureterovaginal**. These fistulas are usually due to devascularization of the ureter rather than direct injury.

Urethrovaginal fistulas generally occur as complications of surgery for urethral diverticula, anterior vaginal wall prolapse, or SUI.

DIAGNOSIS OF A FISTULA

The usual history of painless and continuous vaginal leakage of urine soon after pelvic surgery is strongly suggestive of this problem. **Instillation of methylene blue dye into the bladder will discolor a vaginal pack if a vesicovaginal fistula is present. Intravenous indigo carmine is excreted in the urine and will discolor a vaginal pack in the presence of a vesicovaginal or ureterovaginal fistula.** In addition, cystourethroscopy should be performed to determine the site and number of fistulas. Most posthysterectomy vesicovaginal fistulas are located just anterior to the vaginal vault. **An intravenous pyelogram or retrograde pyelogram should be undertaken to localize a ureterovaginal fistula.**

FISTULA REPAIR

Most obstetric fistulas can be repaired immediately on detection. For postsurgical fistulas, it is usual to wait some weeks to allow the inflammation to settle. During this waiting period, UTI should be treated and estrogen therapy instituted in postmenopausal women. **Steroids have been advocated to hasten resolution of inflammatory changes and allow early surgical intervention. Their use in this circumstance is controversial.**

Vesicovaginal Fistula

The vaginal approach (**Latzko's operation**) is the procedure of choice. **A bulbocavernosus muscle flap or fat pad (Martius graft) may be interposed between the bladder and vagina to provide support, vascularity, and strength to the suture line, especially in patients who have had multiple previous attempted repairs and in those with a postradiation fistula.** Large radiation-induced fistulas may necessitate urinary conduit for urinary diversion.

Ureterovaginal Fistula

Treatment of ureterovaginal fistula depends on its size and location. **Small fistulas usually close spontaneously after placement of a ureteric stent (double J), provided the tissues have not been irradiated.**

If the fistula is close to the ureterovesical junction, the ureter proximal to the fistula can be reimplanted into the bladder (**ureteroneocystostomy**). If the fistula is several centimeters from the bladder, a **Boari flap** may be useful, a **segment of ileum may be interposed** between the proximal ureter and the bladder, or rarely a **transureteroureterostomy** may be employed.

Although urinary incontinence is a common condition, the evaluation of the patient with urinary incontinence can be challenging.

◼ Urethral Syndrome

The urethral syndrome occurs in a patient with various lower urinary tract symptoms, including acute or chronic pain (see Chapter 21), in the absence of obvious bladder or urethral abnormality, and with no evidence of UTI. **Any combination of symptoms may be** present, the most common being urinary frequency, urgency, dysuria, postvoid fullness, incontinence, and dyspareunia.

Diagnosis is based on a detailed history and physical examination, negative urine cultures, dynamic cystourethroscopy, and urodynamic studies.

TREATMENT

Application of vaginal estrogen cream is effective in patients with atrophic urethritis. Some patients may improve with use of tetracycline for 10 to 14 days. **Internal urethrotomy** and **urethrolysis** have also been employed with variable success.

■ Urinary Tract Infection

UTI is one of the most frequently diagnosed infectious diseases in medical practice. Every year in the United States, about 10% of women are diagnosed with cystitis, and this is associated with direct costs of more than $1.6 billion.

About 20% to 30% of women have at least one UTI during their lifetime, and 20% develop recurrent infections. Ninety-five percent of UTIs are symptomatic, and three fourths of these symptomatic episodes show positive urine cultures. Almost all asymptomatic patients have negative cultures.

TERMINOLOGY

The terminology surrounding UTIs is rather complex and requires some definition.

- **Bacteriuria** means the presence of bacteria in the urine.
- **Significant bacteriuria is generally accepted as a bacterial colony count of 10^5 or more per milliliter of urine in a properly collected clean-catch specimen in an asymptomatic patient. Lower colony counts may be accepted in symptomatic patients.**
- **Asymptomatic bacteriuria** is significant bacteriuria with or without pyuria in a patient without symptoms of UTI.
- **Pyelonephritis** is a bacterial infection of the renal parenchyma and the renal pelvicaliceal system. Acute pyelonephritis is commonly associated with chills and fever, flank pain, costovertebral tenderness, urinary frequency, urgency, and dysuria. Chronic pyelonephritis denotes histologic changes of patchy interstitial nephritis, destruction of tubules, cellular infiltration, and inflammatory changes in the renal parenchyma.
- **Chronic pyelonephritis is not synonymous with chronic UTI, which means only prolonged bacteriuria.**
- **Cystitis** is an inflammation of the urinary bladder. Patients with cystitis usually have symptoms of lower urinary tract irritation, such as dysuria (burning on urination), urgency, frequency with small amounts of voided urine, nocturia, suprapubic discomfort, and at times, urinary incontinence and hematuria.
- **Persistence of bacteriuria** is the presence of microorganisms that were isolated at the start of treatment and continue to be isolated while the patient is receiving therapy. Persistence may be caused by several factors, including the presence of resistant organisms, inadequate drug therapy, and poor patient compliance.
- **Superinfection** is the appearance of a different organism while a patient is still receiving therapy. The new organism may be a different strain or a different serologic type.
- **Relapse** occurs with the recurrence of significant bacteriuria with the same species and serologic strain of organism. Relapse usually appears within 2 to 3 weeks of completion of therapy and most likely represents perineal colonization by the infecting organism.
- **Reinfection** is an infection occurring after cessation of therapy with a different strain of microorganism or a different serologic type of the original infecting strain. Typically, reinfection occurs 2 to 12 weeks after a previous episode of infection and indicates recurrent bladder bacteriuria.
- **Recurrent UTI is diagnosed when** two UTIs occur within 6 months or three or more occur during a single year. Women of blood group B or AB have an increased risk for recurrent UTIs.

INCIDENCE AND PREVALENCE

After the age of 1 year and throughout adulthood, females are affected more frequently than males (10:1 ratio). Asymptomatic bacteriuria increases from an incidence in preschool children of 1% to 5% to a peak of about 10% in postmenopausal women. Urologic abnormalities are found in up to 70% of children with a UTI. Box 23-2 lists the risk factors for UTIs in premenopausal and postmenopausal women.

PATHOGENESIS

Bacteria may gain entry to the urinary tract by three pathways: the ascending route, the descending or hematogenous route, and the lymphatic route.

Ascending Infection

The female is more susceptible because of the short length of the urethra, urethral contamination by rectal pathogens, introital and vestibular colonization by pathogenic bacteria, and decreased urethral resistance after menopause. Sexual intercourse is a major source of bacteriuria within 24 hours, and the relative risk is proportional to the frequency of intercourse in the past 7 days (e.g., **honeymoon cystitis**).

Hematogenous Infection

Urinary infection through the hematogenous route is very uncommon, but it is seen occasionally in elderly, debilitated, or immunosuppressed patients with overwhelming infections in whom kidney infection is only part of the multisystemic involvement. **Renal tuberculosis** is almost always acquired through the hematogenous route.

Lymphatic Infection

Experimental evidence suggests that bacterial infection spreads along lymphatic channels that connect the bowel and the urinary tract.

HOST DEFENSE MECHANISMS

Entrance of bacteria into the urinary tract does not necessarily result in infection. **Natural barriers for invasion**, such as the **"washout" effect of normal periodic voiding**, the **antiseptic properties of the bladder tissues**, and the **high concentration of organic acids in normal urine**, prevent bacterial invasion. Other factors, such as a pH of less than 5 and urea ammonium and organic acid content of the urine, all affect bacterial growth. If invasion takes place, the bacteria may remain in the bladder or may ascend to the kidney. **Transient vesicoureteral reflux seen in association**

BOX 23-2 *Risk Factors for Urinary Tract Infection in Women*

> **Premenopausal**
>
> History of urinary tract infection
> Frequent or recent sexual activity
> Diaphragm use for contraception
> Use of spermicidal agents
> Increasing parity
> Diabetes mellitus
> Obesity
> Sickle cell trait
> Anatomic congenital abnormalities
> Urinary tract calculi
> Medical conditions requiring indwelling or repetitive bladder catheterization
>
> **Postmenopausal**
>
> Vaginal atrophy
> Incomplete bladder emptying
> Poor perineal hygiene
> Rectocele, cystocele, urethrocele, or uterovaginal prolapse
> Lifetime history of urinary tract infections
> Type 1 diabetes mellitus
>
> ---
>
> Data from American College of Obstetricians and Gynecologists (ACOG): Treatment of urinary tract infections in nonpregnant women. Practice Bulletin No. 91. Obstet Gynecol 111:785-794, 2008.

with severe lower UTIs may allow the infected urine to reach the kidneys.

PERPETUATING FACTORS

The following factors encourage and perpetuate UTIs:
1. **Mechanical urinary obstruction.** Ureteropelvic junction obstruction, ureteral stricture, urethral stenosis, and calculi are common to patients with recurrent or chronic UTIs.
2. **Functional urinary obstruction abnormalities.** Incomplete bladder emptying and vesicoureteric reflux encourage stasis of urine and bacterial growth. Pregnancy produces transient functional ureteral obstruction both mechanically and hormonally. Hypospadias may result in repeated infections after coitus (honeymoon cystitis).
3. **Systemic factors.** Diabetes mellitus, gout, sickle cell trait, cystic renal disease, and metabolic disorders, such as nephrocalcinosis, chronic potassium deficiency, and renal tubular defects, increase susceptibility to pyelonephritis.

CLINICAL CLASSIFICATION

From the point of view of pathogenesis and management, UTIs in nonpregnant females can be considered to be either uncomplicated or complicated. **Uncomplicated cases account for 95% of UTIs in women and seldom produce renal damage.** They are either the first episode of infection or an episode far removed in time from a previous urinary infection. Ninety percent of first infections are due to *Escherichia coli.* Seventy-five percent of these infective episodes do not recur for several years. **Complicated UTIs occur in patients with neurologic or obstructive abnormalities or in those with underlying parenchymal disease.**

INVESTIGATIONS

Urinalysis

Microscopic examination of an uncentrifuged, unstained specimen (a drop of urine on the slide covered with a coverslip) provides better than 90% accuracy in detecting significant bacteriuria when one or more bacteria are seen per high-power field. A positive Gram stain almost always correlates with a positive quantitative culture. **A negative Gram stain virtually eliminates significant bacteriuria**.

Pyuria is arbitrarily defined as the presence of five or more white blood cells per high-power field in the centrifuged specimen. The presence of white blood cells (pyuria) and red blood cells along with bacteriuria suggests infection. **Pyuria without significant bacteria may indicate a nonbacterial inflammation or a urinary tract foreign body or tumor. It is a classic finding in urinary tuberculosis. Casts, when present, indicate renal parenchymal disease.**

URINE CULTURE AND MICROBIOLOGY

A quantitative urine culture is the most important laboratory test in the diagnosis and management of complicated or uncomplicated UTIs. *E. coli* **is the predominant organism in 80% to 85% of patients.** The remaining, less common organisms are *Klebsiella, Enterobacter, Proteus, Enterococcus*, and *Staphylococcus* species and group D *Streptococcus*. Anaerobic fecal bacteria do not grow well in urine and are rarely seen in urinary infections. Yeast, such as *Candida albicans* (funguria), may be seen in patients with diabetes mellitus or in individuals receiving immunosuppressive therapy, especially in the presence of foreign bodies or indwelling catheters.

There are three techniques for urine collection: (1) the midstream clean-catch method, (2) urethral catheterization, and (3) suprapubic aspiration. The midstream clean-catch method has an 80% reliability, which increases to 95% if two consecutive specimens show a colony count of 100,000 or more of the same organism. In routine cases of uncomplicated infections, the presence of two or more species of organisms in the same specimen normally suggests contamination. **Urethral catheterization provides an optimal urine specimen.** A positive culture has 95% accuracy, and false-positive cultures are rare.

Suprapubic aspiration, although providing the most reliable specimen, is reserved for those in whom contamination is difficult to avoid (e.g., young children and elderly people).

RADIOLOGIC STUDIES

Imaging can be critical in the evaluation of patients whose recurrences are due to bacterial persistence (e.g., stones or infected congenital anomalies), but it is of almost no value in the 99% of patients with reinfections. Intravenous pyelography and computed tomographic urography are the main studies employed. Cystography and voiding urethrocystography may help to detect ureteric reflux, diverticula, and fistulous tracts in patients with persistent bacteriuria.

ENDOSCOPIC STUDIES

Endoscopic studies such as urethroscopy and cystoscopy may be necessary to detect chronic trigonitis, urethritis, urethral or bladder diverticula, fistulas, foreign bodies, or bladder wall trabeculation.

RENAL FUNCTION TESTS

Renal function tests are not required in a patient with an initial uncomplicated UTI. **If episodes recur, blood urea nitrogen and serum creatinine levels should be obtained.** If renal insufficiency is present, a creatinine clearance is helpful.

MANAGEMENT

Unless physical examination and urinalysis (bacteriuria) clearly indicate urinary infection, it is advisable to withhold definite antimicrobial therapy until culture and sensitivity reports are available. **As a general rule, bacteriuria should be treated, and not pyuria.** General measures in the management of UTIs involve the following:

1. **Rest and hydration.** Hydration promotes dilution of bacterial counts, frequent bladder emptying, and reduction of medullary osmolality, which assists phagocytosis.
2. **Acidification of the urine.** Ascorbic acid (500 mg twice daily), ammonium chloride (12 g/day in divided doses), or apricot, plum, prune, or cranberry juices have been employed to increase the antibacterial activity of urine and to inhibit bacterial multiplication. Grapefruit juice and carbonated drinks, particularly those containing citrates, turn the urine alkaline and should be avoided.
3. **Urinary analgesics.** Agents such as phenazopyridine hydrochloride (Pyridium), 100 mg twice daily for 2 to 3 days, are often helpful in relieving dysuria.

Basic Principles of Antimicrobial Therapy

The drug selected should be readily available, of low cost, rapidly absorbed from the upper gastrointestinal tract with minimal irritation, and selectively excreted in the urinary tract. **A high serum level of antibiotics is undesirable in the treatment of acute cystitis because it tends to alter normal bacterial flora. Nitrofurantoin (Macrodantin)** produces low serum levels with a half-life of only 19 minutes, thereby minimizing the chances of alteration of intestinal and vaginal bacterial flora. Treatment with nitrofurantoin is effective against all uropathogens except *Proteus* species.

Single-dose therapy is an effective alternative to a 3- to 7-day course, especially in patients with acute uncomplicated cystitis. Single-dose therapy fails, however, in more than 50% of patients with an upper tract infection. Table 23-2 lists some common antibiotic regimens for uncomplicated cystitis along with their relative costs.

For pyelonephritis, an antibiotic should be selected that will attain a significant serum level because the badly infected renal tissue is poorly perfused. The cephalosporins are more effective and cause fewer side effects and relapses. Cephalosporins (e.g., Keflex, Duricef) are slowly and effectively excreted in urine, thereby reducing the frequency of daily drug administration (500 to 1000 mg twice daily).

Antibiotics such as **ampicillin, tetracycline,** and **trimethoprim-sulfamethoxazole** (e.g., Septra, Bactrim) alter the intestinal flora, destroy the normal vaginal

TABLE 23-2

COMMON TREATMENT REGIMENS FOR UNCOMPLICATED BACTERIAL CYSTITIS

Antimicrobial Agent	Dose	Relative Cost*
SINGLE-DOSE TREATMENTS		
Ampicillin[†]	2 g	1
Amoxicillin[†]	3 g	1
Nitrofurantoin	200 mg	1
Fosfomycin tromethamine	3 g (powder)	3
THREE-DAY COURSE		
Ampicillin[†]	250 mg 4 times daily	1
Amoxicillin[†]	500 mg 3 times daily	1
Trimethoprim	100 mg twice daily	2
Ciprofloxacin	250 mg twice daily	3
SEVEN- TO 10-DAY COURSE		
Nitrofurantoin	100 mg at bedtime	3
Nitrofurantoin macrocrystals	50-100 mg 4 times daily	4

*Relative cost: 1-4, less to more expensive.
[†]Resistance among more common uropathogens is increasing.

and periurethral flora, and may result in a relapse of the UTI. **Quinolones**, both first- and second-generation (e.g., **ciprofloxacin, norfloxacin**) have been found to be very effective against uropathogens.

The high pH of urine associated with *Proteus* species infection results from the splitting of urea and the subsequent liberation of ammonia. The urine has a characteristic "fishy" smell. If the urine is very alkaline (pH > 8.0), trimethoprim-sulfamethoxazole should be prescribed.

For patients with renal insufficiency, ampicillin, trimethoprim-sulfamethoxazole, and doxycycline have been shown to reach adequate levels in the urine without toxic levels in serum. Nitrofurantoin should be avoided because high serum levels may lead to peripheral neuropathy. Similarly, tetracycline may lead to

BOX 23-3 *Principles for Bladder Drainage*

- Avoid nonessential catheterization
- Remove catheters promptly
- Use correct sterile procedure for catheterization to avoid introducing bacteria
- Maintain closed drainage
- Disconnect the drainage system only when there is an obstruction
- Avoid prophylactic antibiotics
- Use suprapubic catheterization for prolonged bladder drainage

severe hepatic damage. **Dosages of aminoglycosides should be adjusted in accordance with creatinine clearance, and the serum levels should be monitored.**

RECURRENT URINARY TRACT INFECTIONS

Patients with recurrent infections demonstrate abnormal vaginal biologic factors. Colonization of vaginal and urethral epithelium usually precedes bacteriuria. Bacterial adherence to squamous cells and lack of vaginal antibody to *E. coli* probably lead to vaginal colonization. Women resistant to *E. coli* carry specific antibodies to their own *E. coli.*

The benefit of long-term administration (6 to 18 months) of antimicrobials in women with recurrent UTIs has been demonstrated. Trimethoprim-sulfamethoxazole has been found to be effective and is the only antibacterial agent known to be excreted in vaginal fluid. Sulfonamides, tetracycline, and ampicillin are not effective prophylactically because of the rapid emergence of resistant fecal strains. Recurrent infections tend to occur in clusters. Prolonged remissions often occur between these clusters, and the timing of the clusters cannot be predicted. **Prophylactic therapy should be initiated when the patient has had two infections within 6 months because she faces a 65% chance of another infection within the next 6 months.**

For women who are able to relate the frequently recurring infections to sexual activity, a single dose of an antimicrobial drug immediately after coitus has been shown to prevent bacteriuria and symptomatic infection.

Prevention of hospital-acquired UTIs in patients is important.

Sixty percent of hospital-acquired infections in gynecologic patients involve the urinary tract and occur particularly in association with catheterization. The principles shown in Box 23-3 should be employed when drainage of the urinary bladder is performed.

SUGGESTED READING

American College of Obstetricians and Gynecologists (ACOG): Pelvic organ prolapse. Practice Bulletin No. 85. Washington, DC, ACOG, September 2007.

American College of Obstetricians and Gynecologists (ACOG): Urinary incontinence in women. Practice Bulletin No. 63. Washington, DC, ACOG, June 2005.

American College of Obstetricians and Gynecologists (ACOG): Treatment of urinary tract infections in nonpregnant women. Practice Bulletin No. 91. Obstet Gynecol 111:785-794, 2008.

Bhatia NN, Bradley WE: Neuroanatomy and neurophysiology of the lower urinary tract: Female incontinence. *In* Raz S (ed:) Female Urology. Philadelphia, WB Saunders, 1983, pp 12-32 .

Rahn DD, Marker AC, Corton MM, et al: Does supracervical hysterectomy provide more support to the vaginal apex than total abdominal hysterectomy? Am J Obstet Gynecol 197:650e1-650e4, 2007.

Chapter 24

Ectopic Pregnancy

MOUSA SHAMONKI • ANITA L. NELSON • JOSEPH C. GAMBONE

An ectopic pregnancy is a gestation that implants outside the endometrial cavity. Despite recent advances in earlier detection, it continues to represent a serious hazard to women's health and their future reproductive potential. An ectopic pregnancy is estimated to occur in 1 of every 80 spontaneously conceived pregnancies. More than 95% of ectopic pregnancies implant in various anatomic segments of the fallopian tube, including the ampullary (75% to 80%), isthmic (12%), infundibular and fimbrial (6% to 11%), and interstitial (2%). Other, less common sites of ectopic implantation are the ovary, uterine cervix, and a rudimentary uterine horn. Rarely, an ectopic pregnancy may be intraligamentous or in the peritoneal cavity (abdominal pregnancy). With in vitro fertilization (IVF) and other assisted reproductive technologies (ARTs), the risk for ectopic pregnancy increases substantially, and the location of those ectopic implantations changes (Figure 24-1). Importantly, the risk for heterotropic implantations (one intrauterine and one ectopic) may rise to 1 in 100 with IVF. Other risk factors for an ectopic pregnancy include a history of a previous ectopic pregnancy, a pregnancy after tubal ligation or with an intrauterine device (IUD) in place, and a history of pelvic inflammatory disease (PID).

■ Epidemiology and Etiology

Even though the mortality rates for ectopic pregnancy have dropped as a result of early diagnosis, this condition still causes 4% to 6% of maternal deaths in the United States and is the most common cause of maternal mortality in the first trimester.

In the past two decades, there was a significant increase in diagnosed ectopic pregnancy rates because of the following:

1. Improved technology, which has allowed for earlier and more complete recognition of early ectopic pregnancies, including ectopic pregnancies that would previously have gone undetected
2. Rising incidence of acute and chronic salpingitis, especially related to *Chlamydia trachomatis*
3. Increasing number of tubal surgeries, such as tubal ligation and tubal reconstruction
4. Increase in ARTs, especially IVF

The key to the successful management of ectopic pregnancy is early diagnosis. A high index of suspicion and vigorous efforts at early diagnosis are needed, so "think ectopic!" is a sign that should be in every emergency room.

The etiology of ectopic pregnancy is not always clear but often is associated with known risk factors (Box 24-1). As many as half of cases result from an alteration of tubal transport mechanisms because of damage to the ciliated surface of the endosalpinx caused by infections, such as chlamydia and gonorrhea. Other etiologies include delayed fertilization, possible transmigration of the oocyte to the contralateral tube, and slowed tubal transport, which delays passage of the morula to the endometrial cavity. Chromosomal abnormalities of the fetus are not a cause of ectopic pregnancy.

■ Natural History of Untreated Tubal Ectopic Pregnancy

Tubal pregnancies rapidly invade the tubal mucosa, eroding into the tubal vessels, which are enlarged and engorged. The segment of the affected tube distends

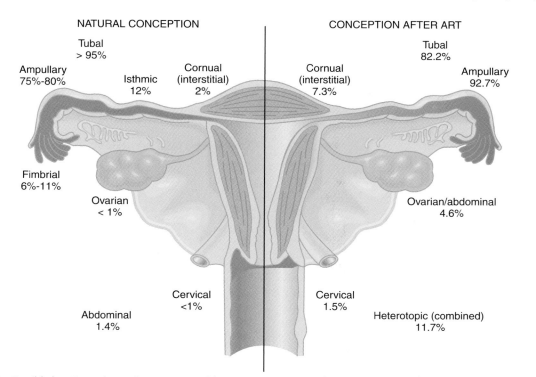

NATURAL CONCEPTION

Tubal
> 95%

Ampullary
75%-80%

Isthmic
12%

Cornual
(interstitial)
2%

Fimbrial
6%-11%

Ovarian
< 1%

Cervical
<1%

Abdominal
1.4%

CONCEPTION AFTER ART

Tubal
82.2%

Cornual
(interstitial)
7.3%

Ampullary
92.7%

Ovarian/abdominal
4.6%

Cervical
1.5%

Heterotopic (combined)
11.7%

FIGURE 24-1   Possible locations of ectopic pregnancy with spontaneous conception vs pregnancies that result from assisted reproductive technologies (ART) such as in vitro fertilization (IVF). *(Modified from Pisarska MD and Carson SA: Incidence and risk factors for ectopic pregnancy. Clin Obstet Gynecol 42[1]:2-8,1999.)*

BOX 24-1   *Risk Factors for Ectopic Pregnancy*

- History of tubal infection
- Cigarette smoking (increased relative risk, 1.26)
- Prior ectopic pregnancy
- History of tubal sterilization within the past 1 to 2 years (higher incidence if cauterization was used)
- History of tubal reconstructive surgery
- Pregnancy with current intrauterine device, depot medroxyprogesterone acetate, or emergency contraceptive pill use
- Infertility due to tubal factors
- Use of assisted reproductive technology

as the pregnancy grows and as blood from the eroded vessels dissects along the tubal wall. Women may have vaginal bleeding or spotting because the pregnancy hormones do not adequately support the endometrial lining and because bleeding from the tube may spill into the uterus as well as into the abdominal cavity. The most common outcomes of established tubal pregnancies include the following:
1. **Tubal rupture,** with resulting intraperitoneal hemorrhage
2. **Pregnancy resorption,** as a result of the restricted blood supply
3. **Tubal abortion into the peritoneal cavity**

Symptoms and Clinical Diagnosis of Ectopic Tubal Pregnancy

The classic triad of symptoms of ectopic pregnancy consists of prior missed menses, vaginal bleeding, and lower abdominal pain. Clinical presentations represent a continuum: (1) acutely ruptured ectopic pregnancy, (2) probable ectopic pregnancy in a symptomatic woman, and (3) possible ectopic pregnancy. Each of these is discussed separately.

ACUTELY RUPTURED ECTOPIC PREGNANCY

The patient who has experienced rupture of her ectopic pregnancy most likely has intraperitoneal hemorrhage and presents with severe abdominal pain and dizziness. She may also complain of ipsilateral shoulder pain from phrenic nerve irritation caused by the blood in her upper abdomen. There may be signs of hemodynamic instability with tachycardia, diaphoresis, hypotension, and even loss of consciousness. Her abdomen may be distended and acutely tender, with guarding and rebound tenderness. The patient usually has cervical motion tenderness and a slightly enlarged, globular uterus. However, she may not have a palpable adnexal mass. The diagnosis is facilitated by a positive urine pregnancy test.

This clinical scenario represents a surgical emergency. Although other tests are often not necessary, an ultrasound would reveal an empty uterus and significant amounts of free fluid in the cul-de-sac. It is critical to establish large-bore intravenous lines and to start fluid resuscitation. Transfusion is important but should not delay emergency surgical intervention (usually by laparotomy, although laparoscopy may be appropriate when a patient is hemodynamically stable).

PROBABLE ECTOPIC PREGNANCY

Women who present with lower pelvic pain and vaginal spotting or bleeding, with or without amenorrhea, can be rapidly tested for pregnancy. The differential diagnosis includes threatened abortion or ectopic pregnancy. The patient generally has other clinical signs, such as tenderness of the abdomen with adnexal or cervical motion tenderness. **The diagnosis of ectopic pregnancy may be confirmed by the absence of intrauterine pregnancy (IUP) on ultrasound in a woman with a level of human chorionic gonadotropin (hCG) that is sufficiently high to guarantee visualization of a normal IUP** (see "Diagnostic Tests" later). There may be a variable amount of free fluid in the cul-de-sac detected by ultrasound. Only occasionally will the ectopic pregnancy be seen on ultrasound as a "double-ring sign" in the adnexa, but a corpus luteum cyst is often present. In such symptomatic women, even though they have stable vital signs, surgical exploration is generally recommended. Conservative surgical procedures, which preserve the fallopian tube, are generally indicated in women desiring future fertility (see "Management" later).

POSSIBLE ECTOPIC PREGNANCY

The most common clinical presentation is that of a possible ectopic pregnancy. Because her symptoms are so mild and nonspecific, **a patient with an ectopic pregnancy may be seen at more than one visit before the diagnosis is confirmed.**

Lower abdominal pain is present in most cases, although it may be mild. Amenorrhea or a history of an abnormal last menstrual period is obtained in 75% to 90% of ectopic pregnancies. Abnormal vaginal bleeding is seen in more than half of patients and ranges from spotting to the equivalent of a normal menstrual period. This spotting or bleeding results from an abnormally low production of hCG by the ectopic trophoblastic tissue. Distinguishing patients with ectopic pregnancy from those with an early threatened abortion or a spontaneous abortion can be challenging.

On physical examination, most patients are afebrile, and less than half have a discernable adnexal mass on pelvic examination. Often, the mass is palpated on the side opposite to the ectopic pregnancy and represents a corpus luteum in the contralateral ovary. The uterus

is soft and is either of normal size or slightly enlarged. On ultrasound, there is a thickened endometrial stripe representing the visible sign of an Arias-Stella reaction, the histologic changes in the endometrial epithelium due to hCG stimulation. There may be a small amount of fluid seen in the cul-de-sac representing some slight intraperitoneal hemorrhage. Rarely is the ectopic pregnancy actually visualized.

DIFFERENTIAL DIAGNOSIS

Many gynecologic and nongynecologic disorders have symptoms in common with ectopic pregnancy and are listed in Box 24-2. A diagnostic algorithm for ectopic pregnancy is illustrated in Figure 24-2.

▣ *Diagnostic Tests*

The diagnosis of early ectopic pregnancy is facilitated by quantitative hCG testing and transvaginal ultrasonography. Office curettage can also be used.

The rapidly dividing fertilized egg begins to produce hCG even before pregnancy occurs, but communication with the maternal circulation to allow detection in maternal serum starts with implantation. The sensitivity of the current methods for detection of hCG in the maternal serum may allow for the confirmation of pregnancy before a missed period.

An accurate diagnosis of ectopic pregnancy requires knowledge of the dynamics of hCG. In the first trimester of normal pregnancies, serum titers of hCG increase exponentially following a nonlinear model. The doubling time of hCG in the serum varies from 1.2 days shortly after implantation to 3.5 days at 2 months after the last menstrual period. Healthy, normally developing pregnancies generally can be detected by a normal rate of increase of maternal serum hCG levels. More than 66% of normal pregnancies show doubling of hCG levels every 48 hours in the first few weeks of pregnancy. However, a normal range exists, and the slowest rise for a normal pregnancy in 2 days is 53%. **If the hCG levels rise by less than 53%, the differential diagnosis includes an abnormal IUP or an**

BOX 24-2   *Differential Diagnosis for Ectopic Pregnancy*

Gynecologic Problems
Threatened or incomplete abortion
Ruptured corpus luteum cyst
Acute pelvic inflammatory disease
Adnexal torsion
Degenerating leiomyoma (especially in pregnancy)

Nongynecologic Problems
Acute appendicitis
Pyelonephritis
Pancreatitis

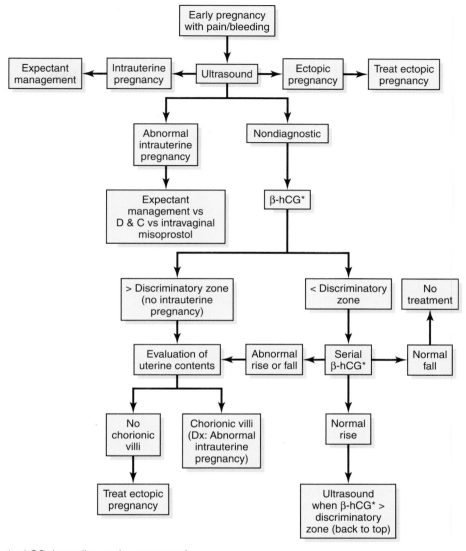

FIGURE 24-2   Diagnostic algorithm for ectopic pregnancy. β-hCG, β-subunit human chorionic gonadotropin; D&C, dilation and curettage; Dx, diagnosis. *(Seeber BE, Barnhart KT: Suspected ectopic pregnancy. Obstet Gynecol 107[2 Part 1]:399-413, 2006.)*

*or hCG depending on the assay used

ectopic pregnancy. **After a spontaneous pregnancy loss, the minimal decline in hCG is 21% to 35% in 2 days. Therefore, if the hCG levels are declining more slowly than 20%, an ectopic pregnancy is likely. Lower levels of hCG (<500) clear from the circulation more slowly than do higher levels.**

There are a number of different assays available today, most of which use at least two separate antibody binding sites to detect the presence or measure the concentration of hCG. **Until there is greater standardization of laboratory testing, it is important to compare over time only titers that are obtained from the same laboratory.** Technically, the **correct test to order today is "hCG,"** but many institutions use the designation "β-hCG" to

determine serial titers of the pregnancy hormone even when the entire molecule is being measured.

Additional tests are often needed to assist in the diagnosis if the patterns in serial hCGs do not give complete results. Transvaginal ultrasound is helpful in diagnosing an ectopic pregnancy by failure to identify an IUP after the hCG levels are adequately high. Although some IUPs may be seen at lower hCG levels, every IUP should be visualized by the time the hCG levels reach the so-called discriminatory zone. The discriminatory zone, or DZ, is defined as the titer of hCG at which an intrauterine sac should reliably be seen with transvaginal ultrasonography in a normal pregnancy. DZ titers differ among institutions, but on

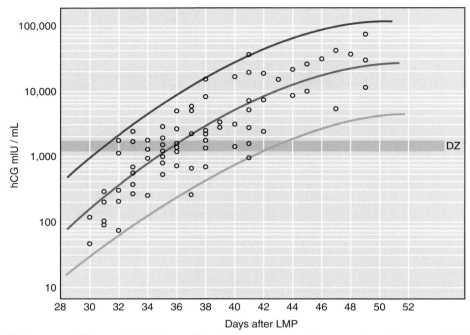

FIGURE 24-3 Distribution curve of human chorionic gonadotropin (hCG) in normal pregnancies with an example of a discriminatory zone (DZ) in *shaded area*. The range of hCG levels (usually 1500 to 2000 mIU/mL per gestation, using the Third International Standard) represents the possible range of the DZ. Every institution should establish a DZ level based on variation in laboratory measurement and the interpretive skill of their ultrasonographer. This DZ level then is recognized as the hCG level above which ultrasound evidence of an intrauterine pregnancy should be seen. LMP, last menstrual period. *(Modified from Pittaway DE, Reisch RL, Wentz AC: Doubling times of human chorionic gonadotropin increase in early variable intrauterine pregnancies. Am J Obstet Gynecol 152:299, 1985.)*

average are equal to 1500 to 2000 mIU/mL of hCG for a singleton pregnancy and 3000 mIU/mL for a twin gestation (Figure 24-3).

An abnormally rising hCG level above 2000 with no gestational sac seen on ultrasound is diagnostic of ectopic pregnancy. However, if the hCG level is below the DZ, an endometrial aspiration with a manual vacuum extractor can be performed. If the hCG levels are not changing appropriately and no products of conception are found on "stat" (immediate) histologic study of the aspirate, the diagnosis of ectopic pregnancy is secure.

Serum progesterone levels greater than 25 ng/mL can reliably indicate a normal IUP, and levels less than 5 ng/mL are consistent with an abnormal pregnancy. However, the value of progesterone testing for ectopic pregnancy is limited by the fact that it requires almost 24 hours to obtain a result and most of the progesterone levels that would be obtained in this situation fall into the gray zone between 5 and 25 ng/mL.

Management

The management of ectopic pregnancy depends on the stability of the patient, the availability of resources, and the desire for future fertility.

SURGICAL MANAGEMENT

Laparotomy is the preferred surgical approach for women who are hemodynamically unstable because rapid access to the bleeding site is critical. Laparotomy is also appropriate whenever it is anticipated that laparoscopy would not be successful, such as when the patient has significant intraperitoneal adhesions from prior surgeries, infection, or endometriosis. **For hemodynamically stable patients, laparoscopy (when available) is the preferred surgical approach because after laparoscopic surgery, patients require fewer days of postoperative hospitalization, suffer less postoperative pain, and recover more quickly.** Laparoscopy also offers the potential to reduce overall treatment costs. If it is determined intraoperatively that laparoscopy is not possible, the surgery can always be converted to laparotomy. Laparoscopy is discussed further in Chapter 30. Figure 24-4 shows a tubal ectopic pregnancy viewed through the laparoscope.

Regardless of the surgical approach, the surgery performed on the fallopian tube itself depends on the amount of tubal damage and the patient's wishes for future fertility. The options include salpingectomy, partial salpingectomy, salpingotomy, and salpingostomy.

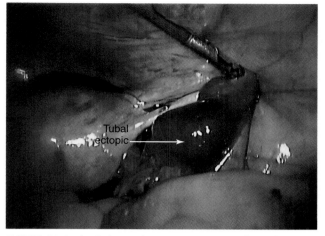

FIGURE 24-4 A tubal ectopic pregnancy as seen through the laparoscope. *(Courtesy of B. Beller, MD, Eugene, Oregon.)*

Salpingectomy (removal of the entire fallopian tube) is recommended when there has been significant damage to the tube, when removal of the damaged elements would leave in place less than 6 cm of functional tube, or when a patient who previously has been sterilized verifies that she still does not desire future fertility. Figure 24-5A illustrates a laparoscopic salpingectomy. **Partial salpingectomy** (removal of a portion of the fallopian tube) is generally performed only if the ectopic pregnancy is implanted in the mid-ampullary portion. The remnants of the tube may be reapproximated in the future. Figure 24-5B illustrates a laparoscopic Endoloop partial salpingectomy. **Salpingotomy** and **salpingostomy** are both procedures in which the ectopic pregnancy site is identified and vasoconstrictive agents are injected beneath the implantation site prior to an incision. With salpingotomy, the incision is closed, whereas it is left open in salpingostomy. An incision is made parallel to the axis of the tube along its antimesenteric border over the site of implantation. The products of conception are removed by gentle dissection or hydrodissection (the use of injected fluid to separate tissues). Bleeding is controlled by judicious use of electrocoagulation. The tube and pelvis are copiously irrigated. Figure 24-5C illustrates a laparoscopic linear salpingostomy. **Most studies have shown that salpingostomy (incision left open), compared with salpingotomy, results in better long-term tubal function.**

There is a 10% to 20% risk for residual trophoblastic tissue whenever the products of conception are dissected from the tube (i.e., when salpingostomy or salpingotomy are performed). Women who do not have resection of the affected tubal areas should have repeat hCG titers 3 to 7 days postoperatively to confirm that no hormone-producing cells remain behind to reinvade the tube. **If repeat hCG titers fail to decline appropriately, methotrexate (MTX) therapy can be** started (see later). The risk for incomplete trophoblastic tissue removal is greatest when the ectopic is "milked" through the tube to extrude through the fimbria. This technique should never be used, even when it appears that the pregnancy is spontaneously aborting through the fimbria. **If there is any concern about significant tubal damage or a high likelihood of retained products of conception, salpingectomy should be performed.**

MEDICAL MANAGEMENT WITH METHOTREXATE

Ambulatory diagnosis and management of women with early, unruptured ectopic pregnancies has replaced surgical diagnosis and treatment in most cases. The most commonly used agent is MTX, which is a folic acid antagonist that inhibits DNA synthesis and cell reproduction. Because of the side effects of MTX and the potential for tubal rupture, careful guidelines for patient selection are required, as shown in Box 24-3.

A suitable patient may be administered MTX in divided doses of 50 mg/m^2 intramuscularly (half of the dose into each buttock). She should return on days 4 and 7 for repeat hCG determinations. If the hCG titers fall at least 15% between those days, the patient can be followed at weekly intervals to verify at least a 15% decline every 7 days until the titers are undetectable (usually <5 mIU/mL). If the titers plateau or fall too slowly, another divided dose of MTX may be given if all the other criteria continue to be met. **If the patient becomes more symptomatic or if hCG titers increase during therapy, surgical intervention is required.** Some centers routinely recommend multiple doses of MTX to reduce treatment failures. Similar outcomes have been shown between single and multidose regimens, and multidose regimens have the disadvantage of needing leucovorin rescue to avoid the significant side effects of relative folate deficiency.

After injection and throughout treatment, patients should be instructed to avoid folate-containing vitamins, nonsteroidal antiinflammatory agents, and alcoholic beverages. Pelvic rest is required. **Effective contraception should be initiated and continued for at least 3 months** after the decrease in hCG titers is observed.

OTHER THERAPEUTIC INTERVENTIONS

When ectopic pregnancy is diagnosed at the time of laparoscopy, **MTX, prostaglandins, or hyperosmolar glucose may be injected into the amniotic sac by a technique called *salpingocentesis*.** The intention is to destroy the ectopic pregnancy without the need for any other procedure. This technique can also be performed transvaginally using ultrasonographic guidance in patients who have not had laparoscopy. The potential advantage of this technique is that it is a one-time injection that reduces systemic side effects. Because information about long-term reproductive function

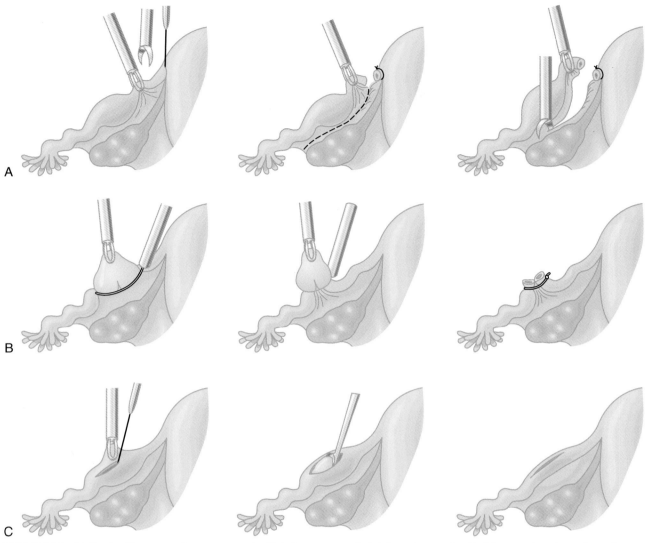

FIGURE 24-5 Methods of laparoscopic management of tubal pregnancy. **A:** Salpingectomy using Endoloop and cautery scissors for isthmic tubal pregnancy. **B:** Partial salpingectomy with Endoloop. **C:** Linear salpingostomy for an ampullary ectopic pregnancy.

after this technique has not yet been reported, its use is still considered experimental.

EXPECTANT MANAGEMENT

Selected patients may qualify for expectant management if they are stable and the diagnosis of ectopic pregnancy is not yet certain or if their symptoms are spontaneously resolving. They must be carefully followed with serial hCG testing and monitoring. As many as 80% of ectopic pregnancies with hCG levels of 1000 mIU/mL or less will not rupture spontaneously or bleed profusely but will undergo spontaneous resolution. Unfortunately, the 20% who experience severe sequelae are not identifiable in advance. **Expectant management is generally reserved for reliable, relatively asymptomatic patients in whom the hCG titers are low enough to make rupture very unlikely (<200 mIU/mL and declining).**

IMPORTANT THERAPEUTIC CONSIDERATIONS

All Rh-negative, unsensitized women who have ectopic pregnancies should receive anti-Rh immunoglobulin (Rh$_O$-GAM). After an ectopic gestation, pregnancy should be avoided for at least 3 months to permit the architecture of the fallopian tube to normalize and to allow complete elimination of MTX, if that agent has been given. Highly effective contraception should be provided as soon as the ectopic pregnancy starts to resolve.

BOX 24-3 *Criteria for Medical Management of Ectopic Pregnancy with Methotrexate*

Indications

Absolute

Hemodynamically stable without active bleeding or signs of hemoperitoneum
Nonlaparoscopic diagnosis
Patient desires future fertility
General anesthesia poses a significant risk
Patient is able to return for follow-up care
No contraindications to methotrexate

Relative

Unruptured mass ≤ 3.5 cm at its greatest dimension
No fetal cardiac motion detected
Patients whose human chorionic gonadotropin level does not exceed a predetermined value (6000-15,000 mIU/mL)

Contraindications

Absolute

Breastfeeding
Overt or laboratory evidence of immunodeficiency
Alcoholism, alcoholic liver disease, or other chronic liver disease
Preexisting blood dyscrasias, such as bone marrow hypoplasia, leukopenia, thrombocytopenia, or significant anemia
Known sensitivity to methotrexate
Active pulmonary disease
Peptic ulcer disease
Hepatic, renal, or hematologic dysfunction

Relative

Gestational sac ≥ 3.5 cm
Embryonic cardiac motion

Data from American College of Obstetricians and Gynecologists (ACOG): Medical management of tubal pregnancy. Practice Bulletin No. 3. Washington, DC, ACOG, December 1998.

Treatment of Uncommon Types of Ectopic Pregnancies

An ovarian ectopic pregnancy produces the same symptoms as a tubal pregnancy. The treatment is aimed at removing the pregnancy and preserving as much normal ovarian tissue as possible. When ovarian preservation is not possible, usually because of profuse bleeding, oophorectomy is indicated. If identified early enough, ovarian ectopic pregnancies may be successfully treated with MTX.

Cervical pregnancy usually presents with profuse vaginal bleeding, and attempts at removal of the pregnancy are often unsuccessful. **MTX and arterial embolization are used to manage cervical pregnancy if the patient is not actively bleeding.** An alternative is to aspirate the cervical ectopic using an oocyte aspiration needle traversing the cervical stroma. Hysterectomy is reserved for large cervical ectopic pregnancies not amenable to nonsurgical intervention and for actively bleeding cervical pregnancies that cannot be controlled conservatively. All patients with cervical ectopic pregnancies should be typed and crossmatched for blood products before surgical intervention is undertaken.

Pregnancies rarely implant in the abdominal cavity (e.g., on the omentum, bowel, or parietal or visceral peritoneum), but if they do so, they may proceed to full term. **At the time of laparotomy in advanced gestations, the placenta presents a major technical difficulty.** Vital organs may be entirely or partially covered by the firmly attached placenta, and any attempt at removal may cause massive bleeding. Partial bowel resection may be required if the bowel is involved. **In most cases, it is best to leave the placenta attached,** especially if the pregnancy is in the second or third trimester, anticipating eventual spontaneous reabsorption. MTX treatment may also be useful to accelerate and enhance placental resorption.

Implications for Future Fertility

Patients who have experienced an ectopic pregnancy are at increased risk for subsequent ectopic pregnancies and problems with infertility. One study demonstrated that the pregnancy rate is just over 80% after either medical or surgical treatment for ectopic pregnancy, with a mean time to conception of 9 to 12 months. Fertility rates are similar after expectant management or surgical intervention. Having one ectopic pregnancy increases the risk for a future ectopic pregnancy by 7- to 13-fold. There is about a 50% to 80% chance that the next pregnancy will be intrauterine and a 10% to 25% chance that it will be ectopic. All patients with recent ectopic pregnancies should receive counseling about this increased risk before attempting another pregnancy.

SUGGESTED READING

American Society for Reproductive Medicine Practice Committee: Revised Practice Committee report on medical treatment of ectopic pregnancy. Fertil Steril 86(Suppl 1):S96-S102, 2006.

Hajenius PJ, Mol F, Mol BW, et al: Interventions for ectopic pregnancy. Cochrane Database Syst Rev 1. CD000324, 2007.

Lipscomb GH: Medical therapy for ectopic pregnancy. Semin Reprod Med 25:93-98, 2007.

Menon S, Colins J, Barnhart KT, et al: Establishing a human chorionic gonadotropin cutoff to guide methotrexate treatment of ectopic pregnancy: A systematic review. Fertil Steril 87:481-484, 2007.

Seeber BE, Barnhart KT: Suspected ectopic pregnancy. Obstet Gynecol 107(2 Pt 1):399-413, 2006.

Chapter 25

Endometriosis and Adenomyosis

JOSEPH C. GAMBONE

Endometriosis and adenomyosis often present difficult diagnostic challenges. In the case of endometriosis, few gynecologic conditions require such difficult surgical dissections.

Endometriosis

Endometriosis is a benign condition in which endometrial glands and stroma are present outside the uterine cavity and walls. Endometriosis is important in gynecology because of its frequency, distressing symptomatology, association with infertility, and potential for invasion of adjacent organ systems, such as the gastrointestinal or urinary tracts.

OCCURRENCE

The prevalence of endometriosis in the general population is not known, but **it is estimated that 5% to 15% of women have some degree of the disease.** At least one third of women with chronic pelvic pain have visualized endometriosis, as do a significant number of infertile women. Interestingly, endometriosis is noted in 5% to 15% of women undergoing gynecologic laparotomies, and it is an unexpected finding in about half of these cases.

 The typical patient with endometriosis is in her 30s, nulliparous, and infertile. However, in practice, many women with endometriosis do not fit the classic picture. Occasionally, endometriosis may occur in infancy, childhood, or adolescence, but at these early ages, it is usually associated with obstructive genital anomalies such as a uterine or vaginal septum. Although endometriosis should regress after menopause unless estrogens are prescribed, 5% of new cases develop in that age group. In addition, the scarifying involution from preexisting lesions may result in obstructive problems, especially in the gastrointestinal and urinary tracts.

PATHOGENESIS

The pathogenesis of endometriosis is not completely understood. Genetic predisposition clearly plays a role. The following three hypotheses have been used to explain the various manifestations of endometriosis and the different locations in which endometriotic implants may be found:

1. **The retrograde menstruation theory** of Sampson proposes that endometrial fragments transported through the fallopian tubes at the time of menstruation implant and grow in various intraabdominal sites. Endometrial tissue, which is normally shed at the time of menstruation, is viable and capable of growth in vivo or in vitro. To explain some rare examples of endometriosis in distant sites, such as the lung, forehead, or axilla, it is necessary to postulate hematogenous spread.

2. **The müllerian metaplasia theory** of Meyer proposes that endometriosis results from the metaplastic transformation of peritoneal mesothelium into endometrium under the influence of certain generally unidentified stimuli.

3. **The lymphatic spread theory** of Halban suggests that endometrial tissues are taken up into the lymphatics draining the uterus and are transported to the various pelvic sites where the tissue grows ectopically. Endometrial tissue has been found in the pelvic lymphatics of up to 20% of patients with the disease.

Most authorities today believe that several factors are involved in the initiation and spread of endometriosis, including retrograde menstruation, coelomic metaplasia, immunologic changes, and genetic predisposition. A fundamental question is why all menstruating women do not develop endometriosis given that most if not all women have retrograde flow into the pelvis during menstruation. The amount of exposure to retrograde flow and the woman's immunologic response appear to be critical. Researchers have identified differences in the chemical composition and biologic pathways of endometrial cells from women with endometriosis compared with unaffected women. They have also found significant differences in the inflammatory factors and growth factors in the peritoneal fluid of affected women. A clearer understanding of the pathophysiology of endometriosis would provide insights into more effective strategies for prevention and treatment.

SITES OF OCCURRENCE

Endometriosis occurs most commonly in the dependent portions of the pelvis. Specifically, implants can be found on the ovaries, the broad ligament, the peritoneal surfaces of the cul-de-sac (including the uterosacral ligaments and posterior cervix), and the rectovaginal septum (Figure 25-1). Quite frequently, the rectosigmoid colon is involved, as is the appendix and the vesicouterine fold of peritoneum. **Endometriosis is occasionally seen in laparotomy scars,** developing especially after a cesarean delivery or myomectomy when the endometrial cavity has been entered. It is probable that endometrial tissue is seeded into the surgical incision. **Two of three women with endometriosis have ovarian involvement.**

PATHOLOGY

Islands of endometriosis respond cyclically to ovarian steroidal hormone production. The implants proliferate under estrogenic stimulation and slough when support from estrogen and progesterone is removed with involution of the corpus luteum. The sloughed material induces a profound inflammatory response resulting immediately in pain and fibrosis in the long term. The macroscopic appearance of endometriosis depends on the site of the implant, activity of the lesion, day of the menstrual cycle, and time since implantation.

Lesions may be raised and flat with red, black, or brown coloration; fibrotic scarred areas that are yellow or white in hue; or vesicles that are pink, clear, or red (Figure 25-2). The color of the implant is generally determined by its vascularity, the size of the lesion, and the amount of residual sloughed material. Newer implants tend to be red, blood-filled active lesions. Older lesions tend to be much less active hormonally, scarred and blue-gray in color with a puckered appearance. These older inactive lesions have been called the "tattooing of endometriosis."

Endometriomas of the ovary are cysts filled with thick, chocolate-colored fluid that sometimes has the black color and tarry consistency of crankcase oil.

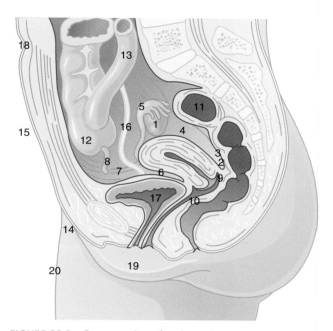

FIGURE 25-1 Common sites of endometriosis in decreasing order of frequency: (1) ovary, (2) cul-de-sac, (3) uterosacral ligaments, (4) broad ligaments, (5) fallopian tubes, (6) uterovesical fold, (7) round ligaments, (8) vermiform appendix, (9) vagina, (10) rectovaginal septum, (11) rectosigmoid colon, (12) cecum, (13) ileum, (14) inguinal canals, (15) abdominal scars, (16) ureters, (17) urinary bladder, (18) umbilicus, (19) vulva, and (20) peripheral sites.

This characteristic fluid represents aged, hemolyzed blood and desquamated endometrium. Usually, endometrial glands and stroma are present in the cyst wall. Sometimes, however, the pressure of the enclosed fluid destroys the endometrial lining of the endometrioma, leaving only a fibrotic cyst wall infiltrated with large numbers of hemosiderin-laden macrophages. Generally, ovarian implants are associated with significant scarring of the ovary to the pelvic side wall or broad ligament. Histologically, two of four characteristics must be found in the endometrioma specimen to confirm the diagnosis—endometrial epithelium, endometrial glands, endometrial stroma, and hemosiderin-laden macrophages.

Although endometriosis is a benign process, it shares many characteristics with malignancy. It is locally infiltrative, invasive, and widely disseminated. It is also curious that cyclic hormones tend to induce growth, whereas continuous hormonal exposure, especially in high doses, generally induces significant regression.

STAGING

The American Society of Reproductive Medicine employs a staging protocol in an attempt to correlate fertility potential with a quantified stage of endometriosis. This staging, which was initially based on the

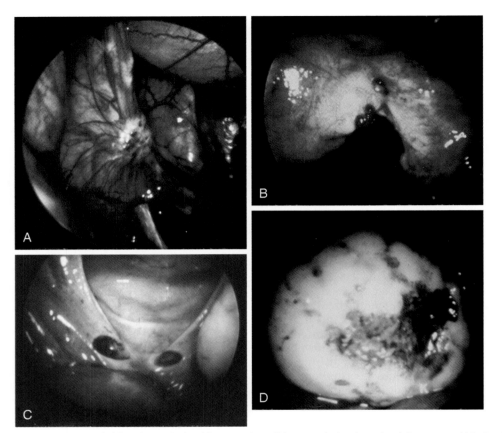

FIGURE 25-2 **A** to **D**: Appearance of old endometriosis with "tattooing" (blue-gray lesions), and red, brown, and black raised lesions of active endometriosis at the time of laparoscopy.

allocation of points depending on the sites involved and extent of visualized disease (Figure 25-3), was modified to include a description of the color of the lesions and the percentage of surface involved in each lesion type, as well as a more detailed description of any endometrioma.

SYMPTOMS

The characteristic triad of symptoms associated with endometriosis is dysmenorrhea, dyspareunia, and dyschezia. The pain that women suffer with endometriosis varies with the time since initiation. Early in the clinical course, women tend to have cyclic pelvic pain, which starts 1 to 2 days before the menstrual flow and resolves at the end of the menses. This secondary dysmenorrhea is thought to be related to the premenstrual swelling and extravasation of blood and menstrual debris, which induces an intense inflammatory reaction in the surrounding tissue mediated by prostaglandins and cytokines that are more directly responsible for triggering the pain sensation. Deep, infiltrating implants, especially those in the retroperitoneal space, are associated with more pain than are superficial lesions. Over time, the pain may become more chronic, with exacerbations at the time of the menses. Interestingly, **there is no clear relationship between the stage of endometriosis and the frequency and severity of pain symptoms.**

Dyspareunia is generally associated with deep-thrust penetration during intercourse and occurs mainly when the cul-de-sac, uterosacral ligaments, and portions of the posterior vaginal fornix are involved. Deep-thrust dyspareunia can also result from uterine immobility due to significant internal scarring caused by endometriosis. Endometriomas in these sites are usually exquisitely tender to palpation.

Dyschezia is experienced with uterosacral, cul-de-sac, and rectosigmoid colon involvement. As the stool passes between the uterosacral ligaments, the characteristic dyschezia is experienced. **Premenstrual and postmenstrual spotting is a characteristic symptom of endometriosis.** Menorrhagia is uncommon, the amount of menstrual flow usually diminishing with endometriosis. If the ovarian capsule is involved with endometriosis, ovulatory pain and midcycle vaginal bleeding often occur. Rarely, as other organ systems are involved, menstrual hematochezia, hematuria, and other forms of endometriotic sloughing become evident.

American Society for Reproductive Medicine
Revised Classification of Endometriosis

Patient's name _____ Date _____

Stage I (minimal)   — 1 – 5
Stage II (mild)   — 6 – 15
Stage III (moderate) — 16 – 40   Laparoscopy _____ Laparotomy _____ Photography _____
Stage IV (severe)   — > 40   Recommended treatment _____

Total _____   Prognosis _____

	Endometriosis	<1 cm	1-3 cm	>3 cm
Peritoneum	Superficial	1	2	4
	Deep	2	4	6
Ovary	R Superficial	1	2	4
	Deep	4	16	20
	L Superficial	1	2	4
	Deep	4	16	20

Posterior cul-de-sac obliteration	Partial		Complete	
	4		40	

	Adhesions	<1/3 Enclosure	1/3 –2/3 Enclosure	>2/3 Enclosure
Ovary	R Filmy	1	2	4
	Dense	4	8	16
	L Filmy	1	2	4
	Dense	4	8	16
Tube	R Filmy	1	2	4
	Dense	4*	8*	16
	L Filmy	1	2	4
	Dense	4*	8*	16

*If the fimbriated end of the fallopian tube is completely enclosed, change the point assignment to 16.
Denote appearance of superficial implant types as red [(R), red, red-pink, flamelike, vesicular blobs, clear vesicles], white [(W), opacifications, peritoneal defects, yellow-brown], or black [(B), black, hemosiderin deposits, blue]. Denote percent of total described as R__%, W__%, and B__%. Total should equal 100%.

FIGURE 25-3   Modified from the revised American Fertility Society classification of endometriosis. *(Reprinted with permission from the American Society for Reproductive Medicine. Fertil Steril 67:819–820, 1996.)*

The association between mild to moderate endometriosis and infertility is not clear. When endometriosis distorts the pelvic structures, its role in infertility is more predictable.

SIGNS

Endometriosis presents with a wide variety of signs varying from the presence of a small, exquisitely tender nodule in the cul-de-sac or on the uterosacral ligaments to a huge, relatively nontender, cystic abdominal mass. Occasionally, a small, tender mulberry-like spot may be seen in the posterior fornix of the vagina.

Characteristically, a tender, fixed adnexal mass is appreciated on bimanual examination. The uterus is fixed and retroverted in a substantial number of women with endometriosis. **Occasionally, no signs at all are appreciated on physical examination.**

DIFFERENTIAL DIAGNOSIS

The main differential diagnoses in the acute phase of endometriosis are (1) chronic pelvic inflammatory disease or recurrent acute salpingitis, (2) hemorrhagic corpus luteum, (3) benign or malignant ovarian neoplasm, and occasionally, (4) ectopic pregnancy.

DIAGNOSIS

The diagnosis of endometriosis should be suspected in an afebrile patient with the characteristic triad of pelvic pain, a firm, fixed, tender adnexal mass, and tender nodularity in the cul-de-sac and uterosacral ligaments. The characteristic sharp, firm, exquisitely tender "barb" (from barbed wire) felt in the uterosacral ligament is the diagnostic sine qua non of endometriosis, but this finding is generally present only in severe cases. An ultrasonic evaluation may indicate an adnexal mass of complex echogenicity, with internal echoes consistent with old blood. Serum levels of the cancer antigen CA 125 are frequently elevated in women with endometriosis. However, the positive predictive value of CA 125 for detecting endometriosis is low (about 20%), and this test should not used to diagnose endometriosis.

The definitive diagnosis is generally made by the characteristic gross and histologic findings obtained at laparoscopy or laparotomy. Unfortunately, even the most experienced surgeon may fail to identify endometriotic implants visually because the older implants may have a very subtle appearance and the deeper infiltrating lesions may not be visible at the surface. Biopsy of any suspicious lesions improves diagnostic accuracy.

MANAGEMENT

The management of endometriosis depends on certain key considerations: (1) the certainty of the diagnosis, (2) the severity of the symptoms, (3) the extent of the disease, (4) the desire for future fertility, (5) the age of the patient, and (6) the threat to the gastrointestinal or urinary tract or both.

Treatment is indicated for endometriosis associated pelvic pain, dysmenorrhea, dyspareunia, abnormal bleeding, ovarian cysts, and infertility due to gross distortion of tubal and ovarian anatomy. Surgical intervention is required for an endometrioma larger than 3 cm, gross distortion of pelvic anatomy, involvement of bowel or bladder, and adhesive disease. Surgery may improve fertility for women with severe endometriosis. Medical therapy is generally the first line to treat other symptomatic women. **There is no convincing evidence that treatment significantly improves fertility in women with mild endometriosis.**

Surgical Treatments

The most comprehensive surgery includes total abdominal hysterectomy, bilateral salpingo-oophorectomy with destruction of all peritoneal implants, and dissection of all adhesions. Usually, an appendectomy is also performed. Because of extensive adhesions, surgery for endometriosis is often technically challenging. If endometriosis involves the cul-de-sac or uterosacral ligaments, the proximity to the ureter, bladder, and sigmoid colon must be considered. If endometriosis obstructs the ureter, resection and ureteroplasty may be necessary to preserve renal function. **Nearly 25% of kidneys are lost when endometriosis blocks the ureter.** Obstruction of the rectosigmoid and even obstruction of the small intestine may require resection of the involved intestinal segment. The surgical risks must be carefully explained to the woman, as well as her subsequent need for treatment for loss of ovarian steroids. She also needs to understand that postoperatively, there is a 20% recurrence rate for endometriosis, usually involving the bowel.

Often the desire for future fertility precludes this surgical option. In this situation, laparoscopic or open surgery is designed to destroy all endometriotic implants and remove all adhesive disease. This usually involves excision (not lysis) of all adhesions and laser ablation or electrocautery of suspected implants. **Large endometriomas (>3 cm) are amenable only to surgical resection.** Because of extensive adhesive disease that generally surrounds these cysts, cystectomy is not always possible; oophorectomy may be necessary. Extensive tubal disease with or without ovarian involvement may be treated with removal of the affected organs but with uterine preservation for in vitro fertilization. **Preoperative treatment with medical agents, such as gonadotropin-releasing hormone (GnRH) agonists for 3 to 6 months can improve surgical success.**

The role of medical therapy postoperatively remains controversial, although it is indicated to treat women who have known residual disease diagnosed at surgery. **There is a risk for recurrence of endometriosis throughout a woman's life**, so measures should be taken to reduce her risk for retrograde menstruation or cyclic ovarian sex steroid production. Depot medroxyprogesterone acetate (DMPA), continuous oral contraceptives, and the levonorgestrel-releasing intrauterine device (IUD) are all attractive long-term options.

Medical Treatments

Therapy should be targeted toward relieving the patient's individual complaints and toward reducing the risk for disease progression. Asymptomatic women found incidentally to have endometriosis may not require any therapy. Dysmenorrhea due to endometriosis can be approached as outlined in Chapter 21, using nonsteroidal antiinflammatory drugs (NSAIDs) and reduction of menstrual flow with hormonal regimens such as low-dose oral contraceptives.

For relief of non-cyclic pelvic pain, short-term medical treatment may be used. NSAIDs, oral contraceptives, and progestins (e.g., medroxyprogesterone acetate) should be considered the appropriate first-line medical treatments for symptomatic endometriosis. When an inadequate response occurs, second-line medical treatment with either a GnRH agonist, higher-dose progestins, or danazol appears to be equally effective.

Cost, individual response, and potential side effects generally guide selection of one agent or the other.

Danazol is an androgenic derivative that may be used in a "pseudomenopause" regimen to suppress symptoms of endometriosis if fertility is not a present concern. It is given over a period of 6 to 9 months, and doses of 600 to 800 mg daily are generally necessary to suppress menstruation. Through its weak androgenic properties, danazol decreases the plasma levels of sex hormone–binding globulin. The resulting increase of free testosterone may cause hirsutism and acne. **Three years after cessation of danazol, 40% of patients have a recurrence of endometriosis. After a full course of danazol therapy, use of a cyclic oral contraceptive may help to delay or prevent such recurrence.**

GnRH agonists cause a temporary medical castration, thereby bringing about a marked, albeit temporary, regression of endometriosis. Treatment of women with endometriosis with GnRH agonists usually produces relief of pain and involution of implants. The disadvantages of these agonists are related to cost, hot flashes, and side effects, including vaginal dryness. They also cause calcium loss from bone and an unfavorable lipid profile. If treatment with a GnRH agonist is effective in relieving chronic pelvic pain and surgery is not indicated, low-dose estrogen-progestin add-back therapy can permit longer-term use of GnRH agonists by mitigating the adverse impact of estrogen deficiency without reducing the efficacy of GnRH agonists.

Oral contraceptives and oral medroxyprogesterone acetate are more effective in treating endometriosis-associated pelvic pain than placebos. The levonorgestrel-releasing intrauterine system reduces dysmenorrhea and may be helpful for inducing regression of cul-de-sac implants without diminishing circulating estrogen levels in the serum.

Surgical and medical treatment options for endometriosis are summarized in Box 25-1.

PREVENTION OF ENDOMETRIOSIS

Whenever severe dysmenorrhea occurs in a young patient, the possibility of varying degrees of obstruction to the menstrual flow must be considered. The possibility of a blind uterine horn in a bicornuate uterus or an obstructing uterine or vaginal septum should be kept in mind. **In more than half of patients who are noted to develop endometriosis during childhood and adolescence, varying degrees of genital tract obstruction may be found.** Whenever a congenital abnormality of the urinary or intestinal tract is detected, the genital tract should be investigated for an obstructive lesion. Infants with genital tract obstruction have been noted to develop endometriosis even in the first year of life. **In all women, minimization of menstrual flow and suppression of ovarian cycling can reduce the risk for endometriosis.**

BOX 25-1 *Treatment Options for Endometriosis*

Surgical

Most definitive: Total abdominal hysterectomy with bilateral salpingo-oophorectomy (TAH-BSO) with destruction and removal of all peritoneal endometriotic implants and adhesions.
NOTE: As is the case with all treatments for endometriosis, there is always a risk for recurrence, even with "definitive" treatment.
Fertility preserving: Laparoscopic or open surgery (laparotomy) with destruction and removal of all peritoneal endometriotic implants and adhesions.
NOTE: Any endometriomas >3 cm in diameter should be removed surgically. Preoperative treatment for 3 to 6 months can improve surgical success.

Medical

First-line: Nonsteroidal antiinflammatory drugs, low-dose oral contraceptives, or progestins (e.g., medroxyprogesterone acetate)
NOTE: This treatment should be given an adequate trial of 3 to 6 months before initiating second-line therapy.
Second-line: Higher doses of progestins (e.g., medroxyprogesterone acetate, or Megace), danazol, or gonadotropin-releasing hormone analogues appear to be equally effective.
NOTE: Laparoscopic confirmation of the diagnosis of endometriosis before initiation of second-line treatment may be performed but is not required.

Adenomyosis

Adenomyosis is defined as the extension of endometrial glands and stroma into the uterine musculature more than 2.5 mm beneath the basalis layer. Often this is an incidental finding on pathologic examination when it is seen in up to 60% of women in their 40s. **About 15% of patients with adenomyosis have associated endometriosis.** Islands of adenomyosis do not participate in the proliferative and secretory cycles induced by the ovary.

PATHOLOGY

Generally, the gross appearance of the uterus consists of diffuse enlargement with a thickened myometrium containing characteristic glandular irregularities, with implants containing both glandular tissue and stroma (Figure 25-4). The endometrial cavity is also enlarged. Occasionally, the adenomyosis may be confined to one portion of the myometrium and take the form of a fairly well-circumscribed adenomyoma. Contrary to the picture in a uterine myoma, no distinct capsular margin can be detected on cut section between the adenomyoma and the surrounding myometrium. The distinction between adenomyosis and uterine leiomyoma may not always be clear on ultrasonic examination. Figure 25-5 illustrates the typical gross appearance of an enlarged uterus with extensive adenomyosis.

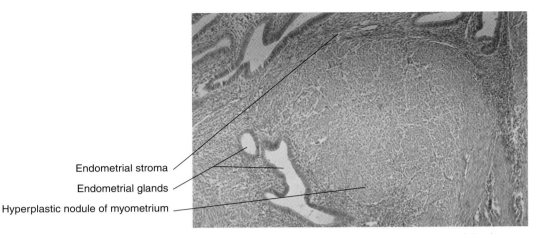

Endometrial stroma

Endometrial glands

Hyperplastic nodule of myometrium

FIGURE 25-4   Histologic illustration of adenomyosis causing the enlargement of the uterus. A hyperplastic nodule of myometrium is seen. Note the endometrial glands and stroma.

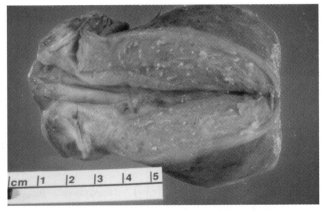

FIGURE 25-5   Enlarged uterus cut open to demonstrate homogeneous enlargement due to adenomyosis. A diagnosis of leiomyomas may be incorrectly made at the time of pelvic examination. *(Courtesy of Dr. Sathima Natarajan, Ronald Reagan–UCLA Medical Center.)*

SYMPTOMS

Although many women are asymptomatic, those who suffer from this condition typically complain of severe secondary dysmenorrhea and menorrhagia. Even though the islands do not cycle in response to ovarian hormonal stimulation, there is still prostaglandin release and local inflammatory changes that can induce pain and tenderness and may disrupt the vasoconstriction of the arterial arcade supplying the endometrium. Deep-thrust dyspareunia, especially premenstrually, can be caused by adenomyosis.

SIGNS

On pelvic examination, the uterus is generally symmetrically enlarged and somewhat boggy and tender if the examination is conducted premenstrually. Occasionally, it may enlarge asymmetrically, which makes it very difficult to distinguish adenomyosis from a myomatous uterus. The consistency of the enlarged adenomyomatous uterus is generally softer than that of a uterine myoma.

TREATMENT

The treatment of adenomyosis depends entirely on the symptoms and the possibility of other diagnoses. Any history of new onset or worsening menorrhagia, particularly in a woman with risk factors for endometrial cancer, should be investigated by endometrial biopsy or fractional dilation and curettage with or without hysteroscopy to rule out malignancy. **Conservative management with NSAIDs and hormonal control of the endometrium are mainstays of therapy.** Combination oral contraceptives or hormone-containing patches and vaginal rings may be used to reduce cyclic blood loss and menstrual pain. DMPA, levonorgestrel IUD, and continuous oral contraceptive pills can be used to try to achieve amenorrhea. If the woman is not a candidate for any of these medical interventions or if medical treatments do not sufficiently control her symptoms, **hysterectomy may be indicated. Endometrial ablation to control the bleeding is another option.**

SUGGESTED READING

D'Hooghe TM, Hill JA: Endometriosis. *In* Berek JS (ed): Berek & Novak's Gynecology, 14th ed. Philadelphia, Lippincott Williams & Wilkins, 2007, pp 1137-1184.

Gambone JC, Mittman BS, Munro MG, et al: Consensus statement for the management of chronic pelvic pain and endometriosis: Proceedings of an expert-panel consensus process. Fertil Steril 78:961-972, 2002.

Stratton P, Sinaii N, Segars J, et al: Return of chronic pelvic pain from endometriosis after raloxifene treatment: A randomized controlled trial. Obstet Gynecol 111:88-96, 2008.

Wen D, Guo SW: The search for genetic variants predisposing women to endometriosis. Curr Opin Obstet Gynecol 19: 395-401, 2007.

Chapter 26

Family Planning

REVERSIBLE CONTRACEPTION, STERILIZATION, AND ABORTION

ANITA L. NELSON

Family planning plays a critical role in promoting the personal health of women, and it uniquely optimizes both maternal health and fetal well-being by allowing couples to plan and prepare for the pregnancies they desire. As such, family planning also has major public health implications.

Condoms and oral contraceptives (OCs) were recognized by the U.S. Centers for Disease Control and Prevention (CDC) as among the 10 most important public health inventions of the 20th century. Considering that this was the century in which vaccinations and treatments for smallpox, polio, yellow fever, and many other diseases that had plagued humans for eons were developed, such recognition highlights the magnitude of the contributions these birth control methods have made. Every year, 600,000 women die worldwide from pregnancy and pregnancy-related causes, and another 3 million women suffer significant permanent disabilities.

Many contraceptive methods also help reduce the spread of some sexually transmitted infections (STIs). For example, even though only 13% of married African women use effective barrier methods of contraception, it has been estimated that, in 2002, those birth control methods prevented 173,000 cases of human immunodeficiency virus (HIV) infection in sub-Saharan Africa.

As effective as modern contraceptives have been, they have not yet achieved their full potential. **Nearly half of pregnancies in the United States are classified as "unintended,"** meaning that the woman electively aborts the pregnancy, or continues with a pregnancy that she did not plan. Many unintended pregnancies occur in women who are using contraception but are not using their chosen method correctly. Nearly 1 million pregnancies occur every year in women taking OCs. More than half of OC users miss three or more pills

each cycle, and many do not refill their prescriptions on a timely basis. Pregnancies that are categorized as "intended" include planned and prepared pregnancies as well as pregnancies to which women are indifferent.

When birth control methods in sexually active women are grouped into tiers based on their efficacy with typical use (Table 26-1), it becomes obvious that the most efficient methods are those that are long-term, convenient, and do not require any ongoing action from the woman (Tier 1). For example, the **intrauterine devices (IUDs) and progestin implants provide the highest level of pregnancy protection, with first-year failure rates in typical use of less than 1%** (Table 26-2). Other hormonal methods, such as the once-every-3-months injection, monthly vaginal rings, weekly patches, and daily pills are in tier 2. Each of these hormonal methods has the potential for very low pregnancy rates (1%), but in typical use, they have first-year failure rates of 7% to 8%. **Tier 3 contraceptive methods are the barrier and behavioral methods.** Here the differential between the potential that the method offers and what is really seen is widest. For example, male condoms have a less than 2% failure rate if used correctly and consistently with every episode of intercourse. However, in real life, the pregnancy rate is 17.4%. Female barrier methods (diaphragms, cervical caps, shields, and female condoms) have higher pregnancy rates. Interestingly, **behavioral methods such as coitus interruptus and fertility awareness methods have rates that are almost equivalent to many barrier methods in typical use.**

The mechanisms of action vary among method of family planning. Contrary to prevailing opinion, the primary action of virtually all methods of birth control is contraception (the prevention of fertilization). Abortion is the disruption of an established pregnancy. Interception is defined as an action that blocks

TABLE 26-1

TIERS OF EFFICACY	
Tier	**Method of Contraception**
1: Longer term	Progestin implants and intrauterine devices
2: Combined hormonal	Depot medroxyprogesterone acetate injections Vaginal rings, transdermal patches Oral contraceptive pills
3: Barrier and behavioral	Male condoms, diaphragms Caps, female condoms, shield Spermicides Withdrawal, fertility awareness method, natural family planning

TABLE 26-2

CONTRACEPTIVE FAILURE RATES COMPARING TYPICAL USE AND PERFECT USE		
	Percent Failure within First Year of Use	
Contraceptive Method	*Perfect Use*	*Typical Use*
No method	85	85
Male sterilization	0.10	0.15
Female sterilization	0.5	0.5
Copper ParaGard T 380A IUD	0.6	0.8
Levonorgestrel-releasing IUD	0.1	0.1
DMPA	0.3	6.7
OC—combined	0.3	8.7
OC—progestin only	0.5	8.7
Diaphragm with spermicide	6	16
Condom—male, latex	2	17.4
Cervical cap—parous	26	32
Cervical cap—nulliparous	9	16
Spermicides	15	29
Fertility awareness	19	25.3
Withdrawal	—	18.4

DMPA, depot medroxyprogesterone acetate; OC, oral contraceptive.
1. Kost K, Singh S, Vaughan B, Trussell J, Bankole A. Estimates of contraceptive failure from the 2002 National Survey of Family Growth. Contraception. 2008;77(1):10-21.
2. Hatcher RA, Trussell J, Nelson AL, Cates W Jr, Stewart FH, Kowal D. *Contraceptive Technology*, 19th ed. New York, Ardent Media, Inc. 2007

implantation (i.e., one that works after fertilization but before pregnancy is established 7 days later).

The safety of all methods of family planning is well established. In selecting options for an individual woman, the requirement is that any method offered must be safer to the woman's health than pregnancy. It is from that perspective that the World

Health Organization (WHO) has developed its Medical Eligibility Criteria (MEC; Table 26-3), which rates the appropriateness of each major contraceptive method in a variety of medical circumstances. Recommendations are made on a 1 to 4 scale, in which a rating of 1 indicates approval and 4 represents an absolute contraindication. This rating often differs from the labeling for individual products, which generally reflects theoretical concerns and desires by the manufacturers to protect themselves from product liability. Prescribers should act on evidence-based recommendations such as the WHO MEC.

Contraception

TIER 1 CONTRACEPTIVE OPTIONS

Intrauterine contraceptives and implants are the most effective, reversible methods available to women at risk for pregnancy. Typical failure rates closely correspond to those seen with correct use (see Table 26-2). Each is also very safe and can be used by women with serious medical conditions for whom pregnancy may be very dangerous.

Contraceptive Implants

In the United States, only one implant is currently available—a single-rod system called **Implanon**. The contraceptive rod measures 4 cm in length and 2 mm in diameter. The progestin, **etonogestrel**, is mixed into the matrix of the plastic rod. The rate at which etonogestrel is released is controlled by a releasing membrane that surrounds the rod. **This rod is indicated for up to 3 years of use.** In clinical trials around the world, involving the experience of more than 58,000 women-cycles, not a single woman became pregnant when the rod was in place. Because **some women conceived within 2 weeks of removal**, those pregnancies are included as possible method failures, bringing the first-year failure rate in the United States to 0.38%.

The implant is placed in the subcutaneous tissue of the inner aspect of a woman's upper nondominant arm. **Placement is done in the office** in a 1-minute procedure. Virtually every woman is a candidate for this convenient, rapidly reversible method. Only women who have had breast cancer within the last 5 years have an absolute contraindication to use of the contraceptive rod. Women who use anticonvulsants, such as phenobarbital or dilantin, which increase cytochrome P-450 enzyme activity, will have higher failure rates, as will women using nonprescription therapies, such as St. John's Wort.

The contraceptive rod was designed to release etonogestrel at levels adequate to suppress ovulation. With detailed ultrasonic and laboratory testing, it was demonstrated that no woman with the rod ovulated during the first 30 months of use, and during the last

TABLE 26-3

WORLD HEALTH ORGANIZATION MEDICAL ELIGIBILITY FOR INITIATING CONTRACEPTION: ABSOLUTE AND RELATIVE CONTRAINDICATIONS

Condition	Qualifier for Condition	Risk Level*					
		Estrogen-Progestin: Pill, Patch, Ring	Progestin-Only: Pill	Progestin-Only: Injection	Progestin-Only: Implant	Progestin IUD	Copper IUD
Anemia	Thalassemia	1	1	1	1	1	2
	Sickle cell disease	2	1	1	1	1	2
	Iron-deficiency anemia	1	1	1	1	1	2
Breast cancer	Family history of cancer	1	1	1	1	1	1
	Current	4	4	4	4	4	1
	In past, no evidence of disease for >5 yr	3	3	3	3	3	1
Breast problems, benign	Undiagnosed mass	2	2	2	2	2	1
	Benign breast disease	1	1	1	1	1	1
Cervical cancer	Cervical intraepithelial neoplasia	2	1	2	2	2	1
	Awaiting treatment	2	1	2	2	4	4
Cervical ectropion		1	1	1	1	1	1
Depression		1	1	1	1	1	1
Diabetes mellitus (DM)	History of gestational DM only	1	1	1	1	1	1
	DM without vascular disease	2	2	2	2	2	1
	DM with end-organ damage or >20 years duration	3	2	3	2	2	1
Drug interactions	Antiretrovirals	2	2	2	2	2	2
	Certain anticonvulsants	3	3	2	3	1	1
	Griseofulvin	2	2	1	2	1	1
	Rifampin	3	3	2	3	1	1
	ALL OTHER ANTIBIOTICS	1	1	1	1	1	1
Endometrial cancer		1	1	1	1	4	4
Endometriosis		1	1	1	1	1	2
Gallbladder disease	Asymptomatic gallstones	2	2	2	2	2	1
	Symptomatic gallstones, without cholecystectomy	3	2	2	2	2	1
	Gallstones treated with cholecystectomy	2	2	2	2	2	1
	Pregnancy-related cholestasis in past	2	1	1	1	1	1
	Hormone-related cholestasis in past	3	2	2	2	2	1
Headaches	Nonmigrainous	1	1	1	1	1	1
Headaches: migraines	Without aura, age <35 yr	2	1	2	2	2	1
	Without aura, age >35 yr	3	1	2	2	2	1
	With aura, any age	4	2	2	2	2	1
HIV infection	High risk	1	1	1	1	2	2
	HIV infected	1	1	1	1	2	2
	AIDS (without drug interactions)	1	1	1	1	3	3

*Risk levels are as follows: (1) method can be used without restriction; (2) advantages generally outweigh theoretical or proven risks; (3) method not usually recommended unless other, more appropriate methods are not available or not acceptable; (4) method not to be used. These contraceptive methods do not protect against sexually transmitted infections (STIs). Condoms should be used to protect against STIs. For more information, see http://www.who.int/reproductive-health/publications/mec/mec.pdf.

Continued

TABLE 26-3

WORLD HEALTH ORGANIZATION MEDICAL ELIGIBILITY FOR INITIATING CONTRACEPTION: ABSOLUTE AND RELATIVE CONTRAINDICATIONS—cont'd

Condition	Qualifier for Condition	Estrogen-Progestin: Pill, Patch, Ring	Progestin-Only: Pill	Progestin-Only: Injection	Progestin-Only: Implant	Progestin IUD	Copper IUD
Hypertension	During prior pregnancy only—now resolved	2	1	1	1	1	1
	Well controlled	3	1	2	1	1	1
	Systolic 140-159 mm Hg or diastolic 90-99 mm Hg	3	1	2	1	1	1
	Systolic >160 mm Hg or diastolic >100 mm Hg	4	2	3	2	2	1
	With vascular disease	4	2	3	2	2	1
Ischemic heart disease	Past or current	4	2	3	2	2	1
Liver disease	Cirrhosis—mild	3	2	2	2	2	1
	Cirrhosis—severe	4	3	3	3	3	1
	Tumors—benign	4	3	3	3	3	1
	Tumors—malignant	4	3	3	3	3	1
	Viral hepatitis—carrier	1	1	1	1	1	1
	Viral hepatitis—active	4	3	3	3	3	1
Obesity	BMI >30 kg/m^2	2	1	1	1	1	1
Ovarian cancer		1	1	1	1	3	3
Ovarian cysts and benign tumors		1	1	1	1	1	1
Pelvic inflammatory disease	Past, with subsequent pregnancy	1	1	1	1	1	1
	Past, without subsequent pregnancy	1	1	1	1	2	2
	Current	1	1	1	1	4	4
Postpartum, not breast-feeding	<48 hr	3	1	1	1	3	2
	2-21 days	3	1	1	1	3	3
	3-4 wk	1	1	1	1	3	3
	>4 wk	1	1	1	1	1	1
Postpartum and breast-feeding	<6 wk postpartum	4	3	3	3	Same as postpartum, not breastfeeding	
	6 wks to 6 mo postpartum	3	1	1	1	1	1
	> 6 mo postpartum	2	1	1	1	1	1
Postabortion	First trimester	1	1	1	1	1	1
	Second trimester	1	1	1	1	2	2
	Immediately after septic abortion	1	1	1	1	4	4
Sexually transmitted infections	Vaginitis	1	1	1	1	2	2
	High risk	1	1	1	1	3	3
	Current gonorrheal culture, chlamydia, purulent cervicitis	1	1	1	1	4	4
Smoking	Age < 35 yr	2	1	1	1	1	1
	Age > 35 yr, < 15 cigarettes/day	3	1	1	1	1	1
	Age > 35 yr, >15 cigarettes/day	4	1	1	1	1	1
Seizure disorder	Without drug interactions	1	1	1	1	1	1

TABLE 26-3

WORLD HEALTH ORGANIZATION MEDICAL ELIGIBILITY FOR INITIATING CONTRACEPTION: ABSOLUTE AND RELATIVE CONTRAINDICATIONS—cont'd

Condition	Qualifier for Condition	Risk Level*					
		Estrogen-Progestin: Pill, Patch, Ring	Progestin-Only: Pill	Progestin-Only: Injection	Progestin-Only: Implant	Progestin IUD	Copper IUD
Stroke		4	2	3	2	2	1
Surgery	Minor, without prolonged immobilization	1	1	1	1	1	1
	Major, without prolonged immobilization	2	1	1	1	1	1
	Major, with prolonged immobilization	4	2	2	2	2	1
Thyroid disorders	Simple goiter, hyperthyroidism, hypothyroidism	1	1	1	1	1	1
Uterine fibroids	Without distortion of uterine cavity	1	1	1	1	1	1
	With distortion of uterine cavity	1	1	1	1	4	4
Valvular heart disease	Uncomplicated	2	1	1	1	1	1
	Complicated	4	1	1	1	2	2
Varicose veins		1	1	1	1	1	1
Venous thrombosis	Family history (first-degree relatives)	2	1	1	1	1	1
	Superficial thrombophlebitis	2	1	1	1	1	1
	Past DVT	4	2	2	2	2	1
	Current DVT	4	3	3	3	3	1

*Risk levels are as follows: (1) method can be used without restriction; (2) advantages generally outweigh theoretical or proven risks; (3) method not usually recommended unless other, more appropriate methods are not available or not acceptable; (4) method not to be used. These contraceptive methods do not protect against sexually transmitted infections (STIs). Condoms should be used to protect against STIs. For more information, see http://www.who.int/reproductive-health/publications/mec/mec.pdf.

BMI, body mass index; DVT, deep venous thrombosis; IUD, intrauterine device.

From http://www.reproductiveaccess.org/contraception/WHO_chart.htm#top and http://www.rhedi.org/contraception/who_chart.php. Reprinted with permission of the Reproductive Health Access Project.

6 months of use, only three ovulations occurred. Pregnancy was prevented in the latter cases presumably because the thickened cervical mucus blocked sperm entry into the upper genital tract. The progestin released also affects the endometrium. These endometrial changes do not contribute in any meaningful way to pregnancy protection but do alter bleeding patterns, which become "unpredictably unpredictable." Women can alternate among amenorrhea, oligomenorrhea, and regular menses. Women should be advised to carry light-day panty liners to be prepared for the unscheduled bleeding and spotting. Return to fertility is rapid after removal of the implant. Removal may be accomplished as an office procedure in less than 3 minutes.

Other contraceptive implants are available outside the United States. The original **Norplant-6,** with six capsules filled with levonorgestrel powder, and the **Jadelle 2 implant system** each provide almost equivalent pregnancy protection for up to 5 years.

Intrauterine Contraceptives

There are two intrauterine contraceptives available in the United States: **the copper T 380A intrauterine device** (Copper-T-IUD) and the **levonorgestrel-releasing intrauterine system** (LNG-IUS). They both offer pregnancy protection equivalent to sterilization and should be seriously considered as an alternative in any woman considering that procedure.

The Copper T-380A IUD (Figure 26-1) is approved by the U.S. Food and Drug Administration for 10 years of use, but studies show it remains very effective for at least 20 years. This IUD provides excellent pregnancy protection that is convenient and rapidly reversible. First-year failure rates are 0.7%, and cumulative 10- to 12-year pregnancy rates are 1.4% to 1.9%. Most women are candidates for IUD use, including those with serious medical problems such as hypertension, morbid obesity, diabetes, stroke, myocardial infarction, and cancer.

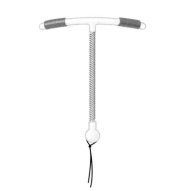

FIGURE 26-1 Copper T 380A intrauterine device.

The only absolute contraindications to immediate IUD placement are active infection or cancer in the cervix or uterus, distortion of the uterine cavity, or a uterine cavity that is not the correct size (6 to 9 cm in depth) to accommodate the device.

The copper IUD works as a contraceptive by immobilizing and killing sperm. Women using this IUD should check their tail strings monthly to verify that their device is still in place. They should be advised that their menses may be heavier and longer.

For women who have heavy or painful menses, the LNG-IUS is generally a better choice. This system is effective for at least 5 years. With first-year failure rates of 0.14%, the LNG-IUS prevents conception by thickening the cervical mucus to prevent sperm entry into the upper genital tract. Over time, the high doses of progestin profoundly change the endometrium, which is reflected in the user's bleeding patterns. Women generally experience frequent episodes of unscheduled bleeding and spotting in the early months, following which bleeding becomes rare. **By 12 months, 20% of women have no bleeding or spotting, and the most common pattern seen is 1 to 3 days of spotting a month.** Hence, hemoglobin levels rise.

In virtually every country, the LNG-IUS is approved for both contraception and for treatment of heavy, prolonged vaginal bleeding. It is at least as effective as endometrial ablation in this regard.

TIER 2 CONTRACEPTIVES: COMBINED HORMONAL PRODUCTS AND PROGESTIN-ONLY INJECTIONS AND PILLS

All these methods work primarily by thickening cervical mucus and by blocking the luteinizing hormone surge to prevent ovulation. Each of these hormonal methods has about the same failure rate in typical use (8%), and each has the potential for much higher efficacy if used correctly and consistently (0.3% to 2%).

Barriers to successful use must be removed to help women achieve more success with these methods. Quick-start protocols should be followed to allow women immediate access to protection. Any of these methods can be started any day of a woman's cycle as long as she is not pregnant, uses emergency contraception (EC) if she had unprotected intercourse in the prior 5 days, and uses condoms for 7 to 9 days afterward until her hormonal method can reliably protect her. **Routine provision of EC in advance of need** provides backup for inevitable lapses in ongoing contraceptive use.

Combined Hormonal Products

Combined hormonal contraceptives with synthetic estrogens and progestins are available as once-daily pills, once-a-week transdermal patches, and once-a-month vaginal rings. Combined oral contraceptives are available with different progestins and varying doses of estrogen to enable clinicians to find formulations that will work well for different women. Formulations are available for extended cycle use to eliminate or minimize the number of scheduled bleeding episodes induced by placebo pills. This scheduled bleeding is not medically indicated but may be desired by some women for personal reasons.

Many other health benefits accrue to women who use combined hormonal contraceptives. Three formulations are approved for the **treatment of acne**, and one is approved for treatment of **premenstrual dysphoric disorder. Bleeding episodes with hormonal methods are less heavy, shorter, less painful, and more predictable** than spontaneous menses. **The risk for ovarian and endometrial cancer is reduced,** and these health benefits increase the longer a woman uses the hormonal contraception.

For healthy reproductive-aged women, combined hormonal contraceptives are very safe. The only measurable risk is the **slightly increased incidence of venous thromboembolism** (VTE)—deep venous thrombosis and pulmonary embolism. This risk is overshadowed by the risk for VTE during pregnancy. **Benign hepatic tumors** are an extremely rare problem, and symptomatic cholelithiasis and mild hypertension may be slightly increased. **Modern lower-dose hormonal contraceptives do not increase the risk for breast cancer, cholelithiasis, fibroids, or heart attacks in healthy women.** Women with preexisting medical problems such as hypertension or diabetes and older women who smoke or are obese face higher risks and require individualized recommendations. The WHO MEC in Table 26-3 provides guidance.

Certain medical conditions are absolute contraindications to the use of combined hormonal methods because their use presents more risks than would pregnancy. These include a history of heart attack, stroke, breast cancer, labile hypertension, advanced diabetes, hepatic failure, migraine with aura, or unexplained abnormal uterine bleeding.

Although most patients believe that combined hormonal contraceptives have numerous side effects, the incidence of "hormonally related" side effects is not increased in placebo-controlled trials. The only exception is the risk for melasma. There are transient changes that do occur in the first 3 months, including unscheduled bleeding or spotting and breast tenderness. There are also women who are more sensitive to certain compounds, but the availability of a wide range of products and delivery systems helps tailor the method to the needs of the individual woman.

Progestin-Only Pills and Injections

Progestin-only methods can be used by virtually every woman, with the exception of women who have had breast cancer in the past 5 years. Women using drugs that increase cytochrome P-450 are not good candidates for progestin-only pills (POPs) but are still candidates for depot medroxyprogesterone acetate (DMPA) injections. **Each of these progestin-only methods thickens cervical mucus, but DMPA also profoundly suppresses gonadotropins to inhibit ovulation.**

POPs are immediately reversible. Return to ovulation with DMPA takes a median time of 10 months. With POPs, women usually continue to experience their own cycles but have less blood loss. With DMPA, there is initially a significant amount of unscheduled bleeding, but with time, most women achieve amenorrhea. Some women gain weight using DMPA. The noncontraceptive benefits with DMPA are impressive, including a reduced incidence of menorrhagia, dysmenorrhea, pain from endometriosis, endometrial cancer, and acute sickle cell crises.

TIER 3 CONTRACEPTIVES: BARRIER AND BEHAVIORAL METHODS

The advantage of this tier of contraceptives is that they need to be used only at the time of intercourse, which is also the feature that most profoundly decreases their utilization and increases their failure rates in typical use.

Barrier Methods

When used correctly and consistently, male condoms have a failure rate of 2%, but in typical use, they are only slightly more effective than withdrawal (17.4%). **Latex condoms also have great potential to reduce all sexually transmitted infections**, but with episodic use, this protection is compromised. To encourage the use of latex condoms, they are now available in a range of different sizes (from snug fitting to roomier from base to head) and different shapes. An array of features has been added to appeal to users, including different textures, flavors, and scents. They also come with a wide variety of accessories, including freshening wipes and vibrating rings to reward condom use.

For couples with latex allergies or women using petroleum-based vaginal products, polyurethane condoms are available. The polyurethane transmits body heat and is impermeable to viruses and bacteria. Animal cecum condoms are not recommended. Condom use should always be advised to minimize STI risk in combination with other methods, but **spermicidal lubricated latex condoms offer no additional protection against STIs or pregnancy.**

Female barrier methods include diaphragms, a vaginal shield, a cervical cap (Femcap), and female polyurethane condoms; vaginal spermicides are also included in this category. Each of the female barriers works best if used with spermicidal gel. Male latex condoms can be combined with all female barrier methods except the female condom. With cleansing, the diaphragm, shield, and cap are reusable for up to 1 year. Spermicides are available as immediately active foams gels and sponges (after hydration) and delayed-acting suppositories and films. Spermicide use is not recommended for multiple applications in a 24-hour period because multiple uses may increase the transmission of HIV.

Behavioral Methods

Withdrawal or coitus interruptus is the most effective behavioral method. The male superior coital position allows the man to move his penis away from the woman's genitals before ejaculation.

For recently breastfeeding women, **lactational amenorrhea is very effective.** When women exclusively breastfeed on demand and have no menses for the first 6 months postpartum, the failure rate is 2%. After 6 months, it is prudent to add another method.

Fertility awareness methods employ a variety of techniques to detect at-risk days. Once those days are identified, couples can practice periodic abstinence or use another behavioral or barrier method at that time. The historical "rhythm method" has been replaced by other methods of natural family planning including the standard days method with its Cycle Beads, urine testing (for luteinizing hormone and estrogens that predict ovulation), sophisticated computing machines, and the Billings technique for detecting cervical secretions on the introitus that change before ovulation.

Other sexual practices that couples use to avoid genital contact to reduce pregnancy may include "outercourse," oral-genital pleasuring, mutual masturbation, or rectal intercourse. These practices may not reduce the risk for STIs.

Emergency Contraception

EC pills containing levonorgestrel or norgestrel are intended to be a backup method for use after unprotected intercourse. It is one of the most important innovations in contraception. In the United States, availability is limited to people aged 18 years and older.

TABLE 26-4

METHODS OF TUBAL STERILIZATION		
Surgical Approach	**Technique**	**Surgical Procedure**
Laparotomy	Pomeroy	Ligature around a "knuckle" (or loop) of tube; excision distally
	Madlener	Crushing and ligature of loop of tube
	Irving	Double ligation, excision between; proximal end buried in myometrium; distal end buried in broad ligament
	Uchida	Tubal serosa stripped from muscular coat; tubal segment excised; proximal end ligated and buried in broad ligament
	Fimbriectomy	Ligation of distal end of tube and mesosalpinx; excision of fimbriated end
Laparoscopy	Electrocoagulation	Electrical "burn" of two adjacent segments with or without transection
	Falope ring	Loop of tube drawn into applicator tube; plastic ring placed around both limbs of loop
	Hulka clip	Plastic crushing clip placed across tube (not a loop); kept closed by steel spring
	Filshie clip	Titanium clip placed across the tube; associated with increased risk for infection
Minilaparotomy	Pomeroy ligation; electrocoagulation	As above
Transcervical	Insertion of tubal plug	Placement of plug through a hysteroscopic transcervical approach that causes fibrosis over time

Virtually every woman can use the levonorgestrel EC (marketed as Plan B). Product labeling advises that the two doses be taken 12 hours apart, but a single dose of two pills is at least as effective. Use within 72 hours of exposure is advisable, so clinicians should provide women at risk for unscheduled intercourse with a prescription in advance. EC is not an abortifacient, and it has no teratogenic effect if inadvertently administered during pregnancy. It works only by suppressing ovulation. Various combinations of routine OCs with levonorgestrel or norgestrel plus estrogen can be offered if LNG-EC is not available.

Sterilization

Permanent sterilization is the most common method of birth control used by U.S. women older than 30 years. Common methods of fallopian tube sterilization are listed and described in Table 26-4.

Vasectomy (interruption of the vas deferens) can be done under local anesthesia in an office setting ("no scalpel" vasectomy) or as an outpatient surgical procedure. Interestingly, there are no data available about long-term efficacy of vasectomy. Once a man has achieved azoospermia following 6 to 10 ejaculations after the procedure, he is considered sterile. **There are no long-term hormonal, metabolic, or autoimmune effects associated with vasectomy.**

Fallopian tube procedures are most commonly used for female sterilization, although hysterectomy performed for other indications also sterilizes a woman. Tubal interruption can be done through a mini-laparotomy incision, using a laparoscope or hysteroscopically. Usually, **mini-laparotomy techniques** with suture ligation and interruption of the tube (the **Pomeroy technique**; Figure 26-2) **are performed** through a small subumbilical incision immediately postpartum. Laparoscopic approaches are usually performed as interval procedures in nonpregnant women when the woman's uterus lies in the pelvis. The fallopian tubes can be interrupted with cautery, clips, or rings (Figure 26-3). **With the hysteroscope, small plugs can be anchored in the proximal portions of the tube** to incite fibrosis and, over time, cause the tube to occlude.

Reversibility of sterilization procedures varies by technique and by the amount of fallopian tube destroyed by the initial procedure. The range of success varies from 30% to 70%. The convenience of tubal ligation is obvious, but the cost and the surgical and anesthetic risks (e.g., hemorrhage, infection, damage to intraperitoneal structures, and even death) need to be considered.

Ten-year follow-up studies demonstrate that **all sterilization methods are less effective in younger women** (up to 5.4% failure rates in women younger than 28 years), but that postpartum sterilization procedures have the lowest 10-year failure rates.

Long-term complication rates are low. However, because at least 6% to 10% of women consider reversal and many more regret having been sterilized, it is critical to encourage women to consider all their reversible options first.

Abortion

Abortion is the interruption (spontaneous or induced) of an established pregnancy before 20 weeks' gestation. The term *miscarriage* is usually used by the lay public to describe spontaneous pregnancy loss. *Elective* and *therapeutic abortion* are terms used to describe induced pregnancy termination.

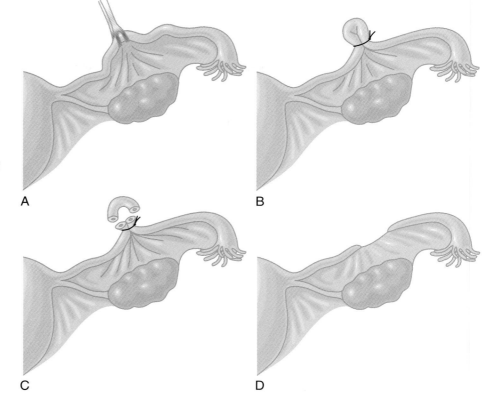

FIGURE 26-2   Pomeroy method of tubal ligation. **A:** Tube is grasped with Babcock forceps. **B:** A loop is ligated. **C:** The loop is excised. **D:** Several months later, the fibrosed ends of the tube separate.

A

B

C

D

Under the 1963 *Roe v. Wade* U.S. Supreme Court decision, induced abortion is a legal procedure until fetal "viability" is achieved, usually described as 24 weeks of gestational age, unless a fetal anomaly inconsistent with extrauterine life is identified to permit later pregnancy termination. **Maternal mortality rates decrease significantly whenever abortion is legalized** and provided by medically trained personnel. Every pregnant woman needs to be made aware of all her options, including continuing the pregnancy, abortion, and adoption. Decisions in these areas are extremely difficult and personal. In some states, women are required to wait 24 hours between giving consent and undergoing the termination. In some states, a teen's parental

FIGURE 26-3   Tubal occlusion with the Hulka clip (**A**) and Falope ring (**B**). The ring causes a portion of tube to undergo necrosis, and the end result resembles the illustrated tube in Figure 26-2D. Cautery procedures use electric energy to acutely destroy portions of each fallopian tube.

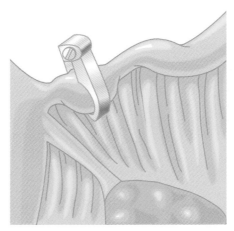

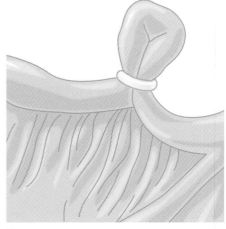

A

B

notification or approval is required before abortion. Access to abortion services may become increasingly difficult because **more than half of the counties in the U.S. have no abortion providers.**

Early in pregnancy (less than 49 days), both medical and surgical procedures can be offered. Mifepristone (an antiprogestin) can be administered and followed later by **misoprostol** (a prostaglandin) to induce uterine contractions expelling the products of conception. This approach has been proved effective (96%). Other agents, such as methotrexate, can be used to induce abortion, but methotrexate is less effective and generally requires a longer time to complete the process.

Aspiration with a manual vacuum or suction curettage is more than 99% effective in early pregnancy after cervical dilation has been achieved with misoprostol or laminaria (Figure 26-4). This type of procedure can be performed either under local anesthesia (paracervical block) or under sedation with the patient awake. Complication rates are very low, but the patient must understand that hemorrhage, infection, uterine perforation, retained products of conception, and anesthetic complications are possible. **Early pregnancy termination is safer than continuing the pregnancy or undergoing tonsillectomy.** There are no long-term adverse effects on women's reproductive health with uncomplicated procedures.

Second-trimester abortions are generally performed because prenatal diagnosis has revealed a serious genetic abnormality or because of an intrauterine fetal demise. Here, the role of medical abortion has been pivotal. Prostaglandin or misoprostol intravaginal suppositories are used to induce contractions, and the fetus is delivered vaginally. Occasionally, follow-up curettage may be needed to remove an undelivered placenta. Some patients prefer surgical procedures such as dilation and evacuation for elective termination.

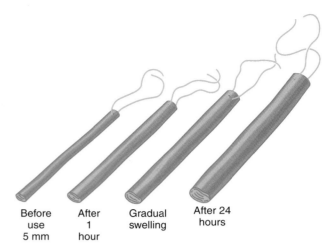

Before use 5 mm   After 1 hour   Gradual swelling   After 24 hours

FIGURE 26-4   Laminaria tents (osmotic dilators) used to gradually dilate the uterine cervix by absorbing body fluid.

This surgical procedure may be needed to treat women with infected pregnancies (septic abortions).

Although early abortion is an extremely safe procedure from a maternal safety perspective, most experts and patients would agree that pregnancy prevention is clearly preferable.

SUGGESTED READING

Abbott J: Transcervical sterilization. Curr Opin Obstet Gynecol 19:325-330, 2007.

Hatcher RA, Trussell J, Nelson AL, et al: Contraceptive Technology. 19th ed. New York, Ardent Media, 2007.

Hatcher RA, Zieman M, Cwiak C, et al: A Pocket Guide to Managing Contraception. Tiger, GA, Bridging the Gap Foundation, 2005.

Speroff L, Darney PD: A Clinical Guide for Contraception. 4th ed. Baltimore, MD, Lippincott Williams & Wilkins, 2005.

Chapter 27

Sexuality and Female Sexual Dysfunction

JOSEPH C. GAMBONE

Sexuality refers to how individuals express themselves as sexual beings. Physically, sexuality encompasses sexual intercourse and other forms of sexual contact. Often patients may have medical concerns about their sexual feelings and behavior and how these activities may affect or be affected by disease. Obstetrician-gynecologists should be familiar with the physiology of human sexual response and the types of sexual dysfunction that women may experience. Because female sexuality is most often expressed with another individual, usually male, it is important for healthcare professionals who take care of women to know the more important aspects of the male sexual response. The sociologic aspects of human sexuality and sexual behavior, such as cultural, ethical, moral, religious, or legal, are beyond the scope of this chapter.

Sexual Development

Although sexuality and sexual expression rarely begins before puberty, gender identity is experienced much earlier, at about age 3 to 4 years. Children who are unable to identify with their assigned birth-gender have **gender identity disorder** (GID) and may develop transgender issues later in life. **The diagnosis of GID can be made in an individual who has a strong and persistent cross-gender identity and a discomfort about the assigned gender.**

During puberty, many teens begin exploring their bodies as well as experiencing sexual activity with others. Many teens, especially males, have early intercourse and are not well educated about contraception, the risks for pregnancy, or sexually transmitted infections (STIs). Young girls often have intercourse because of feelings of love, whereas boys are usually driven by curiosity. It is especially important for physicians to discuss sexuality with teens and to educate them about contraception and STI prevention. Teens are often apprehensive about discussing these issues and may fear parental discovery. They are usually more receptive to open-ended questions.

The early reproductive years are often the time when sexuality is explored and reproduction or its prevention becomes a priority. Infertility may be an issue in this age group, and many emotions may be evoked in infertile patients, often leading to sexual problems.

With increasing age and especially after menopause, the frequency and satisfaction with intercourse may decline. Decreased estrogen production causes progressive vaginal atrophy, which in turn leads to decreased vaginal lubrication, dyspareunia, and more difficulty in achieving orgasm. The decreased estrogen also decreases the acidity of the vaginal secretions, predisposing the woman to vaginal infections.

In many older couples, the frequency of intercourse declines because of the male partner's inability to have erections. Illnesses or increased use of medications may also affect sexual functioning. A better understanding of the causes and more effective treatment for male erectile dysfunction are changing sexual behavior for many older individuals.

Variation in Sexual Expression

Human sexual expression is varied and often controversial. Health-care professionals must be knowledgeable and nonjudgmental about healthy and legal sexual expression and lifestyles to facilitate open and comfortable communication.

Heterosexuals are individuals who engage in sexual activity with the opposite sex. Most individuals engage in heterosexual behavior, which is considered "normal." **Homosexuals are those who engage in sexual**

activities with members of the same sex. Men who are homosexual are referred to as gay, whereas homosexual women are referred to as gay or lesbian. Although gay men tend to engage in more physical relationships and may have multiple partners, lesbians are generally inclined to be monogamous.

The reported incidence of homosexuality ranges from 6% to 20% in men and 3% to 18% in women. Several theories on homosexuality have been proposed, including a genetic predisposition, the maternal use of prenatal hormones, and other environmental factors. A multifactorial cause is likely.

Many homosexuals feel a need to conceal their sexuality for fear of loss of family, friends, or jobs. Familiarity with homosexuals has been shown to decrease the prejudice, and recently many homosexuals have "come out," revealing their identities and expecting equal rights.

Bisexuals are those who engage in sexual activity with both men and women, either concomitantly or at different phases of their life. The reported incidence of bisexuality is 1% to 7% of men and 1% to 2% of women. Many individuals briefly explore same-sex activity at some time in their life but do not consider themselves bisexual.

Transgender or transsexual individuals are often confused with homosexuals. **They have a strong belief from childhood that they were born into a body with the wrong sex. Most are heterosexual to their identified gender** (i.e., men who believe they are women are attracted to men), and few are homosexual. **Children with ambiguous genitalia who are assigned a particular gender may later show regret toward their assignment.** Some experts recommend that these children be given a name that is appropriate to both genders to allow them to decide their gender for themselves later in life. Female-to-male transsexuals (FTM) are women that grow up as "tomboys" and often cross-dress. Male-to-female transsexuals (MTF) are men that grow up dressing as women. Transgender surgery is difficult to perform, especially FTM, and it is only performed in certain areas of the United States and the world. Box 27-1 lists some other variations in human sexual expression along with their definitions.

▨ Sexual Response

The process of sexual response was fully described by Masters and Johnson in 1966 based on extensive research. They delineated the female and male physical sexual response cycles. Although other modifications have been published, their version remains the classic description of human sexual response. The female cycle is divided into four phases, whereas in men, five phases are described. Generally, clitoral tissue is the most sexually sensitive anatomic area for women.

BOX 27-1 *Other Forms of Sexual Expression and Their Definitions*

Transvestism: Sexual excitement or gratification from wearing clothing of and enacting the opposite sex
Fetishism: Sexual excitement or gratification associated with an inanimate object (i.e., underwear) or body part (i.e., feet)
Pedophilia: Sexual excitement or gratification from children
Zoophilia: Sexual excitement or gratification through intercourse with animals
Exhibitionism: Sexual excitement or gratification from exposing one's body, especially the genitals
Voyeurism: Sexual excitement or gratification from watching others
Masochism: Sexual excitement or gratification from enduring physical or physiologic pain; may be self-inflicted
Sadism: Sexual excitement or gratification from inflicting physical or physiologic pain onto others; also cruelty not associated with sexual behaviors

---

Most women need to experience a caring relationship and nongenital physical stimulation before satisfactory sexual arousal can occur.

FEMALE SEXUAL RESPONSE CYCLE

The Excitement Phase

This phase starts with physical or psychological stimulation and may last minutes or hours. There is a sex flush, accompanied by erection of the nipples and engorgement of the breasts. A sex flush is an erythematous morbilliform skin change over the chest, neck, and face that occurs to a noticeable degree in 75% of women. In addition, the uterus elevates, and vaginal lubrication begins. The clitoris and labia enlarge, and the heart rate and blood pressure increase. Most muscles become tense (Figure 27-1A).

The Plateau Phase

During this phase, the breasts continue to enlarge, and the clitoris may elevate and retract under its hood. The Bartholin's glands may secrete fluid near the vaginal opening, and there is tenting of the uterus to allow easier passage of sperm. The vagina and labia become more engorged, and there is increased blood pressure, heart rate, respiratory rate, and muscle tension (see Figure 27-1B).

The Orgasmic Phase

During this phase, there is release of sexual tension. The orgasmic phase is possible without actual physical stimulation. This phase is concentrated in the clitoris, vagina, and uterus. There is contraction of vaginal, uterine, lower abdominal, and anal muscles, usually 5 to 12

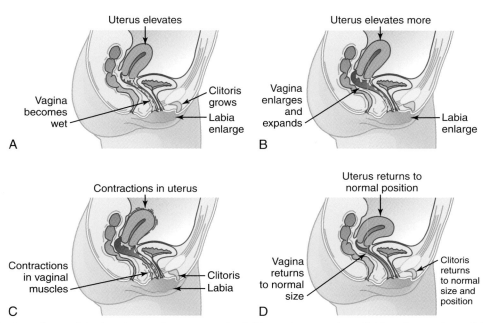

FIGURE 27-1 The four phases of the female sexual response cycle. **A:** The excitement phase. **B:** The plateau phase. **C:** The orgasmic phase. **D:** The resolution phase.

synchronized contractions 1 second apart. The first few contractions are the strongest and the closest together. Blood pressure, heart rate, and respiratory rate peak in this phase, and there is usually loss of voluntary muscle tone (e.g., most women curl their toes at orgasm). Women can have multiple orgasms before they enter the resolution phase (see Figure 27-1C).

The Resolution Phase

During this phase, the nipples and breasts decrease in size, and the vagina, clitoris, and uterus return to normal size and position. The sex flush disappears, and the blood pressure, heart rate, and respiratory rate also return to normal (see Figure 27-1D).

MALE SEXUAL RESPONSE CYCLE

The Excitement Phase

This phase begins with physical or psychological stimulation and may last minutes or hours. The nipples and penis become erect, and there is increased heart rate and blood pressure. The muscles become tense, and there is blood pooling in the extremities with vasocongestion in the penis and scrotum with testicular swelling and elevation (Figure 27-2A).

The Plateau Phase

The testicles enlarge by 50%, and the prostate and penis also enlarge. There is increased blood flow, and the bulbourethral or Cowper's gland secretes pre-ejaculatory fluid, which may contain sperm. There is

increased blood pressure, heart rate, respiratory rate, and muscle tension. There is generally chest sex flushing (see Figure 27-2B).

The Orgasmic Phase

During the orgasmic phase, there is release of sexual tension; this phase is possible without actual physical stimulation. There are rhythmic contractions of the seminal vesicles, vas deferens, and prostate. The ejaculatory ducts push semen into the urethra, and ejaculation occurs with urethral contractions. The first few contractions are the strongest and the closest together. During this phase, the anal sphincter contracts. The *point of imminence* occurs a few seconds before ejaculation and refers to the point when a man knows an orgasm is inevitable (see Figure 27-2C).

The Resolution Phase

In the resolution phase, the genitals and penis decrease in size and return to a flaccid state. The testes descend, and the sex flush disappears. The blood pressure, heart rate, and respiratory rate return to normal (see Figure 27-2D).

The Refractory Phase

The refractory phase (not illustrated) occurs only in men. Because of this phase, men are not able to have multiple orgasms. During this phase, no amount of stimulation will cause another ejaculation. This phase lasts minutes in young men and hours to days in older men.

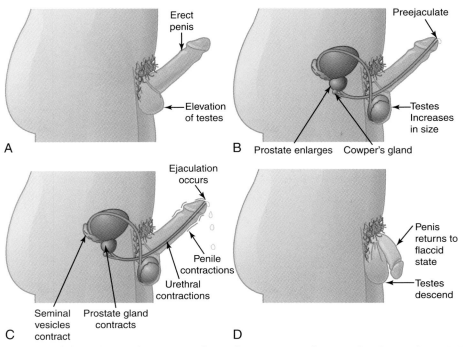

FIGURE 27-2   The five phases of the male sexual response cycle. **A:** The excitement phase. **B:** The plateau phase. **C:** The orgasmic phase. **D:** The resolution phase. **E:** The refractory phase (not illustrated).

The similarity between the male and female cycles is apparent. Although the average time spent in each phase may differ (due primarily to learned behaviors), the elements of each cycle are the same. Because different neuronal circuits mediate each of these phases, sexual dysfunction may affect some phases without affecting the others.

Sexual Dysfunction

The overall prevalence of sexual dysfunction is not known, but female sexual dysfunction is common. It has been estimated that one third of women experience decreased libido in situations in which the decrease is not desired. Comorbid conditions such as diabetes or obesity often play a causative role in sexual dysfunction, and not all women who lack interest in sexual activity are troubled by it.

EVALUATION OF SEXUAL FUNCTION

The assessment of sexual functioning should be an integral part of a complete medical evaluation, especially for the obstetrician-gynecologist. Skills for taking a sexual history are often overlooked in medical schools and sometimes ignored by physicians. It is more difficult to inquire about a patient's sexuality if the physician is uncomfortable with the topic or is judgmental about sexual orientation. Clinicians may also be concerned about a patient's answers, not knowing what to say or do if a history of sexual trauma is revealed. They may also feel untrained to deal with problems and solutions for sexual inadequacies. Often, they worry that the patients will misunderstand or be offended by the questions.

In taking a history, it is helpful to follow a routine pattern of questioning: (1) age of menarche, (2) menstrual patterns, (3) pregnancy history, (4) contraception use, (5) STI prevention, (6) sexual orientation, and (7) difficulties with sexual relations. Intimate partner violence and sexual abuse questions can then follow. Some sample questions may include the following:
• "Are you currently sexually active, and if so, with men, women, or both?"
• "Are you having any difficulties with sexual relations?"
• "Have you ever been in a situation in which you have experienced unwanted or harmful sexual activity?"
There are several factors that may affect taking a sexual history, including the physician's own sexuality. A gay physician may be more thorough or may be afraid to inquire about a patient's sexual orientation. At times, clinicians of both sexes may find themselves attracted to patients. In these instances, acceptance of the feelings as normal is appropriate, so long as behavior is unaffected and a professional relationship is maintained. Some patients may be seductive or even

BOX 27-2   *American Foundation of Urologic Disease Consensus Classification of Female Sexual Dysfunction*

Sexual Desire/Interest Disorders*

Hypoactive sexual desire disorder
Sexual aversion disorder

Sexual Arousal Disorder*

Female sexual arousal disorder*

Sexual Orgasmic Disorder*

Sexual Pain Disorders*

Dyspareunia
Vaginismus
Other sexual pain disorder (genital pain from noncoital
    stimulation)

*Each disorder can be subtyped as lifelong vs acquired, generalized vs situational, and by origin (organic, psychogenic, mixed, or unknown).

BOX 27-3   *Some Drugs that Can Diminish Sexual Functioning in Women*

- Antihypertensive agents: reserpine, propranolol, methyldopa, atenolol, spironolactone
- Antidepressant medications: tricyclics or selective serotonin reuptake inhibitors
- Hypnotic agents: alcohol, barbiturates, tranquilizers, or diazepam
- Narcotics: heroin or methadone
- Antipsychotic agents: fluphenazine or chlorpromazine
- Stimulants: cocaine or amphetamines
- Hallucinogens: lysergic acid or mescaline
- Diuretics: acetazolamide

make sexual advances, but the physician must make it clear to the patient that the relationship is professional and not personal.

Appropriate boundaries of behavior during a physical examination must be maintained, and caution should be used with inappropriate language or overly friendly conversations. The patient may feel uncomfortable, especially with a doctor of the opposite sex, and fearful about potentially embarrassing discoveries, especially during the examination of the breasts and genitals. Drapes should be used to cover all the private body parts that are not being examined, and the physician should tell the patient what he or she is doing at all times. **A nursing assistant or chaperone should be present during the examination.**

FEMALE SEXUAL DYSFUNCTION

Sexual dysfunction is categorized by the Sexual Function Health Council of the American Foundation of Urologic Disease by failure of one or more of the phases of the sexual response cycle. Sexual dysfunction also includes pain disorders (Box 27-2).

Female sexual dysfunction is a common condition and often increases with age. Sexual dysfunction can be subdivided into three different categories, depending on whether it is **primary** (realistic sexual expectations have never been met under any circumstances), **secondary** (all phases have functioned in the past, but one or more no longer does), **or situational** (the response cycle functions under some circumstances, but not others). When a patient complains of hypoactive sexual desire, it is important to determine what her preferences are in contrast to those of her partner. A woman who desires intercourse twice a week may be perfectly normal but may not function well in a relationship in which her partner desires coitus daily. Sexual

dysfunction can occur in homosexual or heterosexual relationships, or even in masturbatory situations.

ETIOLOGY OF SEXUAL DYSFUNCTION

As a general rule, primary problems are predominantly psychogenic and tend to be of longer duration. Secondary problems are often associated with the onset of a disease process or the use of a pharmacologic agent. If such an association cannot be established, deterioration in the patient's relationship or some other chronologically related change in the patient's life experience should be sought. It is important to consider **psychological causes**, such as depression or anxiety; **organic causes**, such as atherosclerosis, diabetes, or genital infections; and **pharmacologic causes** (Box 27-3). Factors initiating a problem may be different from those maintaining it. For example, drugs may precipitate a problem, but if anxiety and fear of failure sustain the difficulty, discontinuation of the drug alone may not rectify the problem.

SEXUAL FUNCTION DISORDERS

Sexual Desire and Interest Disorders

Sexual desire appears to be an appetite similar to hunger, controlled by a dopamine-sensitive excitatory center, in balance with a serotonin (5-hydroxytryptamine)-sensitive inhibitory center. **In both males and females, testosterone appears to be the hormone responsible for initially programming these centers during gestation and for maintaining their threshold of response.** Stimulation and ablation experiments in cats and other mammalian species have located these centers within the limbic system, with significant nuclei in the hypothalamic and preoptic regions. For a woman, desire and interest in sexual activity result from a complex of both biologic and psychological inputs, including her feelings about her partner.

Disorders of sexual desire and interest include hypoactive sexual desire disorder and sexual aversion disorder. Lack of desire involves a decrease or absence of fantasy. **Sexual aversion disorder** may result from prior sex-associated trauma and personal aversion. Often in established relationships, decreased desire may result from sexual activity becoming too predictable and routine. Also, lack of privacy or external stresses, especially stress in the relationship, may initiate this disorder. Another important category of causes of hypoactive desire arises in the context of unrelated disease. Women may fear sex with a partner who has had a heart attack or may have decreased desire themselves following a mastectomy or hysterectomy.

Arousal-Phase Disorder

Sexual arousal disorder is defined as the inability to attain or maintain sufficient sexual excitement, expressed as a lack of subjective excitement or somatic response such as genital lubrication. Estrogen is the hormone responsible for maintaining the vaginal epithelium and allowing transudation and lubrication to occur. Its deficiency (with breastfeeding or after menopause) is by far the most common cause of excitement phase dysfunction in women. Extragenital changes during the excitement phase include an increase in heart rate and blood pressure, enhanced muscle tension throughout the body, an increase in breast size, nipple erection, and engorgement of the surrounding areolae, and a sex flush. Some women do not recognize these symptoms as excitement and may experience difficulty and even failure on that basis.

Orgasmic-Phase Disorder

During the orgasmic phase, a series of reflex clonic contractions of the levator sling and related genital musculature occur, mediated primarily by the sympathetic nervous system.

Orgasmic disorder is characterized by difficulty with or failure to attain orgasm following sufficient sexual stimulation and arousal. Anorgasmia may be situational. Many women experience orgasm only with manual or oral clitoral stimulation but not with penile thrusting alone. If they are willing to increase direct clitoral stimulation before, during, or after penile penetration, they may achieve a wholly satisfactory sexual adaptation. Women who have been orgasmic in the past but have lost that capacity should be screened for organic or pharmacologic causes, and changes in their relationship or relationships should be carefully explored.

Most women with primary anorgasmia have had minimal or no effective stimulation from self or partner. These patients should be encouraged to learn how to achieve orgasm through self-stimulation, and then to share this new information with their partners. Increasing the intensity of stimulation should increase the intensity of response.

Sexual Pain Disorders

Dyspareunia is genital pain associated with sexual intercourse. It is helpful to categorize dyspareunia into three groups for easier diagnosis and treatment: (1) **pain with intromission** (often due to vestibulitis, vaginismus, fissures, or other vulvar lesions); (2) **mid-vaginal pain** (often due to lack of lubrication, surgical scars, or urethral diverticulosis); and (3) **deep-thrust dyspareunia** (often due to endometriosis, interstitial cystitis, pelvic adhesions, or neoplasms).

Vaginismus is defined as severe pain or involuntary spasm of the distal vaginal and pelvic floor muscles during attempted penetration. Examination reveals no organic condition, but the pubococcygeal muscles are tight, and vaginal penetration by speculum or examining finger is painful and difficult, if not impossible. Often affected women harbor fantasies about the inadequacy of their vaginas to accommodate a speculum or penis and fear that penetration will damage them. These women respond remarkably well to education and reassurance. Others may have been traumatized by early sexual or other abuse and require more intensive psychological therapy. One important issue is whether they are motivated to participate with their partners in a stepwise **desensitization program.** This involves the slow, gentle vaginal insertion of dilators of gradually increasing size under the patient's own control. Once sufficient progress has been made, the partner's fingers and, ultimately, his penis may be substituted for the dilators. Alleviation of the problem is usually accomplished in 3 to 6 months.

Noncoital sexual pain disorder is pain that is induced by noncoital sexual stimulation.

MANAGEMENT OF SEXUAL DYSFUNCTION

Hormonal therapy is valuable in a limited number of situations. Estrogen (orally or vaginally) may improve desire, arousal, and orgasm by decreasing dyspareunia due to vaginal atrophy. **Testosterone may improve desire and arousal but should be used only in hypoandrogenic women, especially after surgical menopause.** Sildenafil (Viagra), used mostly in men with erectile dysfunction, inhibits cyclic guanosine monophosphate (cGMP) breakdown, therefore increasing clitoral and vaginal smooth muscle relaxation as well as improving lubrication. cGMP functions as a messenger in the nitric oxide–mediated relaxation of genital smooth muscle,. **The use of sildenafil in women has not been as effective as in men.**

A clitoral vacuum device (the EROS-CTD) has **been approved by the U.S. Food and Drug Administration** and is said to improve clitoral blood flow and engorgement. **Fantasy therapy is helpful for hypoactive desire,** and **sensate-focusing therapy is helpful for excitement-phase defects.**

TREATMENT SUCCESS

As a group, orgasmic difficulties appear to respond to treatment most readily. For example, primary orgasmic difficulties may be resolved by means of guided masturbatory training and cognitive behavioral sex therapy. Secondary anorgasmia is more often associated with emotional or psychiatric disorders and relationship issues, so treatment is less effective. **Excitement-phase dysfunctions do not have such positive outcomes, although problems with lubrication can nearly always be resolved satisfactorily. Lack of desire is the most resistant to treatment.** Persons with little desire often have little internal motivation to seek more frequent sexual activity or to pursue help. Fewer than half of such patients show definite improvement. When the relationship is poor, behavioral approaches directed toward the sexual problem are rarely successful. Studies using medical and pharmacologic interventions for female arousal or orgasmic disorders, in contrast to those for erectile disorder and premature ejaculation in males, are still ongoing but show some promise.

SUGGESTED READING

Berman JR, Goldstein I: Female sexual dysfunction. Urol Clin North Am 28:405-416, 2001.

Esposito K, Giugliano F, Ciotola M, et al: Obesity and sexual dysfunction, male and female. Int J Impot Res Jul-Aug; 20(4):358-365, 2008. Epub 2008: April 10.

Frank JE, Mistretta P, Will J: Diagnosis and treatment of female sexual dysfunction. Am Fam Physician 77:635-642, 2008.

Hayes RD, Dennerstein L, Bennett CM, et al: Risk factors for female sexual dysfunction in the general population: Exploring factors associated with low sexual function and sexual distress. J Sex Med Jul; 5(7):1694-1701, 2008.

Palha AP, Esteves M: Drugs of abuse and sexual functioning. Adv Psychosom Med 29:131-149, 2008.

Chapter 28

Family and Intimate Partner Violence, and Sexual Assault

BRUCE B. ETTINGER • JOSEPH C. GAMBONE

▨ Intimate Partner Violence and Family Violence

Family violence refers to abuse of children and older individuals in addition to violent behavior directed against a current or former intimate partner. Intimate partner violence (formerly known as domestic violence) is defined as intentionally abusive or controlling behavior by a person who is in an intimate or close relationship with the victim.

The focus of the first part of this chapter is on intimate partner violence because the obstetrician-gynecologist is most likely to deal with the effects of abusive behavior directed against an intimate domestic partner. Intimate partner violence can include verbal abuse, intimidation, social isolation, and physical assault, such as a punch, a kick, a threat, a severe beating, an act of sexual assault, or even murder. It occurs in every age group, in all ethnic groups, in every occupation, and in every socioeconomic group. Although the obstetrician-gynecologist may be called to see a patient with acute injuries from partner violence or sexual assault, he or she is more likely to have to deal with the nonacute clinical manifestations of abuse (Box 28-1). Although most often perpetrated by a man against a woman, the gender relationship may occasionally be reversed. Intimate partner violence can also occur between same-sex partners.

EPIDEMIOLOGY

The prevalence and incidence of intimate partner violence is not known, but it is considerable. It has been estimated that as many as 2 million women are abused every year by someone they know. Any estimate of prevalence is likely to be understated owing to the likelihood that a significant number of victims are fearful of disclosing abuse against them. One study of the incidence of partner abuse found that of all women seeking care in an emergency room (ER), 54% said they had been threatened or injured at some time in their lives by a partner, and 24% said they had been injured by a current partner. One in three women presenting to an ER with injuries has symptoms related to partner violence. More than 20% of violent crimes against women and 30% of female murders are committed by intimate partners. Estimates of the number of pregnant women who are victims of partner abuse range from less than 1% to 20%.

Other forms of family violence are prevalent. The level of child abuse is epidemic, and it is estimated that nearly 500,000 elderly persons in domestic settings in the United States are abused or neglected. Seventy percent of cases of abuse of the elderly are perpetrated by a family member, including adult children.

In all cases of ongoing family or intimate partner abuse, the key enabling feature is some form of victim vulnerability, which the victim cannot or will not attempt to overcome.

ADVERSE EFFECTS OF INTIMATE PARTNER VIOLENCE

The impact of intimate partner abuse and violence includes significant health, social, and economic effects. Nearly one third of female intimate partner violence victims have physical injuries that require medical attention. Many victims develop posttraumatic stress disorder with all of its chronic symptoms and increased risk for suicide. Women who are "battered" and abused have lower overall health status and more depression and disability.

Social services for women who are victims of intimate partner abuse are inadequate. Nearly one third of battered women who request refuge are turned away because of a lack of space. Those turned away and their children often must return to a violent home. **Many become homeless and involved in substance abuse** as an escape mechanism or because they are forced into use and addiction by their partners.

The overall societal cost of intimate partner violence has been estimated to be in excess of $6 billion annually, and individual costs are increased because of higher insurance premiums paid by victims.

The abuser often provides for and is periodically in a caring and loving relationship with the victim, who may still love the abuser despite the abuse. Other obstacles to leaving the abuser include (1) fear of more abuse, (2) loss of economic support, (3) fear of social isolation, (4) feelings of failure, (5) promises of change, (6) previously unanswered calls for help, and in many cases (7) fear of loss of child custody. Figure 28-1 illustrates the cycle of violence that exists in these abnormal relationships.

ADDRESSING INTIMATE PARTNER AND FAMILY VIOLENCE

Healthcare providers may have difficulty bringing up the topic of possible intimate partner violence. Because of the alarming frequency of this problem, **it is important to ask all women, when alone with them, if they feel safe in their own home.** This should be a *routine practice* in taking a social history. Even without a suspicion of physical abuse, the woman should be asked directly if a partner has ever hit, kicked, hurt, or threatened her. If a positive response is obtained, it is important to document any physical findings. Pictures and drawings should be used.

It is helpful and reassuring to tell the victim that she is not alone, that help is available to her, and that her partner's behavior is unacceptable. Nearly every victim will believe that she is the only person to suffer such abuse because of the isolating nature of abusive behavior. The perpetrator most likely will have convinced the victim that she is at fault and responsible for the abuse.

In addition to the need to comply with any reporting requirements (some states mandate reporting to appropriate authorities if there are acute injuries), social workers and other professionals should always be consulted when abuse is acknowledged, or even if it is just suspected. Box 28-2 lists the responsibilities that health-care providers have in addressing intimate partner and domestic violence.

BOX 28-1   *Clinical Manifestations of Possible Intimate Partner Violence**

- Inadequately explained injuries such as bruises and abrasions
- Unusual difficulty during a gynecologic examination, such as excessive distress, discomfort, or avoidance behaviors
- Chronic and unexplained pelvic pain, urinary symptoms, sexual dysfunction, or irritable bowel syndrome
- Persistent or recurrent vaginitis or sexually transmitted infections despite appropriate treatment
- Persistent vague complaints, such as headache, backache, palpitations, and digestive, sleep, or eating disorders
- Complaints or signs of depression, anxiety, phobias, panic attacks, feelings of shame or worthlessness
- Unintended pregnancy
- Suicidal ideation

*No single presentation can confirm intimate partner or family violence.

Data from American College of Obstetricians and Gynecologists (ACOG): Special Issues in Women's Health-Intimate Partner and Domestic Violence. Washington, DC, ACOG, 2005.

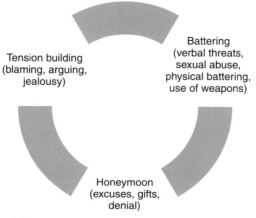

FIGURE 28-1   Cycle of violence. Elements of the cycle occur on a repetitive, unpredictable, and frequent basis. Verbal and emotional abuse is the most common form of assault. An alternating kindness followed by abuse in an unpredictable manner contributes to the emotional distress and long-term psychological morbidity of victims. *(Reprinted from Obstetrics and Gynecology Clinics of North America, 34(3), Gunter J, Intimate Partner Violence, 367-388, Copyright 2007, with permission from Elsevier.)*

BOX 28-2 *Medical Professionals' Responsibilities in Addressing Intimate Partner and Family Violence*

- Implement a universal screening program
- Acknowledge any trauma
- Assess immediate safety of the patient and any children
- Help to establish a safety plan
- Review options
- Offer educational materials and toll-free hotline information (see Box 28-3)
- Provide referrals
- Document interactions
- Provide ongoing support at subsequent visits
- Inform authorities when appropriate (state medical societies can inform about legal requirements)

Data from American College of Obstetricians and Gynecologists (ACOG): Special Issues in Women's Health-Intimate Partner and Domestic Violence. Washington, DC, ACOG, 2005.

Sexual Assault and Rape

Sexual assault and rape have different technical or legal definitions depending on the state or country involved. However, **any sexual act performed on a person without his or her consent is classified as sexual assault.** Sexual assault includes any unwanted genital, anal, or oral penetration by a part of the attacker's body or by any object. **Rape**, on the other hand, **is generally a violent attack** that may or may not stem from the perpetrator's sexual desire. Very often, the perpetrator uses sex as a means of control over another person. Whatever the rapist's intent, rape is definitely not a welcomed sexual experience for the victim. During any act of rape, the victim's predominant feeling is one of fear for her life or fear of mutilation.

Women of all ages, ethnicities, and socioeconomic groups can be victims of sexual assault, although the very young, the mentally and physically disabled, and the elderly are more vulnerable. **Nearly 75% of assaults are perpetrated by someone known to the victim,** such as husbands (marital or partner rape), boyfriends (date rape), fathers (incest), mothers' boyfriends, other relatives, or work associates. The American Medical Association reports that 20% of women younger than 21 years have been sexually assaulted. Other estimates are that 41% of women (of all ages) have been victims of actual or attempted sexual assault and that 50% of these have been victims more than once. **Death occurs in about 1% of sexual assaults (including rapes), and serious injury occurs in 4%.**

MEDICAL CARE FOR SEXUAL ASSAULT

The medical consultation should proceed only after a supportive, caring relationship has been established. The adult or adolescent woman should be actively involved in the consultation so that she may regain a feeling of control over what has happened to her. **The purposes of the consultation are threefold: (1) to provide her acute medical care, (2) to gather evidence, and (3) to transition her into the long-term care she will need for psychological recovery from the extreme loss of control and great fear of death that nearly every rape victim suffers.** These objectives should be explained to her, and she should be allowed to dictate the pace of the questioning and the order of the examination.

During the interview and examination phases, a chaperone or patient advocate should be present. Careful attention must be paid to the rules governing the chain of evidence to maintain the legal integrity and utility of all the specimens, photos, and other materials collected. The woman should be asked about the detailed specifics of her assault in order to direct the collection of needed evidence and to address any risk for injury or infection. Information about her recent menstrual history, use of medications, recent immunizations, contraceptive use, and past medical and surgical history is important.

A thorough physical examination is needed to evaluate possible injuries because **40% of all women who are sexually assaulted sustain injuries.** If possible, photographs or sketches should be obtained of the injured areas. The Centers for Disease Control and Prevention recommend routine testing for **gonorrhea** and **chlamydia** from specimens collected from any site of penetration or attempted penetration. Wet mount and culture for **trichomonas** are routine, and a microscopic evaluation for **bacterial vaginosis** and **candidiasis** is prudent in a woman with a vaginal discharge. Serum tests for **human immunodeficiency virus** (HIV), **hepatitis B**, and **syphilis** are needed for baseline evaluation. Positive HIV status can be another clue to identifying victims of abuse.

Prophylaxis is suggested as preventive therapy. This includes hepatitis B vaccination (if previously unvaccinated) and appropriate antibiotics for sexually transmitted infections (see Chapter 22). **It is critical to provide any woman at risk for pregnancy with emergency contraception** (see Chapter 26). If prophylaxis for HIV is considered necessary, consultation with an HIV specialist is recommended. **Tetanus toxoid** should be administered to an unprotected, injured woman.

PSYCHOLOGICAL SEQUELAE OF SEXUAL ASSAULT

Sexual assault is almost always associated with both immediate and long-term effects on victims. These effects have been termed the *rape trauma syndrome* and involve the following two phases:

1. **Acute and disorganization phase:** This phase lasts days to weeks. **Immediately after the experience, victims frequently appear calm, although preoccupied**

and **inattentive.** They are anxious, have difficulty sleeping, and commonly express shock, disbelief, fear, guilt, and shame. The **psychological problems** that may result are varied and can mimic those seen in the aftermath of other kinds of traumatic experiences. Among those expected in the acute phase of adjustment are **irritability, tension, anxiety, depression, fatigue, and persistent ruminations. Somatic symptoms** of a general nature may occur, such as **headaches or irritable bowel syndrome,** or symptoms may be more specific to the reproductive system, such as **vaginal irritation or discharge. Behavioral problems,** such as **overeating and alcohol or substance abuse,** may also surface, particularly when such problems have been evident in the past. **Long-term sequelae** include **changes in lifestyle, the occurrence of disturbing dreams and nightmares, and the persistence of phobic reactions. Fear persists as the predominant feeling.** These reactions often make it difficult for the victim to concentrate effectively on everyday activities and relationships.

2. **Integration and resolution phase**: During this phase, victims begin to accept the assault, but problems at work or with relationships may persist.

The management of the sexual assault victim in the acute phase influences long-term adjustment. Many rape victims may manifest **posttraumatic stress disorder.** The likelihood of this disorder developing is high, owing to the abrupt nature of the crime, its violence, the passivity and helplessness imposed on the victim, and the high probability of receiving physical as well as psychological trauma. **The lifetime prevalence of posttraumatic stress disorder in rape victims is about 50%.**

In addition to attending to immediate physical and emotional needs, the initial evaluation provides an opportunity to prepare the victim for the long-term psychological impact of the experience. This preparation is intended to diminish the long-term consequences and to enable the woman to recognize the common psychosocial sequelae when they occur, thus enabling her to seek professional help at an early stage.

Longer-term reactions involve nightmares, phobic reactions, and sexual fears. Stimuli associated with the rape, such as a similar-looking man or similar surroundings, may be associated with flashbacks. **Flashbacks may also occur during pelvic examinations.** Reactions to the sexual assault may result in problems with sexual behavior and functioning. **Loss of libido is a common response to stressful or traumatic circumstances of any kind. Other complaints include vaginismus, impaired vaginal lubrication, and loss of orgasmic capacity.** These problems may be even more likely if the assault occurred at home while the woman was asleep. Preparing the woman for these eventualities can be extremely helpful in preventing sexual

BOX 28-3 *Key Telephone Numbers for Medical Professionals and Victims of Family Violence and Sexual Assault*

National Domestic Violence Hotline: 1-800-799-SAFE (7233 or 7234) TTY 1-800-787-3224 (hearing impaired)
RAINN (Rape, Abuse, Incest National Network) Hotline: 1-800-656-HOPE
National Child Abuse Hotline: 1-800-4-A-CHILD (1-800-422-4453)
Elder Abuse Hotline: 1-800-922-2275
Disabled Person Abuse Hotline: 1-800-426-9009

dysfunction from developing or persisting. **Giving permission for a lower-than-usual sexual drive** during the period following the assault may remove some performance anxiety. **Explaining how anxiety and stress can inhibit sexual responsiveness** and providing ways in which this can be overcome are also important.

AFTERCARE PLANNING

Careful follow-up must be arranged. If the patient used the prophylactic therapies, a return visit is needed in 1 week to review the initial laboratory results and to monitor her progress. Repeat testing is needed only if the woman is symptomatic. If she did not receive prophylaxis, repeat testing for gonorrhea, chlamydia, and trichomonas should be performed in 2 weeks and for syphilis in 6 weeks. Repeat serum tests for HIV should be performed 6, 12, and 24 weeks after the assault, regardless of whether prophylactic measures were taken.

Before discharging the patient, it is important to ensure that she has a safe place to go and a suitable means of transportation. She should also be given (in writing) the names, addresses, and phone numbers of resources available in the community to meet her medical, legal, and psychosocial needs related to the assault (Box 28-3).

SUGGESTED READING

American College of Obstetricians and Gynecologists (ACOG): Special Issues in Women's Health: Intimate Partner and Domestic Violence. Washington DC, ACOG, 2005.

American College of Obstetricians and Gynecologists (ACOG): Special Issues in Women's Health: Sexual Assault. Washington DC, ACOG, 2005.

Centers for Disease Control and Prevention: Intimate partner violence prevention. Retrieved April 12, 2008, from http://www.cdc.gov/ncipc/dvp/IPV/default.htm.

Ellsberg M, Jansen Ha, Heise L, et al, for the WHO Multi-country Study on Women's Health and Domestic Violence against Women Study Team: Intimate partner violence and women's physical and mental health in the WHO Multi-country Study on Women's Health and Domestic Violence: An observational study. Lancet 371:1165-1172, 2008.

Karch DL, Lubell KM, Friday J, et al: Centers for Disease Control and Prevention (CDC) surveillance for violent deaths. MMWR Surveill Summ 57(3):1-45, 2008.

Chapter 29

Breast Disease: A Gynecologic Perspective

NEVILLE F. HACKER • MICHAEL L. FRIEDLANDER

It is important that gynecologists be expert in breast examination, diligent about screening asymptomatic women for breast cancer, familiar with common benign and malignant disorders of the breast, and conversant with the various therapeutic options. In a number of centers in the world, gynecologic oncologists treat breast cancer.

Screening of the Breast in Asymptomatic Women

SELF-EXAMINATION

Many breast cancers are detected by women themselves, and monthly breast self-examination should be promoted. Written information should be supplemented by practical training. There is no solid evidence that breast self-examination reduces breast cancer mortality, but it is reasonable to assume that a woman's increased awareness of her own breasts may lead to an earlier diagnosis.

Breast Self-Examination Technique

The patient may be invited to perform the examination after each menstrual period. She should commence the technique in the upright position, carefully inspecting the breasts initially with her arms by her sides and then with her arms raised above her head. She should palpate the supraclavicular and axillary regions for the presence of nodes. The patient should then lie down and systematically palpate each quadrant of the breast against the chest wall, using the flat of her fingers. Finally, she should palpate the areolar areas and then compress the nipples for evidence of secretion.

Breast Examination by Physician

A complete breast examination should be performed by a physician at least annually. The breasts are first inspected with the patient in an upright position. The contour and symmetry are observed, and any skin changes or nipple retraction is noted. **Skin retraction, because of tethering to an underlying malignancy, may be highlighted by having the patient extend her arms over her head.**

Palpation of the breast, areola, and nipple is performed with the flat of the hand. If any mass is palpated, its fixation to deep tissues should be determined by asking the patient to place her hands over her hips and contract her pectoral muscles. Each axilla is then carefully examined while the patient's arm is supported. The supraclavicular fossae are also palpated for lymphadenopathy. **After palpation in the upright position, the examination is repeated in the supine position.**

MAMMOGRAPHY

Radiologic examination of the breast is an important component of the screening process carried out in asymptomatic women and should be performed in conjunction with a thorough physical examination. **Densities and fine calcifications constitute suspicious findings, and clinically inapparent malignancies less than 1 cm in diameter may be detected.**

Mammograms of high quality can be made with about 0.3 cGy or less of radiation, so there is little, if any, risk for this technique causing breast cancer.

In the Breast Cancer Detection Demonstration Project carried out by the American Cancer Society and the National Cancer Institute, **89% of 3557 cancers were correctly identified by mammography, 42% of which were not clinically detectable.**

The American Cancer Society recommends annual mammograms starting at age 40 years.

ULTRASONOGRAPHY

Ultrasonography can differentiate cystic from solid masses and may demonstrate solid tissue that is potentially malignant within or adjacent to a cyst. It is also useful for imaging palpable focal masses in women younger than 30 years, reducing the need for x-ray studies in this population.

MAGNETIC RESONANCE IMAGING

Magnetic resonance imaging is a useful adjunct in breast imaging. Reported advantages include improved staging and treatment planning, enhanced evaluation of the augmented breast, better detection of recurrences, and possibly improved screening of high-risk women.

◼ Diagnosis of Breast Lesions

Physiologic nodularity and cyclic tenderness caused by the changing hormonal milieu must be distinguished from benign or malignant pathologic changes. **Definitive diagnosis of breast neoplasms may be made by open biopsy or by fine-needle (22-gauge) aspiration cytology.**

FINE-NEEDLE BIOPSY

Fine-needle aspiration biopsy of the palpably suspicious lump in the breast can be performed in the outpatient clinic. Smears are prepared from the aspirate to allow cytologic evaluation. In experienced hands, the test is both sensitive and specific. **A negative result should never be accepted as definitive when there are clinical or mammographic indications that the lesion may be malignant.** In the presence of a palpable lump, fine-needle aspiration cytology should make it possible to diagnose breast cancer without formal excisional biopsy in about 90% of cases, allowing the definitive management of the patient to be discussed preoperatively.

OPEN BREAST BIOPSY

Small masses may undergo **excisional biopsy,** whereas large masses should undergo **incisional biopsy,** or occasionally core-cutting needle biopsy. Absolute indications for open breast biopsy are listed in Box 29-1. Relative indications for breast biopsy include those women with a clinically benign mass but a positive family or personal history of breast cancer, a history of atypical hyperplasia, or an equivocal finding on mammography or cytology.

BOX 29-1   *Absolute Indications for Open Breast Biopsy*

- Clinically suspicious (dominant) mass that persists through a menstrual cycle, regardless of mammographic findings; if fine-needle aspiration cytology is unequivocally positive, most surgeons proceed directly to definitive treatment.
- Cystic mass that does not completely collapse on aspiration (residual solid component) or that contains bloody fluid.
- Spontaneous serous or serosanguineous nipple discharge; in the absence of a mass, a "trigger point" should be demonstrable.

Open breast biopsy may be performed as an outpatient procedure under local anesthesia or as an inpatient procedure under general anesthesia. Women with large breasts who have small, deeply situated lesions are not good candidates for outpatient biopsies, nor are those who have a nonpalpable lesion detected by mammography.

◼ Common Benign Breast Disorders

FIBROCYSTIC CHANGES

The earlier term *fibrocystic disease* has little clinical value, and the term was abandoned by the College of American Pathologists in 1985. Lesions formerly grouped together under the designation of fibrocystic disease represent a pathologically heterogeneous group of diseases that can be divided into three separate histologic categories: nonproliferative lesions, proliferative lesions (hyperplasia) without atypia, and atypical hyperplasias.

HYPERPLASIA

Hyperplasia is the most common benign breast disorder and is present in about 50% of women. Histologically, the hyperplastic changes may involve any or all of the breast tissues (lobular epithelium, ductal epithelium, and connective tissue). **When the hyperplastic changes are associated with cellular atypia, there is an increased risk for subsequent malignant transformation.**

It is postulated that the hyperplastic changes are caused by a relative or absolute decrease in production of progesterone or an increase in the amount of estrogen. Estrogen promotes the growth of mammary ducts and the periductal stroma, whereas progesterone is responsible for the development of lobular and alveolar structures. Patients with hyperplasia improve dramatically during pregnancy and lactation because of the large amount of progesterone produced by the corpus luteum and placenta and the increased production of estriol, which blocks the hyperplastic changes produced by estradiol and estrone.

The disorder usually occurs in the premenopausal years. Clinically, the lesions are usually multiple and bilateral and are characterized by pain and tenderness, particularly premenstrually.

Treatment depends on the age of the patient, the severity of the symptoms, and the relative risk for the development of breast cancer. Women older than 25 years should undergo baseline mammography to exclude carcinoma. **Cysts may be aspirated to relieve pain** (Figure 29-1). If the fluid is clear and the lump disappears, careful follow-up only is indicated. **Open biopsy is required if the fluid is bloody or if there is any residual mass following aspiration.**

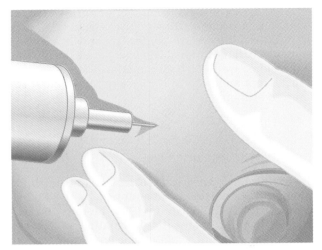

FIGURE 29-1   Aspiration of a breast cyst. Ultrasound may be used to differentiate a solid from a cystic breast mass.

FIBROADENOMA

Composed of both fibrous and glandular tissue, the fibroadenoma is the most common benign tumor found in the female breast. Clinically these tumors are sharply circumscribed, freely mobile nodules that may occur at any age but are common before the age of 30 years. They usually are solitary and generally are removed when they reach 2 to 4 cm in diameter, although **giant forms up to 15 cm in diameter occasionally occur and have malignant potential.** Pregnancy may stimulate their growth, and regression and calcification usually eventuate postmenopausally. These larger tumors require surgical excision for definitive diagnosis and cure.

INTRADUCTAL PAPILLOMA

Papillary neoplastic growths may develop within the ducts of the breast, most commonly just before or during menopause. They are rarely palpable and are usually diagnosed because of a bloody, serous, or turbid discharge from the nipple. **Mammography and cytologic examination of the fluid are helpful in investigating nipple discharge. Excisional biopsy of the lesion and involved duct is the treatment of choice.**

Histologically there is a spectrum of lesions ranging from those that are clearly benign to those that are anaplastic and give evidence of invasive tendencies.

GALACTOCELE

A galactocele is a cystic dilation of a duct that is filled with thick, inspissated, milky fluid. It presents during or shortly after lactation and implies some cause for ductal obstruction, such as inflammation, hyperplasia, or neoplasia. Often multiple cysts are present. **Secondary infection may produce areas of acute mastitis**

TABLE 29-1

ESTABLISHED RISK FACTORS FOR BREAST CANCER	
Risk Factor	**Relative Risk**
Age (≥50 vs <50 yr)	6.5
Family history of breast cancer	
First-degree relative	1.4-13.6
Second-degree relative	1.5-1.8
Age at menarche (<12 vs ≥14 yr)	1.2-1.5
Age at menopause (≥55 vs <55 yr)	1.5-2.0
Age at first live birth (>30 vs <20 yr)	1.3-2.2
Benign breast disease	
Breast biopsy (any histologic finding)	1.8-10.5
Atypical hyperplasia	4.0-4.4
Hormone replacement therapy	1.0-1.5

Data from Armstrong K, Eisen A, Weber B: Assessing the risk of breast cancer. N Engl J Med 342:564-571, 2000.

or abscess formation. Needle aspiration is usually curative. If the fluid is bloody or the mass does not disappear completely, excisional biopsy is required.

◾ Breast Cancer

Breast cancer is the most common female malignancy, accounting for 26% of malignancies in women. It is second only to lung cancer as the leading cause of cancer deaths in women. More than 175,000 new cases are diagnosed annually in the United States, and about 40,000 of these women die from the disease. **In the United States, there is a 1 in 8 chance that a woman will develop breast cancer during her lifetime, if she lives to 90 years of age.**

ETIOLOGY

Established risk factors for breast cancer are shown in Table 29-1, but 75% of women develop the disease despite having no apparently increased susceptibility.

The incidence and mortality rates for breast cancer are about 5 times higher in North America and northern Europe than they are in many Asian and African countries. Migrants to the United States from Asia (principally Chinese and Japanese) do not experience a substantial increase in risk, but their first-generation and second-generation descendants have rates approaching those of the white population in the United States. The difference may be related to dietary customs.

Menopausal hormone replacement therapy appears to produce a small increased risk for breast cancer, and the estrogen-progestin regimen increases the risk beyond that associated with estrogen alone.

About 5% to 10% of breast cancer cases are hereditary, resulting from mutations in the *BRCA1* or *BRCA2* gene. These genetic mutations also increase the risk

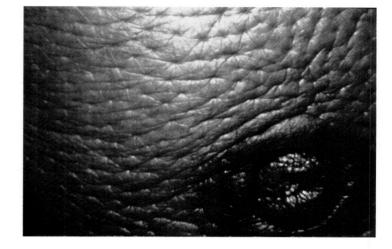

FIGURE 29-2 Carcinoma of the breast. Note the nipple retraction and the peau d'orange appearance. *(From Swartz MH: Textbook of Physical Diagnosis, 5th ed. Philadelphia, Saunders, 2006.)*

for ovarian cancer. Hereditary breast cancer is particularly common in premenopausal women. Women with a mutated *BRCA1* or *BRCA2* gene have up to a 70% risk for developing breast cancer by 65 years of age.

TUMOR TYPES

The mammary epithelium gives rise to a wide variety of histologic tumor types. **About 80% of all breast cancers are nonspecific infiltrating ductal carcinomas.** These tumors usually induce a significant fibrotic response and are stony hard to clinical palpation. **Less common types include lobular, medullary, mucinous, tubular, and papillary.** In many tumors, several patterns coexist.

Paget's disease of the breast occurs in about 3% of breast cancer patients. It represents a specialized form of intraductal carcinoma that arises in the main excretory ducts of the breasts and extends to involve the skin of the nipple and areola, producing an eczematoid appearance. **The underlying carcinoma, although invariably present, can be palpated clinically in only about two thirds of patients.**

Inflammatory breast cancer represents 1% to 4% of cases and is often seen in pregnancy. It is characterized clinically by warmth and redness of the overlying skin and induration of the surrounding breast tissues. Biopsies of the erythematous areas reveal malignant cells in subdermal lymphatics, causing an obstructive lymphangitis. Inflammatory cells are rarely present. **Most patients have signs of advanced cancer at the time of diagnosis, including palpable regional lymph nodes and distant metastases.**

TUMOR SPREAD

Breast cancer spreads by local infiltration as well as by lymphatic or hematogenous routes. Locally, the tumor infiltrates directly into the breast parenchyma, eventually involving the overlying skin or the deep pectoral fascia.

Lymphatic spread is mainly to the axillary nodes, involvement of which occurs in up to 50% of patients with symptomatic breast cancer and in 10% to 20% of patients with screen-detected breast cancers. The second major area for lymph node metastases is the internal mammary node chain. These nodes are most likely to be involved when the primary lesion is medially or centrally situated. **The supraclavicular nodes are usually involved only after axillary node involvement.**

Hematogenous spread occurs mainly to the lungs and liver, but other common sites of involvement include bone, pleura, adrenals, ovaries, and brain.

STAGING

Several systems of staging for cancer of the breast have been recommended. The one recommended by the American Joint Committee on Cancer is available at http://www.cancerstaging.org.

CLINICAL FEATURES

Carcinoma of the breast is usually painless and may be freely mobile. A serous or bloody nipple discharge may be present. With progressive growth, the tumor may become fixed to the deep fascia. **Extension to the skin may cause retraction and dimpling, whereas ductal involvement may cause nipple retraction. Blockage of skin lymphatics may cause lymphedema and thickening of the skin, a change referred to as** *peau d'orange* (Figure 29-2) due to its "orange peel" appearance.

TREATMENT

With increasing awareness of the likelihood of early hematogenous spread and an increasing number of early lesions being diagnosed, the present trend is toward a more conservative surgical approach to breast cancer in conjunction with adjuvant radiation and, if necessary, chemotherapy or hormonal therapy.

Surgery

Radical mastectomy, as first described in 1894 by Halsted and Meyer, was for many years the standard operation for operable breast cancer. The procedure consists of an en bloc dissection of the entire breast, together with the pectoralis major and minor muscles and the contents of the axilla. At present, breast-conserving surgery is increasingly practiced. **Survival rates after conservative surgery are equal to those after radical mastectomy.** Although the size of the primary carcinoma is not a limiting factor for breast conservation, if the breast is small, breast conservation is unsatisfactory even for small tumors and is impractical for large tumors.

Routine axillary lymph node dissection has progressively been replaced by lymphatic mapping and sentinel lymph node resection as a less morbid means of determining the tumor status in the axilla. Routine examination of the sentinel node should include hematoxylin and eosin staining. If the node is negative, ultrastaging should be performed, using serial sectioning and immunohistochemical staining for cytokeratin. If the sentinel node is negative, the remaining nodes will be negative with an accuracy of about 95%, so axillary dissection may be avoided. If the node is positive, axillary dissection should be performed.

Breast reconstruction after mastectomy is an integral part of the treatment of breast cancer. It should be available to any woman who desires it, provided that her general condition allows for operation and her expectations for reconstruction are realistic. The procedure may be performed at the time of the mastectomy or may be delayed.

Radiation Therapy

Conservative surgery is always performed in conjunction with radiation therapy to the breast. This approach gives equivalent outcomes to radical mastectomy, and functional and cosmetic results are improved. External-beam therapy is used, with 4500 to 5000 cGy delivered to the entire breast. **The ipsilateral supraclavicular and internal mammary nodes may be treated if there are multiple positive axillary nodes. The axilla is not routinely irradiated after an axillary node dissection because of the high incidence of lymphedema.**

ADJUVANT THERAPY

Adjuvant systemic therapy is used for most patients with early breast cancer, regardless of lymph node status. **Overall, adjuvant therapy reduces the risk for relapse by about one third, and reduces the risk for death by 25%.**

Current recommendations for adjuvant chemotherapy and hormonal therapy are as follows:
- Premenopausal patients with estrogen-receptor (ER)-negative tumors should receive adjuvant chemotherapy.
- Premenopausal patients with ER-positive tumors should be considered for hormonal therapy in addition to chemotherapy.
- Postmenopausal patients with ER-positive tumors who have negative nodes should be treated with adjuvant tamoxifen for 2 years followed by an aromatase inhibitor (such as anastrazole) for 3 years or an aromatase inhibitor for 5 years. Those with positive nodes should receive both hormonal therapy and chemotherapy.
- Postmenopausal patients with ER-negative tumors should receive adjuvant chemotherapy.

An added bonus of tamoxifen is a 70% reduction in the risk for cancer in the contralateral breast.

Chemotherapy usually consists of anthracycline-based regimens (e.g., four cycles of doxorubicin [Adriamycin] and cyclophosphamide; six cycles of 5-fluorouracil, doxorubicin, and cyclophosphamide; or six cycles of 5-fluorouracil, epirubicin, and cyclophosphamide), with or without the addition of taxanes (paclitaxel or docetaxel).

In patients with established metastases, symptoms may be palliated with combination chemotherapy. Partial responses are obtained in 40% to 60% of patients, and complete clinical responses are obtained in 5% to 15%. The median duration of response is 5 to 15 months, but responses can last for some years.

Trastuzumab (Herceptin), a humanized monoclonal antibody directed against HER2/neu (human epidermal growth factor receptor 2, also referred to as c-erbB-2), has been approved by the U.S. Food and Drug Administration for patients with early breast cancer in conjunction with chemotherapy and also for the treatment of patients with metastatic breast cancer. Its efficiency is predicted by either HER2/neu protein overexpression or gene amplification.

PROGNOSIS

Although prognosis is related to the stage of the disease and the age of the patient (older patients have a better prognosis), **the status of the axillary lymph nodes is the single most important prognosticator.** ER status is also of independent prognostic significance; patients with ER-negative tumors have a poorer prognosis.

In the National Surgical Adjuvant Breast Project, patients with negative lymph nodes had an actuarial 5-year survival rate of 83%, compared with 73% for patients with one to three positive nodes, 45% for those with four or more positive nodes, and 28% for those with more than 13 positive nodes.

BREAST CANCER IN PREGNANCY

About 3% of breast cancers occur during pregnancy, complicating about 1 in every 3000 pregnancies. Diagnosis is usually delayed because small masses are more difficult to palpate in hypertrophied breasts. Needle aspiration or open biopsy, however, should be performed promptly on any suspicious mass.

The surgical treatment is essentially the same as for the nonpregnant patient. Postoperative irradiation is delayed until after delivery. **For patients with nodal metastases, abortion is advisable in the first trimester of pregnancy because of the teratogenic risks of the adjuvant chemotherapy.** Adjuvant chemotherapy can be administered in the second and third trimesters of pregnancy. In the third trimester, chemotherapy should be delayed until after delivery, although surgery should occur promptly after diagnosis.

Stage for stage, prognosis for pregnant patients is not much worse than that for nonpregnant patients. There is no indication to advise against subsequent pregnancy for breast cancer patients who have no evidence of recurrence.

SUGGESTED READING

Bonadonna G, Valagussa P, Veronesi U: Lessons from the initial adjuvant cyclophosphamide, methotrexate, and fluorouracil studies in operable breast cancer. J Clin Oncol 26:342-344, 2008.

Clarke M, Coates AS, Darby SC, et al, for the Early Breast Cancer Trialists' Collaborative Group (EBCTCG): Adjuvant chemotherapy in oestrogen-receptor-poor breast cancer: Patient-level meta-analysis of randomised trials. Lancet 371:29-40, 2008.

Del Mastro L, Dozin B, Aitini E, et al: Timing of adjuvant chemotherapy and tamoxifen in women with breast cancer: Findings from two consecutive trials of Gruppo Oncologico-Ovest-Mammel; a Intergruppo (GONO-MIG) Group. Ann Oncol 19:299-307, 2008.

Goldhirsch A, Wood WC, Gelber RD, et al, for the 10th St. Gailen Conference: Progress and promise: Highlights of the International Expert Consensus on the Primary Therapy of Early Breast Cancer 2007. Ann Oncol 18:1133-1144, 2007.

Mansel R, Locker G, Fallowfield L, et al: Cost-effectiveness analysis of anastrozole vs tamoxifen in adjuvant therapy for early stage breast cancer in the United Kingdom: The 5-year completed treatment analysis of the ATAC ("Arimidex," Tamoxifen Alone or in Combination) trial. Br J Cancer 97:152-161, 2007.

Chapter 30

Gynecologic Procedures

JOSEPH C. GAMBONE

Gynecologic procedures are becoming less invasive and safer, and advances in surgical technique are resulting in more effective and efficient reproductive healthcare for women. Smaller and more flexible instrumentation for endoscopic procedures and the development of robotic techniques are examples of these recent advances.

The gynecologic surgeon should have a high level of training during residency, followed by an ongoing commitment to retraining and retooling as effective procedures are added or substituted for outdated ones. Training methods now include computer-assisted simulations of procedures, providing for greater patient safety while learning and retraining. All facilities should have an active quality assessment program to continuously evaluate the safety and appropriateness of gynecologic care, including surgery.

It is not the purpose of this chapter to qualify the reader as a gynecologic surgeon. It is, however, essential that students and residents become familiar with the basic principles of common gynecologic surgical procedures so that they can properly assist in the operating room and carry out perioperative care.

Appropriateness of Gynecologic Procedures

Before any procedure or surgery begins, the most appropriate option (when more than one exists) for an individual patient must be selected, with optimal patient involvement in the decision-making process preceding informed consent.

At least 80% of gynecologic surgical procedures are considered to be elective; that is, there are other alternative treatments to be considered. The appropriateness of performing these procedures should be evaluated by physician and patient on an individual basis (Box 30-1). **The trend toward minimal invasiveness in gynecologic surgery should not lead to minimal or questionable indications**.

Credentialing, Privileging, and Ongoing Training

The rapid introduction of new technology can present a challenge to the surgeon, who will need to keep up with the most advanced procedures, and to the institution, which is required to be certain that those who are granted surgical privileges have been properly trained and are currently qualified.

After a surgeon's credentials (diplomas, training certificates, and licenses) have been properly verified, a useful classification for the purpose of privileging stratifies procedures into the following levels: **level 1**, procedures not requiring additional training after

BOX 30-1   *The PREPARED Checklist**

P is the procedure
R is the reason or rationale
E is the expectation
P is the preference that the patient may have (e.g., to avoid surgery, or the side effects of medication)
A is the alternative(s)
R is the risk(s)
E is the expense (hospital costs and surgeon's fees)
D is the decision to perform or not to perform the procedure

---

*PREPARED is a useful mnemonic checklist to assess preoperatively the appropriateness of a health-care procedure, including elective gynecologic surgery. An analysis of each gynecologic or other health-care procedure can be carried out and the patient completely and efficiently counseled using this format.

residency (e.g., dilatation and curettage [D&C], cervical conization', adnexal excision, and abdominal or vaginal hysterectomy); **level 2,** procedures requiring additional training (e.g., laparoscopic myomectomy); and **level 3,** procedures requiring advanced training and special skills generally acquired during subspecialty training (e.g., radical hysterectomy, tubal anastomosis, or oocyte harvesting).

As new procedures are incorporated into basic residency training, they can be reclassified.

Informed Consent and General Risks Associated with Procedures

The patient should be thoroughly counseled about surgical risks as part of the process of informed consent (see Chapter 1). In general, risks fall into three categories: risks of anesthesia, intraoperative risks, and postoperative complications. Risks of anesthesia depend on the type of anesthesia used (awake sedation, regional anesthesia, or inhalation agents). Regional anesthesia carries the risk for infection, postprocedure spinal headache, and failure, in which case an inhalation agent must be added to the regional anesthetic. Inhalation agents may be associated with the risk for aspiration pneumonia, allergic reaction to the agent, and damage to teeth or airways if intubation is necessary. Stroke, myocardial infarction, and death can result. The intraoperative risks include excessive bleeding and unintended damage to organs or tissue. Postoperative risks include infection, persistent bleeding, and thrombosis, all of which can lead to significant morbidity or even mortality. The specific risks of each procedure are given later.

Endometrial Sampling Procedures

One of the most common minor gynecologic surgical procedures is D&C: dilation of the cervix and curettage of the endometrium. Recent advances in office-based instrumentation for diagnosis (hysteroscopy, endometrial sampling [Figure 30-1], and ultrasonic evaluation of endometrial thickness) have resulted in an appropriate decrease in the use of D&C. **However, if cancer of the cervix or endometrium is suspected, a thorough fractional curettage may be the best procedure to confirm its presence.**

INDICATIONS

D&C may be a diagnostic or a therapeutic procedure. A diagnostic D&C is performed for irregular menstrual bleeding, heavy menstrual bleeding, or postmenopausal bleeding, unless an endometrial biopsy has already revealed a diagnosis of malignancy. Irregularities in the contour of the endometrial cavity, either congenital (e.g., uterine septum) or acquired (e.g., submucous

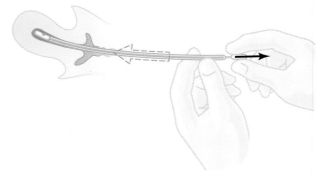

FIGURE 30-1   Endometrial sampling using the Pipelle instrument. A flexible hollow plastic tube is inserted and held in the uterine cavity as the stylet is withdrawn, creating a vacuum and resulting in aspiration of tissue.

myomas), are sometimes determined during the operation. The finding of a thin endometrium on a transvaginal ultrasound (generally <5 mm) may eliminate the need for biopsy or D&C in some women. In patients younger than 40 years with irregular bleeding, hormonal manipulation preceded by office endometrial sampling frequently obviates the need for curettage.

The D&C may have a therapeutic effect in patients with heavy or irregular bleeding from endometrial hyperplasia, endometrial polyps, or small, pedunculated submucous myomas. Unwanted first-trimester pregnancies are usually evacuated by dilation and suction curettage, although nonsurgical techniques are now available.

TECHNIQUE

The operation is performed with the patient in the dorsal lithotomy position. Most D&Cs are now performed on an outpatient basis. Paracervical blocks and local anesthesia are frequently employed.

A pelvic examination is done under anesthesia, and after sterile preparation, a weighted speculum is placed in the posterior vagina. The cervix is grasped with a single-toothed or double-toothed tenaculum. A Kevorkian curette is used for curettage of the endocervical canal. The depth of the uterine cavity is determined with a uterine sound, and the cervix is then dilated with a set of graduated dilators. A small polyp or ovum forceps is introduced through the dilated cervix and gently rotated to remove any endometrial polyps. A thorough curettage is done with a sharp curette, proceeding with each stroke in either a clockwise or a counterclockwise manner to ensure that the entire uterine cavity has been covered.

COMPLICATIONS

The most common surgical complications of D&C are hemorrhage, infection, perforation of the uterus, and laceration of the cervix. **Perforation of the uterus, even in experienced hands, is a not uncommon**

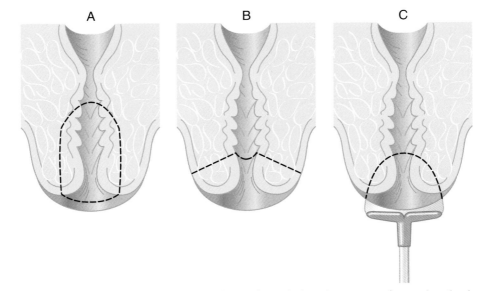

FIGURE 30-2 Cone biopsy of the cervix. **A:** Diagnostic conization performed when the squamocolumnar junction is not fully visualized colposcopically. **B:** Therapeutic conization performed for disease involving the ectocervix and distal endocervical canal. **C:** Loop electrosurgical excision procedure. The goal of the procedure is to remove the cervical tissue to just above the squamocolumnar junction, including any visible lesions.

complication and occurs particularly with a retroverted uterus, during pregnancy, or in postmenopausal patients with endometrial cancer. As long as no bowel or large blood vessels are injured, careful observation and antibiotics may be all the therapy that is required.

Except in an acute emergency, such as an infected incomplete abortion, D&C should be done reluctantly in the presence of infection.

Cervical Procedures

Conization of the cervix is a procedure in which a cone-shaped portion of the cervix is removed for diagnostic or occasionally therapeutic purposes. The section of the tissue surrounding the external os represents the base of the removed specimen. The apex is either close to the internal os (Figure 30-2A) or close to the external os (Figure 30-2B). Conization may also be performed in an office setting using loop electrosurgical excision (Figure 30-2C) or large loop excision of the transformation zone of the cervix. **Loop excision should not be performed before identification of a cervical intraepithelial lesion that requires treatment by colposcopically directed punch biopsy.**

The technique of cryoablation is commonly used to treat condylomas of the cervix, vagina, and vulva. These procedures almost always are office based, and little if any anesthesia is required.

Laser instruments are sources of intense beams of light energy. The letters in the acronym *laser* stand for light amplification by the stimulated emission of radiation. When used in surgery, this radiant energy is converted inside the cell to thermal or acoustic energy, resulting in controlled vaporization or coagulation of tissue. Lasers come in longer wavelengths (carbon dioxide [CO_2]) or shorter wavelengths (neodymium–yttrium-aluminum-garnet [Nd:YAG], potassium-titanyl-phosphate [KTP], and argon) that can be propagated along flexible optical fibers. This allows delivery of energy for cutting, vaporization, and coagulation to tissues in locations unreachable by a CO_2 laser.

Because of the additional expense of laser equipment and the lack of evidence for improvements in outcome, **the use of this technology has been decreasing in recent years.** Nevertheless, laser technology has been applied to conization of the cervix, removal of leiomyomas (myomectomy), and destruction of the ectopic endometrial implants of endometriosis.

Pelvic Endoscopy

Gynecologic endoscopy (laparoscopy and hysteroscopy) is widely used for the diagnosis and treatment of reproductive organ disease and dysfunction. Laparoscopy and hysteroscopy have largely moved from the hospital operating room to the freestanding surgical outpatient unit, and with smaller instruments (needlescopes) and more refined fiberoptic technology, even into the office setting. **Because of the expense involved, the value of these techniques must be considered in terms of outcome, particularly the long-term health and functional status of the patient.**

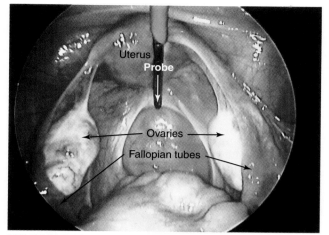

FIGURE 30-3   Laparoscopic view of female pelvis. *(Courtesy of B. Beller, MD, Eugene, Oregon.)*

Laparoscopy

The laparoscope is an instrument for viewing the peritoneal cavity. Both pelvic and upper abdominal structures can be inspected. The attachment of a video camera on the lens of the laparoscope allows more than one surgeon to view the operative site on a video screen and assist during procedures (Figure 30-3). Multiple puncture sites through the skin and into the abdominal cavity provide for the insertion of small rigid or flexible instruments directed toward the pelvis. Procedures that were once performed by laparotomy are now routinely carried out less invasively.

The indications for laparoscopy are both diagnostic and therapeutic. **Laser technology can be applied to operative laparoscopic procedures both to excise and to vaporize areas of pathology.**

Absolute contraindications to laparoscopy include bowel obstruction and large hemoperitoneum with hypovolemic shock. In patients who have had multiple previous laparotomies, a history of peritonitis, previous bowel surgery, or a lower midline abdominal incision, open laparoscopy is preferable. In these conditions, the peritoneal cavity is opened through a small subumbilical incision under direct vision before introduction of the trocar and sheath.

INDICATIONS

The following are indications for laparoscopy:
1. **Tubal sterilization.** The most common indication for the use of the laparoscope in gynecology is sterilization.
2. **Ectopic pregnancy.** The laparoscope is commonly used for the removal of tubal pregnancies that do not meet the criteria for medical therapy.
3. **Pelvic infection.** Although it is not routinely used for diagnosis of pelvic inflammatory disease (PID), the laparoscope can provide confirmation of a diagnosis when there is a diagnostic dilemma.
4. **Infertility.** Routine laparoscopic evaluation of the infertile woman is widely recommended but controversial because of a lack of controlled evidence of improved outcome. Advanced assisted reproductive techniques, such as in vitro fertilization (IVF) and gamete intrafallopian transfer (GIFT), may involve laparoscopic procedures, although the aspiration of oocytes for IVF is now most commonly performed transvaginally using ultrasonic guidance (see Chapter 34).
5. **Pelvic pain.** Acute and chronic pelvic pain can be investigated using the laparoscope.
6. **Endometriosis.** The laparoscope has become a widely used intervention for the diagnosis, staging, and treatment of ectopic endometrial tissue in both overtly symptomatic (pelvic pain) and silently symptomatic (infertility) patients. Laser coagulation, thermal vaporization, excision of endometriosis, and aspiration of endometriomas results in consistent, but sometimes temporary, improvement of pain and moderate improvement in fertility potential. Repeated procedures and the need for medical adjuvant treatment are common.
7. **Ovarian neoplasms.** Because of the need to rule out pelvic malignancies, the laparoscope can be used as a less invasive procedure to evaluate a persistent small adnexal mass. Laparoscopic ovarian cystectomy or salpingo-oophorectomy allows a tissue diagnosis to be made. **Laparoscopic aspiration of cysts can be dangerous and may result in dissemination of an unsuspected ovarian cancer. Ovarian biopsy is seldom indicated, and in premenopausal patients with simple cystic enlargement, a trial of hormonal suppression or observation is indicated instead of immediate surgical intervention.** Most such lesions are functional cysts that spontaneously regress. The laparoscope in expert hands has been advocated for staging and second-look procedures in patients with ovarian cancer. These procedures have become feasible since the advent of laparoscopic lymphadenectomy, but port-site recurrences are a potential problem.
8. **Myomectomy.** Laparoscopic myomectomy remains controversial because of the possibility that smaller leiomyomas will be removed because they *can* be rather than because they *should* be. **Advocates of the procedure recommend that fibroids larger than 6 cm not be removed using the laparoscope.**
9. **Urogynecologic procedures.** Urethropexy can be performed laparoscopically, with reported success rates comparable to procedures performed percutaneously (see Chapter 23).
10. **Hysterectomy.** The laparoscope has been used by some to replace an abdominal procedure

(laparoscopic hysterectomy), to assist in a vaginal hysterectomy, and to convert an abdominal hysterectomy to a vaginal hysterectomy. Adoption of laparoscopic hysterectomy has been limited, with fewer than 10% of hysterectomies performed with the use of this instrument.

TECHNIQUE

The procedure is performed with the patient in a modified dorsal lithotomy position (i.e., with knee crutches), usually under general anesthesia. An intrauterine manipulator is inserted to help in the visualization of the pelvic organs. A pneumoperitoneum is created by inserting a spring-loaded needle, such as a Veress needle, into the peritoneal cavity through the subumbilical fold, and insufflation with either CO_2 or nitrous oxide. The trocar and surrounding sheath are then inserted through a small subumbilical incision.

The lighted telescope is inserted into the sheath and advanced slowly. With the patient in the Trendelenburg position (tilted with the upper body lower than the pelvis), visualization of pelvic organs confirms that the peritoneal cavity has been entered. Gas may be added intermittently and automatically to maintain a sufficient pneumoperitoneum. To perform a second puncture, which is sometimes necessary, especially in laparoscopic surgical procedures, the abdominal wall is transilluminated to identify the position of the inferior epigastric vessels, and a 4- to 6-mm trocar and sheath are inserted under laparoscopic guidance through a small incision at the pubic hairline. A probe or other surgical instrument (e.g., surgical scissors) is passed through the second sheath.

On completion of the procedure, hemostasis is checked, the gas is released from the peritoneal cavity, and the instruments are withdrawn. The small skin incisions are closed with a clip or single subcuticular suture.

COMPLICATIONS

Insufflation of the abdominal wall may occur from failure to enter the peritoneal cavity with the Veress needle. Perforation of a viscus, especially adherent bowel, may occur at the time of insertion of the trocar and sheath. Once the instruments have been successfully introduced into the peritoneal cavity, lack of adequate hemostasis or coagulation burns of a viscus may occur. A poor pneumoperitoneum increases the risk for these complications.

Bowel burns during fulguration are the most serious complication of laparoscopy, although the most common complications are related to the anesthesia. Bowel burns result either from direct contact with the bowel or from a unipolar spark and are usually not detected at the time of the procedure. Several days later, bowel perforation with peritonitis may become

evident. **The increased use of bipolar instruments has diminished the occurrence of this serious complication.** There is an increased risk for anesthetic complications in a patient with a pneumoperitoneum.

■ *Hysteroscopy*

INDICATIONS AND USES

During the past 100 years, the hysteroscope has seen progressive improvements in light sources, optical systems, distending media, and electronic equipment, and the instrument now has a wide variety of indications and benefits in clinical gynecology. Hysteroscopy has substantially improved accuracy when compared with x-ray hysterography, and in some cases it may be more effective than diagnostic D&C in detecting intrauterine pathology such as endometrial polyps or submucous myomata.

HYSTEROSCOPIC INSTRUMENTATION

The hysteroscope (Figure 30-4) is a telescope consisting of light bundles and a sheath through which the telescope is inserted. For pure diagnostic use, the telescope is inserted alone, whereas for operative capabilities, it is inserted in conjunction with other instruments.

Two different types of telescopes are used today: rigid and flexible fiberoptic. Rigid telescopes are most commonly 1 to 5 mm in diameter for diagnostic procedures, and operative hysteroscopes typically range from 8 to 10 mm in diameter and contain a working element through which operative instruments are inserted.

Operating instruments such as rigid or flexible scissors, graspers, biopsy forceps, or even laser fibers are inserted through operating channels, which may be part of the outer sheath, or through separate devices interposed between the telescope and the outer sheath, which are called *bridges*. In addition to the standard operating instruments, some bridges have attachable electrodes and finger-controlled mechanisms to allow the performance of precision intrauterine surgery.

The uterine cavity needs distention for adequate visualization through the hysteroscope. Different distention media such as carbon dioxide gas and both low- and high-viscosity fluid may be used. It is critically important for the surgeon to know which media are compatible with electrosurgical or laser energy sources and which are prone to fluid overload or anaphylactic shock during the procedure.

OFFICE-BASED VS HOSPITAL-BASED HYSTEROSCOPY

Telescopes have become progressively narrower and can now be safely inserted into the cervical canal with minimal pain. Several manufacturers have small office-based telescopes that use physiologic low-viscosity distention fluids such as saline or Ringer's lactate. These

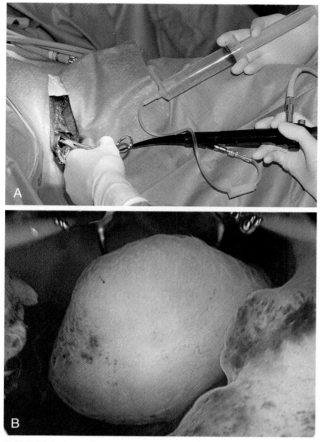

FIGURE 30-4 **A:** Surgeon preparing to insert a hysteroscope (in right hand) through the vagina. **B:** View of an intrauterine polyp (center) as seen through the hysteroscope. These lesions can be removed during the procedure. (**A,** From Goldberg JM, Falcone T: *Atlas of Endoscopic Techniques in Gynecology. London, WB Saunders, 2000, p 185; **B,** from Goldberg JM, Falcone T: Atlas of Endoscopic Techniques in Gynecology. London, WB Saunders, 2000.*)

allow the performance of hysteroscopy with little more than a paracervical block in patients who are bleeding, and they do not cause the shoulder pain and uterine spasm that often accompany use of carbon dioxide as a distention medium. **At present, a significant number of hysteroscopies are performed as office procedures.**

OPERATIVE PROCEDURES

Infertility

When abnormalities such as intrauterine synechiae or septa are found, hysteroscopic correction is associated with a high rate of success. Synechiae, almost always the result of trauma such as curettage or other uterine surgery, may vary from mild to severe, obliterating only a small part or almost all of the endometrial cavity. **One third of patients with intrauterine synechiae have no apparent menstrual abnormalities.** Hysteroscopic

scissors are most commonly used for incision of the adhesions, although lasers or electrical knife electrodes may also be used. **In infertile patients, conception rates up to 60% and a reduction of pregnancy wastage by 50% may be expected after incision of synechiae.**

Probably the most rewarding of all hysteroscopic procedures is the excision of an intrauterine septum, a congenital anomaly that occurs in up to 1% of women. Usually performed as an outpatient procedure, excision of the septum is a relatively short procedure, with minimal bleeding and minimal risks. It is best performed with mechanical scissors as opposed to electrical or laser devices to limit the spread of thermal injury to adjacent healthy myometrium.

In most cases, it is desirable to monitor the depth of incision by concomitant laparoscopy or ultrasonography to reduce the risk for uterine perforation.

Abnormal Uterine Bleeding

The hysteroscopic evaluation of the patient with abnormal uterine bleeding frequently uncovers the presence of submucous myomas or endometrial polyps.

Small endometrial polyps can be removed easily using hysteroscopic scissors or grasping forceps inserted through an accessory channel of the operating hysteroscope, or they can be removed blindly with a polyp forceps followed by hysteroscopic reinspection to ensure complete removal. Because the endocervical canal is rarely dilated larger than 10 mm to accommodate the operating instruments, polyps or myomas that are significantly larger than this must be morcellated before removal. The use of mechanical methods for morcellation (scissors) is almost impossible, owing to their delicate construction and their small size. **The urologic resectoscope has been used to morcellate or vaporize all or part of such lesions.** Electrodes composed of thin wires, roller balls, roller cylinders, and grooved vaporization tips, coupled with continuous (cutting) electrical waveforms, allow simple removal of such lesions.

Endometrial Ablation

Endometrial ablation is the destruction of the uterine lining for the treatment of chronic menorrhagia. It is performed when more conservative treatments, such as hormonal therapy and curettage, are unsuccessful and when the more radical alternative of hysterectomy is undesirable or contraindicated.

Two general methods of endometrial ablation have emerged. The first type requires hysteroscopic visualization and employs electrical or laser energy to shave, vaporize, or coagulate the endometrial surface.

After a preoperative drug regimen to suppress the endometrial thickness (danazol or leuprolide), hysteroscopic laser surgery can be performed on an outpatient basis under general or regional anesthesia in about 1 hour. A hysteroscope is introduced into the uterus and a fiberoptic delivery system is passed through the operating channel. Resectoscopic endometrial ablation has become a more popular technique than laser ablation, and it appears to be at least as effective; its advantages are a significantly shorter operating time and much less expensive equipment.

Amenorrhea occurs in up to 70% of patients after resectoscopic ablation, whereas hypomenorrhea occurs in more than 90% of cases. Continued excessive bleeding is believed to be more likely when multiple myomas or severe adenomyosis exists.

A more recent method of endometrial ablation does not require hysteroscopic visualization. These techniques use either a reservoir for the delivery of heat to the endometrial surface or microwave energy directed at the endometrium to render it unresponsive to hormonal stimulation. Because they are narrower than operative hysteroscopes and their attachments and can be inserted blindly into the uterine cavity, these methods are intended for office use and for use by surgeons who may not have the experience or skills needed for laser or resectoscopic surgery.

COMPLICATIONS OF OPERATIVE HYSTEROSCOPY

Operative hysteroscopy generally comprises procedures that are relatively simple and safe, resulting in few complications. The overall complication rate is about 2%, with major complications (perforation, hemorrhage, fluid overload, bowel or urinary tract injury) occurring in less than 1% of procedures. **The most significant risks of operative hysteroscopy are perforation of the uterus, excessive bleeding, and distention medium hazards (e.g., gas embolism, fluid overload, anaphylactic shock).** Much less frequent and less serious complications include infections (e.g., endometritis, pelvic inflammatory disease), traumatic cervical lacerations, and postoperative cervical stenosis.

Hysterectomy

Hysterectomy is the most commonly performed major gynecologic operation and among the top five most commonly performed major surgical procedures in the United States. It can be performed either abdominally or vaginally. Although some indications for hysterectomy remain controversial, high patient satisfaction levels and increasing safety for the procedure have been reported.

Table 30-1 provides a useful list of indications for abdominal or vaginal hysterectomy.

ABDOMINAL HYSTERECTOMY

A total abdominal hysterectomy is the most commonly performed procedure for benign uterine disease and involves the "simple" excision of the uterine corpus

---

TABLE 30-1

HYSTERECTOMY: INDICATION LIST WITH CRITERIA

ACUTE CONDITION

A-1*	Pregnancy catastrophe (e.g., severe hemorrhage)
A-2	Severe infection (e.g., ruptured tubo-ovarian abscess)
A-3*	Operative complication (e.g., uterine perforation)

BENIGN DISEASE

B-1	Leiomyomas
	  Symptomatic (e.g., bleeding, pressure)
	  Asymptomatic (≥12 wk size, confuses adnexal evaluation)

B-2	Endometriosis (distinct endometriosis, unresponsive to hormonal suppression or conservative surgery)
B-3	Adenomyosis (with symptomatic menometrorrhagia unresponsive to treatment)
B-4	Chronic infection (e.g., recurrent pelvic inflammatory disease)
B-5	Adnexal mass (e.g., ovarian neoplasm)
B-6	Other (operator defined, criteria specified)

CANCER OR SIGNIFICANT PREMALIGNANT DISEASE

C-1	Invasive disease of reproductive organs
C-2	Significant preinvasive disease of the uterus (CIN-3 or adenomatous hyperplasia of the endometrium with cellular atypia)
C-3	Cancer of adjacent or distant organ (gastrointestinal, genitourinary, or breast cancer)

DISCOMFORT (NO CONFIRMING TISSUE PATHOLOGY EXPECTED)

D-1*	Chronic pelvic pain (negative laparoscopy and nonsurgical treatment attempted)
D-2*	Pelvic relaxation (symptomatic)
D-3*	Recurrent uterine bleeding (unresponsive to hormone regulation, curettage, or endometrial ablation—normal-sized uterus)
D-4*	Other (operator defined, criteria specified)

EXTENUATING CIRCUMSTANCES (NOT SPECIFICALLY INDICATED BUT POSSIBLY JUSTIFIED—REQUIRES PREOPERATIVE PEER REVIEW)

E-1*	Sterilization (extenuating circumstances)
E-2*	Cancer prophylaxis (e.g., recurrent CIN after cone biopsy or persistent adenomatous hyperplasia of the endometrium without atypia)
E-3*	Other—listing extenuating circumstances

*Denotes indications for which tissue pathology is not expected to confirm the preoperative diagnosis.

CIN, cervical intraepithelial neoplasia.

Data from Gambone JC, Lench JB, Slesinski MJ, et al: Validation of hysterectomy indications and the quality assurance process. Obstet Gynecol 73:1045, 1989.

---

and cervix. **It may be performed intrafascially,** in which case the surgeon stays safely within the endopelvic fascia that surrounds the cervix and upper vagina, **or extrafascially,** in which case the investing fascia of the cervix and upper vagina is removed with the specimen. **A subtotal hysterectomy excises the uterine corpus,** usually at the level of the internal cervical os. **A radical hysterectomy involves the wide excision of the parametrial tissue laterally** (Figure 30-5), **along with the uterosacral ligaments posteriorly,** after the rectum is

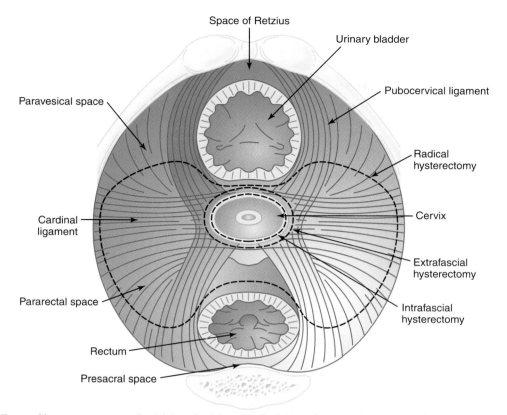

FIGURE 30-5   Types of hysterectomy: extrafascial, intrafascial, and radical. Note the extensive amount of parametrial tissue that is removed in a radical hysterectomy.

dissected free and after each ureter is dissected out of its tunnel beneath the uterine artery.

Indications

The indications for **total abdominal hysterectomy** may include such benign conditions as uterine myomas, endometriosis, chronic PID, stage I endometrial cancer, and uterine bleeding that is unresponsive to more conservative measures. In some cases, a subtotal hysterectomy may be preferred if the bladder is densely adherent to the front of the cervix. Some women may request a subtotal hysterectomy because of possible involvement of the cervix in the sexual response.

A **radical hysterectomy** is indicated for stage Ib and occasionally stage IIa cervical cancer. Endometrial cancer with gross cervical involvement may also be managed by radical hysterectomy.

In women who undergo hysterectomy at or after menopause, the uterine adnexa (fallopian tubes and ovaries) are usually removed. However, there are few studies weighing the risks and benefits of removing these normal organs. Before menopause, the option of preserving the ovaries at the time of hysterectomy

vs the expense and possible dangers of hormonal replacement therapy must be thoroughly discussed with the patient preoperatively. In general, the ovaries are preserved at hysterectomy for benign disease before menopause unless there is a strong family history of breast or ovarian cancer. The choice of incidental oophorectomy, along with incidental appendectomy, awaits a thorough, prospective quality-of-life analysis (economic and medical) to guide gynecologic surgeons and their patients.

Technique

Abdominal hysterectomy is carried out with the patient in the supine position, usually under general anesthesia. First, a thorough pelvic and abdominal examination under anesthesia is carried out and recorded. The choice of incision depends on the indication for the procedure. A vertical incision is advisable in patients who have had several prior abdominal operations, are extremely obese, or in whom extensive adhesions or endometriosis is anticipated. In patients with restricted benign disease, incisions along the lines of Langer (transverse in the lower abdomen) achieve a better cosmetic result. The various lower abdominal incisions and their anatomy are discussed in Chapter 3 and depicted in Figure 3-12.

After making the abdominal incision into the peritoneal cavity, the upper abdomen is manually explored with special reference to the liver, gallbladder, stomach, spleen, and para-aortic lymph nodes, and a reference to each must be recorded in the operative note. The intestines are inspected in cases of cancer with careful attention to mesenteric lymph nodes and the vermiform appendix. The patient is then placed in the Trendelenburg position, and the abdominal viscera are packed out of the pelvis with laparotomy tapes.

Each round ligament is clamped, incised, and ligated. The peritoneum on both sides is incised lateral to the infundibulopelvic ligament. This allows entry to the retroperitoneum between the leaves of the broad ligament exposing the ureter and pelvic vessels. The vesicouterine fold of the peritoneum is incised transversely between the incised round ligaments, and the bladder (adherent to the peritoneum) is reflected inferiorly off the fascia of the lower uterine segment, cervix, and upper vagina.

If the adnexa are to be removed, the ureters are identified, and the infundibulopelvic ligaments with the ovarian vessels are clamped, cut, and tied. The medioposterior leaf of the broad ligament is incised toward the uterus, thus exposing the uterine artery and veins as they course superiorly toward the utero-ovarian vascular anastomosis just below the ovarian ligament. If the uterine adnexa are to be preserved, the ovarian ligaments are clamped, incised, and ligated on each side.

The uterine vessels thus exposed are stripped of their adventitial tissue (skeletonized), clamped at the level of the internal cervical os, incised, and securely ligated bilaterally. The ligated uterine vessels are reflected laterally, allowing access to the cardinal ligament (of Mackenrodt). Staying medial to the ligated uterine vessels, the cardinal ligament on either side is clamped, incised, and ligated with a transfixion ligature. It may take several bites to free the cardinal ligaments from the lower cervix and upper vagina.

The peritoneum just below the posterior surface of the cervix is incised transversely between the utero-sacral ligaments, and the rectum is reflected from the posterior aspect of the cervix and upper vagina. The uterosacral ligaments are clamped, incised, and ligated, which frees them from the cervix and upper vagina. The total uterus (corpus and cervix) is removed by cutting across the vagina just below the cervix, with care taken to sufficiently reflect the urinary bladder and rectum inferiorly to avoid injury. **The vaginal cuff is normally closed with absorbable sutures,** incorporating the cardinal and uterosacral ligaments into each lateral angle of the vagina to preclude the later development

of a vaginal vault prolapse. If the uterosacral ligaments are widely separated, they may be plicated to prevent the formation of an enterocele. **Progressive circular sutures (of Moschowitz) may be placed to obliterate a particularly large pouch of Douglas, which also portends an increased risk for enterocele.**

Three points in the procedure present a particular risk for injury to the ureter: (1) as the infundibulopelvic ligaments are clamped and incised, (2) as the uterine vessels are ligated, and (3) as the cardinal ligaments are clamped if the urinary bladder is not sufficiently reflected inferiorly. **Use of the retroperitoneal approach, with identification of the ureters bilaterally and careful reflection of the bladder inferiorly, prevents ureteric injury.**

VAGINAL HYSTERECTOMY

Vaginal hysterectomy, if feasible, is preferable to the abdominal approach because it avoids a visible scar, is associated with less pain, affords an opportunity to correct pelvic relaxation, and generally requires less postoperative hospitalization and disability.

Indications

Ideally, vaginal hysterectomy is elected for benign disease when the uterus is mobile, is less than 12 gestational weeks in size, is characterized by some pelvic relaxation, and is expected to contain few or no adhesions from endometriosis, PID, or multiple prior lower abdominal operations. The procedure is most commonly performed in association with the correction of uterine prolapse, cystocele, rectocele, or enterocele in postmenopausal women.

The advent of laparoscopically assisted vaginal hysterectomy has greatly expanded the indications for the vaginal approach by freeing up adnexal adhesions, facilitating simultaneous removal of the tubes and ovaries, and identifying conditions that would not safely be managed at the time of vaginal hysterectomy.

Technique

The principles of the operation are similar to those of abdominal hysterectomy except that ligation of the ligaments and vessels proceeds in the reverse order. The patient is placed in the dorsolithotomy position after induction of anesthesia. The bladder is emptied, and a thorough pelvic examination is performed. A weighted vaginal retractor is placed in the vagina, a tenaculum is placed on the cervix, and the uterus is drawn down toward the vaginal introitus and tested for descent and mobility. A transverse incision is made through the vaginal epithelium between the uterosacral ligaments at the posterior junction of the cervix and vagina. The peritoneum of the cul-de-sac is bluntly mobilized and sharply entered. Adhesions of the cul-de-sac and posterior uterine wall are excluded by finger exploration. The uterosacral ligaments are clamped, cut, and ligated, allowing additional descent of the uterus.

At this point, the vaginal epithelial incision is extended circumferentially around the cervix, and the bladder is advanced superiorly along the anterior uterine wall, exposing the anterior uterovesical fold of the peritoneum, which is sharply entered. The pubocervical ligaments (bladder pillars) containing the ureters are bluntly displaced laterally and the cardinal ligaments are clamped, cut, and ligated, allowing further descent of the uterus.

An angle retractor (e.g., Heaney, Deaver) is placed into the opening of the anterior vesicouterine fold of the peritoneum, and the urinary bladder is retracted anteriorly. The uterine vessels are clamped, usually with a Heaney clamp, ensuring that the tips of the clamp include the peritoneal edge both anteriorly and posteriorly and that the tips are snug against the lateral uterine wall to include all the uterine vessels. The clamped vessels are cut and securely ligated.

Downward traction on the uterus should allow full exposure of the round ligaments, fallopian tubes, ovarian ligaments, and utero-ovarian vascular anastomoses, and these structures are clamped as a group on each side, cut free of the uterus, and securely ligated. Because these pedicles are quite bulky, especially in premenopausal patients, it is wise to double clamp and ligate them, first with a loop hemostatic ligature and then with a transfixion ligature.

If the adnexa are to be removed, the suspensory ligament of the ovary is addressed instead of the ovarian ligament. With Allis clamps, the fimbriated end of the fallopian tube and ovary are drawn inferiorly into the operative field, which brings the suspensory ligament of the ovary into full view, allowing it to be clamped, cut, and ligated, while taking special care to avoid the adjacent ureter. To visualize the ureter more clearly, the round ligament may be initially and separately clamped and ligated, which opens up the lateral extraperitoneal space. This phase of the procedure may be quite difficult in a premenopausal primigravida with good pelvic support, and is most readily achieved laparoscopically.

The peritoneum is then closed with a pursestring suture or one or more transverse U-sutures, leaving the pedicles in an extraperitoneal position. As with an abdominal hysterectomy, the uterosacral ligaments may be plicated with one or more sutures to avoid an enterocele. The ovarian and round ligaments may be sutured together in the midline, but this is optional because they add little or no pelvic support. The cardinal ligaments, however, should each be sutured to the lateral aspect of the vaginal cuff to provide vaginal support, to increase vaginal depth, and to prevent the later development of a vaginal vault prolapse. The cardinal ligaments should not be sutured together across the midline because that might shorten the vagina.

The vaginal epithelium is then closed with interrupted absorbable sutures. If the bladder pillars have been plicated to correct a cystocele or if a urethropexy has been employed to correct stress incontinence, catheter drainage of the bladder may be employed for 24 to 48 hours postoperatively.

COMPLICATIONS OF HYSTERECTOMY

Complications associated with any abdominal or pelvic surgery include anesthetic complications, hemorrhage, atelectasis, wound infection, urinary tract infection, thrombophlebitis, and pulmonary embolism. **Atelectasis occurs most commonly in the first 24 to 48 hours** and can be prevented and treated with aggressive pulmonary toilet. **Wound infection usually occurs about 5 days postoperatively** and is associated with redness, tenderness, swelling, and increased warmth around the wound.

Treatment may require systemic antibiotics, opening the incision, draining the discharge, local débridement, and wound care. **Urinary tract infection can occur at any time in the postoperative period,** and urine for microscopy and culture should be obtained from any patient with a postoperative fever. **Thrombophlebitis (with possible subsequent pulmonary embolism) is manifested by fever and leg swelling or pain; it usually occurs 7 to 12 days postoperatively.** Pulmonary embolism may occur even in the absence of signs of thrombophlebitis. **Wound disruption after abdominal hysterectomy with evisceration of intestines is generally heralded by a profuse serous discharge from the wound (peritoneal fluid) 4 to 8 days after surgery.** When evisceration is suspected, the wound should be explored in the operating room.

The most common intraoperative complication of abdominal or vaginal hysterectomy is bleeding from the infundibulopelvic or utero-ovarian pedicles, the uterine vascular pedicle, or the vaginal cuff. When postoperative hemorrhage occurs, bleeding from the vaginal cuff can sometimes be identified and controlled vaginally. **If bleeding is sufficient to cause hypotension, laparotomy may be required to tie off the bleeding vascular pedicle.**

Infection is common to both procedures and is manifested by fever and lower abdominal pain. Examination often reveals tenderness and induration of the vaginal cuff, which is indicative of pelvic cellulitis. This can usually be treated with antibiotic therapy. **Administration of prophylactic cephalosporin perioperatively has proved beneficial in controlling infection in vaginal hysterectomies performed in premenopausal patients.**

Injury to the ureter is the most serious complication of hysterectomy and usually occurs during the abdominal procedure, particularly during a difficult dissection for PID, endometriosis, or pelvic cancer.

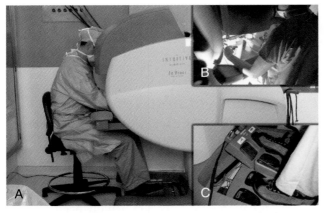

FIGURE 30-6   **A** to **C:** The da Vinci computer-assisted robotic surgical system. Note the console from which the surgeon directs the movement of the instruments. *(From Townsend CM, et al.: Sabiston Textbook of Surgery, 18th ed. Philadelphia, Saunders, 2008.)*

Ureteral injury can also occur during a vaginal hysterectomy. If not detected intraoperatively, fever and flank pain can develop postoperatively, and a ureterovaginal fistula or urinoma may become apparent 5 to 21 days after surgery. **If noted intraoperatively, a ureteral injury can be repaired by implanting the proximal cut end of the ureter into the bladder or by anastomosing the proximal and distal ends of the transected ureter over a ureteric stent.**

Intraoperative injury to the rectum or bladder, if recognized, should be repaired immediately. If a bladder repair is necessary, an indwelling catheter (suprapubic or transurethral) should be left on free drainage for 5 to 7 days. On rare occasions it may be necessary to protect the repair of an extensive rectal injury with a temporary loop colostomy.

■ *Robotic Surgery in Gynecology*

The role of computer-assisted or robotic surgery in gynecology is evolving. Prospective studies are needed to compare the efficacy of this technology to conventional methods. In 2005, the da Vinci surgical system (Intuitive Surgical, Sunnyvale, Calif) received U.S. Food and Drug Administration approval (Figure 30-6). As this new technology is introduced to improve surgical performance, its limitations (such as lack of tactile feedback and increased cost) will need to be addressed. Robotic-assisted instrumentation is being used for hysterectomy, pelvic reconstructive surgery, and gynecologic oncology.

SUGGESTED READING

Abstracts of the Global Congress of Minimally Invasive Gynecology, 36th Annual Meeting of the American Association of Gynecologic Laparoscopists, Washington, DC. J Minim Invasive Gynecol 14(6 Suppl):S1-S154, 2007.
Advincula AP, Song A: The role of robotic surgery in gynecology. Curr Opin Obstet Gynecol 19:331-336, 2007.
American College of Obstetricians and Gynecologists (ACOG): Technology Assessment in Obstetrics and Gynecology, Hysteroscopy. Washington, DC, ACOG, 2005, pp 350-353.
Hart R, Karthigasu B, Drishnan A: The benefits of virtual reality simulator training for laparoscopic training. Curr Opin Obstet Gynecol 19:297-302, 2007.
Reich H: Total laparoscopic hysterectomy: Indications, techniques and outcomes. Curr Opin Obstet Gynecol 19:337-344, 2007.

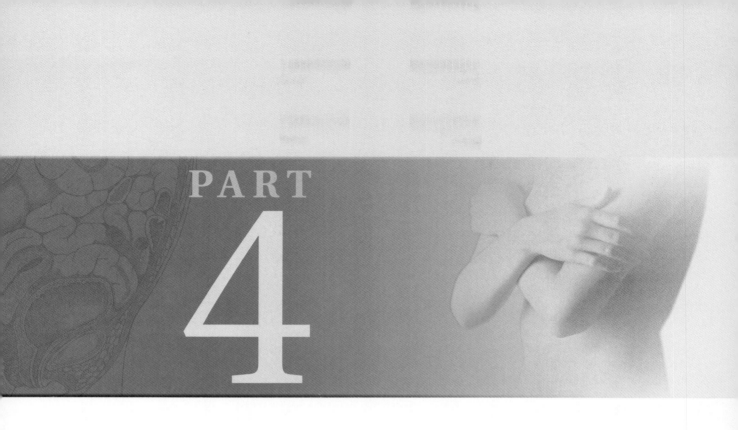

PART 4

REPRODUCTIVE ENDOCRINOLOGY AND INFERTILITY

Chapter 31

Puberty and Disorders of Pubertal Development

MARGARETA D. PISARSKA • CAROLYN J. ALEXANDER •
RICARDO AZZIZ • RICHARD P. BUYALOS, JR.

This part of *Essentials* (Chapters 31 through 36) deals with the normal and abnormal hormonal influences on the female reproductive system. The sequence of events is an excellent example of the "Life-Course Perspective" for women's health and health care introduced in Chapter 1. This series of events begins with endocrine changes in the fetus, the neonate, and then into childhood and pubertal development, then is followed by the early reproductive years, continuing on through the female climacteric, over the life course of a woman's reproductive years. This section of the book concludes with a chapter on other common disorders that are *influenced* by normal and abnormal hormonal changes during the menstrual cycle.

Puberty encompasses the development of secondary sexual characteristics and the acquisition of reproductive capability. During this transition, usually between 10 and 16 years of age, a variety of physical, endocrinologic, and psychological changes accompany the increasing levels of circulating sex steroids.

The onset of pubertal changes is determined primarily by genetic factors, including race, **and is also influenced by geographic location** (girls in metropolitan areas, at altitudes near sea level, or at latitudes close to the equator tend to begin puberty at an earlier age) and **nutritional status** (obese children have an earlier onset of puberty, and those who are malnourished or who have chronic illnesses associated with weight loss have a later onset of menses). **Excessive exercise** relative to the caloric intake can also delay the onset of puberty. **It has been proposed that an "invariant mean weight" of 48 kg (106 lb) is essential for the initiation of menarche** in healthy girls and that leptin, a peptide secreted by adipose tissue, may be the link between weight and initiation of menarche. **Psychological factors**, severe neurotic or psychotic disorders, and chronic isolation may

interfere with the normal onset of puberty through a mechanism similar to adult hypothalamic amenorrhea.

In the United States and Western Europe, a decrease in the age of menarche (age at first menses) was noted between 1840 and 1970. This trend has plateaued in the past 30 years (Figure 31-1). **Presently, the mean age of menarche is about 12.4 years in the United States.**

Endocrinologic Changes of Puberty

FETAL AND NEWBORN PERIOD

The fetal hypothalamic-pituitary-gonadal axis is capable of producing adult levels of gonadotropins and sex steroids. By 20 weeks' gestation, levels of gonadotropins—follicle-stimulating hormone (FSH) and luteinizing hormone (LH)—rise dramatically in both male and female fetuses (Figure 31-2). **The female fetus acquires the lifetime peak number of oocytes by mid-gestation,** and she experiences a brief period of follicular maturation and sex steroid production in response to elevated gonadotropin levels in utero. This transient increase in serum estradiol (a sex steroid) acts on the fetal hypothalamic-pituitary unit, resulting in a reduction of gonadotropin secretion (negative feedback effect), which in turn reduces estradiol production. This indicates that the inhibitory effect of sex steroids on gonadotropin release is operative before birth.

In both male and female fetuses, serum estradiol is primarily of maternal and placental origin. With birth and the acute loss of maternal and placental sex steroids, the negative feedback action on the hypothalamic-pituitary axis is lost, and gonadotropins are once again released from the pituitary gland, reaching adult or near adult concentrations in the early neonatal period. **In the female infant, peak serum levels of gonadotropins are**

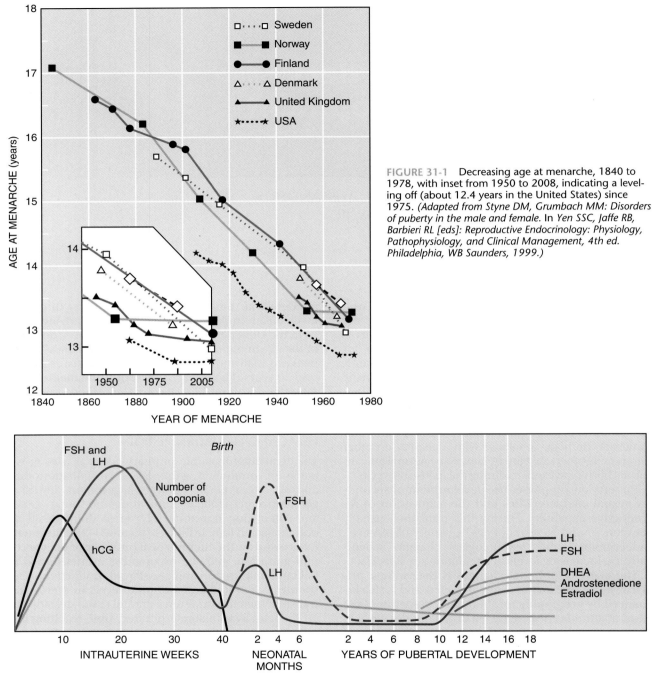

FIGURE 31-1 Decreasing age at menarche, 1840 to 1978, with inset from 1950 to 2008, indicating a leveling off (about 12.4 years in the United States) since 1975. *(Adapted from Styne DM, Grumbach MM: Disorders of puberty in the male and female. In Yen SSC, Jaffe RB, Barbieri RL [eds]: Reproductive Endocrinology: Physiology, Pathophysiology, and Clinical Management, 4th ed. Philadelphia, WB Saunders, 1999.)*

FIGURE 31-2 Changes in the concentration of gonadotropins (LH and FSH), sex steroids (DHEA, androstenedione, and estradiol), and the number of oogonia throughout fetal life and pubertal development. hCG, human chorionic gonadotropin; LH, luteinizing hormone; FSH, follicle-stimulating hormone; DHEA, dehydroepiandrosterone. *(Adapted from Speroff L, Fritz M: Neuroendocrinology. In Speroff L, Fritz M [eds]: Clinical Gynecologic Endocrinology and Infertility, 7th ed. Baltimore, Williams & Wilkins, 2005.)*

generally seen by 3 months of age and then slowly decline until a nadir is reached by the age of 4 years. In contrast to gonadotropin levels, sex steroid concentrations decrease rapidly to prepubertal values within 1 week after birth and remain low until the onset of puberty.

CHILDHOOD

The hypothalamic-pituitary-gonadal axis in the young child is suppressed between the ages of 4 and 10 years. The hypothalamic-pituitary system regulating gonadotropin release has been termed the ***gonadostat.*** Low levels of gonadotropins and sex steroids during this prepubertal period are a function of two mechanisms: maximal sensitivity of the gonadostat to the negative feedback effect of the low, circulating levels of estradiol present in prepubertal children, and intrinsic central nervous system inhibition of hypothalamic gonadotropin-releasing hormone (GnRH) secretion. These mechanisms occur independent of the presence of functional gonadal tissue. This is clearly demonstrated in children with gonadal dysgenesis. Agonadal children display elevated gonadotropin concentrations during the first 2 to 4 years of life, followed by a decline in circulating FSH and LH levels by 6 to 8 years of age. By 10 to 12 years of age, gonadotropin concentrations spontaneously rise once again, eventually achieving castration levels. This pattern of gonadotropin secretion in early childhood is similar to that of children with normal gonadal function. These data suggest that an intrinsic central nervous system regulator of GnRH release is the principal inhibitor of gonadotropin secretion from 4 years of age until the peripubertal period.

LATE PREPUBERTAL PERIOD

In general, androgen production and differentiation by the zona reticularis of the adrenal cortex are the initial endocrine changes associated with puberty.

Serum concentrations of dehydroepiandrosterone (DHEA), dehydroepiandrosterone sulfate (DHEA-S), and androstenedione rise between the ages of 8 and 11 years. This rise in adrenal androgens induces the growth of both axillary and pubic hair and is known as *adrenarche* or *pubarche*. This increase in adrenal androgen production occurs independent of gonadotropin secretion or gonadal steroid levels, and the mechanism of its initiation is not understood at this time. Recent studies indicate that girls who undergo premature pubarche are more likely to develop polycystic ovary syndrome (PCOS) as adults.

PUBERTAL ONSET

By about the 11th year of life, there is a gradual loss of sensitivity by the gonadostat to the negative feedback of sex steroids (Figure 31-3). As a consequence of this reduced negative feedback effect, GnRH pulses (with their mirroring pulses of FSH and LH) increase in amplitude and frequency. The factors that reduce the sensitivity of the gonadostat are incompletely understood. Some studies indicate that a rise in the concentration of leptin, a hormone produced by adipocytes (fat cells) that mediates appetite satiety, precedes and is necessary for this change. This, in turn, supports the connection between minimum weight or total body fat and the onset of puberty. A further decrease in sensitivity

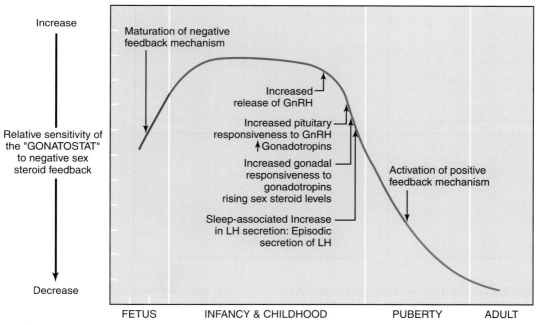

FIGURE 31-3   Changes in set point of the hypothalamic-pituitary unit (gonadostat) (*solid lines*) and the maturation of the negative and positive feedback mechanisms from fetal life to adulthood in relation to the normal changes of puberty. This figure does not illustrate the change in the sex steroid–independent intrinsic central nervous system inhibitory mechanism that is observed from late infancy to puberty. GnRH, gonadotropin-releasing hormone; LH, luteinizing hormone. (*Adapted from Styne DM, Grumbach MM: Disorders of puberty in the male and female. In Yen SSC, Jaffe RB [eds]: Reproductive Endocrinology: Physiology, Pathophysiology, and Clinical Management, 2nd ed. Philadelphia, WB Saunders, 1991.*)

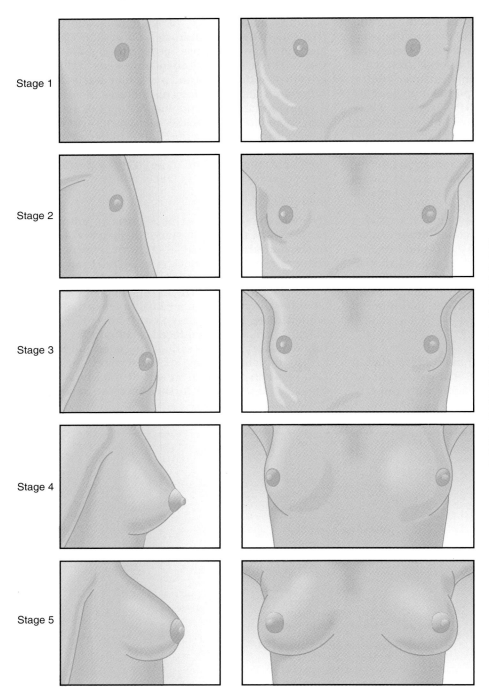

Stage 1

Stage 2

Stage 3

Stage 4

Stage 5

FIGURE 31-4 Stages of breast development as defined by Marshall and Tanner. *Stage 1:* Preadolescent; elevation of papilla only. *Stage 2:* Breast bud stage; elevation of breast and papilla as a small mound with enlargement of the areolar region. *Stage 3:* Further enlargement of breast and areola without separation of their contours. *Stage 4:* Projection of areola and papilla to form a secondary mound above the level of the breast. *Stage 5:* Mature stage; projection of papilla only, resulting from recession of the areola to the general contour of the breast. *(Adapted from Marshall WA, Tanner JM: Variations in pattern of pubertal changes in girls. Arch Dis Child 44:291, 1969.)*

of the gonadostat, combined with the loss of intrinsic central nervous system inhibition of hypothalamic GnRH release, is heralded by sleep-associated increases in GnRH secretion. This nocturnal-dominant pattern gradually shifts into an adult-type secretory pattern, with GnRH pulses occurring every 90 to 120 minutes throughout the 24-hour day.

The increase in gonadotropin release promotes ovarian follicular maturation and sex steroid production, which induces the development of secondary sexual characteristics. By mid to late puberty, maturation of the positive-feedback mechanism of estradiol on LH release from the anterior pituitary gland is complete, and ovulatory cycles are established.

■ *Somatic Changes of Puberty*

Physical changes of puberty involve the development of secondary sexual characteristics and the acceleration of linear growth (gain in height). The classification of breast and pubic hair development by Marshall and Tanner is employed for descriptive and diagnostic purposes (Figures 31-4 and 31-5).

STAGES OF PUBERTAL DEVELOPMENT

The first physical sign of puberty is usually breast budding (thelarche), followed by the appearance of pubic or axillary hair (pubarche or adrenarche). Unilateral breast development is not uncommon in early puberty and may last up to 6 months before the development of the contralateral breast. **Maximal growth or peak height velocity is usually the next stage, followed by menarche (the onset of menstrual periods).** The final somatic changes are the appearance of adult pubic hair distribution and adult-type breasts. In about 15% of normal girls, the development of pubic hair occurs before breast development. The sequence of pubertal changes generally occurs over a period of 4.5 years, with a normal range of 1.5 to 6 years (Figure 31-6).

Race plays a role in determining the age of the onset of puberty. African American girls begin puberty earlier than other racial groups (on average between the ages of 8 and 9 years), followed by Mexican Americans and whites (Table 31-1). In African American girls, thelarche and adrenarche can occur as early as 6 years of age, whereas in whites, they can occur as early 7 years of age.

A useful acronym used to remember the usual chronologic order of the stages of female pubertal development is T-A-P-M (thelarche, adrenarche, pubarche, and menarche).

ADOLESCENT GROWTH SPURT

In general, the pubertal girl's growth spurt is seen 2 years earlier than in boys. Growth hormone, estradiol, and insulin-like growth factor I (formerly somatomedin-C) are

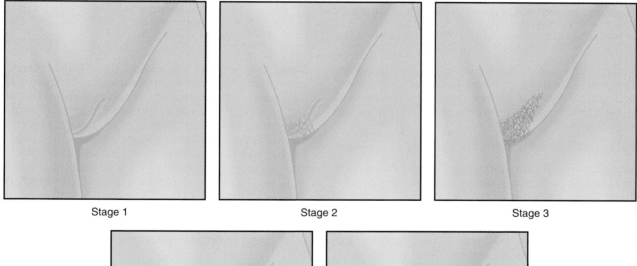

Stage 1 Stage 2 Stage 3

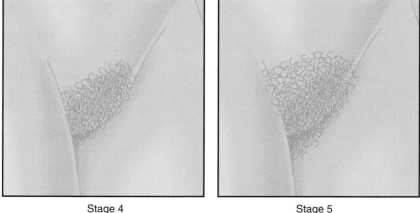

Stage 4 Stage 5

FIGURE 31-5 Stage of female pubic hair development according to Marshall and Tanner. *Stage 1:* Preadolescent; absence of pubic hair. *Stage 2:* Sparse hair along the labia; hair downy with slight pigment. *Stage 3:* Hair spreads sparsely over the junction of the pubes; hair is darker and coarser. *Stage 4:* Adult-type hair; there is no spread to the medial surface of the thighs. *Stage 5:* Adult-type hair with spread to the medial thighs assuming an inverted triangle pattern.

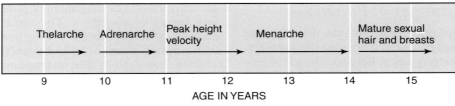

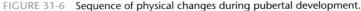

FIGURE 31-6   Sequence of physical changes during pubertal development.

TABLE 31-1

PUBERTY MILESTONES IN FEMALES

Puberty Milestone	Mean Age (yr)		
	Non-Hispanic White Females	*Black Females*	*Mexican American Females*
Pubic hair*	10.5	9.5	10.3
Breast development*	10.3	9.5	9.8
Menarche*	12.7	12.1	12.2
Menarche†	12.7	12.3	12.5

*Estimated with application of weights for the examination sample of The Third National Health and Nutrition Examination Survey and using probit model for the status quo data of the puberty measurements.
†Estimated using failure time model for the recalled age at menarche.
Data from Wu T, Mendola P, Buck GM: Ethnic differences in the presence of secondary sex characteristics and menarche among US girls: The Third National Health and Nutrition Examination Survey (NHANES III), 1988-1994. Pediatrics 110:752-757, 2002.

involved in the adolescent growth spurt. Peak height velocity occurs about 1 year before the onset of menarche. There is limited linear growth after menarche because gonadal steroid production accelerates fusion of the long-bone epiphyses.

BODY COMPOSITION AND BONE AGE

There are no significant differences in skeletal mass, lean body mass, or percentage of body fat between prepubertal boys and prepubertal girls. After attaining sexual maturity, girls generally have less skeletal and lean body mass and a greater percentage of body fat than boys.

Bone age correlates well with the onset of secondary sexual characteristics and menarche. Bone age is determined by using radiographs of the left (or nondominant) hand and wrist, elbow, or knee and comparing them with an index population. Osseous maturation is particularly useful in the evaluation of adolescents with delayed onset of puberty. Bone maturation, chronologic age, and height can also be used to predict the final adult stature from standardized nomograms.

▦ *Precocious Puberty*

Precocious puberty refers to the development of any sign of secondary sexual maturation at an age earlier than 2.5 standard deviations less than the expected age of pubertal onset. In North America, these ages are 8 years for girls and 9 years for boys. The incidence of precocious puberty is 1 in 10,000 children in

North America, and it is about 5 times more common in girls. **In 75% of cases of precocious puberty in girls, the cause is idiopathic.** A thorough evaluation to eliminate a serious disease process and to arrest potential premature osseous maturation that may affect the normal growth pattern is mandatory.

The early development of secondary sexual characteristics may promote psychosocial problems for the child and should be carefully addressed. **Typically, these girls are taller than their peers as children but ultimately are shorter as adults owing to the premature fusion of the long-bone epiphyses.** A classification system for female precocious puberty is shown in Box 31-1.

Precocious puberty may be divided into two major subgroups: **heterosexual precocious puberty (development of secondary sexual characteristics opposite those of the anticipated phenotypic sex) and isosexual precocious puberty (premature sexual maturation that is appropriate for the phenotype of the affected individual).**

Investigations for females with precocious puberty are shown in Box 31-2.

HETEROSEXUAL PRECOCITY

In females, heterosexual precocity results from virilizing neoplasms, congenital adrenal hyperplasia, or exposure to exogenous androgens.

Androgen-secreting neoplasms in females are either ovarian (most commonly Sertoli-Leydig cell) or adrenal in origin and are exceedingly rare in childhood.

They are diagnosed by abdominal physical and radiologic examinations and are treated by surgical removal.

Congenital adrenal hyperplasia most commonly results from a defect of the adrenal enzyme 21-hydroxylase leading to excessive androgen production. More severe forms of this defect cause the birth of a female with ambiguous genitalia. If untreated, progressive virilization during childhood and short adult stature will result. The treatment of this disorder includes replacement of cortisol with a related glucocorticoid and surgical correction of any anatomic abnormalities in the first few years of life. A less severe form of this defect, referred to as nonclassic (late-onset adrenal hyperplasia), can cause premature pubarche and an adult disorder resembling PCOS.

ISOSEXUAL PRECOCIOUS PUBERTY

Complete isosexual precocious puberty results in the development of the full complement of secondary sexual characteristics and increased levels of sex steroids. It may arise from premature activation of the normal process of pubertal development involving the hypothalamic-pituitary-gonadal axis, which is called **true isosexual precocity.** Exposure to estrogen, independent of the hypothalamic-pituitary axis (such as from an estrogen-producing tumor), is called **pseudoisosexual precocity.**

True Isosexual Precocity

In females, 75% of cases are constitutional. It may be diagnosed by the administration of exogenous GnRH (a GnRH stimulation test) with a resultant rise in LH levels equivalent to that seen in older girls who are undergoing normal puberty. **In about 10% of girls with the true form of precocious puberty, a central nervous system disorder is the underlying cause.** This includes tumors, obstructive lesions (hydrocephalus), granulomatous diseases (sarcoidosis, tuberculosis), infective processes (meningitis, encephalitis, or brain abscess), neurofibromatosis, and head trauma. It is postulated that these conditions interfere with the normal inhibition of hypothalamic GnRH release. **Children with precocious puberty secondary to organic brain disease often exhibit neurologic symptoms before the appearance of premature sexual maturation.** Evaluation of true isosexual precocity should include magnetic resonance imaging of the head for lesions.

BOX 31-1 *Classification of Female Precocious Puberty*

Heterosexual Precocious Puberty

Virilizing neoplasm
   Ovarian
   Adrenal
Congenital adrenal hyperplasia (adrenogenital syndrome)
Exogenous androgen exposure

Isosexual Precocious Puberty

Incomplete Isosexual Precocious Puberty

Premature thelarche
Premature adrenarche
Premature pubarche

Complete Isosexual Precocious Puberty

True isosexual precocious puberty
   Constitutional (idiopathic)
   Organic brain disease
      Central nervous system tumors
      Head trauma
      Hydrocephalus
      Central nervous system infection (abscess, encephalitis, meningitis)

Pseudoisosexual Precocious Puberty

Ovarian neoplasm
Adrenal neoplasm
Exogenous estrogen exposure
Advanced hypothyroidism
McCune-Albright syndrome
Peutz-Jeghers syndrome

Data from Brenner PF: Precocious puberty in the female. *In* Mishell DR Jr, Davajan V (eds): Infertility, Contraception and Reproductive Endocrinology, 3rd ed. Cambridge, MA, Blackwell Scientific Publications, 1991, p 349.

BOX 31-2 *Laboratory Tests Used Selectively to Evaluate Female Precocious Puberty*

Radiologic

Serial bone age (isosexual precocity)
Magnetic resonance imaging (MRI) or computed tomography (CT) of the brain with optimal visualization of hypothalamic region and sella turcica (true isosexual precocity)
MRI, CT, or ultrasonography of the abdomen, pelvis, or adrenal gland (heterosexual precocity, pseudoisosexual precocity)

Laboratory

Luteinizing hormone (LH) and follicle-stimulating hormone (FSH)

Dehydroepiandrosterone sulfate (DHEA-S), testosterone (heterosexual precocity)
17-OH progesterone, 11-deoxycortisol (suspected congenital adrenal hyperplasia [CAH] causing heterosexual precocity)
Thyroid function tests [TSH, free T_4] (isosexual precocious puberty)
Gonadotropin-releasing hormone (GnRH) stimulation test: LH measurement after 100 μg of GnRH given intravenously (to differentiate gonadotropin-dependent from gonadotropin-independent isosexual precocity)

Pseudoisosexual Precocity

Pseudoisosexual precocity occurs when estrogen levels are elevated and cause sexual characteristic maturation without activation of the hypothalamic-pituitary axis. In these girls, a GnRH stimulation test does not induce pubertal levels of gonadotropins. Causes include ovarian tumors and cysts, exogenous estrogenic compound use, McCune-Albright syndrome, severe prolonged hypothyroidism, and Peutz-Jeghers syndrome. Curiously, when the initial cause of pseudoisosexual precocity is eliminated, some girls go on to develop true isosexual precocity.

Some ovarian tumors can be felt on abdominal examination and are usually unilateral. Other lesions may require radiologic imaging for diagnosis. Treatment of these lesions is surgical.

The McCune-Albright syndrome (polyostotic fibrous dysplasia) **represents 5% of cases of female precocious puberty** and consists of sexual precocity, multiple cystic bone defects that fracture easily, café au lait spots with irregular borders (most frequently on the face, neck, shoulders, and back), and adrenal hypercortisolism. Hyperthyroidism and acromegaly may also occur in this syndrome. The pathophysiology involves a somatic mutation in affected postzygotic tissues, which causes them to function independent of their normal stimulating hormones.

Prolonged severe hypothyroidism has been hypothesized to cause pituitary gonadotropin release in response to the persistently elevated secretion of thyroid-releasing hormone (TRH). Concomitant elevated prolactin levels may also occur with the development of galactorrhea. Ovarian cysts may occasionally develop, and bone age may be retarded. This is the only form of precocious puberty associated with delayed bone age. Treatment is with thyroid replacement therapy.

The Peutz-Jeghers syndrome has been associated with a rare sex cord tumor with annular tubules, which may be estrogen secreting. Because this syndrome of gastrointestinal tract polyposis and mucocutaneous pigmentation has also been reported in association with a granulosa-theca cell tumor, children with this disorder should be screened for the development of gonadal neoplasms.

Incomplete isosexual precocity is the early appearance of a single secondary sexual characteristic. These conditions include **premature thelarche,** the isolated appearance of breast development before the age of 4 years (unilateral or bilateral) that resolves spontaneously within months and that is probably secondary to transient estradiol secretion; **premature adrenarche,** the isolated appearance of axillary hair before the age of 7 years that is the result of premature androgen secretion by the adrenal gland; and **premature pubarche,** the isolated appearance of pubic hair in girls before 8 years of age.

In general, premature thelarche and premature adrenarche are associated with appropriate sexual maturation, although they may be associated with the development of nonclassic adrenal hyperplasia and perhaps polycystic ovary syndrome. Therapy for these conditions is not required. Both conditions are more common in girls than in boys. It is not possible to diagnose an incomplete form of sexual precocity on a single evaluation, and interval examinations of **bone age** are necessary to rule out true precocious puberty.

TREATMENT OF TRUE ISOSEXUAL PRECOCIOUS PUBERTY

About 75% of cases of precocious puberty in girls prove to have a constitutional or idiopathic cause, and these patients are candidates for GnRH agonist (e.g., leuprolide acetate) therapy. These girls require treatment to prevent further sex steroid release and accelerated epiphyseal fusion. **If the condition is left untreated, fewer than 50% of girls with idiopathic precocity will attain an adult height of 5 feet.**

GnRH agonists are the most effective therapy for idiopathic precocity. Long-term GnRH agonist treatment suppresses pituitary release of LH and FSH, resulting in the decline of gonadotropin levels to prepubertal concentrations and arrest of gonadal sex steroid secretion. Clinically, normal gonadotropin release, sex steroid production, and pubertal maturation resume 3 to 12 months after discontinuation of GnRH agonist therapy.

The final adult stature of girls with GnRH-dependent causes of precocious puberty is strongly influenced by their chronologic age at diagnosis and initiation of treatment. When GnRH agonist treatment is initiated before the chronologic age of 6 years, the final adult height is increased by 2% to 4% (Figure 31-7). In contrast, the final adult height is usually not affected when the chronologic age at diagnosis and treatment is greater than 6 years of age.

Most children with sexual precocity have few significant behavioral problems, but emotional support is important in these children. **Behavioral expectations by family members and teachers should be based on the child's chronologic age, which determines psychosocial development, and not on the presence of secondary sexual characteristics.**

▓ Delayed Puberty

Although there is a wide variation in normal pubertal development, most girls in the United States begin pubertal maturation by the age of 13 years. **Failure to undergo thelarche by age 14 years requires evaluation.** A physiologic delay in the onset of puberty occurs

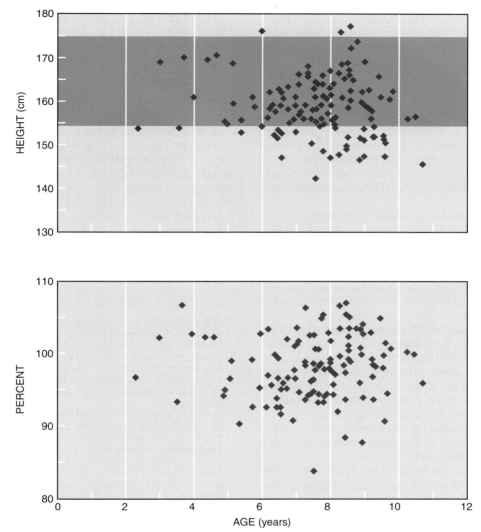

FIGURE 31-7   Scatter diagram of final height vs age at diagnosis of girls with gonadotropin-releasing hormone (GnRH)–dependent precocious puberty who were treated with GnRH agonist therapy *(top)*. The *shaded area* represents the range of normal adult height for North American women. *Bottom,* Percentage target height (final target height/target height × 100) vs the age at diagnosis. *(Modified from Kletter GD, Kelch RP: Effects of gonadotropin-releasing hormone analogue therapy on adult stature in precocious puberty. J Clin Endocrinol Metab 79:333, 1994.)*

BOX 31-3   *Radiologic and Laboratory Tests Used to Evaluate Female Delayed Puberty*

Radiologic

Magnetic resonance imaging (MRI) or computed tomography (CT) of the brain with optimal visualization of hypothalamic region and sella turcica (hypogonadotropic hypogonadism)

Laboratory

Follicle-stimulating hormone (FSH)
Karyotype (delayed puberty, ambiguous genitalia)
Progesterone (delayed puberty secondary to 17-hydroxylase [P450c17] deficiency)
Prolactin (hypogonadotropic hypogonadism)

in only 10% of girls with delayed puberty, and exclusion of other diagnoses is necessary. **Physiologic delays in puberty tend to be familial.** A careful history must be taken, with special attention to the patient's past general health, height, dietary habits, and exercise patterns. Details about the pubertal development of the patient's siblings and parents should be obtained. Box 31-3 lists tests that should be performed to evaluate girls with delayed puberty.

In general, the causes of delayed onset of puberty can be subdivided into two categories: hypogonadotropic hypogonadism and hypergonadotropic hypogonadism. Disorders resulting in hypogonadotropic hypogonadism that may cause primary or secondary amenorrhea are discussed in Chapter 32. Of note, **anorexia nervosa**, which **can result in hypogonadotropic hypogonadism** and delayed puberty, can affect 0.5% to 1.0% of young women. It is important to recognize this disorder in the evaluation of these patients. **Chromosomal abnormalities or injury to the ovaries by surgery, chemotherapy, or radiation may cause hypergonadotropic hypogonadism.** When the patient's abnormal karyotype includes the presence of a Y chromosome, gonadectomy is recommended to prevent potential malignant neoplastic transformation.

A growing list of single gene disorders resulting in delayed or absent female puberty is being documented in the literature.

Kallmann syndrome presents with hypogonadotropic hypogonadism and anosmia or hyposmia. It may result from a mutation of the *KAL* gene on the X chromosome or from autosomal mutations that prevent the embryologic migration of GnRH neurons into the hypothalamus. These individuals may have other anomalies of midline structures of the head. One in 50,000 females is affected.

Mutations of the GnRH receptor gene in females have resulted in low gonadotropin levels with primary amenorrhea or delayed puberty.

FSH β-subunit gene mutations and **FSH receptor gene mutations** have been associated with primary amenorrhea and varying degrees of incomplete development of secondary sexual characteristics.

Females with **aromatase deficiency** present at puberty with progressive virilization, absence of thelarche, and primary amenorrhea.

17-Hydroxylase (P450c17) deficiency interferes with production of the androgenic and estrogenic steroids, resulting in deficient or absent pubertal development. The accumulation of progesterone before the block leads to excessive synthesis of the mineralocorticoid, 11-deoxycorticosterone, that generally causes hypertension and hypokalemia.

Leptin and leptin receptor gene mutations are associated with retarded pubertal development and childhood morbid obesity.

Mutations in the steroidogenic acute regulatory (*StAR*) gene result in complete loss of adrenal steroidogenesis and delayed puberty, which is called *congenital lipoid adrenal hyperplasia.* The StAR protein is necessary in the transport of cholesterol from the outer mitochondrial membrane to the inner mitochondrial membrane, which is the rate-limiting step in steroidogenesis.

Adolescents who present with permanent hypoestrogenism require estrogen therapy as described in Chapter 32, **to complete the development of secondary sexual characteristics.** Hormone therapy with estrogen plus a progestin or with a low-dose oral contraceptive after establishment of secondary sexual characteristics is required to avoid menopausal symptoms and to prevent osteoporosis. To further maximize bone mineral accretion, 1500 mg of elemental calcium and 400 mg of vitamin D daily are recommended. This should be combined with regular weight-bearing exercises.

SUGGESTED READING

Carr B, Blackwell R, Azziz R: Disorders of puberty and amenorrhea. *In* Carr B, Blackwell R, Azziz R (eds): Essential Reproductive Medicine, 1st ed. New York, McGraw-Hill, 2005.

Feldman Witchel S, Plant TM: Puberty: Gonadarche and adrenarche. *In* Strauss JF, Barbieri RL (eds): Yen and Jaffe's Reproductive Endocrinology: Physiology, Pathophysiology, and Clinical Management, 5th ed. Philadelphia, WB Saunders, 2004.

Jaffe RB: Disorders of sexual development. *In* Strauss JF, Barbieri RL (eds): Yen and Jaffe's Reproductive Endocrinology: Physiology, Pathophysiology, and Clinical Management, 5th ed. Philadelphia, WB Saunders, 2004.

Pigneur B, Trivin C, Brauner R: Idiopathic central precocious puberty in 28 boys. Med Sci Monit 14:CR10-14, 2008.

Speroff L, Fritz M: Abnormal puberty and growth problems. *In* Speroff L, Fritz M (eds): Clinical Gynecologic Endocrinology and Infertility, 7th ed. Baltimore, Williams & Wilkins, 2005.

Speroff L, Fritz M: Normal and abnormal sexual development. *In* Speroff L, Fritz M (eds): Clinical Gynecologic Endocrinology and Infertility, 7th ed. Baltimore, Williams & Wilkins, 2005.

Chapter 32

Amenorrhea, Oligomenorrhea, and Hyperandrogenic Disorders

CAROLYN J. ALEXANDER • RUCHI MATHUR •
LARRY R. LAUFER • RICARDO AZZIZ

Amenorrhea, or the absence of menses, is a common symptom of several pathophysiologic states. This condition traditionally has been divided into **primary amenorrhea**, in which menarche (the first menses) has not occurred, and **secondary amenorrhea**, in which menses has been absent for 6 months or more. A more functional or clinical division of menstrual disorders based on initial history and physical examination would be as follows: primary amenorrhea with sexual infantilism, primary amenorrhea with breast development and müllerian anomalies, and amenorrhea and oligomenorrhea with breast development and normal müllerian structures. The last group includes disorders causing primary as well as secondary amenorrhea, oligomenorrhea, and the hyperandrogenic states (Table 32-1).

▓ Primary Amenorrhea

The diagnosis of primary amenorrhea is made when no spontaneous uterine bleeding has occurred by the age of 16 years. The workup should be initiated earlier if there is no evidence of breast development (thelarche) by age 14 years or if the patient has failed to menstruate (menarche) spontaneously within 2 years of thelarche. The presence of normal breast development confirms gonadal secretion of estrogen but not necessarily the presence of ovarian tissue. The presence of normal amounts of pubic and axillary hair confirms gonadal or adrenal secretion of androgens as well as the presence of functional androgen receptors.

PRIMARY AMENORRHEA WITH SEXUAL INFANTILISM

Patients with primary amenorrhea and no secondary sexual characteristics (sexual infantilism) display the absence of gonadal hormone secretion. The differential diagnosis is based on whether the defect is the result of a lack of gonadotropin secretion (**hypogonadotropic hypogonadism**) or an inability of the ovaries to respond to gonadotropin (**hypergonadotropic hypogonadism due to gonadal agenesis or dysgenesis**). The distinction can be made by the measurement of a basal serum follicle-stimulating hormone (FSH).

Hypogonadotropic Primary Amenorrhea and Sexual Infantilism

Patients with hypogonadotropic hypogonadism have low FSH levels, whereas patients with hypergonadotropic hypogonadism (e.g., gonadal dysgenesis) have elevated FSH levels in the menopausal range (>20 or 40 mIU/L, depending on the assay used). The measurement of serum luteinizing hormone (LH) is of limited additional diagnostic value. The absence of breast development is indicative of inadequate secretion of estrogen.

Hypogonadotropic hypogonadism may be caused by lesions of the hypothalamus or pituitary gland or by functional disorders that result in inadequate gonadotropin-releasing hormone (GnRH) synthesis and release. Because patients with sexual infantilism caused by hypogonadotropic hypogonadism may have

The views expressed in this chapter are those of the authors and do not reflect the official policy or position of the Department of the Navy, Department of Defense, or the United States Government.

TABLE 32-1

CLINICAL CLASSIFICATION OF MENSTRUAL DISORDERS

Disorder	Notable Diagnostic Findings	Examples	Notable Clinical Features
PRIMARY AMENORRHEA WITH SEXUAL INFANTILISM			
Hypogonadotropic hypogonadism	Low FSH and LH, low estrogen; screening for other pituitary hormones is indicated; MRI of the hypothalamic-pituitary area is recommended	Central nervous system or pituitary tumor, constitutionally delayed puberty, Kallmann syndrome	Exclude serious causes before diagnosing constitutional delay; anosmia/hyposmia with Kallmann syndrome
Hypergonadotropic hypogonadism	Elevated FSH and LH, low estrogen; karyotype indicated to rule out Y chromosome	Gonadal agenesis/dysgenesis including Turner syndrome (45 XO) and pure gonadal dysgenesis (46 XX or 46 XY)	May rarely present as secondary amenorrhea; streak gonads, short stature, and webbing of the neck with Turner syndrome
17-Hydroxylase (P450c17) deficiency	Low sex steroids (estrogens and androgens)		Hypertension and hypokalemia due to mineralocorticoid excess (see Figure 32-1)
PRIMARY AMENORRHEA WITH BREAST DEVELOPMENT AND MÜLLERIAN ANOMALIES			
Androgen insensitivity (46 XY)	Male levels of androgens in serum	Androgen insensitivity syndrome (formerly called *testicular feminization syndrome*)	Internal testicles, vaginal dimple, no uterus and breast development with smaller areola/nipples
Normal female karyotype (46 XX)	Female levels of androgens in serum		
Imperforate hymen	Hematocolpos on abdominal ultrasound		Bulge at introitus, cyclic pain with absent vaginal bleeding
Transverse vaginal septum	Obstruction visible on MRI		Cyclic lower abdominal pain without menses, hematometra, lowered fertility potential
Cervical agenesis	Cervix absent on MRI		Hysterectomy likely
Müllerian agenesis/ dysgenesis	Intravenous pyelogram indicated	Meyer-Rokitansky- Küster-Hauser syndrome	Vaginal dimple only, absent uterus on rectal
AMENORRHEA/OLIGOMENORRHEA WITH BREAST DEVELOPMENT AND NORMAL MÜLLERIAN STRUCTURES			
Pregnancy	Positive pregnancy test		
Uterine defects	Intrauterine scarring on hysterosalpingogram	Asherman's syndrome	Fertility problems
Hypoestrogenism	Low serum estrogen levels		
Hypopituitary dysfunction	Low FSH, LH, and prolactin; other hormone deficiencies should be ruled out	Excessive exercise (runner's amenorrhea); anorexia nervosa	Lean body mass; anorexia nervosa is primarily a psychiatric disorder with significant mortality
Premature ovarian failure	Elevated serum FSH, low serum estrogen, karyotype indicated if age < 30 yr	Autoimmune premature ovarian failure	Age <40 yr
Hyperprolactinemia	Elevated serum prolactin	Pituitary adenoma; empty sella syndrome; hypothyroidism; drugs; others (see Box 32-2)	Galactorrhea
Normal estrogen and amenorrhea	Normal hormone levels	Mild hypothalamic amenorrhea; exercise, nutrition, stress, hypothyroidism	
Hyperandrogenism	Elevated androgens (variable)	Congenital adrenal hyperplasia; polycystic ovary syndrome; HAIR-AN syndrome; others (see Box 32-2)	Hirsutism, acne, insulin resistance, virilization

FSH, follicle-stimulating hormone; HAIR-AN, hyperandrogenic insulin resistance and acanthosis nigricans; LH, luteinizing hormone.
Modified from Gambone JC: Student Manual. University of California—Los Angeles, David Geffen School of Medicine, 2003.

a craniopharyngioma or other central nervous system tumor, magnetic resonance imaging (MRI) or computerized tomography (CT) of the hypothalamic-pituitary area is recommended.

Hypogonadotropic hypogonadism resulting in primary amenorrhea and sexual infantilism may also be the result of lesions of the pituitary, including prolactin-secreting adenomas, or a general process of pituitary failure. These patients should be screened for other pituitary hormonal deficiencies by testing for thyroid-stimulating hormone (TSH), growth hormone, and adrenocorticotropic hormone (ACTH).

Finally, apparent hypogonadotropic hypogonadism may actually represent constitutionally delayed

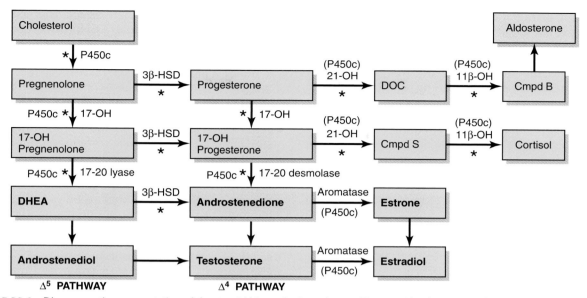

FIGURE 32-1   Diagrammatic representation of the steroid biosynthetic pathways. The *asterisk* refers to specific enzyme defects that result in congenital adrenal hyperplasia. Cmpd B, corticosterone; Cmpd S, II-deoxycortisol; DHEA, dehydroepiandrosterone; DOC, desoxycorticosterone; HSD, hydroxysteroid dehydrogenase; OH, hydroxylase; P450c, cytochrome P450.

puberty. This delay in the normal onset of puberty is generally attributed to undefined hereditary factors because there is commonly a history of late puberty in family members. Constitutional delay of puberty is a diagnosis of exclusion.

Hypergonadotropic Primary Amenorrhea and Sexual Infantilism

Patients with hypergonadotropic hypogonadism have some form of failed gonadal development or premature gonadal failure and will have elevated FSH levels. These patients may have gonadal agenesis (the absence or early disappearance of the normal gonad). Examples in males who may appear to be female in some cases are **pure gonadal dysgenesis**, or the **testicular regression syndrome**. These patients have an apparently normal 46 XY karyotype but lack testicular development. If fetal testicular regression occurs between 8 and 10 weeks of gestation, they may have female external genitalia with or without ambiguity in addition to a lack of gonads, a hypoplastic uterus (secondary to absent secretion of antimüllerian hormone), and rudimentary genital ducts (Swyer syndrome). Regression of the testes after 12 to 14 weeks results in variable development of male external genitalia. Anorchia, or streak gonads, occurs with testicular regression syndrome.

Other individuals with hypergonadotropic primary amenorrhea and sexual infantilism may have gonadal dysgenesis, or the presence of an abnormally developed gonad due to chromosomal defects. The differential diagnosis includes 45 XO (Turner syndrome), a structurally abnormal X chromosome, mosaicism with or without a Y chromosome, and pure gonadal dysgenesis (46 XX and 46 XY). Although most affected patients show no signs of secondary sexual characteristics, occasionally an individual with mosaicism or Turner syndrome will have sufficient ovarian follicular activity and secrete enough estrogen to cause breast development, menstruation, ovulation, and rarely even pregnancy.

In individuals with the presence of a Y chromosome, there is a risk for developing a gonadoblastoma (a benign germ cell tumor of the gonad) and eventually dysgerminoma (a malignant germ cell tumor). All patients with hypergonadotropic hypogonadism should have a karyotype performed. Because it is important to identify mosaicism, a greater number of white blood cells (>35) should be karyotyped.

Rarely, some patients with primary amenorrhea and sexual infantilism have a defect of estrogen and androgen production. One example of this is a 17-hydroxylase (P450c17) deficiency, which prevents the synthesis of these sex steroids (Figure 32-1). These individuals have hypertension and hypokalemia caused by mineralocorticoid excess. Other patients, such as those with a 46 XY karyotype and Leydig cell agenesis, may lack the cells necessary for sex steroid production. Because the Leydig cells in the testicle are responsible for producing testosterone, these individuals are born with female external genitalia.

Patients with sexual infantilism may be treated to stimulate breast development by very gradually

increasing estrogen doses. One commonly used regimen is to start with 0.3 mg conjugated estrogen every other day and slowly increase over 3- to 6-month intervals. This treatment should be guided by the presence or absence of mastalgia and the rate of breast development. The estrogen can be safely increased to 0.6 mg or more daily if necessary.

Individuals with persistent hypogonadotropic hypogonadism who seek fertility require either human menopausal gonadotropin injections or pulsatile GnRH administered by an infusion pump. Patients with gonadal dysgenesis and 17-hydroxylase deficiency who have a normal uterus and cervix can achieve pregnancy only by in vitro fertilization using donor oocytes.

PRIMARY AMENORRHEA WITH BREAST DEVELOPMENT AND MÜLLERIAN ANOMALIES

Patients with primary amenorrhea, breast development, and some defect of müllerian structures fall into two categories: those with complete androgen insensitivity syndrome (AIS), formerly called *testicular feminization,* **and those with müllerian dysgenesis or agenesis.** The distinction between these two diagnoses can be made by the measurement of a serum testosterone level and determination of the karyotype.

Androgen Insensitivity Syndrome

Patients with complete androgen insensitivity syndrome have a defect in the androgen receptor. Their karyotype is 46 XY, and they demonstrate male levels of testosterone, although usually on the lower side of normal. They may also have mildly elevated FSH and LH levels because their testes are located within the abdominal wall or cavity (cryptorchic). This location, with greater body heat, typically does not allow for normal male hormonal secretion. Breast development (with smaller nipples and areolae than normal genotypical females) is caused by the testicular secretion of estrogens and by the conversion of circulating androgen to estrogens in the liver and elsewhere. **The testicles of individuals with AIS secrete normal male amounts of antimüllerian hormone; therefore, patients have only a vaginal dimple and no uterus.** Treatment should consist of gonadal resection to avoid neoplasia (i.e., gonadoblastomas and dysgerminomas) once puberty is complete. The creation of a neovagina when the patient is prepared for sexual activity is possible by surgical and nonsurgical methods. Psychological counseling is an important component in the care of these patients.

Müllerian Dysgenesis or Agenesis

Patients with primary amenorrhea, breast development, and a 46 XX karyotype have levels of testosterone appropriate for females. This clinical diagnosis may be caused by müllerian defects that cause obstruction of the vaginal canal (e.g., imperforate hymen or a transverse vaginal septum) or by the absence of a normal cervix or uterus and normal fallopian tubes. An imperforate hymen should be suspected in adolescents who report monthly dysmenorrhea in the absence of vaginal bleeding (see Figure 18-7, pg 237). Clinically, these patients often present with a vaginal bulge and a midline cystic mass on rectal examination. Ultrasonography confirms the presence of a normal uterus and ovaries with a hematocolpos. These patients should be treated with hymenectomy.

Alternatively, women may present with similar symptoms but without a vaginal bulge. When ultrasonography confirms a normal uterus and ovaries, **a transverse, obstructing vaginal septum (see Figure 18-8, pg 237) or cervical agenesis should be suspected.** MRI is the diagnostic procedure of choice in these patients. If the MRI scan confirms a transverse septum, surgical correction is indicated. Surgical construction of a functional cervix is extremely difficult. In general, it is recommended that these women undergo hysterectomy.

Finally, **rectal examination and ultrasonography may be a sign of the absence of a uterus indicating müllerian agenesis or Meyer-Rokitansky-Küster-Hauser syndrome.** This syndrome is characterized by a failure of the müllerian ducts to fuse distally and to form the upper genital tract. These patients may have unilateral or bilateral rudimentary uterine tissues (anlagen), fallopian tubes, and ovaries. It is uncommon to have functional endometrial tissue within the anlagen. On occasion, the ovaries are not visible on ultrasonography because they have not descended into the pelvis. In these cases, CT or MRI may identify them well above the pelvic brim. **Currently, the pathophysiology leading to müllerian dysgenesis defects is not known.**

Creation of a neovagina can be accomplished using one of two general approaches. **The Frank method of vaginal dilation** uses dilation of the vaginal pouch with vaginal forms (usually thermoplastic acrylic resin [Lucite] dilators) over the course of weeks to months. Alternatively, a **McIndoe vaginoplasty,** which involves the surgical creation of a neovaginal space using a split-thickness skin graft, may be performed. Both of these methods should be initiated and performed close to the time when the patient anticipates having vaginal intercourse.

Congenital anatomic abnormalities of the uterus or vagina, or both, are often associated with renal abnormalities such as a unilateral solitary kidney or a double renal collecting system, among others. **Therefore, these patients should have an intravenous pyelogram or other diagnostic study to confirm a normal urinary system.**

Amenorrhea and Oligomenorrhea with Breast Development and Normal Müllerian Structures

Disorders in which the patient has breast development and a demonstrable cervix and uterine fundus on physical examination may cause primary as well as secondary amenorrhea, or may present as oligomenorrhea (menstrual cycles at greater than 35- to 45-day intervals).

All patients with menstrual bleeding disorders should be tested for pregnancy. Once pregnancy has been excluded, these individuals can be characterized as shown in Table 32-1. Initial history taking should include questions about the timing of thelarche, pubarche, and menarche. The timing and development of the menstrual disorder (present since puberty or new), significant weight change, strenuous exercise activities, dietary habits, sexual activity, concomitant illnesses or complaints, abnormal facial or body hair growth, scalp hair loss, acne, and the presence or absence of hot flashes and vaginal dryness should be noted. A comprehensive list of medications and dietary supplements taken should be obtained.

In addition to a pregnancy test, the initial investigation of the amenorrheic patient should include an FSH level and a progestin challenge test. Failure of the patient to have withdrawal bleeding after receiving a progestational agent indicates significant hypoestrogenism or hyperandrogenism, a uterine defect, or pregnancy. The absence of a withdrawal bleed after the administration of a progestational agent due to a uterine defect can be ruled out by the presence of withdrawal bleeding following sequential estrogen and progestin therapy. Progestogens used include medroxyprogesterone acetate, 5 to 10 mg/day orally for 5 to 14 days; norethindrone acetate, 2.5 to 5 mg/day orally for 5 to 14 days; oral micronized progesterone, 100 to 300 mg/day for 5 to 14 days; or progesterone in oil, 100 mg intramuscularly. Some clinicians prefer to order a serum estradiol (E2) instead of a progestin challenge to evaluate estrogen status.

UTERINE DEFECTS

Women who do not have withdrawal bleeding after a hormonal challenge test and who have a history of uterine instrumentation, particularly a dilation and curettage, following vaginal delivery or pregnancy termination may have Asherman's syndrome. This interesting syndrome is characterized by intrauterine scarring (synechiae), and these patients may have normal ovulatory cycles with cyclic premenstrual symptoms. Patients with Asherman's syndrome should be evaluated by hysterosalpingography or sonohysterography. Hysteroscopic treatment with excision of the synechiae and normalization of the uterine cavity is the treatment of choice.

AMENORRHEA AND OLIGOMENORRHEA ASSOCIATED WITH HYPOESTROGENISM

The differential diagnosis for patients with amenorrhea associated with low levels of estrogen includes hypothalamic-pituitary dysfunction (hypothalamic amenorrhea), premature ovarian failure, and hyperprolactinemia. Women in the first group have low FSH and prolactin levels, women in the second group have high FSH and normal prolactin levels, and women in the third group have high prolactin and low FSH levels.

Hypothalamic-Pituitary Dysfunction

Patients with hypothalamic amenorrhea include women experiencing severe weight loss, women undergoing excessive exercise resulting in low body fat, and women experiencing severe psychological stress. Also included are women with physical wasting from severe systemic diseases such as disseminated malignancies and patients with pituitary or central nervous system lesions. In its most severe and life-threatening form, women may have pituitary failure or anorexia nervosa. All patients with hypogonadotropic hypogonadism and hypothalamic-pituitary dysfunction should be evaluated for the status of the other pituitary hormones. Evaluation should also include an MRI of the hypothalamus and pituitary gland to exclude neoplastic and other lesions if it is uncertain whether the patient has one of the functional disorders described previously.

When hypothalamic-pituitary dysfunction cannot be resolved by identifying a modifiable underlying cause (e.g., excessive exercise), estrogen and progestin therapy, usually in the form of a combined oral contraceptive pill, is prescribed to reduce the risk for osteoporosis. This therapy is also recommended to maintain normal vaginal and breast development. In patients with anorexia nervosa, ovarian hormone therapy without weight gain will not totally prevent osteoporosis.

Premature Ovarian Failure

Premature ovarian failure is defined as ovarian failure before the age of 40 years (see Chapter 35). **When it occurs in patients younger than 30 years of age, ovarian failure may be caused by a chromosomal disorder. A karyotype is performed to exclude mosaicism (i.e., some cells bearing a Y chromosome).** If cells with a Y chromosome are present, a gonadectomy to prevent malignant transformation is indicated.

Other causes of premature ovarian failure include ovarian injury from surgery, radiation, or chemotherapy; galactosemia; carrier status of the fragile X syndrome; and autoimmunity. When premature ovarian failure is secondary to autoimmunity, other endocrine organs may be affected as well. Because there are no specific laboratory tests available to diagnose autoimmune ovarian failure, all patients with unexplained ovarian failure should be screened for diabetes (fasting glucose), hypothyroidism (TSH and free thyroxine [T_4]), hypoparathyroidism (serum calcium and phosphorus), and hypocortisolism (fasting morning cortisol or cortisol response to ACTH stimulation). It is not unusual for patients with premature ovarian failure to have episodes of normal ovarian and menstrual function. **Patients with premature ovarian failure require hormonal therapy (estrogen and a progestin) to reduce the risk for osteoporosis.**

AMENORRHEA AND OLIGOMENORRHEA WITH HYPERPROLACTINEMIA AND GALACTORRHEA

The principal action of prolactin is to stimulate lactation. Hypersecretion of prolactin leads to gonadal dysfunction by interrupting the secretion of GnRH, which inhibits the release of LH and FSH and, in turn, impairs gonadal steroidogenesis. The primary influence on prolactin secretion is tonic inhibition of dopamine input from the hypothalamus. Any event disrupting this inhibition can result in a rise in prolactin levels.

The consequences of hyperprolactinemia that are clinically significant include menstrual disturbances and galactorrhea. About 10% of women with amenorrhea have elevated prolactin levels, and a prolactin

BOX 32-1   *Causes of Elevated Prolactin*

- Pregnancy (10-fold rise from baseline)
- Excessive exercise
- Postprandial states
- Stimulation of the chest wall or nipple
- Medications
- Metoclopramide
- Phenothiazines
- Butyrophenones
- Risperidone
- Monoamine oxidase inhibitors
- Tricyclic antidepressants
- Serotonin reuptake inhibitors
- Verapamil
- Reserpine
- Methyldopa
- Estrogens
- Craniopharyngiomas
- Granulomatous infiltration of the pituitary or hypothalamus
- Acromegaly
- Severe head trauma
- Prolactinomas
- Pituitary stalk compression
- Hypothyroidism
- Chronic renal failure
- Marijuana or narcotic use

level should be measured in all cases of amenorrhea of unknown cause. Potential causes of elevated serum prolactin are noted in Box 32-1. Normal serum prolactin levels are less than 20 ng/dL, depending on the laboratory used. In patients with prolactin-secreting tumors, levels are usually more than 100 ng/dL. An elevated prolactin level should be confirmed by a second test, preferably in the fasting state because food ingestion may cause transient hyperprolactinemia. At the same time that the repeat prolactin level is drawn, a TSH level should be obtained to test for hypothyroidism because hyperprolactinemia may be seen in hypothyroid conditions.

A biologically inactive complex of prolactin and immunoglobulin, called *big prolactin,* can give a physiologically insignificant elevation. Therefore, the presence of a clinical abnormality should initiate the decision to test for hyperprolactinemia. **If clinically significant hyperprolactinemia is not explained by hypothyroidism or drug use, CT or MRI of the sella turcica should be performed.**

Galactorrhea is the most frequently observed abnormality associated with hyperprolactinemia. The secretion of milk may occur spontaneously or only after breast manipulation. Both breasts should be examined gently by palpating the gland moving from the periphery to the nipple. To confirm galactorrhea, a smear may be prepared and examined microscopically for the presence of multiple fat droplets (indicating milk). **Besides galactorrhea, hyperprolactinemia frequently causes oligomenorrhea or amenorrhea.**

Prolactinomas

Pituitary adenomas may cause hyperprolactinemia and make up about 10% of all intracranial tumors. Their etiology is unknown. Prolactinomas can be divided into two categories: macroadenomas ($\geq$10 mm in diameter) or microadenomas (<10 mm in diameter). This distinction is important because microadenomas are unlikely to cause new problems due to additional growth. About half of patients with hyperprolactinemia have radiographic changes in the sella turcica consistent with an adenoma. Most patients have normal or low baseline levels of FSH.

Other Central Nervous System Lesions Affecting Prolactin

About 60% of **pituitary adenomas** do not produce prolactin but may cause hyperprolactinemia by compression of the pituitary stalk. Another interesting lesion, **the empty sella syndrome,** is caused by a herniation of the subarachnoid membrane into the pituitary sella turcica through a defective or incompetent sella diaphragm. An empty sella may coexist with a prolactin-secreting pituitary adenoma. **Hypothalamic tumors** may also cause hyperprolactinemia by damaging the hypothalamus or by compression of the pituitary stalk, thereby interfering with the production or transport of dopamine. **Craniopharyngiomas are the most common of these lesions**.

Pharmacologic Agents Affecting the Secretion of Prolactin

A number of drugs may cause hyperprolactinemia and nonphysiologic galactorrhea (see Box 32-1). The mechanism of drug-induced hyperprolactinemia is secondary to reduced hypothalamic secretion of dopamine, depriving the pituitary of a natural inhibitor of prolactin release. When clinically indicated, patients with hyperprolactinemia caused by medications should be encouraged to discontinue the medication for at least 1 month. If hyperprolactinemia persists, or if the patient cannot interrupt the medication, a complete evaluation is indicated.

Miscellaneous Causes of Hyperprolactinemia

Patients with **acute or chronic renal failure** may have hyperprolactinemia because of delayed clearance of the hormone. These patients rarely require treatment other than for their renal failure. Patients with scars from previous chest surgery, including breast implantation, may have galactorrhea caused by **peripheral nerve stimulation**. Herpes zoster of the area including the breasts, as well as other forms of breast stimulation, can cause galactorrhea and sometimes hyperprolactinemia by the same mechanism. In about 3% to 5% of patients with galactorrhea and hyperprolactinemia, **primary hypothyroidism is the underlying cause**. These patients have a low serum free thyroxine (T_4) level. Consequently, they lack negative feedback on the hypothalamic-pituitary axis, resulting in increased secretion of thyrotropin-releasing hormone (TRH). TRH, in turn, stimulates elevated levels of TSH and prolactin. **Patients with primary hypothyroidism should be given T_4 replacement therapy.** Rarely cancers such as bronchogenic carcinoma or hypernephroma can result in elevated prolactin levels.

Treatment of Galactorrhea and Hyperprolactinemia

The objectives of therapy include the elimination of lactation, the establishment of normal estrogen levels, and the induction of ovulation when fertility is desired. The recommended forms of management are periodic observation, medical therapy, and surgery.

OBSERVATION. Periodic observation is indicated in normally menstruating women with galactorrhea who have either normal serum prolactin levels or idiopathic elevations of prolactin. **As long as the galactorrhea is not socially embarrassing and the patient has regular menses (confirming normal estrogen levels), there is no need to institute treatment.** Patients with oligomenorrhea who do not desire fertility should be treated with periodic progestins or, if contraception is needed, with combined hormonal contraceptives, to induce regular uterine bleeding. Failure to induce withdrawal bleeding with progestins is suggestive of hypoestrogenism. When verified by low serum levels of estradiol (<30 pg/mL) and a negative pregnancy test, cyclic hormonal therapy (estrogen and a progestin) should be initiated. **Long-term treatment with bromocriptine** (for hyperprolactinemia) **in women with normal estrogen levels is not indicated**.

Observation can be extended to some women with radiologic evidence of a pituitary microadenoma (<10 mm in diameter). **Because the growth rate of microadenomas is slow, an annual measurement of serum prolactin is appropriate in patients with normal estrogen levels.** Macroadenomas (≥10 mm in diameter) require further evaluation by periodic pituitary scanning and possible treatment.

MEDICAL THERAPY. Patients with hyperprolactinemia may have galactorrhea and anovulation with resulting infertility. In more severe cases, they may be hypoestrogenic, which places them at risk for developing osteoporosis. **Anovulatory patients without demonstrable tumors by MRI, and for whom the only issues are prevention of osteoporosis and menstrual cycle regulation, may be treated medically with combination hormonal contraceptives.**

The ergot compounds, bromocriptine and cabergoline, act as dopamine agonists to reduce prolactin secretion and allow for the restoration of cyclic, physiologic estrogen secretion. Bromocriptine has a high initial incidence of side effects such as headache, nausea, and orthostatic hypotension. As a consequence, it should be started at a dose of 1.25 to 2.5 mg at bedtime and slowly increased in divided doses to tolerance and restoration of normal prolactin levels. Some patients tolerate bromocriptine better when it is given vaginally. Cabergoline is taken in twice-weekly doses beginning at 0.25 mg and increasing to a maximum of 1 mg twice weekly. It is better tolerated and more convenient to take than bromocriptine, but it is also more expensive.

Ninety-five percent of women without radiographic evidence of an adenoma require 5 mg/day of bromocriptine, whereas about 50% of patients with adenomas require higher doses to resume regular menses. **Bromocriptine normalizes the secretion of prolactin in 82% of women with microadenomas and restores menses and fertility in more than 90%.** Usually, menses resume, and galactorrhea resolves after about 6 weeks of bromocriptine therapy in women without adenomas. If an adenoma is present, it takes another 3 or 4 weeks for bromocriptine to become effective. Return of ovulation requires an average of 10 weeks without a tumor and 16 weeks with a microadenoma. Restoration of normal menstrual cycles and pregnancy may occur without complete normalization of the serum prolactin level. Discontinuation of therapy usually results in the return of hyperprolactinemia, leading to galactorrhea and amenorrhea.

Patients with macroadenomas (≥10 mm diameter) should have visual field testing and screening for other pituitary hormone deficiencies. A repeat MRI is done 6 months after the full therapeutic dose of bromocriptine is reached. As long as shrinkage of the adenoma is demonstrated, bromocriptine therapy is continued. **Surgery should be performed for patients with significant visual field defects or symptoms that cannot be relieved by medical therapy.**

Bromocriptine therapy is usually discontinued as soon as a pregnancy is confirmed. The risk for symptomatic enlargement of a microadenoma during pregnancy is only about 1%. When a macroadenoma is confined to the sella turcica, it is also unlikely to enlarge significantly during pregnancy. If there is extension of a macroadenoma beyond the sella turcica, there is a 15% to 30% risk for enlargement during pregnancy. If possible, these larger lesions should be debulked before conception, and bromocriptine treatment should be initiated. Pregnant patients with macroadenomas should have visual fields evaluated in each trimester. When abnormalities in visual fields develop, bromocriptine treatment should be reinstituted or increased and maintained for the rest of the pregnancy. There is no increase in fetal malformations as a result of bromocriptine treatment, and the drug can be discontinued after the completion of pregnancy to allow for breastfeeding. Cabergoline has not been adequately evaluated for use in pregnancy.

SURGERY. When surgery is required, the transsphenoidal route for the microsurgical exploration of the sella turcica gives the best results. Recurrence rates for microadenomas after surgery approach 30%, and this increases to 90% for macroadenomas. For this reason, medical management is preferred, with surgery reserved for cases with expansion outside of the sella turcica or for compressive symptoms, such as visual defects. Women who do not tolerate pharmacologic therapy may need surgery. Fifty percent of patients followed for 5 to 10 years after successful resection of an adenoma have recurrence of hyperprolactinemia without radiologic evidence of tumor.

Amenorrhea and Oligomenorrhea with Normal Estrogen Levels

Patients with amenorrhea or oligomenorrhea who consistently have normal levels of estrogen have a mild form of hypothalamic anovulation that may be caused by low body weight and exercise issues, psychological stress, recent pregnancy, or lactation. They may also have been treated with Depo Provera or combined hormonal contraceptives in the recent past. These iatrogenic causes usually resolve spontaneously within 6 months. Some women with amenorrhea or oligomenorrhea and normal estrogen levels may have a subclinical androgen excess disorder, such as a mild form of polycystic ovary syndrome (PCOS).

When contraception is not required in these anovulatory women and fertility is not desired, periodic progestin withdrawal to confirm normal estrogen levels and protect their endometrium is appropriate. When fertility is not desired, combination hormonal contraception is appropriate.

Amenorrhea and Oligomenorrhea with Hyperandrogenism

Hyperandrogenism is the clinical manifestation of elevated levels of male hormones in women. Features may range from mild unwanted excess hair growth and acne to alopecia (hair loss), more extensive hirsutism, and masculinization and virilization. Hirsutism is the presence of male-like hair growth caused by conversion of vellus to terminal hairs in areas such as the face, chest, abdomen, or upper thighs. Figure 32-2 illustrates a scoring system for hirsutism. Signs of masculinization include loss of female body fat and decreased breast size. **Virilization is the addition of temporal balding, deepening of the voice, and enlargement of the clitoris** to any of the previous signs of excess male hormone. Androgens in women are normally produced in the ovaries and the adrenal glands (see Figure 32-1, pg 357). Hyperandrogenic disorders may be divided into functional and neoplastic disorders of the adrenal or ovary (Box 32-2).

NORMAL ANDROGEN METABOLISM

The formation of androgens results from the metabolism of cholesterol via the Δ^5 or Δ^4 pathway (see Figure 32-1). The stimulus for ovarian androgen production is LH.

About half of serum testosterone and androstenedione originates in the ovary, whereas the other half arises from the adrenal gland. Dehydroepiandrosterone (DHEA), and its sulfate DHEA-S, are primarily products of the adrenal and serve as markers for the secretion of adrenal androgens. **Most androgens are bound in the circulation to specific proteins, such as albumin and sex hormone–binding globulin (SHBG). In the bound form, androgens are biologically inactive.** The biologically active or free fraction represents only about 1% to 2% of total circulating testosterone.

When androgens reach a target tissue, they are further metabolized, which results in more potent

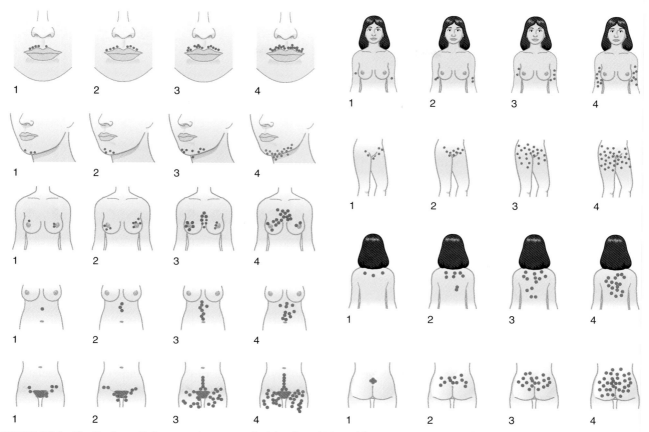

FIGURE 32-2   The Ferriman-Gallwey scoring system for hirsutism. *(Adapted from American Journal of Obstetrics and Gynecology, 140[5], Hatch R, 815-830, Copyright 1981, with permission from Elsevier.)*

BOX 32-2   *Hyperandrogenic Disorders*

Adrenal Disorders

Congenital adrenal hyperplasia (CAH)
Cushing's syndrome
Adrenal adenomas and carcinomas

Ovarian Disorders

Polycystic ovary syndrome (PCOS)
HAIR-AN syndrome
Ovarian neoplasms
Sertoli-Leydig cell tumors
Hilus cell tumors
Lipoid cell tumors

Idiopathic Hirsutism

HAIR-AN, hyperandrogenic insulin resistance and acanthosis nigricans.

---

intracellular hormones. **Testosterone is converted (by 5α-reductase) to dihydrotestosterone (DHT), which possesses greater biologic potency.** The skin, particularly its pilosebaceous unit, is capable of this conversion. Frequently, hirsutism is accompanied by oily skin and acne. Alternatively, testosterone may be aromatized to estrogens, changing its androgenic effect.

Hyperandrogenic Disorders

In general, hyperandrogenic disorders can be attributed to excessive secretion of androgens by the ovaries, by the adrenals, or both.

ADRENAL DISORDERS

Congenital Adrenal Hyperplasia

Congenital adrenal hyperplasia (CAH) is a general term used to describe an assortment of disorders that arise from inborn glandular enzyme deficiencies associated with the overproduction of steroids. **The most common cause of CAH is 21-hydroxylase deficiency.** CAH represents a spectrum of disorders, ranging from the severe salt-wasting form, to simple virilizing CAH, to nonclassic CAH. Both salt-wasting and simple-virilizing CAH are called *classic* because symptoms (e.g., salt loss or ambiguous genitalia in female newborns) are present at birth or shortly thereafter. Alternatively, the nonclassic form (also called *late onset*) presents later in life, generally at the time of puberty or later. These patients do not present with genital abnormalities, although they may develop hirsutism, acne, and menstrual and ovulatory irregularities.

Because 21-hydroxylase is responsible for the conversion of 17-hydroxyprogesterone to 11-deoxycortisol (compound S), a deficiency in 21-hydroxylase results in an excessive accumulation of 17-hydroxyprogesterone. As a result, this enzyme disorder is marked by an elevated serum 17-hydroxyprogesterone level as well as increases in its Δ^4 metabolites androstenedione and testosterone (see Figure 32-1). **This disease is inherited as an autosomal recessive trait.**

Cushing's Syndrome

Another major adrenal disorder leading to excessive androgen production is Cushing's syndrome or persistent hypercortisolism. Characteristic cushingoid signs include truncal obesity, moon-like faces, hypertension, easy bruisability, impaired glucose tolerance, muscle wasting, osteoporosis, abdominal striae, and supraclavicular and cervical spinal fat pads. Other manifestations include hirsutism, acne, and irregular menses. This disorder may arise from a cortisol-producing tumor of the adrenal gland or from an ACTH-producing pituitary adenoma (Cushing's disease). This is a rare cause of menstrual dysfunction in women.

Adrenal Neoplasms

Adrenal tumors causing hyperandrogenism without symptoms and signs of glucocorticoid excess are rare. Adenomas, which produce androgens only, generally secrete large amounts of DHEA-S. Adrenal carcinomas may produce large amounts of both glucocorticoids and androgens.

OVARIAN DISORDERS

Polycystic Ovary Syndrome

Six to 10% of women of reproductive age have some form of PCOS. This syndrome is a chronic condition that has been defined as anovulation or oligo-ovulation with clinical or laboratory evidence of hyperandrogenism and without evidence of any other underlying condition. Its onset is usually at the time of puberty. **There is a heritable aspect to PCOS** with an increased chance that first-degree female relatives are affected.

Clinically, the most common signs of PCOS are hirsutism (90%), menstrual irregularity (90%), and infertility (75%). Hirsutism is less likely in women who have used combined hormonal contraceptives for most of their postpubertal lives and for women of East Asian ethnicity. Although many patients with PCOS demonstrate abdominal obesity, the prevalence of obesity varies widely by country of origin, with the United States having the highest prevalence of obesity in women with PCOS (about 60%).

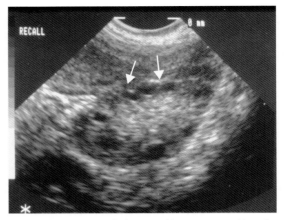

FIGURE 32-3 Transvaginal ultrasound in a woman with polycystic ovarian disease. The multiple subcapsular cysts, with their "string of pearls" appearance (*arrows*), are common in this syndrome.

In most patients with PCOS, **the ovaries contain multiple follicular cysts that are inactive** and arrested in the mid-antral stage of development. The cysts are located peripherally in the cortex of the ovary (Figure 32-3). The ovarian stroma is hyperplastic and usually contains nests of luteinized theca cells that produce androgens. About 20% of hormonally normal women may also have polycystic-appearing ovaries.

The hyperandrogenism of PCOS results from an overproduction of male hormones by the ovary and often the adrenal gland. It is not clear what the ultimate underlying pathophysiology of PCOS is or even whether it is a single clinical entity. **Patients with PCOS exhibit increased LH pulse frequency, usually resulting in higher circulating levels of LH.** It is likely that these patients exhibit increased LH levels because of increased GnRH secretion from the hypothalamus and increased pituitary sensitivity to GnRH.

The increased LH level promotes androgen secretion from ovarian theca cells, leading to elevated levels of ovarian-derived androstenedione and testosterone. This then leads to atresia of many developing follicles and interferes with the normal development of a dominant or preovulatory ovarian follicle much of the time. Peripheral conversion of androgen to estrogen results in tonic estrogen levels that are higher than those found normally in the early follicular phase and that suppress FSH release from the pituitary gland. The normal pattern of stimulated estrogen rise is disrupted, and the midcycle LH surge does not occur with resulting anovulation and progesterone production. **Some PCOS patients have excessive androgen production from the adrenal glands as well as the ovaries.** The mechanism for the excess adrenal androgen production in PCOS is unclear.

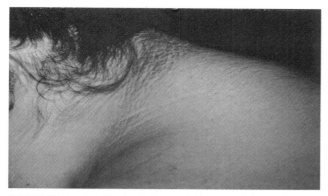

FIGURE 32-4 Acanthosis nigricans of the nape of the neck. These gray-brown velvety areas of the skin can be seen on the neck, groin, abdomen, or axillae and are markers of insulin resistance and hyperinsulinemia. *(Courtesy of Ricardo Azziz, MD, MPH, MBA, Cedars-Sinai Medical Center.)*

In women with PCOS there is an association between abnormal androgen production and insulin resistance with hyperinsulinism. In about 60% to 70% of patients with PCOS, insulin sensitivity is decreased, leading to insulin hypersecretion. This hyperinsulinemia results from direct insulin stimulation of theca cells resulting in androgen secretion. **Elevated androgen and insulin levels in PCOS also reduce the hepatic production and secretion of SHBG.** When SHBG production is suppressed, the amount of free testosterone may be dramatically increased, even though the overall increase in total testosterone is moderate or small. Thus, the physical manifestations of hyperandrogenism in PCOS may seem dramatic in relation to the level of total testosterone.

In the long term, the insulin resistance associated with PCOS may lead to an increased risk for metabolic syndrome (diabetes and heart disease). The unopposed estrogens in women with PCOS may cause hyperplasia of the endometrium and occasionally endometrial carcinoma.

The diagnosis of PCOS continues to be somewhat controversial because of disagreement about diagnostic criteria. PCOS is a diagnosis of exclusion. It is also a syndrome, rather than a distinct and readily definable disease. **The European Society for Human Reproduction and Embryology defines PCOS as being present when patients demonstrate irregular ovulation (usually with clinically evident oligomenorrhea), signs of hyperandrogenism, or polycystic ovaries, after other causes of these signs have been ruled out.**

Hyperandrogenic Insulin Resistance and Acanthosis Nigricans Syndrome

Hyperandrogenic insulin resistance and acanthosis nigricans (HAIR-AN) syndrome is an inherited hyperandrogenic disorder of severe insulin resistance, distinct from PCOS. HAIR-AN syndrome is characterized by extremely high circulating levels of insulin (>80 µU/mL basally or >500 µU/mL following an oral glucose challenge) due to severe insulin resistance. Because insulin is also a mitogenic hormone, these extremely elevated insulin levels result in hyperplasia of the basal layers of the epidermal skin, leading to the development of acanthosis nigricans, a velvety, hyperpigmented change of the crease areas of the skin (Figure 32-4). In addition, because of the effect of insulin on ovarian theca cells, the ovaries of many patients with the HAIR-AN syndrome are hyperthecotic. Patients with this disorder can be severely hyperandrogenic and even present with virilization. In addition, these patients are at significant risk for dyslipidemia, type 2 diabetes mellitus, hypertension, and cardiovascular disease. These patients are particularly difficult to treat, although the use of long-acting GnRH analogues has been promising.

Ovarian Neoplasms

Androgen-producing ovarian tumors are extremely uncommon, occurring in about 1 in 500 hirsute women and include Sertoli-Leydig, hilus, and lipoid cell tumors and virilizing conditions associated with hyperplasia of the stroma surrounding non–hormone-producing ovarian neoplasms. These tumors include cystic teratomas, Brenner's tumors, serous cystadenomas, and Krukenberg's tumors (see Chapter 20).

IDIOPATHIC HIRSUTISM

Some women exhibit mild to moderate hirsutism without a measurable elevation in the circulating levels of androgens or irregular ovulation, a condition referred to as *idiopathic hirsutism*. This condition has also been erroneously referred to as *constitutional hirsutism*. Idiopathic hirsutism may occur as a result of increased tissue conversion of testosterone to the more biologically active DHT. Almost all conditions resulting in hirsutism (e.g., PCOS, HAIR-AN syndrome, or CAH), have an inherited or familial component. True hirsutism (male-pattern terminal hairs) is rarely constitutional and almost always signals an underlying androgenic disorder in women.

Evaluation of Patients with Signs of Hyperandrogenism

HISTORY

Functional disorders such as PCOS or late-onset CAH often first appear during puberty and tend to progress slowly. In these disorders, the signs of androgen excess develop over several years. In contrast, **neoplastic disorders can occur at any time.** They most often arise years after puberty, and their manifestations appear abruptly. Progression is rapid, and these patients frequently present with the recent onset of virilization. There is some overlap with functional disorders in that 15% of patients with HAIR-AN syndrome can also exhibit signs of virilization, particularly severe hirsutism, temporal balding, and even some clitoral enlargement.

PHYSICAL EXAMINATION

The degree of hirsutism (see Figure 32-2), acne, or androgenic alopecia should be assessed and the thyroid palpated for enlargement. Patients should be expressly asked about excess facial hair because they may conceal their hirsutism by waxing or electrolysis and be too embarrassed to volunteer the information. Evidence of cushingoid features should be noted. Acanthosis nigricans (see Figure 32-4) is a frequent marker of insulin resistance and hyperinsulinemia. A bimanual pelvic examination may identify ovarian enlargement. Asymmetric ovarian enlargement associated with the rapid onset of virilization can indicate a rare androgen-producing tumor.

LABORATORY EVALUATION

The laboratory evaluation of patients with virilization or significant hirsutism, or both, is aimed primarily at exclusion of serious disorders.

A basal 17-hydroxyprogesterone level is useful to exclude 21-hydroxylase–deficient CAH. With concentrations greater than 2 ng/mL, ACTH stimulation testing measuring 17-hydroxyprogesterone is the definitive method of diagnosis. When Cushing's syndrome is suspected, either a 24-hour measurement of free urinary cortisol or an overnight dexamethasone suppression test should be performed. For the latter test, 1 mg of dexamethasone is given orally at bedtime, and serum cortisol is measured in an 8:00 AM fasting specimen; normal values are less than 5 g/dL.

Measurement of prolactin and TSH levels excludes hyperprolactinemia with or without thyroid dysfunction. In patients with unclear signs of hyperandrogenism, the measurement of **serum levels of total and free testosterone and DHEA-S may be helpful. Confirmed values of DHEA-S in excess of 7000 ng/mL or total testosterone in excess of 200 ng/dL is highly suspicious for an adrenal or ovarian androgen-producing tumor. However, the best predictor of an androgen-secreting neoplasm, rare as it is, is the clinical presentation. Signs of virilization are present in 98% of patients with tumors, regardless of the peripheral level of testosterone.**

A pelvic ultrasound should be obtained whenever any high-risk features are present to exclude an ovarian tumor. Androgen-secreting tumors of the adrenal gland can be detected by **CT or MRI.** If clinical or laboratory findings indicate the presence of an androgen-secreting tumor, and it cannot be located by imaging

studies, **selective venous catheterization** may be carried out and androgens measured in the venous blood from each adrenal gland and ovary.

In patients with PCOS and the HAIR-AN syndrome, evaluation of their metabolic status should be performed. Although a fasting glucose level is adequate screening for diabetes mellitus in many women, in patients with PCOS, optimal screening should include a 2-hour oral glucose tolerance test, measuring both glucose and insulin. Lipid levels should be measured in patients with PCOS, at least in those over the age of 35 years, and in younger patients with evidence of metabolic dysfunction (e.g., HAIR-AN syndrome).

TREATMENT OF HYPERANDROGENISM

Treatment should be guided by the nature of the underlying disease, the severity of clinical symptoms and signs, and the desires of the patient. **In the rare instance that an ovarian or adrenal neoplasm exists, surgical removal of the tumor is indicated.** In premenopausal women, unilateral salpingo-oophorectomy is sufficient for an ovarian tumor and preserves future childbearing potential. In postmenopausal women, the treatment is usually a total abdominal hysterectomy and bilateral salpingo-oophorectomy. **In patients with Cushing's syndrome, treatment is surgical removal of the source of excess cortisol or ACTH** (adrenal or pituitary tumor).

PCOS is by far the most common functional ovarian disorder causing hyperandrogenism, and the management of PCOS depends on the patient's presentation and desires. **The therapy for the hirsutism in PCOS patients is ovarian suppression, which is usually achieved by administration of a combination contraceptive.** This estrogen-progestin treatment suppresses gonadotropins (LH and FSH), which allows regression of the overproduction of testosterone and androstenedione by the ovary. Estrogen also stimulates SHBG production, which decreases free testosterone levels.

The treatment of hirsutism is best accomplished by the addition of an **androgen blocker. The most commonly used drug for hirsutism in women in the United States is spironolactone.** This aldosterone antagonist competes for testosterone-binding sites, thereby exerting a direct antiandrogenic effect at the target organ. In addition, spironolactone interferes with steroid enzymes and decreases testosterone production. Because this medication opposes the action of aldosterone, serum potassium levels may rise and should be monitored. Other drugs that block the binding of androgens to its receptor include **flutamide** and **cyproterone acetate**, whereas **finasteride** blocks the conversion of testosterone to its more potent metabolite, dihydrotestosterone. It may take up to 6 months to begin to observe a cosmetic improvement in hirsutism, and maximum effect may not be seen for up to 2 years.

Suppression of abnormal androgen production or action generally suppresses future hair growth but does not immediately cause the existing hirsutism to disappear. **To obtain good cosmetic results, some local hair removal is usually required in addition to the biochemical treatment.** Local methods include shaving, depilatory creams, electrolysis, and laser hair removal. Plucking of individual hairs should be discouraged because growth of surrounding hair follicles may be stimulated by this technique.

All patients with PCOS and chronic anovulation are at risk for the development of endometrial hyperplasia and endometrial cancer. Hence, management of patients not taking combined oral contraceptives should always include scheduled progestin-induced withdrawal of the endometrium to reduce this risk. This may be accomplished with 10 mg of oral medroxyprogesterone acetate daily, 100 mg of oral micronized progesterone twice daily, or 5 mg of norethindrone acetate daily, for 12 to 14 days every other month.

The underlying insulin resistance and hyperandrogenism of many patients with PCOS may have a significant effect on their risk for diabetes mellitus and possibly cardiovascular morbidity. Women with PCOS have a threefold to sevenfold higher risk for developing type 2 diabetes mellitus. Women with PCOS and hyperandrogenism also tend to have increased levels of low-density lipoprotein cholesterol (LDL cholesterol) and reduced levels of high-density lipoprotein cholesterol

(HDL cholesterol) and are at increased risk for developing hypertension. Thus, patients with PCOS and chronic anovulation should be counseled regarding weight loss, nutrition, exercise, and other lifestyle changes that will reduce their risk for developing diabetes mellitus and cardiovascular disease.

Patients with functional adrenal hyperandrogenism, such as CAH, are treated by the administration of glucocorticoids (e.g., 0.25 mg dexamethasone every other day at bedtime). However, many of these women (like those with PCOS) also require suppression of ovarian androgen secretion using combination oral contraceptives and antiandrogens.

SUGGESTED READING

American College of Obstetricians and Gynecologists (ACOG): Polycystic ovary syndrome. ACOG Technical Bulletin No. 41. Washington, DC, ACOG, December 2002.

Azziz R: The evaluation and management of hirsutism. Obstet Gynecol 101:995-1007, 2003.

Azziz R, Carmina E, Dewailly D, et al, for the Androgen Excess Society: Criteria for defining polycystic ovary syndrome as a predominantly hyperandrogenic syndrome: An Androgen Excess Society guideline. Position Statement. J Clin Endocrinol Metab 91:4237-4245, 2006.

Azziz R, Carmina E, Sawaya ME: Idiopathic hirsutism. Endocr Rev 21:347-362, 2000.

Azziz R, Dewailly D, Owerbach D: Non-classic adrenal hyperplasia: Current concepts. J Clin Endocrinol Metab 78:810-815, 1994.

Patel SS, Bamigboye V: Hyperprolactinemia. J Obstet Gynaecol 27:455-459, 2007.

Chapter 33

Dysfunctional Uterine Bleeding

JOSEPH C. GAMBONE

Dysfunctional uterine bleeding (DUB) is defined as abnormal uterine bleeding (AUB) in women between menarche and menopause that cannot be attributed to medications, blood dyscrasias, systemic diseases, trauma, uterine neoplasms, or pregnancy. This form of AUB is almost always caused by aberrations in the hypothalamic-pituitary-ovarian hormonal axis resulting in anovulation. The diagnosis of DUB is made by excluding other treatable causes of AUB.

The bleeding is generally from a proliferative, or discordant (mixed), endometrium. In most cases, it is associated with anovulatory or oligo-ovulatory ovarian cycles (e.g., polycystic ovary syndrome), and estrogen levels are frequently unopposed by progesterone. On occasion, it occurs with apparently normal ovulatory cycles. It is one of the most common problems dealt with in the gynecologic clinic or private office.

Abnormal bleeding patterns are defined in Box 33-1. Taken together, these abnormal patterns are sometimes designated as menometrorrhagia.

Most DUB occurs during the years around the menarche (11 to 14 years of age) or menopause (45 to 50 years of age). During the perimenopausal years, the anovulatory bleeding is mainly caused by the declining functional capacity of the ovary. In adolescence, the anovulatory bleeding may be caused by a failure of the hypothalamic-pituitary system to respond to the positive feedback effect of estrogen.

Abnormalities of menstrual bleeding are thought to be associated with alterations in endometrial vascular homeostasis. A normally efficient menstrual cycle is discussed in detail in Chapter 4, and the normal events are briefly summarized as follows.

First, gradually increasing estrogen levels support and maintain the growth of endometrium during the proliferative phase of the cycle. The proliferative phase is variable in length, but it generally lasts 13 days from the onset of menses to the luteinizing hormone surge. The increasing level of estrogen supports growth, prevents breakthrough bleeding, and stimulates an increase in endometrial progesterone receptors.

Second, about 24 hours after the luteinizing hormone surge, ovulation occurs, and the corpus luteum forms. It produces estrogen and progesterone in increasing amounts and lasts for about 14 days unless an intervening pregnancy prolongs it by secretion of human chorionic gonadotropin (hCG). With the demise of the corpus luteum, the levels of estrogen and progesterone fall precipitously, and the decidual portion of the endometrium desquamates.

Third, during the luteal phase of the endometrial cycle, there is a marked increase in tissue levels of prostaglandin $F_{2\alpha}$, which is a powerful vasoconstrictor, and this eventually leads to endometrial ischemia. The process allows for a complete sloughing of the outer two thirds of the endometrium and avoids prolonged menstruation. **During anovulatory cycles, the resulting nonsecretory endometrium contains less**

BOX 33-1   *Common Abnormal Bleeding Patterns*

- **Polymenorrhea:** abnormally frequent menses at intervals of <24 days
- **Menorrhagia (hypermenorrhea):** excessive and/or prolonged menses (>80 mL and >7 days) occurring at normal intervals
- **Metrorrhagia:** irregular episodes of uterine bleeding
- **Menometrorrhagia:** heavy and irregular uterine bleeding
- **Intermenstrual bleeding:** scant bleeding at ovulation for 1 or 2 days

BOX 33-2 *Nondysfunctional Causes of Abnormal Uterine Bleeding*

Iatrogenic
Exogenous estrogen (e.g., oral contraceptives)
Aspirin
Heparin, sodium warfarin (Coumadin)
Tamoxifen
Intrauterine device

Dyscrasias
Thrombocytopenia
Increased fibrinolysins
Autoimmune disease
Leukemia
Von Willebrand's disease

Systemic Disorders
Hepatic disease (impaired metabolism of estrogens)
Renal disease (hyperprolactinemia)
Thyroid disease

Trauma
Laceration
Abrasion
Foreign body

Organic Conditions
Complications of pregnancy
Uterine leiomyomas
Malignancies of cervix or corpus
Endometrial polyp
Adenomyosis
Endometritis
Endometrial hyperplasia

BOX 33-3 *Evaluation of a Patient Who May Have Dysfunctional Uterine Bleeding*

Laboratory Evaluation*
Complete blood count
Platelet count
Serum iron and iron-binding globulin
Coagulation studies (prothrombin time and partial thromboplastin time)
Bleeding time
Urinary human chorionic gonadotropin assay
Thyroid function studies
Serum progesterone
Liver function studies
Prolactin levels
Serum follicle-stimulating hormone levels

Diagnostic Procedures*
Cervical cytology (Papanicolaou smear)
Endometrial biopsy
Pipelle (flexible syringe suction curette)
Office curette (Novak, Randall type)
Vacuum (Vabra) curette
Pelvic ultrasonic imaging
Hysteroscopy, hysterosonogram, and/or dilation and curettage

*Used selectively based on history and physical examination.

prostaglandin and is less apt to initiate an efficient menstrual period of short duration. The unopposed estrogenic effect is likely to result in cycles of irregular duration and prolonged menses. With repeated cycles of unopposed estrogen, endometrial hyperplasia or even cancer may develop.

Diagnosis

The diagnosis of DUB is usually made by excluding other causes of AUB. **A possible unexpected pregnancy should always be ruled out initially**. Box 33-2 lists possible causes of AUB to be considered. A **pelvic examination** must be performed to verify that the source of bleeding is uterine and not the result of a cervical, rectal, vaginal, vulvar, or urethral lesion. **Iatrogenic causes** such as oral contraceptive–induced breakthrough bleeding or bleeding associated with an intrauterine device should be considered. **Dyscrasias of the blood** such as von Willebrand's disease should be ruled out. **Systemic diseases** such as liver, renal, or thyroid conditions may represent treatable causes of AUB. **Trauma**, although unusual, is an occasional cause of vaginal

and even uterine bleeding and should be considered at the time of the pelvic examination. **Organic causes** of AUB include tumors, infections, and complications of pregnancy. **Benign tumors and growths** include endocervical and endometrial polyps, leiomyomas (uterine fibroids), adenomyosis, and endometrial hyperplasia. **Malignant neoplastic conditions** include cervical and uterine cancers. **Infections** that may cause AUB include cervicitis, endometritis, and pelvic inflammatory disease.

Two investigations are most useful for confirming DUB: a pelvic ultrasound and an endometrial biopsy. If they are both normal and show nothing more than a nonsecretory endometrium, a presumptive diagnosis of DUB is highly likely. Other tests and procedures that may be useful to exclude other causes of AUB are listed in Box 33-3.

Management

The management of DUB becomes relatively clear once other, more serious causes of bleeding have been excluded, particularly endometrial or cervical cancer. For less significant bleeding, observation and expectant management may be reasonable. Box 33-4 lists the appropriate hormonal management of significant DUB.

Heavy endometrial hemorrhage from menarche through the perimenopause may require high-dose estrogens (sometimes given intravenously) to support

BOX 33-4 *Hormonal Management of Dysfunctional Uterine Bleeding*

Massive Intractable Bleeding

Administer 25 mg IV of conjugated estrogens.

Continued Management after Massive Bleeding Has Abated

Administer conjugated estrogens, 2.5 mg orally daily for 25 days.* May double the dose if bleeding recurs or increases.

Add 10 mg of medroxyprogesterone acetate (MPA)† for the last 10 days of treatment.

Allow 5 to 7 days for withdrawal bleeding.

Administer the Mirena intrauterine system, which releases levonorgestrel through an intrauterine device.

Management of Moderate Menometrorrhagia

Estrogen-Progestin Combination

Administer conjugated estrogen,* 1.25 mg orally each day for 25 days with 10 mg MPA† orally for the last 10 days of the estrogen treatment.

Administer oral contraceptive (e.g., Brevicon)‡ for 21 days, with a 7-day withdrawal.

Cyclic Progestin

Administer MPA†, 10 mg orally each day for 10 to 15 days each month, usually for a 3-month trial; a 5- to 7-day period of menstrual withdrawal should follow cessation of the MPA each month.

Mirena Intrauterine System with Levonorgestrel-Releasing Intrauterine Device

---

*May substitute other oral estrogen (e.g., ethinyl estradiol, 0.02 mg).
†May substitute other progestin (e.g., Megace, 5 mg).
‡May substitute other combined oral contraceptives and may increase dose up to 4 tablets daily for heavier bleeding.

the endometrium and diminish bleeding. If the bleeding substantially abates, lower-dose oral estrogen followed by, or in combination with, a progestin can then be initiated. If the bleeding is unremitting, dilation and curettage may be necessary.

The more common and less urgent type of DUB is best managed by cyclic estrogens with a progestin added in the latter 10 to 15 days of the 25-day estrogen cycle (see Box 33-4). A 5- to 7-day withdrawal bleed is expected each month as the medications are withdrawn on the 21st or 25th day. The cycle is repeated each month for 3 to 6 months, after which a normal

pattern may be spontaneously established. Oral contraceptives should not be used for women in their 40s who are smokers, because of the high content of estrogens and their association with thrombophlebitis and myocardial infarction. **Cyclic progestins alone may be used for younger patients who are likely to have sufficient endogenous estrogens to prime the endometrial progesterone receptors.** The Mirena intrauterine system, which releases levonorgestrel, has been reported to be useful for treating DUB. It has a 55% 5-year continuation rate and a 30% early discontinuation rate in women being treated for DUB. These drugs are unlikely to be effective after prolonged bleeding. Only when these measures are ineffective should a dilation and curettage or hysteroscopy and biopsy be performed.

For older patients who do not respond to medical therapy and who do not anticipate later pregnancies, more radical and potentially permanent therapeutic measures may be considered. Endometrial ablation at the time of hysteroscopy provides an amenorrhea rate of up to 75% and relief of excessive bleeding in most of the remainder. However, about 10% continue to have bleeding problems. **Vaginal hysterectomy** may be appropriate for women who have associated problems such as pelvic relaxation or severe dysmenorrhea or for patients who are refractory to endometrial ablation.

Although DUB is annoying or even distressing, it is seldom life-threatening. Conservative treatment, after a thorough evaluation, is generally successful, although it may extend over several months, and the problem may recur.

It is important rule out unsuspected pregnancies and genital tract cancers, reserving hysterectomy for those patients with significant precancerous lesions or refractory problems.

SUGGESTED READING

Association of Professors of Gynecology and Obstetrics: Clinical Management of Abnormal Uterine Bleeding, Educational Series on Women's Health Issues. Boston, Jespersen and Associates, 2002.

Hillard PJA: Benign diseases of the female reproductive tract. *In* Berek JS (ed): Berek and Novak's Gynecology, 14th ed. Philadelphia, Lippincott Williams & Wilkins, 2007, pp 461-467.

Mukherjee K, Jones K: The treatment of DUB with Mirena IUS: A survival analysis. Gynecol Surg 2:251-254, 2005.

Chapter 34

Infertility and Assisted Reproductive Technologies

DAVID R. MELDRUM

It is estimated that 10% to 15% of couples in the United States are involuntarily infertile. Newer reproductive technologies such as in vitro fertilization (IVF) and embryo transfer are increasing the success of treatment for this condition.

A couple is considered infertile after unsuccessfully attempting to achieve pregnancy for 1 year. Infertility is termed *primary* **when it occurs without any prior pregnancy and** *secondary* **when it follows a previous conception.** Some conditions, such as azoospermia, endometriosis, and tubal occlusion, are more common in women with primary infertility, but virtually all conditions occur in both settings, making the distinction of little clinical significance.

■ *Physiology of Conception*

Conception requires the juxtaposition of the male and female gametes at the optimal stage of maturation, followed by transportation of the conceptus to the uterine cavity at a time when the endometrium is supportive of its continued development and implantation (see Chapter 4). For these events to occur, the male and female reproductive systems must be both anatomically and physiologically intact, and coitus must occur with sufficient frequency and at the proper time (preferably a few hours before) to the release of the oocyte from the follicle. **Even when fertilization occurs, it is estimated that more than 70% of resulting embryos are abnormal and fail to develop or become nonviable shortly after implantation.**

Considering the vast complexity of the reproductive process, it is remarkable that **80% of couples achieve conception within 1 year.** More precisely, 25% conceive within the first month, 60% within 6 months, 75% by 9 months, and 90% by 18 months. The steadily decreasing rate of monthly conception demonstrated by these figures most likely reflects a spectrum of fertility extending from highly fertile couples to those with relative infertility. After 18 months of unprotected sexual intercourse, the remaining couples have a low monthly conception rate without treatment, and many may have absolute defects preventing fertility (sterility).

■ *General Principles of Evaluation*

Conception requires adequate function of multiple physiologic systems in both partners. Infertility may result from either one major deficiency (e.g., tubal occlusion) or multiple minor deficiencies. Failure to realize this important dictum may lead the inexperienced practitioner to overlook additional factors that might be more amenable to treatment than the one that has been identified. **Infertility in about 40% of infertile couples has multiple causes.** Therefore, in general, a complete infertility evaluation should be performed on each couple.

Age substantially decreases the rate of conception because of lower embryo quality, reduced ovulation, and possibly decreased coital frequency. From a large study of donor insemination, the strictly age-related reduction appears to be about one third for women aged 35 to 45 years. It is reasonable to begin the basic evaluation at 6 months in older patients and to consider starting treatment for unexplained infertility earlier in women older than 35 years of age.

■ *Basic Evaluations*

Evaluation and therapy may be started earlier when obvious defects are identified, or they may be delayed, for instance, when a correctable factor, such as infrequent intercourse, is identified.

TABLE 34-1

COMMON INFERTILITY FACTORS

Factor	Incidence (%)	Basic Investigations
Male, coital	40	Semen analysis Postcoital test
Ovulatory	15-20	Urinary luteinizing hormone self-test*; serum progesterone*
Cervical	5	Postcoital test
Uterine, tubal	30	Hysterosalpingogram Laparoscopy
Peritoneal	40	Laparoscopy

*Investigations only when menses are regular (every 22 to 35 days); oligomenorrhea generally requires treatment.

In general, the first 6 to 8 months of evaluation involve relatively simple and noninvasive tests and the performance of a radiologic evaluation of tubal patency (hysterosalpingography, or HSG), which can sometimes have a therapeutic effect. **In some studies, use of an oil-based dye about doubled the success rate after HSG.** Operative evaluation by laparoscopy is thus reserved for the small proportion of couples who have not conceived after 18 to 24 months or who have specific abnormalities or indications of a probable pelvic factor.

To keep the status of the evaluation in mind, it is helpful to arrange the workup under a series of five categories that can be mentally reviewed at each visit. Table 34-1 shows the approximate incidence and the tests involved in the evaluation of each category. Box 34-1 summarizes the treatment options for infertility. **In 5% to 10% of couples, no explanation can be found (idiopathic infertility).**

◼ Etiologic Factors

MALE COITAL FACTOR

History

The history from the male partner should cover any pregnancies previously sired; any history of genital tract infections, such as prostatitis or mumps orchitis; surgery or trauma to the male genitalia or inguinal region (e.g., hernia repair); and any exposure to lead, cadmium, radiation, or chemotherapeutic agents. Excessive consumption of alcohol or cigarettes or unusual exposure to environmental heat should be elicited. **Some medications, such as furantoins and calcium channel blockers, reduce sperm quality or function.**

Physical Examination

Physical examination is done on referral to a urologist when semen analysis is abnormal. The normal location of the urethral meatus should be ensured. Testicular size should be estimated by comparison with a set of

BOX 34-1   *Treatment Options for Infertility*

Male Factor Problems

Avoidance of alcohol and
Scheduled intercourse without toxic lubricants
Ligation of venous plexus for significant varicocele
   and low semen quality
IUI with washed sperm
Intracytoplasmic sperm injection combined with IVF
Donor sperm insemination (frozen and thawed from
   tested donor)

Ovulatory Factor Problems

Clomiphene citrate without or with hCG to trigger
   ovulation
Gonadotropins (hMG)—combination of LH and FSH,
   or pure FSH; low-dose regimen decreases risk for
   multiple pregnancies
IVF and embryo transfer
Donor egg IVF and embryo transfer for unresponsive
   age-related infertility

Cervical Factor Problems

Treatment of any lower reproductive tract infection
IUI with washed sperm

Uterine-Tubal Factor Problems

Tuboplasty (microsurgical technique more effective)
Tubal anastomosis for sterilization reversal; good results
   with laparoscopic technique
IVF

Peritoneal Factor Problems

Laparoscopic treatment of endometriosis or adhesions
   (see Chapter 25)
Medical treatment for endometriosis (see Chapter 25)
IVF

Unexplained Infertility

Trial of COS with or without IUI
IVF

COS, controlled ovarian hyperstimulation; FSH, follicle-stimulating hormone; hCG, human chorionic gonadotropin; hMG, human menopausal gonadotropin; IUI, intrauterine insemination; IVF, in vitro fertilization.

standard ovoids. The presence of a varicocele should be elicited by asking the patient to perform Valsalva's maneuver in the standing position.

Investigations

A semen analysis should be performed following a 2- to 4-day period of abstinence. The entire ejaculate should be collected in a clean, nontoxic container. Until relatively recently, the full range of normal variation was not appreciated. Characteristics of a normal semen analysis are shown in Table 34-2.

An excessive number of leukocytes (more than 10 per high-power field) may indicate infection, but special

TABLE 34-2

CHARACTERISTICS OF NORMAL SEMEN ANALYSIS	
Characteristics	**Quantity**
Semen volume	2-5 mL
Sperm count	Greater than 20 million/mL
Sperm motility	Greater than 50%*
Normal forms	Greater than 30% standard morphology or greater than 14% "strict" morphology
White blood cells	Fewer than 10 per high-power field or 1×10^6/mL

*At least 25% A motility or 40% A plus B motility.

stains are required to differentiate polymorphonuclear leukocytes from immature germ cells. Semen quality varies greatly with repeated samples. **An accurate appraisal of abnormal semen requires at least three analyses.** Periodic reassessment is necessary.

Endocrine evaluation of the male with subnormal semen quality may uncover a specific cause. Hypothyroidism can cause infertility, but there is no place for the empirical use of thyroxine. **Low levels of gonadotropins and testosterone may indicate hypothalamic-pituitary failure. An elevated prolactin concentration may indicate the presence of a prolactin-producing pituitary tumor. An elevated level of follicle-stimulating hormone (FSH) generally indicates substantial parenchymal damage to the testes,** as inhibin, produced by the Sertoli cells of the seminiferous tubules, provides the principal feedback control of FSH secretion. A response to any treatment is unlikely in the presence of an elevated level of FSH. However, the level of FSH is not helpful in predicting whether sperm will be recovered with testicular sperm extraction.

Treatment

The couple should be advised to have intercourse about every 1 to 2 days during the periovulatory period (e.g., days 12 through 16 of a 28-day cycle). **Because infrequent coitus is a common contributing factor, firm advice in this regard can be beneficial.** This "scheduled intercourse" can be disruptive and stressful, however, and insemination using husband or partner sperm may relieve considerable pressure on a couple.

The woman should be advised to lie on her back for at least 15 minutes after coitus to prevent rapid loss of semen from the vagina. Lubricants may be toxic to sperm. **A nontoxic lubricant, Preseed, has been developed for infertile couples.**

Smoking should be reduced or stopped, as should intake of alcohol. The use of saunas, hot tubs, or tight underwear should be discouraged, as should exposure to other environments that raise scrotal temperature, because these factors may affect spermatogenesis.

Low semen volume may provide insufficient contact with the cervical mucus for adequate sperm migration to occur. When a high semen volume coexists with a low count, infertility may result because a lower density of sperm contacts the cervical mucus. **At present, these abnormalities of volume are most commonly treated with sperm washing and intrauterine insemination (IUI).**

If low sperm density (oligospermia) or low motility (asthenospermia) is caused by hypothalamic-pituitary failure, injections of human menopausal gonadotropin (hMG) may be effective. The suppressive effects of **hyperprolactinemia** on hypothalamic function **can be reversed by the administration of bromocriptine,** a dopamine agonist. **When low semen quality coexists with a varicocele** (dilation and incompetence of the spermatic veins), **improved semen quality, particularly motility, may occur with ligation of this venous plexus.** Various medications (clomiphene, human chorionic gonadotropin [hCG], testosterone, and hMG) have been tried when no cause is apparent (idiopathic oligoasthenospermia), but none has proved effective. Because about 3 months is required for spermatogenesis and sperm transport to occur, frequent semen checks during treatment are unnecessary and serve only to discourage the patient.

If semen quality cannot be improved, IUI with close timing of the insemination to the precise point of ovulation is effective. By washing and concentrating the sperm into a small volume by centrifugation, large numbers of sperm can be placed into the uterus. Without washing, IUI must be limited to small amounts of semen, owing to marked cramping. Accurate timing may be accomplished either by measurement of daily luteinizing hormone (LH) concentrations or by controlled stimulation of the cycle with clomiphene or hMG, followed by administration of hCG when follicular diameter, as seen by ultrasonography, indicates maturity. Insemination may then be carried out within a few hours of ovulation, which occurs about 36 hours following the onset of the LH surge or hCG injection. When urinary LH testing is used, there is a delay of several hours between the onset of the surge and the positive urine test. It is advisable to test in the afternoon or evening, with insemination the following morning.

IVF is an effective treatment for the male factor because with intracytoplasmic sperm injection (ICSI), only one motile sperm for each egg is required. Finally, insemination with donor sperm is effective when the male factor is refractory to treatment.

OVULATORY FACTOR

History

Most women with regular cycles (every 22 to 35 days) are ovulating, particularly if they have premenstrual molimina (e.g., breast changes, bloating, and mood change). Recent studies indicate reduced fecundity associated with very irregular cycles.

Investigations

The simplest screening tests to confirm reasonably normal ovulation are serial measurement of urinary LH, which assesses the duration of luteal function, and the mid-luteal level of serum progesterone, which assesses the level of luteal function. The interval from the urinary LH surge to the onset of menses should be at least 12 days. An older test of ovulation, the basal body temperature, is now seldom used. A luteal progesterone level of greater than 5 ng/mL indicates ovulatory activity, but mid-luteal concentrations usually exceed 10 ng/mL in cycles in which conception can take place. Because of the marked pulsatile secretion of progesterone, a level between 5 and 40 ng/mL can be found in the normal luteal phase.

Despite ovulation, an inadequate luteal phase may be responsible for infertility. **Endometrial biopsy, considered for many years to accurately reflect luteal function, has been recently shown to be a very imprecise test, causing most practitioners to abandon it as a tool to assess ovulation.**

Treatment

Use of fertility drugs such as clomiphene citrate or gonadotropins will correct any luteal insufficiency in women with unexplained infertility.

In women whose menses are less frequent than every 35 days (oligomenorrhea), it is helpful to induce more frequent ovulation, thus increasing the opportunity for pregnancy and improving the ability to time coitus. Ovulation induction should always be preceded by a thorough workup, as discussed in Chapter 32, because conditions causing anovulation may be worsened by pregnancy or may complicate it. In addition, ovarian failure seldom responds to attempts to induce ovulation.

The choice of the most appropriate technique for ovulation induction is determined by the patient's specific diagnosis. With this approach, regular ovulation can be restored in more than 90% of anovulatory women. Provided that these patients persevere with treatment for an adequate period of time, and no other infertility factors are present, their fertility should approximate that of normal women.

Pituitary insufficiency requires the injection of hMG (follicle-stimulating hormone [FSH] and LH). Hypothalamic amenorrhea is caused by infrequent or absent pulsatile release of gonadotropin-releasing hormone (GnRH). GnRH is highly effective when administered in small pulses subcutaneously or intravenously in these patients every 90 to 120 minutes by a small portable infusion pump. Because this treatment is not currently as available in the United States, hMG

is used, but with a much higher risk for multiple pregnancy. **Hyperprolactinemia and its suppressive effect on the hypothalamus are specifically treated by use of the dopamine agonists bromocriptine (Parlodel) and cabergoline (Dostinex).**

Most of the remaining patients with anovulation have some form of polycystic ovarian syndrome (PCOS) and generally respond to clomiphene, an orally active antiestrogen. Anovulation occurs in patients with polycystic ovaries because of chronic, mild suppression of FSH release. These women often have both increased ovarian and increased adrenal androgen production. Clomiphene, by inhibiting the negative feedback effect of endogenous estrogen, causes a rise of FSH and stimulation of follicular maturation. One of the principal causes of excessive ovarian androgen production is higher circulating insulin concentrations because of insulin resistance. Metformin, which reduces glucose mobilization and increases insulin sensitivity, is currently being used together with clomiphene or gonadotropins to improve response as well as to reduce an excessive response to ovulation induction. Metformin can also be used alone and may result in ovulation and pregnancy.

Other treatments used to induce ovulation in PCOS are laparoscopic "ovarian drilling," in which multiple small craters are created with laser or cautery, and dexamethasone, which increases the ovarian response to clomiphene. Surgery is not often recommended because of the possibility of causing scarring around the ovaries and tubes.

If ovulation does not occur with clomiphene, follicular development may be occurring, but the normal LH surge may fail to occur. This results in lack of follicular rupture. **Assessment by serial pelvic ultrasonography and carefully timed hCG administration may lead to normal ovulation. If follicular maturation is not occurring, ovulation induction will require low-dose FSH or hMG.**

The main complications of ovulation induction are related to excessive stimulation of the ovaries. Substantial enlargement of the ovary with clomiphene citrate can generally be avoided by examining the ovaries before each treatment course and by using the lowest effective dose. Cystic ovarian enlargement is not an uncommon complication of hMG treatment but almost always regresses spontaneously. **The hyperstimulation syndrome is a critical illness associated with marked ovarian enlargement and exudation of fluid and protein into the peritoneal cavity.** The use of serum estradiol measurements, transvaginal ultrasonic scanning, and low-dose gonadotropin has greatly reduced the incidence of hyperstimulation syndrome. When starting at 50 to 75 units and increasing the dose by 25 to 50 units every 7 days if follicular maturation is not detected, there is a marked reduction in the incidence of multifollicular development, hyperstimulation, and multiple pregnancy. **Multiple pregnancy occurs in 6% to 8% of clomiphene citrate conceptions, with less than 1% of cases exceeding twins.** Multiple gestation occurs in 20% to 30% of hMG conceptions, and 5% of these conceptions are multiple births of more than two. Ultrasonic monitoring reduces this risk if the hCG is withheld in the presence of an excessive number of mature follicles. **Current use of a low-dose regimen of hMG or pure FSH reduces the overall risk for multiple pregnancy to about 5%.**

CERVICAL FACTOR

During the few days before ovulation, the cervix produces profuse watery mucus (**spinnbarkeit**) that exudes out of the cervix to contact the seminal ejaculate. To assess its quality, the patient must be seen during the immediate preovulatory phase (days 12 to 14 of a 28-day cycle). Spuriously abnormal results can be reduced by timing the test to the morning after the urinary LH surge.

Investigations

The amount and clarity of the mucus is recorded. **The spinnbarkeit may be tested by touching the mucus with a piece of pH paper and lifting vertically. The mucus should extend in a thread to at least 6 cm.** The pH should be 6.5 or greater. **A postcoital (Sims-Huhner) test is performed 2 to 12 hours after intercourse to assess the number and motility of spermatozoa that have entered the cervical canal.** The number of sperm, however, does not correlate well with semen quality, recovery of sperm from the cul-de-sac, or subsequent fertility. Consequently, the predictive value of this test for fertility is low. Although many practitioners have abandoned this test, treatment for poor mucus may avoid the morbidity and expense of fertility drugs.

Treatment

Any cervical infection is treated by prescribing a 10-day course of doxycycline, 100 mg twice daily, for both partners. Persistent chronic cervicitis may be treated with cryotherapy if antibiotic treatment fails. Poor mucus quality can be treated (bypassed) with **IUI.**

UTERINE OR TUBAL FACTOR

Abnormalities of the uterine cavity are seldom the cause of infertility. Large submucosal myomas or endometrial polyps, as seen in Figure 34-1, may be associated with infertility and first-trimester spontaneous abortions. The role of intramural myomas is not clear, although myomectomy has been associated with conception in 40% to 50% of couples in uncontrolled series, and some studies with IVF have shown reduced conception with intramural myomas. Subserous fibroids do not affect fecundity.

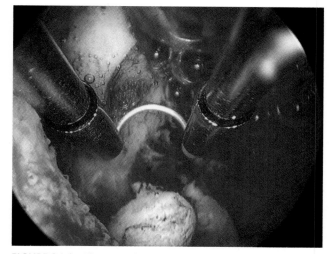

FIGURE 34-1   Photograph of a significant submucous polyp (*bottom center*) seen at the time of hysteroscopy.

Tubal occlusion may occur at three locations: the fimbrial end, the mid-segment, or the isthmus-cornu. Fimbrial occlusion is by far the most common. Prior salpingitis is a common cause of tubal occlusion, although about half of cases are not associated with any such history. Isthmic-cornual occlusion can be congenital or caused by mucus plugs, endometriosis, tubal adenomyosis, or prior infection. Mid-segment occlusion can be seen after surgery or infection with tuberculosis.

Investigations

Tubal abnormalities may be diagnosed by HSG or laparoscopy. To perform HSG, an occlusive cannula is placed in the cervix, and the instillation of a radiopaque dye is followed with image intensification under fluoroscopy. Selected radiographs are taken for permanent documentation (Figure 34-2). Anesthesia generally is not required. A water-soluble dye is used initially to confirm tubal patency because of the adverse effects of sequestration of an oil-based dye within the lumen of an occluded tube. If patency is confirmed, an oil-based dye may then be instilled because of its prominent therapeutic effect in women with unexplained infertility. If only one tube fills with dye, the hysterosalpingogram should be considered normal because this finding is usually, although not invariably, caused by the dye following the path of least resistance.

Serious infections can result from HSG. Confirmation of a normal pelvic examination and prophylactic doxycycline should reduce this risk to a minimum.

Treatment

In most circumstances, microsurgical tuboplasty is more effective than conventional surgical techniques for reversal of tubal occlusion. About 60% to 80% of patients achieve pregnancy after reversal of steriliza-tion using microsurgical techniques. Tubal anasto-mosis may be carried out laparoscopically, with good results in experienced hands.

When performed for fimbrial occlusion, neosal-pingostomy is associated with a success rate of 20% to 30%, although it has reached 40% with long-term follow-up. Most often this is done by laparoscopy. Be-cause a hydrosalpinx reduces the success rate of IVF by about 50%, any hydrosalpinx not repaired should be removed or its communication with the uterus in-terrupted by cautery or clips.

For an isthmic-cornual occlusion caused by dis-ease, clearing the obstruction with oral danazol has been reported when the occlusion coexists with peri-toneal endometriosis. Selective catheterization has restored patency in most proximal occlusions and should be the first line of therapy. Microsurgical resec-tion and reanastomosis are associated with a 50% to 60% pregnancy rate. **If the intramural portion of the tube is occluded, reimplantation is required, with a new opening being made into the endometrial cavity.**

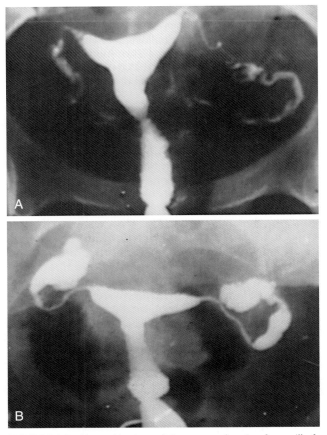

FIGURE 34-2   Normal hysterosalpingogram showing free spill of contrast material (**A**) and bilateral hydrosalpinges (**B**).

A substantially lower rate of success is achieved in this circumstance, a laparotomy is required, and similar success can be achieved with a single cycle of IVF.

At least 10% of conceptions after repair of diseased tubes are ectopic pregnancies. Anastomosis of healthy tubes carries a risk for ectopic pregnancy of about 3% to 5%. This possibility must always be considered in the management of an early pregnancy following tuboplasty.

PERITONEAL FACTOR

Laparoscopy identifies previously unsuspected patho-logic conditions in 30% to 50% of women with unex-plained infertility. Endometriosis is the most common finding. Periadnexal adhesions may be found and may hold the fimbriae away from the ovarian surface or en-trap the released oocyte.

Endometriosis may interfere with tubal motility, cause tubal obstruction, or cause adhesions that di-rectly disturb the pick-up of the oocyte by the fimbriae. Other mechanisms of endometriosis-associated infer-tility must exist as well because even minimal endo-metriosis has some negative effect. In a randomized study of laparoscopic cautery versus no treatment for minimal endometriosis, treatment resulted in one of eight affected women conceiving. These same women, however, may conceive with other treatments used for unexplained infertility. **There is a strong trend toward omitting laparoscopy in women who have no symp-toms indicating pelvic disease and who have a normal pelvic examination, a normal HSG, and a normal pel-vic ultrasound.** A serum titer for antichlamydia anti-bodies may be helpful if this approach is taken, to avoid overlooking occult pelvic adhesions.

Treatment of endometriosis depends on its extent and is discussed further in Chapter 25. **If substantial adhe-sions or endometriomas are present, laparoscopic sur-gery is preferable** because these conditions generally do not respond to medical management. **With advanced operative laparoscopic techniques, most endometrio-sis can be removed or ablated** without laparotomy by using advanced instrumentation, lasers, or fulguration.

Danazol, GnRH agonists, and oral medroxypro-gesterone acetate are effective treatments for symp-tomatic disease, with continuous oral contraception therapy being generally inferior. If minimal disease with scattered implants is found, simple cautery at the time of laparoscopy should suffice.

Periadnexal adhesions may be lysed by operative laparoscopy. Microsurgical techniques diminish ad-hesions. The most effective adjunct in preventing re-current scarring is the placement of an artificial tissue barrier, separating the raw surfaces during the early period of healing.

Because of the current high success rate with IVF, that treatment is often done as an alternative to the above surgeries. It is particularly important to conserve ovarian function as much as possible. **If ovarian reserve is low, IVF is preferable to removal of an endometrioma,** because of the compromised ovarian function that often results from ovarian surgery.

Unexplained Infertility

No cause is found for infertility in 5% to 10% of patients who have documented ovulation, normal semen analyses, and a normal HSG. The problem may be primarily one of sperm transport because IUI with washed sperm appears to increase the rate of conception. Some studies have shown subtle abnormalities of follicular growth and ovulation, partly explaining the increased fecundity with fertility drugs.

In other cases, a defect in the ability of the sperm to fertilize the egg may be present because a lower rate of fertilization is noted in couples with unexplained infertility who undergo IVF compared with couples in whom there is a tubal cause for infertility. **Another male problem that may not be detected by routine evaluation is the presence of antisperm antibodies.**

Other possible mechanisms of unexplained infertility include minimal endometriosis and mildly reduced ovarian reserve (reduced number of normal oocytes without hormonal abnormalities such as elevated FSH levels).

Intrauterine insemination, usually with controlled ovarian stimulation (stimulation of multiple follicles with clomiphene, gonadotropins, or both and hCG timing of insemination), is employed next. The final therapy is IVF.

Assisted Reproductive Technologies

The last resort for infertile couples with any of the aforementioned factors and failure of lesser treatments is the procedure of IVF and embryo transfer (Figure 34-3). In most cases of tubal occlusion in which the rate of success with tubal repair is low (<30%), IVF is preferable to surgery because of the more rapid conception rate and the lower ectopic pregnancy rate. **Even severe male factors can be effectively treated with IVF by using intracytoplasmic sperm injection, with high fertilization rates of injected oocytes and pregnancy rates similar to those of non–male-factor IVF (30% to 35%).**

TECHNIQUE

A GnRH agonist is given to prevent premature LH release. It is commonly started in the mid-luteal phase or overlapped with an oral contraceptive. After ovarian suppression (with GnRH agonist), **the ovaries are stimulated with FSH, hMG, or both,** on the second or third day of the next cycle. Follicle size is assessed by transvaginal ultrasonic scanning.

An injection of hCG (usually 10,000 U) is given based on follicular size and estradiol levels to induce the resumption of meiosis and completion of oocyte maturation. Thirty-five hours after the hCG injection, multiple oocytes are aspirated under transvaginal ultrasonic guidance. After a further period of in vitro maturation, washed sperm are added, or a single sperm is injected (ICSI) into each oocyte. Fertilization may be identified 14 to 18 hours after insemination by the visualization of two pronuclei. The conceptus is then transferred to the uterine cavity 2 to 5 days after oocyte retrieval by means of a tiny catheter. In some cases, the hatching process is aided by making an artificial opening in the zona pellucida ("assisted hatching"). **Surplus embryos not transferred at the time of the IVF treatment can be frozen, stored, and transferred in a later menstrual cycle in the event of failure or for additional pregnancies.**

OUTCOME

The pregnancy rate with IVF has been highly variable from center to center, owing to the complexity of the techniques required, whereas the pregnancy rate with

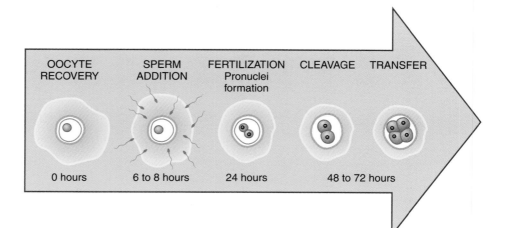

FIGURE 34-3 Approximate time course for in vitro fertilization and embryo transfer.

OOCYTE RECOVERY   SPERM ADDITION   FERTILIZATION Pronuclei formation   CLEAVAGE   TRANSFER

0 hours   6 to 8 hours   24 hours   48 to 72 hours

gamete intrafallopian transfer (GIFT), a technique in which oocytes and washed sperm are mixed and placed into the fallopian tube or tubes, has been more consistent. **The mean live delivery rate per retrieval with IVF currently approximates 30%, with about 1% of clinical pregnancies being ectopic.** Most studies have not shown any significant increase of fetal abnormalities.

EGG DONATION

It is possible to achieve pregnancy with IVF and embryo transfer using donor eggs, with a higher success rate than in regular IVF (about 40%). The eggs generally come from young fertile women (known or anonymous volunteers). The recipient can be programmed for optimal uterine receptivity by replacement doses of estradiol and progesterone. Estradiol and progesterone must be continued until the placenta takes over in the late first trimester. **The excellent success of egg donation mandates the conservation of the uterus whenever future fertility is desired, even if the ovaries must be removed.**

◼ *Overall Success of Infertility Therapy*

Conventional therapies result in conception in 50% to 60% of infertile couples. The application of the newer treatments described here should enable even more couples who are willing to exhaust all measures to reach their goal.

SUGGESTED READING

Gambone JCL: Are adverse pregnancy and fetal outcomes more common with assisted reproductive technologies? What should patients be told? Clin Obstet Gynecol 49:123-133, 2006.
Mayo Clinic: Infertility. Retrieved February 6, 2008, from http://www.mayoclinic.com/health/infertility/DS00310.
Meldrum DR: Low dose follicle-stimulating hormone therapy for polycystic ovarian disease. Fertil Steril 55:1039, 1991.
Meldrum DR: Assisted reproductive technologies: Clinical aspects. *In* Carr BR, Blackwell RF, Azziz R (eds): Essential Reproductive Medicine. New York, McGraw-Hill, 2006, pp 535-560.

Chapter 35

Climacteric
MENOPAUSE AND PERI- AND POSTMENOPAUSE

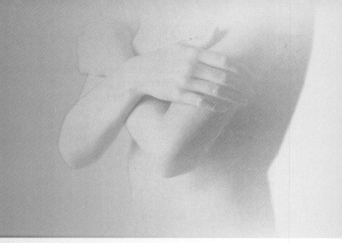

LARRY R. LAUFER • JOSEPH C. GAMBONE

As average life expectancy increases in the United States and elsewhere, women and men are often living well into their ninth decade of life. The preservation of their quality of life in terms of both physical and mental activity is a high priority for them. Many women will live for 30 to 40 years after reproductive function ends.

The *climacteric* **refers to the phase in a woman's reproductive life when a gradual decline in ovarian function results in decreased sex steroid production with its sequelae.** Because this phase is a normal consequence of the aging process, it should not be considered an endocrinopathy.

Menopause literally refers to the last menstrual period. The exact time of menopause is usually determined in retrospect; that is, 1 year without menses. **In most women, menopause occurs between the ages of 50 and 55 years, with an average age of 51.5 years,** but some have their menopause before the age of 40 (premature menopause), whereas a few may menstruate until they are in their 60s.

Women are born with about 1.5 million oocytes (primary ovarian follicles) and reach menarche (first menstruation) with about 400,000 potentially responsive eggs. Most women ovulate about 400 times between menarche and menopause, and during this time, nearly all other oocytes are lost through atresia. When the oocytes either have ovulated or become atretic, the ovary becomes minimally responsive to pituitary gonadotropins, the ovarian production of estrogen and progesterone ends, and ovarian androgen production is reduced. These hormone alterations often result in unpleasant and even harmful physical, psychological, and sexual changes in postmenopausal women and can have a negative impact on their quality of life.

Hormonal Changes

Menopause rarely occurs as a sudden loss of ovarian function. **For some years before menopause, the ovary begins to show signs of impending failure.** Anovulation becomes common, with resulting unopposed estrogen production and irregular menstrual cycles (see Chapter 33). On occasion, heavy menses, endometrial hyperplasia, and increasing mood and emotional changes may occur. In some women, hot flashes (or flushes) and night sweats begin well before menopause is reached. These **perimenopausal symptoms may last 3 to 5 years before there is complete loss of menses and postmenopausal levels of hormones are reached.**

Some women may suffer a more abrupt loss of estrogen. This usually occurs following a surgical intervention that removes or damages the ovaries or their blood supply or, on occasion, following chemotherapy or radiotherapy for cancer. **Women who reach menopause before the age of 40 years are said to have premature menopause or premature ovarian failure.** Other causes of premature ovarian failure include abnormal karyotypes involving the X chromosome, the carrier state of the fragile X syndrome, galactosemia, and autoimmune disorders that may cause failure of a number of other endocrine organs.

Some women continue to produce estrogen indirectly in substantial amounts for many years after menopause. **Androstenedione from the ovary and the adrenal gland is converted in peripheral fat tissues to estrone, which is then capable of maintaining**

The views expressed in this chapter are those of the authors and do not reflect the official policy or position of the Department of the Navy, Department of Defense, or the United States Government.

the vagina, skin, and bone in reasonable cellular tone and reducing the incidence of flashes. Although this unopposed estrogen may be beneficial to women, it may also be responsible for the increased incidence of endometrial or breast cancer, particularly among obese women. For this reason, it is important that postmenopausal women have regular breast examinations and, if abnormal vaginal bleeding occurs, endometrial sampling.

■ *Ovarian Senescence*

The ovary produces a sequence of hormones during a normal menstrual cycle. Under the influence of luteinizing hormone (LH), cholesterol from the liver is used to produce the androgens androstenedione and testosterone in the theca cells of the ovarian follicle. They, in turn, are converted in the granulosa cells immediately surrounding the oocytes into estrogen. Following ovulation, the luteal cells (luteinized granulosa cells) manufacture and secrete progesterone as well as estrogen. The synthesis of these sex hormones depends on the presence of viable follicles and ovarian stroma and the production of follicle-stimulating hormone (FSH) and LH in adequate amounts to induce their biosynthetic activity. The ovarian and adrenal (for comparison) steroid biosynthetic pathways are depicted in Figure 35-1.

ESTROGEN

Following menopause, estradiol (E2) values decline (to only 10 to 50 pg/mL), **but estrone levels may increase.** Estrone (E1) can be produced by peripheral conversion

of androstenedione from the ovary and the adrenal gland. In some women, the amount of postmenopausal estrogen may be considerable.

ANDROGENS

Women normally produce significant quantities of androgens by the metabolic conversion of cholesterol to both androstenedione and testosterone. Although the major portion of androgen is aromatized to estrogen, some androgen circulates. After menopause, there is a decrease in the level of circulating androgens, with androstenedione falling to less than half that found in normal menstruating young women, whereas testosterone gradually diminishes over about 3 to 4 years. **Even though postmenopausal women produce less androgens, they tend to be more sensitive to them because of the lost opposition of estrogen.** This sometimes results in unwelcome changes such as excessive facial hair growth and decreased breast size.

PROGESTERONE

With anovulation during the climacteric and ovarian failure after the menopause, the production of progesterone declines to low levels. The minimal progesterone present is insufficient to induce those cytoplasmic enzymes (estradiol dehydrogenase and estrone sulfuryltransferase) that convert estradiol to the less potent estrone sulfate and to reduce the levels of cellular estrogen receptors. Altogether, this may result in increased estrogen-induced mitosis in the endometrium. The absence of progesterone also prevents the secretory histologic transformation in

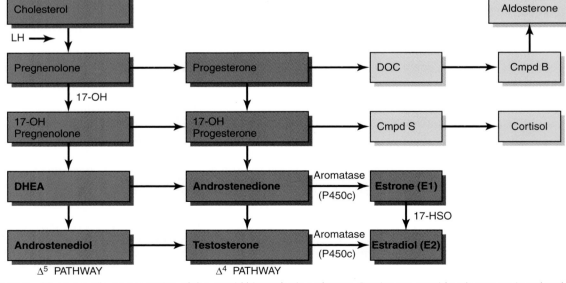

FIGURE 35-1   Diagrammatic representation of the steroid biosynthetic pathways. Ovarian sex steroid pathways are in red and adrenal in blue. Cmpd B, corticosterone; Cmpd S, II-deoxycortisol; DH, hydroxylase; DHEA, dehydroepiandrosterone; DOC, desoxycorticosterone; LH, luteinizing hormone; P450c, cytochrome P450.

the endometrium and its subsequent sloughing. As a consequence, perimenopause is often associated with irregular vaginal bleeding, endometrial hyperplasia and cellular atypia, and an increased incidence of endometrial cancer.

GONADOTROPINS

The two gonadotropins, LH and FSH, are produced in the anterior pituitary gland. **When levels of estrogen are low, the arcuate nucleus and paraventricular nucleus in the hypothalamus are freed from negative feedback and are able to secrete increasing amounts of gonadotropin-releasing hormone (GnRH) into the pituitary portal circulation.** This, in turn, stimulates an increased release of LH and FSH into the circulation. The higher central nervous system neurotransmissions responsible for the increased pulsatile release of GnRH (and subsequent gonadotropin release) are also thought to have parallel effects elsewhere in the hypothalamus, especially the body temperature control region. This leads to sudden induction of increased skin blood flow and perspiration—the hot flash that so characterizes menopause. Typical levels of FSH in postmenopausal women are greater than 20 or 40 IU/L, depending on the assay used.

Clinical Manifestations

Loss of estrogen is associated with urogenital atrophy and osteoporosis (Table 35-1). Although postmenopausal women have a higher incidence of heart disease and of cancer, the relationship between these adverse events and reduced endogenous estrogen production, as well as the effects of hormonal therapy on them, remains unclear and controversial.

GENERAL SYMPTOMS

About 85% of women experience hot flashes as they pass through the climacteric, but about half of these women are not seriously disturbed by them. For about 40% of affected women, the hot flash is a most

TABLE 35-1

CONSEQUENCE OF ESTROGEN LOSS

Symptoms (early)	Hot flushes (flashes) Insomnia Irritability Mood disturbances
Physical changes (intermediate)	Urogenital atrophy Stress (urinary) incontinence Skin collagen loss
Diseases (late)	Osteoporosis Dementia of the Alzheimer's type (possible) Cardiovascular disease (unclear relationship) Cancers, for example, colon (unclear relationship)

distressing experience. Flashes may occur as frequently as every 30 to 40 minutes, but more often they occur about 8 to 15 times daily. There may be associated sweating, dizziness, and palpitations. Often, the hot flash may awaken the woman at night and impair the quality of her sleep. **As a consequence of frequent flashes at night, the woman may experience increased fatigue and irritability.** Women are often given sedatives, hypnotics, or psychotropic drugs in an attempt to relieve these symptoms caused by estrogen deficiency. **Some complain of confusion, loss of memory, lethargy, and inability to cope, as well as mild depression.** In addition, the hypoestrogenic state may be associated with a **loss of the sense of balance**, possibly resulting in an increased risk for falling. Many of these symptoms improve considerably when appropriate hormonal therapy (estrogen and a progestin or estrogen alone) is initiated. **Severe or even sustained moderate depression should never be attributed solely to climacteric hormonal changes.**

UROGENITAL SYMPTOMS

The vagina is sensitive to estrogen, and it responds to this hormone by producing a thick, moist epithelium with an acidic secretion (pH of about 4.0). The absence of estrogen results in a thin, dry epithelium with an alkaline secretion (pH > 7.0). **The postmenopausal vagina shrinks in diameter and splits and tears easily.** Atrophic vaginitis may result in unpleasant dryness, discharge, and severe dyspareunia.

Because the bladder and vagina are derived from the same embryologic tissue, it is not surprising that some postmenopausal women also complain of urinary symptoms such as frequency, urgency, nocturia, and urinary incontinence. Hormonal therapy markedly improves atrophic vaginitis but cannot prevent adequately or treat urinary incontinence.

Osteoporosis

Remodeling of bone continues throughout life, but with estrogen deprivation, osteoclastic activity far exceeds the osteoblasts' ability to lay down bone. Under these conditions, osteopenia and finally osteoporosis occur. An early clinical sign of osteoporosis is a loss of height greater than 1.5 inches because of vertebral compression fracture, which may be accompanied by acute and chronic back pain. Other important osteoporotic events include wrist and hip fractures. **Ten to 15 years after menopause has occurred, women begin to fracture their bones at a rate exceeding that of men by a factor of threefold to fivefold.** About 200,000 women break a hip each year in the United States, and the annual cost of osteoporotic fractures and their complications has been estimated to be in excess of $14 billion. The earlier women are deprived of estrogen in their lives, the earlier osteoporotic bone loss begins. **Most calcium is lost from trabecular bone, and as a consequence, the spinal column and femoral neck are the bones most commonly fractured.**

Risk factors for osteoporosis include a family history of osteoporosis, slender body composition, white or Asian ethnic origin, sedentary lifestyle, alcohol consumption, cigarette smoking, thyroid excess, or use of corticosteroid or anticonvulsant medications. The North American Menopause Society recommends bone mineral density screening for osteoporosis in women with risk factors who are 50 years of age or older and in women without risk factors who are 65 years or older. The preferred screening modality is dual-energy x-ray absorptiometry measurements of the total hip and spine. The results of these studies are expressed in T scores, which are standard deviations (SDs) from the peak bone mineral density of normal young adults. Osteoporosis is defined as a T score of less than –2.5 SD. Drug therapy is recommended in postmenopausal women with a T score of less than –2.5 SD or a T score of –2.0 to –2.5 SD plus an additional risk factor for fracture. If bone mineral density measurements are used to monitor the effects of drug therapy, they should be repeated after at least 6 months of treatment.

Reducing the risk for osteoporotic fracture entails several changes of diet and lifestyle. **Postmenopausal women should consume 1200 to 1500 mg of calcium and 400 to 600 U of vitamin D daily, which are contained in two to three portions of dairy products.** Those who cannot or will not include dairy products in their meals should be encouraged to use calcium and vitamin D supplements. Excessive supplementation should be discouraged to avoid renal complications. **Walking and weight-bearing exercises both help to increase bone mineral mass and reduce the risk for fracture-causing falls.** The risk for falling can be reduced further by elimination of throw rugs in the home, placement of handrails in the bathroom, and minimizing the use of alcoholic beverages. **Smoking should be discouraged** for many other health reasons in addition to osteoporosis prevention. Patients receiving replacement therapy for hypothyroidism should be tested to ensure that they are not receiving an excessive (and potentially bone density–depleting) dose.

Pharmacologic treatments for osteoporosis include estrogen (with or without a progestin), selective estrogen receptor modulators (SERMs), bisphosphonates, calcitonin, and parathyroid hormone. Data from the Women's Health Initiative (WHI) study, sponsored by the National Institutes of Health, demonstrated that combined estrogen and progestin therapy reduced postmenopausal total fractures by 24% compared with controls, with a 34% reduction of hip fractures. This translates to a reduction of the hip fracture rate from 15 to 10 cases per 10,000 postmenopausal women per year. **SERMs, such as raloxifene, have been found to be beneficial for the prevention of vertebral fractures,** but data are lacking regarding the prevention of hip fracture. **Bisphosphonates, such as alendronate, are effective in both preventing and, at higher doses, treating osteoporosis** without requiring long-term, continued use. In general, bisphosphonates have few adverse side effects. However, they must be taken properly (empty stomach, upright position, and with a large glass of water) to minimize the risk for esophagitis and esophageal ulcers. Both calcitonin and parathyroid hormone are second-line adjunctive treatments for osteoporosis.

■ *Ovarian Hormone Therapy*

For four decades, ovarian hormone therapy has been advocated for an expanding set of prophylactic indications. Initially, hormone therapy was provided for the treatment of hot flashes and the symptoms of genitourinary atrophy. Later, increasing evidence revealed that prevention of osteoporosis was a specific benefit of ovarian hormone therapy.

A number of large observational cohort and case-control studies suggested ovarian hormone therapy might prevent or delay the onset of arteriosclerotic heart disease and Alzheimer's disease through a number of diverse mechanisms. On the other hand, observational studies have raised concerns about ovarian hormone therapy and the risks for venous thrombosis, pulmonary embolism, and breast cancer. Although observational studies provide useful information, they are subject to several sources of bias. Table 35-2 lists some of the biases that may occur during observational studies.

Randomized controlled trials tend to minimize the biases of observational studies. However, they are difficult and time-consuming to do when the conditions

TABLE 35-2	
SOME OF THE INHERENT BIASES IN OBSERVATIONAL STUDIES	
Selection bias	Hormone therapy users may be different from nonusers in terms of behaviors and disease risk.
Prescribing bias	Only well women are given hormone therapy.
Prevention bias	Monitoring and treatment are more intensive in women on hormone therapy.
Compliance bias	Women with greater adherence (even to placebo) have better outcomes.
Recall bias	Women who develop a disease have a better recollection of treatments taken.
Prevalence-incidence bias	Early adverse effects of hormone therapy not observed if user dies before becoming part of cohort.

being observed are relatively uncommon. The Women's Health Initiative (WHI) study attempted to sort out the risks and benefits of ovarian hormone therapy. More than 16,000 women were entered into one arm of the study comparing a combined preparation of conjugated estrogens and medroxyprogesterone acetate with placebo. After 5 years of follow-up, this combined ovarian hormone arm was halted in July 2002. **The previously reported protection from osteoporotic fracture was confirmed by the WHI study. In addition, a 37% reduction in the rate of colorectal cancer was found.** This would result in six fewer cases of colorectal cancer (10 vs 16) per 10,000 women per year. **Combined ovarian hormone use, however, was found to increase the risks for coronary artery disease events (by 29%), stroke (by 41%), thromboses (by 100%), and breast cancer (by 26%).** Although most of the risks increased after 1 to 2 years of use, increased risk for breast cancer became apparent only after 4 years of use. There was no significant increase in death rates between treatment and placebo groups (Figure 35-2). Contrary to several previous studies, the WHI found an overall harmful rather than protective effect on cognitive decline and dementia.

In February 2004, the estrogen-only arm of the WHI was halted owing to a significantly increased risk for stroke. It confirmed a protective effect against hip fracture, whereas none of the other significant findings in the combined arm were found to be present. The risk for breast cancer was not increased in the estrogen-only arm of the WHI.

The WHI study has been widely criticized for studying women who, for the most part, were well past the age of menopause when they were entered into the study (average age was 63 years). Laboratory and animal studies have shown an arteriosclerotic protective effect of estrogen after gonadectomy, when begun immediately. Additional analysis of WHI data has failed to confirm increased coronary artery events in subjects who began therapy less than 10 years after the menopause.

Although definite limitations of the WHI study have been identified, **the findings have had a significant effect on clinical practice, and the routine use of hormone therapy after menopause is now viewed with caution. The general consensus is that combined ovarian hormone therapy is indicated primarily for the relief of significant menopausal symptoms such as frequent hot flashes, genitourinary discomfort, and other quality-of-life issues.** The length of treatment should be minimized depending on the individual

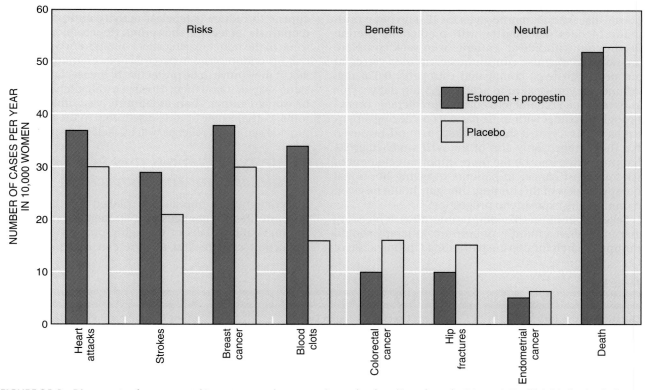

FIGURE 35-2 Disease rates for women taking estrogen plus progestin or placebo. *(Data from the Women's Health Initiative Study Group, 2002.)*

patient's clinical course and preference, after informed consent. On the other hand, most experts recommend that younger hypoestrogenic women, such as those who undergo premature menopause or bilateral oophorectomy, should take hormonal therapy.

A large observational cohort study, the Million Women Study (MWS), is addressing the risks and benefits of hormone therapy after menopause. More than 1 million women have been enrolled in the United Kingdom, and thus far no long-term results have been fully analyzed or reported. After a little more than 4 years of follow-up, however, the MWS reported an increased breast cancer risk with hormone therapy. Table 35-3 lists these results.

The need for prevention and treatment of osteoporosis may be determined by bone densitometry studies rather than ovarian status, **with bisphosphonates or raloxifene as the first line of treatment in the absence of concomitant significant menopausal symptoms.**

Management of Ovarian Hormonal Therapy

Women who still have a uterus should not be given unopposed estrogen for the treatment of menopausal symptoms because of the high risk for developing endometrial hyperplasia and endometrial adenocarcinoma. Concurrent progestin is protective for endometrial disease and may be given for 12 days per month or for 14 days per quarter with predictable uterine bleeding on withdrawal. **Patients who seek complete amenorrhea may use continuous combined estrogen and progestin** (e.g., conjugated estrogens, 0.625 mg, and medroxyprogesterone acetate, 2.5 mg daily). This latter regimen is characterized by unpredictable breakthrough bleeding, with most patients achieving amenorrhea within a year. It should be kept in mind, however, that the estrogen-only arm of the WHI study suggests that progestins may be the more important element of risk for breast cancer in patients receiving hormonal therapy. In view of this finding, thought should be given to minimizing exposure to progestins.

Severe continuous bleeding or intermittent bleeding after more than 4 months of hormonal therapy should prompt a search for uterine pathology. Optimization of menopausal symptom control, while reducing adverse side effects of therapy, may be accomplished by using the lowest effective dose and by substituting continuous transdermal estrogen for oral estrogen preparations when symptoms are not adequately controlled. When the patient's main concerns are with genitourinary symptoms, vaginal estrogen cream, tablets, or rings may be used on an as-needed basis without necessarily adding a progestin.

Selective Estrogen Receptor Modulators

The biologic effect of estrogenic substances is mediated by the translocation of a ligand-estrogen receptor complex into the nucleus where various estrogen-responsive genes are activated or repressed. **At least two estrogen receptors, α and β, are presently known to exist.** They exert different biologic effects and exist in different proportions in different tissues. In addition, different ligands bound in complex with the same receptor manifest different biologic activity. The use of SERMs attempts to take advantage of these facts to produce some of the biologic effects of native estradiol. SERMs in use today include clomiphene, tamoxifen, and raloxifene. Unlike estradiol and other SERMs in current use, **raloxifene does not stimulate endometrial or breast duct epithelial proliferation.** However, **raloxifene does appear to reduce osteoclast activity and prevent osteoporosis (at least in the spine).** Hence, raloxifene has some of the bone-sparing effect of estradiol without the risk for endometrial hyperplasia or carcinoma, and in fact, it may prove to be protective of breast cancer in the same way as tamoxifen. However, **raloxifene appears to worsen rather than ameliorate vasomotor symptoms.** Perhaps new SERMs discovered in the future will provide symptom relief as well as skeletal protection.

Lifestyle Changes and Alternative Treatments for the Climacteric

Increasingly, an emphasis is placed on the importance of lifestyle changes as a strategy for decreasing the inevitable effects of the aging process. **The most important change that anyone can make overall to**

TABLE 35-3		
RELATIVE RISKS (CONFIDENCE INTERVALS) OF BREAST CANCER WITH DURATION OF CURRENT USE OF HORMONES		
Duration of Use (yr)	Current Users of Estrogen Only	Current Estrogen and Progestin Users
<1	0.81 (0.55-1.20)	1.45 (1.19-1.78)
1-4	1.25 (1.10-1.41)	1.74 (1.60-1.89)
5-9	1.32 (1.20-1.46)	2.17 (2.03-2.33)
≥10	1.37 (1.22-1.54)	2.31 (2.08-2.56)

Data from Speroff L: The Million Women Study and breast cancer. Maturitas 46:1-6, 2003.

increase longevity, reduce heart disease, and reduce calcium loss from bone is to stop smoking. Controlling weight, engaging in regular exercise, and eating a healthier, low-fat, and balanced diet should be strongly recommended, especially in women with diabetes, hypertension, or significantly elevated blood lipids. All counseling about the effects of menopause should include a discussion of these issues and recommendations along with any possible medical therapies. In particular, the statin drugs are especially important for postmenopausal women with unfavorable lipid profiles because they significantly reduce the risk for cardiovascular disease and serendipitously protect against osteoporosis.

Phytoestrogens (plant products that are functionally or structurally similar to estrogen) and herbal substances have been marketed to consumers as the "natural" alternative to traditional hormone therapy for the symptoms of perimenopause and menopause. Women should be made aware that even placebos may decrease some of the symptoms, such as hot flashes, and that some herbal preparations have been shown to be ineffective or even harmful. Also, patients should be made aware of the less rigorous evaluation and regulation that these products undergo.

With proper counseling, appropriate screening, and professional care, the signs, symptoms, and sequelae of the climacteric can be managed successfully. Short-term use of hormonal therapy for symptom control, healthy lifestyle changes, appropriate monitoring, and medical or surgical intervention when necessary should provide a safe and effective level of care.

SUGGESTED READING

Million Women Study Collaborators: Breast cancer and hormone replacement therapy in the Million Women Study. Lancet 362:419-427, 2003.

North American Menopause Society: Management of postmenopausal osteoporosis: Position statement. Menopause 9:84-101, 2002.

Shifren JL, Schiff I: Menopause. *In* Berek JS (ed): Berek and Novak's Gynecology, 14th ed. Philadelphia, Lippincott Williams & Wilkins, 2007, pp 1323-1340.

Chapter 36

Menstrual Cycle–Influenced Disorders

LARRY R. LAUFER • JOSEPH C. GAMBONE

The human menstrual cycle is unique as a physiologic process in that it involves mechanisms that change on a daily basis rather than remaining stable. This process of change is carried out through the many intricate hormonal interactions between the hypothalamic region of the brain, the pituitary gland, the ovaries, and to some extent, the adrenal glands and the pancreatic islets of Langerhans (see Chapter 4). To a large degree, the subject matter of reproductive endocrinology deals with disturbances of this interglandular hormonal communication that may result in irregular or absent menstrual cycles.

There is a second group of menstrual cycle–associated disorders, the hallmark of which is regular ovulatory cycles that cause dysfunction of other organ systems. In these menstrual-influenced disorders, the causative factors are not abnormal concentrations of the hormones of the hypothalamic-pituitary-ovarian (HPO) axis, but rather are atypical end-organ responses to normal levels of gonadotropins and sex steroids. A common feature of these disorders is the inability to distinguish between affected women and normal controls by measurement of the traditional HPO hormones. Interestingly, in many cases, relief from the symptoms of these disorders can be obtained by intentionally disrupting or abolishing regular menstrual function. The most typical menstrual cycle–influenced disorder is premenstrual syndrome, or PMS.

Premenstrual Syndrome and Premenstrual Dysphoric Disorder

The acronyms PMS for premenstrual syndrome and PMDD for premenstrual dysphoric disorder refer to the same pathologic process at opposite ends of the symptom spectrum (Figure 36-1). In both PMS and PMDD, patients experience adverse physical, psychological, and behavioral symptoms during the luteal phase of the menstrual cycle. There is a crescendo of symptom intensity up to the time that menses begins, with quick resolution thereafter. Some patients have a brief surge of symptoms at the time of ovulation in midcycle.

As many as 80% of regularly ovulating women experience some degree of physical and psychological premenstrual symptomatology. Those who have mild to moderate symptoms are said to have PMS. In 5% or less of women, these symptoms are so severe that they seriously interfere with usual daily functioning or personal relationships. These women are characterized as having PMDD.

Common symptoms reported by patients include depressed mood, anxiety, affective lability and irritability, decreased interest in regular activity, difficulty concentrating, fatigue, change of appetite, sleep disturbance, and feelings of being overwhelmed. Physical symptoms include breast swelling and tenderness, bloating (a sense of abdominal swelling), weight gain, edema, and headache. The diagnosis of these disorders is confirmed by the predominant occurrence of symptoms in the luteal phase as documented on a menstrual calendar of two consecutive cycles.

A formal set of diagnostic criteria has been proposed in the fourth text revision of the *Diagnostic and Statistical Manual of Mental Disorders (DSM-IV)* of the American Psychiatric Association for PMDD (Table 36-1). Although the *DSM-IV* definition of PMDD specifies that this is not just an exacerbation of another disorder, the dividing line between PMDD and other neuropsychiatric disorders is not so clear cut. For

---

The views expressed in this chapter are those of the authors and do not reflect the official policy or position of the Department of the Navy, Department of Defense, or the United States Government.

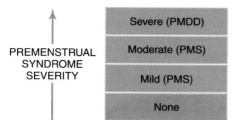

Spectrum of Premenstrual Syndromes

PREMENSTRUAL SYNDROME SEVERITY

- Severe (PMDD)
- Moderate (PMS)
- Mild (PMS)
- None

FIGURE 36-1   Spectrum of premenstrual syndromes. PMDD, premenstrual dysphoric disorder; PMS, premenstrual syndrome.

example, **46% of PMDD patients have a history of a prior major depressive episode.** Moreover, patients with PMDD and clinical depression share similar sleep electroencephalogram alterations, and they are both responsive to the selective serotonin reuptake inhibitor (SSRI) antidepressants.

Although PMS and PMDD patients and controls do not differ in their average cyclic levels of sex steroids, gonadotropins, prolactin, or cortisol, **there exists a strong basis to believe that these disorders have a hormonal rather than purely psychologic basis.** First, abolition of the menstrual cycle with gonadotropin-releasing hormone (GnRH) agonists, pregnancy, menopause, or spontaneous anovulation provides symptomatic relief, whereas sequential ovarian hormone therapy in hypogonadal patients can induce PMS and PMDD symptoms. Second, cycles with higher luteal phase levels of estradiol are associated with more severe symptoms.

The physiologic mechanism that results in the occurrence of PMS and PMDD is not well understood. Evidence exists that the phenomenon arises, in part, from atypical metabolism of progesterone that results in lower levels of the steroid allopregnenolone within the central nervous system. Allopregnenolone is a neuroactive progesterone metabolite that modulates central gamma-aminobutyric acid (GABA) receptors that modify behavior, emotion, subjective perceptions, and response to stress. In addition, the GABA and serotoninergic neurons may be inherently dysfunctional in PMS and PMDD patients, especially in those with severe depressive symptoms—hence the overlap between PMDD and clinical depression. Major depressive disorder (MDD) persists, however, on a daily basis for weeks without a relationship to the menstrual cycle. **MDD, which usually does not have premenstrual physical symptoms, may however be exacerbated during the luteal phase of the menstrual cycle.** In such cases, both PMDD and MDD need to be treated (Table 36-2).

Research performed to determine the best therapy for this disorder is problematic, because of the subjective nature of the condition as well as the wide variation in the severity of the symptoms from one cycle to the next. In addition, external influences at work and at home will affect the severity of the symptoms. Finally, placebo interventions produce significant initial benefits in most PMS and PMDD studies. All these considerations necessitate prolonged studies, which are expensive and infrequently performed.

TABLE 36-1

CRITERIA FOR PREMENSTRUAL DYSPHORIC DISORDER

- Symptoms seriously interfere with usual functioning and relationships.
- Premenstrual timing is confirmed by menstrual calendar in two consecutive cycles.
- Symptoms resolve after the onset of menses.
- Symptoms are not an exacerbation of another disorder.
- At least five premenstrual symptoms:
  1. At least one of the following:
     Depressed mood
     Marked anxiety
     Marked affective lability
     Marked irritability
  2. Other possible symptoms:
     Decreased interest in regular activities
     Difficulty in concentrating
     Lethargy, fatigue
     Appetite change, food cravings
     Sleep disturbance
     Feelings of being overwhelmed
     Physical symptoms (breast swelling and tenderness, bloating, weight gain, edema, or headache)

TABLE 36-2

DISTINGUISHING PREMENSTRUAL DYSPHORIC DISORDER FROM PREMENSTRUAL SYNDROME AND MAJOR DEPRESSIVE DISORDER

	Predominant Mood Symptoms	Premenstrual Physical Symptoms	Marked Social Impairment	Monthly Cyclicity
Premenstrual syndrome (PMS)	–/+	+	–	Yes
Premenstrual dysphoric disorder (PMDD)	+	+	+	Yes
Major depressive disorder (MDD)	+	–	+	No

Treatment

Most women who could be characterized as having PMS should be treated individually and conservatively, with **reassurance and mild diuretics** for symptoms such as bloating. The mild anxiety that frequently occurs with PMS may be treated with an antianxiety agent such as **buspirone.** At present, the most effective therapy studied for women with PMDD is the SSRI class of antidepressants. **Fluoxetine taken at dosages of 20 to 60 mg per day during the luteal phase of the cycle** provides significant symptom improvement in 50% to 60% of patients. **Sertraline at 50 to 150 mg per day** is equally effective. Side effects of the SSRIs are usually self-limited and include insomnia and sexual dysfunction.

Other preparations have been effective in at least one randomized controlled trial. They include **calcium carbonate at 1200 mg per day**, for control of mood and behavioral symptoms; **spironolactone at 100 mg per day**, for mood and bloating; and **buspirone at 25 to 60 mg per day,** for premenstrual anxiety. **Danocrine and bromocriptine** are effective for the treatment of cyclic mastalgia. Pyridoxine (vitamin B_6) at 50 to 100 mg a day has demonstrated mixed results in clinical trials.

GnRH agonists used with estrogen and progestin "add back" to minimize hot flashes are effective in eliminating PMS and PMDD symptoms. However, this is an expensive therapeutic approach.

Treatments that have been **demonstrated to be ineffective** in randomized controlled trials include oral or vaginal progesterone and conventional use of combined oral contraceptives. With the latter, patients have PMS-like symptoms during the placebo week.

Recent studies have shown benefit from the continuous use, or 24- out of 28-day use, of an oral contraceptive containing the progestin drospirenone.

Menstrual Migraine Headaches

Migraine headaches, which are believed to result from sequential intracranial vasoconstriction and vasodilation, are known to be influenced by menstrual cycling. They are 2 to 3 times more common in women than in men. They improve in about 80% of patients during pregnancy but recur postpartum. Usually, migraines resolve after the onset of the menopause. **Sixty percent of women who suffer migraine link the occurrence of their attacks to the menstrual cycle,** and 7% exclusively have migraines on the 2 days before or after the onset of menstruation. Menstrual migraines usually occur without a preceding aura and are more long-lasting and resistant to treatment than migraines occurring at other times in the menstrual cycle.

The link between migraine headaches and the hormonal changes of the menstrual cycle is believed to be the phenomenon of estrogen withdrawal. Evidence for this derives from several observations: first, a small proportion of women with menstrual migraine have an upsurge in headache frequency following the preovulatory estradiol surge; second, exogenous estrogen reduces the incidence of migraines; and third, exogenous progesterone may delay the onset of menstruation without preventing the migraine attacks.

Several mechanisms have been proposed to explain why estrogen withdrawal produces migraine headaches. They include abnormal platelet aggregation, central nervous system endogenous opioid dysregulation, and stimulation of increased synthesis of prostaglandin in the central nervous system.

Standard treatment of migraine headaches includes triptans, nonsteroidal antiinflammatory drugs, and ergotamines. Drugs used for the short-term prophylaxis of menstrual migraines can be taken 3 to 5 days before and after the onset of menses. They include nonsteroidal antiinflammatory drugs and triptans. Monitoring of the menstrual cycle by basal body temperature charting or the use of a luteinizing hormone surge detector kit permits the initiation of these agents for more effective headache prevention.

Several hormonal protocols may also be effective in preventing menstrual migraines. For short-term prophylaxis, 100-μg transdermal estrogen patches begun 48 hours before anticipated menses and continued for 3 to 6 days have been shown to be effective. Continuous oral contraceptive pills for intervals of 2 to 4 months (with symptomatic treatment during withdrawal between intervals) provide long-term prevention of migraines.

Catamenial (Monthly) Epilepsy

Seventy percent of female epileptic patients report an increased incidence of seizures premenstrually. Fourteen percent of female epileptic patients have catamenial epilepsy in which seizures only occur in the perimenstrual phase of the cycle. **This includes all varieties of epilepsy.** In these women, the onset of epilepsy is usually at the time of, or shortly after, menarche. Eight-four percent of catamenial epileptic patients have significant premenstrual syndrome symptoms, in contrast to a 22% incidence of PMS in epileptic patients whose seizures do not correlate with the menstrual cycle.

Two mechanisms are thought to underlie the phenomenon of catamenial epilepsy. The first is a direct effect on the neurons of the brain of the reduced progesterone-to-estradiol ratio. In vitro, estradiol lowers the seizure threshold of many varieties of neurons whereas progesterone raises the threshold, making a seizure more likely. Thus, catamenial epilepsy reflects the effect of a reduced progesterone (and allopregnenolone) concentration or progesterone-to-estradiol ratio during the late luteal phase of the menstrual cycle. This correlates well with several clinical observations: first, some patients with catamenial epilepsy also suffer exacerbations during the preovulatory estradiol surge; second, seizure activity is prone to increase in anovulatory cycles, which may be managed with the use of clomiphene; and third, seizure activity may decrease in incidence after menopause.

A second mechanism explaining this disorder is a reduction in serum levels of anticonvulsants during the late luteal phase. This is believed to be mediated by increased hepatic mono-oxygenase activity resulting directly from reduced sex steroid levels (primarily progesterone). This is the rationale for the treatment option of closely tracking the menstrual cycle and determining anticonvulsant concentrations in the late luteal phase, so that drug dosage may be altered when necessary.

The anticonvulsant effect of progesterone is the basis of using Depo-Provera, progestin-only oral contraceptive pills, or premenstrual progesterone suppositories (50 to 400 mg twice daily) to reduce seizure activity. Ganaxolone, an allopregnenolone analogue taken cycle days 21 through 3 of the next cycle, has also been found to be an effective seizure prophylactic. **GnRH agonist therapy** has been helpful for intractable cases. Combined oral contraceptives have inconsistent effects, with some patients suffering exacerbations during the placebo week. Moreover, pill efficacy is reduced by anticonvulsants, resulting in a higher contraceptive failure rate with low-dose preparations.

Other Menstrual Cycle–Influenced Disorders

PREMENSTRUAL ASTHMA

Eight to 40% of female asthmatic patients report increased symptoms or decreased peak expiratory flow rates in the premenstrual phase of their cycles. Progesterone has bronchodilatory and antiinflammatory effects that may be responsible for this phenomenon. Similar to other maneuvers with menstrual-influenced disorders, monitoring of the cycle to modify glucocorticoid or leukotriene antagonist dosage may be helpful. There is little experience with hormone-based therapies in asthma.

DIABETES MELLITUS

Seventy percent of female type 1 diabetic patients report changes in glycemic control premenstrually. Possible mechanisms for this effect include PMS-induced dietary binges and reduction of physical activity. The suggested management is intensified adherence to diet control, exercise, and glucose measurement. On the other hand, SSRIs, which may be used to treat PMDD, have been found to increase insulin sensitivity.

PREMENSTRUAL ACNE

Although acne is worsened by the increased sebum production associated with androgen excess in conditions such as polycystic ovary syndrome, regularly cycling women have little cyclic variation in androgen levels. **The mechanism of premenstrual acne is unclear,** but it may be secondary to altered immune function or hormone-related constriction of the pilosebaceous ductal orifice in the late luteal phase.

Other Conditions

In some individuals, the following conditions may be influenced by the menstrual cycle: rheumatoid arthritis, irritable bowel syndrome, hereditary angioedema, aphthous ulcers, Behçet's syndrome, acute intermittent porphyria, paroxysmal supraventricular tachycardia, multiple sclerosis, glaucoma, urticaria, erythema multiforme, and myasthenia gravis. Interestingly, in the case of myasthenia gravis, 25% to 50% of female patients improve premenstrually.

SUGGESTED READING

American College of Obstetricians and Gynecologists (ACOG): Practice Bulletin on Premenstrual Syndrome, No. 15. Washington, DC, ACOG, 2000.

Case AM, Reid RL: Menstrual cycle effects on common medical conditions. Compr Ther 27:65-71, 2000.

Kessel B: Premenstrual syndrome: Advances in diagnosis and treatment. Obstet Gynecol Clin North Am 27:625-631, 2000.

Rapkin A, Mikacich J: Premenstrual syndrome: Gynaecology or psychiatry? Reprod Med Rev 9:223-239, 2001.

Stotland NL: Premenstrual syndrome. *In* Berek JS (ed): Berek and Novak's Gynecology, 14th ed. Philadelphia, Lippincott Williams & Wilkins, 2007, pp 358-366.

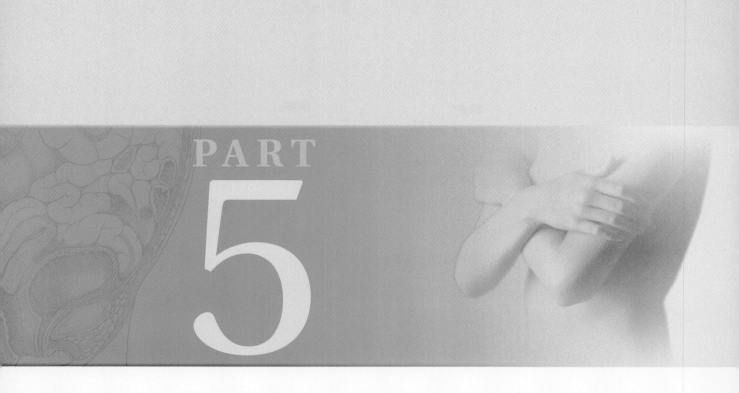

5

GYNECOLOGIC
ONCOLOGY

Chapter 37

Principles of Cancer Therapy

NEVILLE F. HACKER

The standard modalities for the management of gynecologic cancer are surgery, chemotherapy, radiation therapy, and hormonal therapy. In this chapter, the principles of chemotherapy, radiation therapy, and hormonal manipulation are discussed, together with the principles of pain management and end-of-life issues. Targeted therapies and hyperthermia are at present experimental modalities and are not included.

◼ Cellular Biology

The characteristic feature of malignant tumor growth is its uncontrolled cellular proliferation, which requires replication of DNA. There are two distinct phases in the life cycle of all cells: **mitosis** (M phase), during which cellular division occurs; and **interphase,** the interval between successive mitoses.

Interphase is subdivided into three separate phases (Figure 37-1). Immediately following mitosis is the G_1 **phase,** which is of variable duration and is characterized by a diploid content of DNA. DNA synthesis is absent, but RNA and protein synthesis occur. During the shorter **S phase,** the entire DNA content is duplicated. This is followed by the G_2 **phase,** which is characterized by a tetraploid DNA content and by continuing RNA and protein synthesis in preparation for cell division. When mitosis occurs, a duplicate set of chromosomal DNA is inherited by each daughter cell, thus restoring the diploid DNA content. Following mitosis, some cells leave the cycle temporarily or permanently and enter the G_0 **or resting phase.**

The growth fraction of the tumor is the proportion of actively dividing cells. The higher the growth fraction, the fewer the number of cells in the G_0 phase and the faster the tumor-doubling time.

Chemotherapeutic agents and radiation kill cells by first-order kinetics, which means that a constant proportion of cells is killed for a given dosage, regardless of the number of cells present. Both therapeutic modalities are most effective against actively dividing cells because cells in the resting (G_0) phase are better able to repair sublethal damage. Unfortunately, both therapeutic modalities also suppress rapidly dividing normal cells, such as those in the gastrointestinal mucosa, bone marrow, and hair follicles.

◼ Chemotherapy

One of the major advances in medicine since the 1950s has been the successful treatment of certain disseminated malignancies, including choriocarcinoma and germ cell ovarian tumors, with chemotherapy.

CLASSIFICATION OF CHEMOTHERAPEUTIC AGENTS

Chemotherapeutic agents act primarily by disrupting nuclear DNA, thus inhibiting cellular division. They may be subdivided into two categories according to their mode of action relative to the cell cycle:

1. **Cell cycle–nonspecific agents,** such as alkylating agents, cisplatin, and paclitaxel, exert their damage at any phase of the cell cycle. They may damage resting as well as cycling cells, but the latter are much more sensitive.
2. **Cell cycle–specific agents** exert their lethal effects exclusively or primarily during one phase of the cell cycle. Examples include hydroxyurea and methotrexate, which act primarily during the S phase; bleomycin, which acts in the G_2 phase; and the vinca alkaloids, which act in the M phase.

PRINCIPLES OF CHEMOTHERAPY

Chemotherapeutic agents are selected on the basis of previous experience with particular agents for a given tumor. The drugs are usually given systemically so that the tumor can be treated regardless of its anatomic

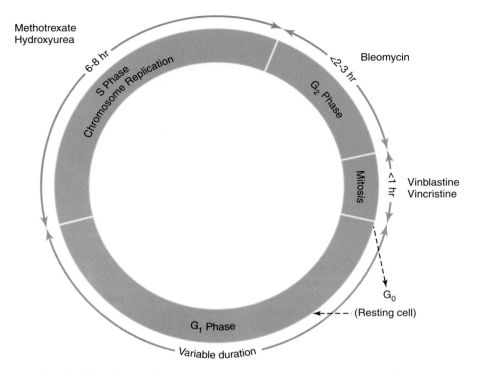

FIGURE 37-1 Phases of the cell cycle and sites of action of cell cycle–specific drugs.

location. To increase the local concentration, certain drugs may occasionally be administered topically, by intraarterial infusion, or by intrathecal or intracavitary instillation (e.g., intraperitoneal therapy for ovarian cancer).

Chemotherapy is generally not administered if the neutrophil count is less than 1500 cells/mm³ or if the platelet count is less than 100,000 cells/mm³. Nadir blood counts are obtained 7 to 14 days after treatment, and subsequent doses may need to be reduced if there is significant myelosuppression or if the patient develops febrile neutropenia. Dosage reduction may also be necessary because of toxicity to other organs, such as the gastrointestinal tract, liver, or kidneys.

Resistance to chemotherapeutic agents may be temporary or permanent. Temporary resistance is mainly related to the poor vascularity of bulky tumors, which results in poor tissue concentrations of the drugs and an increasing proportion of cells in the relatively resistant G_0 phase of the cell cycle. Permanent resistance mainly results from spontaneous mutation to phenotypic resistance and occurs most commonly in bulky tumors. Permanent resistance may also be acquired by frequent exposure to chemotherapeutic agents.

CHEMOTHERAPEUTIC AGENTS

The common agents used in the management of gynecologic malignancies may be classified as shown in Table 37-1. This table also contains a summary of the main indications for and side effects of these drugs.

Alkylating Agents

The cytotoxicity of alkylating agents results from their ability to cause alkylation to DNA, resulting in cross-linkage between DNA strands and prevention of DNA replication. There is cross-resistance among the various alkylating agents.

Antimetabolites

Antimetabolites are compounds that closely resemble normal intermediaries, for which they may substitute in biochemical reactions, and thereby produce a metabolic block; for example, **methotrexate** competitively inhibits the enzyme dihydrofolate reductase, thus preventing the conversion of dihydrofolate to tetrahydrofolate. The latter is required for the methylation reaction necessary for the synthesis of purine and pyrimidine subunits of nucleic acid.

TABLE 37-1

INDICATIONS, SIDE EFFECTS, AND PRECAUTIONS FOR COMMONLY USED CHEMOTHERAPEUTIC AGENTS

Drug	Main Indications	Side Effects	Precautions
ALKYLATING AGENTS			
Chlorambucil	Ovarian carcinoma	Bone marrow depression	
Melphalan	Ovarian and tubal carcinoma	Bone marrow depression, leukemia	Avoid prolonged courses (more than 12 cycles) to avoid leukemia
Cyclophosphamide	Ovarian carcinoma, germ cell tumors, squamous carcinomas, sarcomas	Bone marrow depression, nausea and vomiting, alopecia, hemorrhagic cystitis, sterility	Maintain adequate fluid intake to avoid cystitis
ANTIMETABOLITES			
Methotrexate	Gestational trophoblastic disease	Bone marrow depression, nausea and vomiting, stomatitis, alopecia, liver and renal failure, dermatitis	Ensure normal kidney and liver function
5-Fluorouracil	Vaginal and vulvar intraepithelial neoplasia (topical application)	Pain and ulceration	
Gemcitabine	Ovarian carcinoma	Bone marrow depression, flu-like illness, skin rash	Intravenous infusion
ANTIBIOTICS			
Actinomycin-D	Gestational trophoblastic disease	Bone marrow depression, nausea and vomiting, diarrhea, stomatitis, alopecia, dermatitis, local tissue necrosis	Administer through running intravenous infusion to avoid extravasation
Doxorubicin	Ovarian carcinoma, recurrent endometrial carcinoma, sarcoma	Bone marrow depression, nausea and vomiting, cardiomyopathy, cardiac arrhythmias, alopecia, local tissue necrosis	Administer through running intravenous infusion; do not exceed total dose of 550 mg/m^2 to avoid cardiac toxicity; avoid if significant heart disease is present
Liposomal doxorubicin	Ovarian cancer	Hand-foot syndrome; less cardiotoxic than doxorubicin	Intravenous infusion
Bleomycin	Germ cell tumors, squamous carcinomas	Pneumonitis and pulmonary fibrosis, alopecia, stomatitis, cutaneous reactions	Do not exceed total dose of 400 U; monitor pulmonary function with carbon monoxide diffusion capacity
PLANT ALKALOIDS			
Vinblastine	Germ cell tumors, sarcomas	Bone marrow depression, nausea and vomiting, stomatitis, diarrhea, local tissue necrosis	Administer through running intravenous infusion
Vincristine	Germ cell tumors, sarcomas	Neurotoxicity, constipation, alopecia, local tissue necrosis; bone marrow depression less marked	Administer through running intravenous infusion; prophylactic cathartics may be helpful
Etoposide	Germ cell tumors	Bone marrow depression; nausea and vomiting	Administer slowly intravenously
Paclitaxel	Ovarian carcinoma, breast carcinoma	Myelosuppression, alopecia, allergic reactions, cardiac arrhythmias	Intravenously as a 3- to 24-hr infusion
Docetaxel	Ovarian and breast cancer	Myelosuppression, alopecia, dermatologic reactions	Intravenous infusion, intravenous dexamethasone to reduce fluid retention
OTHER DRUGS			
Cisplatin	Ovarian carcinoma, germ cell tumors, squamous carcinomas	Renal toxicity, ototoxicity, neurotoxicity, severe nausea and vomiting, bone marrow depression less marked, hypokalemia, hypomagnesemia	Administer intravenous fluids to maintain urinary output of 100 mL/hr during infusion; discontinue if creatinine clearance of <35 mL/hr

Continued

TABLE 37-1

INDICATIONS, SIDE EFFECTS, AND PRECAUTIONS FOR COMMONLY USED CHEMOTHERAPEUTIC AGENTS—CONT'D

Drug	Main Indications	Side Effects	Precautions
OTHER DRUGS—CONT'D			
Carboplatin	Ovarian carcinoma, germ cell tumors	Bone marrow depression, less gastrointestinal toxicity, less renal toxicity, less neurotoxicity	Suitable for outpatient therapy because no need for high urinary output
Hexamethylmelamine	Ovarian carcinoma	Bone marrow depression, nausea and vomiting, neurotoxicity, depression	Given orally
Topotecan	Ovarian cancer	Bone marrow depression	Intravenously for 5 days every 3 weeks

Antibiotics

Antibiotics are naturally occurring antitumor agents elaborated by certain species of *Streptomyces*. They have no single, clearly defined mechanism of action, but many agents in this group intercalate between strands of the DNA double helix, thereby inhibiting both DNA and RNA synthesis and causing oxygen-dependent strand breaks.

Plant Alkaloids

The most common plant alkaloids are the **vinca alkaloids,** which are derived from the periwinkle plant. These include vincristine and vinblastine. They are spindle toxins that interfere with cellular microtubules and cause metaphase arrest.

Other plant alkaloids include the **epipodophyllotoxins** such as etoposide (VP16), which are extracts from the mandrake plant, and **paclitaxel** (Taxol), an extract from the bark of the Pacific yew tree. **Docetaxel (Taxotere)** is the first semisynthetic analogue of paclitaxel. Etoposide appears to act by causing single-strand DNA breaks. Paclitaxel binds preferentially to microtubules, which results in their polymerization and stabilization.

Other Drugs

Cisplatin, one of the more important drugs in gynecologic oncology, causes inhibition of DNA synthesis by forming interstrand and intrastrand linkages. Carboplatin is an analogue of cisplatin with a similar mechanism of action and efficacy, but with less gastrointestinal and renal toxicity.

Radiation Therapy

Radiation may be defined as the propagation of energy through space or matter.

TYPES OF RADIATION

There are two main types of radiation: electromagnetic and particulate.

Electromagnetic Radiation

Examples of electromagnetic radiation include the following:
- Visible light
- Infrared light
- Ultraviolet light
- X-rays (photons)
- Gamma rays (photons)

X-rays and gamma rays are identical electromagnetic radiations, differing only in their mode of production. X-rays are produced by bombardment of an anode by a high-speed electron beam; gamma rays result from the decay of radioactive isotopes, such as cobalt-60 (^{60}Co).

X-rays and gamma rays (photons) are differentiated from electromagnetic radiation of longer wavelength by their greater energy, which allows them to penetrate tissues and cause ionization.

Particulate Radiation

Particulate radiation consists of moving particles of matter. Their energy consists of the kinetic energy of the moving particles.

$$\text{Energy} = 0.5\,\text{mass} \times \text{velocity}^2$$

The particles vary greatly in size and include the following:
- Neutrons (no charge)
- Protons (positive charge)
- Electrons (negative charge)

The most commonly used particles are electrons. They may be derived from a linear accelerator, the beam of electrons being directed into the patient without first striking a metal target and producing x-rays. Alternatively, high-energy electrons (called β particles) may be derived from the radiodecay of an unstable isotope, such as phosphorus-32 (^{32}P). Particulate radiation penetrates tissues less than photons but also produces ionization.

UNIT OF RADIATION MEASUREMENT

The Gray (Gy) is equivalent to an absorbed energy of 1 joule per kilogram of absorbing material.

INVERSE SQUARE LAW

The intensity of electromagnetic radiation is inversely proportional to the square of the distance from the source. Thus, the dose of radiation 2 cm from a point source will be 25% of the dose at 1 cm.

BIOLOGIC CONSIDERATIONS

Ionization of Molecules

Radiation damage is caused by the ionization of molecules in the cell, with the production of free radicals. Because about 80% of a mammalian cell is water, most of the cellular radiation damage is mediated by ionization of water and the production of the free radicals H (hydrogen) and OH (hydroxide). **Free radicals may cause irreversible damage to DNA,** making it impossible for the cell to continue replication. Minor or sublethal damage to DNA, which the cell is capable of repairing, may also occur. RNA, protein, and other molecules in the cell are also damaged, but these molecules can be more readily repaired or replaced.

Oxygen Effect

In the absence of oxygen, cells show a twofold to threefold increase in their capacity to survive radiation exposure. This means that **hypoxic cells are less radiosensitive than are fully oxygenated cells.** The enhancement of the lethal effects of radiation by oxygen is presumed to occur because the oxygen will combine with the free radicals split from cell targets by the radiation. This prevents the recombination of the free radicals with the targets, which would restore the integrity of the targets.

The effect of oxygen has important clinical implications. First, **anemic patients should undergo transfusion before radiation therapy.** Second, **bulky tumors are usually poorly vascularized and, therefore, are often hypoxic,** particularly in the center. Such areas are likely to be relatively resistant to radiation so that viable tumor cells may remain despite marked shrinkage of the tumor.

Pharmacologic Modification of the Effects of Radiation

A variety of chemical compounds are capable of enhancing the lethal effects of radiation. A series of randomized clinical trials has demonstrated a significant survival advantage, particularly in terms of local disease control, when cisplatin-containing chemotherapy is given concurrently with radiation for locoregionally advanced cervical cancer. Some of the regimens tested have included 5-fluorouracil in combination with cisplatin. This is called *chemoradiation.*

Time-Dose Fractionation of Radiation

Successful radiation therapy requires a delicate balance between dosage to the tumor and that to the surrounding normal tissues. A dose of radiation that is too high sterilizes the tumor but results in an unacceptably high complication rate because of the destruction of normal tissues.

Most normal tissues, such as gastrointestinal mucosa and bone marrow, have a remarkable capacity to recover from radiation damage by the division of stem cells as well as by repair of sublethal radiation damage. Tumors, in general, have less ability to repair and repopulate. This difference can be exploited by administering the radiation in multiple fractions, thereby allowing some recovery, particularly of normal cells, between fractions.

If the interval between each fraction increases, the total dose must increase to produce the same biologic effect because of the amount of recovery that will occur in the interval. **Cells that survive the acute effects of radiation usually repair sublethal damage within 24 hours;** therefore, conventionally fractioned radiation is usually given in daily increments.

When treating the pelvis with external radiation, each fraction is usually 180 to 200 cGy. In treating the whole abdomen, fractions are decreased to 100 to 120 cGy because the tolerance of normal tissues decreases as the volume irradiated increases. The major factors influencing the outcome of radiation therapy are summarized in Box 37-1.

MODALITIES OF RADIATION THERAPY

The modalities used to deliver radiation therapy are listed in Box 37-2. In general, there are two radiation techniques: teletherapy and brachytherapy. **In teletherapy, a device quite removed from the patient is used, as with external-beam techniques.** Figure 37-2 is a linear accelerator used to deliver external-beam pelvic radiation. In brachytherapy, the radiation source is placed either within or close to the target tissue, as with intracavitary and interstitial techniques. In contrast to external-beam therapy, intracavitary and interstitial techniques allow a high dose of radiation to be delivered to the tumor, whereas dosages to

BOX 37-1 *Major Factors Influencing the Outcome of Radiation Therapy*

Normal tissue tolerance
Malignant cell type
Total volume irradiated
Total dose delivered
Total duration of therapy
Number of fractions
Type of equipment used
Tissue oxygen concentration

External Beams

Kilovoltage ("orthovoltage") (125-400 kV)
Cobalt-60 machine (1.25 MeV)
Linear accelerator (4-35 MeV)
Betatrons (20-42 MeV)
Particle accelerators (e.g., electrons, protons, neutrons)

Intracavitary (Cesium or Iridium)

Afterloading applicators
Low dose rate (^{137}Cs)
High dose rate (^{192}Ir)
Intraperitoneal (e.g., ^{32}P)

Interstitial

Permanent
Seeds (e.g., ^{198}Au, ^{125}I)
Removable
Ribbons (e.g., ^{192}Ir)
Needles (e.g., ^{226}Ra, ^{137}Cs)

BOX 37-3 *Advantages of Megavoltage Therapy*

Skin sparing
Greater dose at deeper depth in tissues
Shorter treatment times
No differential bone absorption (therefore no bone necrosis)
Can treat larger fields easily (e.g., whole abdomen)

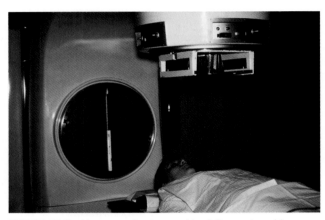

FIGURE 37-2   Linear accelerator used to deliver external-beam pelvic radiation.

surrounding normal tissues are considerably lower and are determined by the inverse square law.

Teletherapy

EXTERNAL-BEAM THERAPY. As the energy of the electromagnetic radiation increases, the penetration of the tissues increases, resulting in a relative sparing of the skin and an increased dosage to deeper tissues. At megavoltage energies (1 million electron volts or greater), there is no differential absorption of energy by bone.

Orthovoltage machines are no longer used except to treat skin cancers. Cobalt machines, developed in the early 1950s, have also been largely replaced by linear accelerators, which have a higher range of energies. The advantages of megavoltage therapy over the earlier orthovoltage machines are listed in Box 37-3.

External radiation allows a uniform dose to be delivered to a given field. The tolerance of the normal

tissues (e.g., bowel, bladder, liver, kidneys) limits the total dosage that can be delivered. External radiation is usually used to shrink a large tumor mass before brachytherapy. When used alone, it is generally useful only when there is small residual macroscopic or microscopic disease following surgery. With highly radiosensitive tumors (e.g., dysgerminoma), external radiation alone may sterilize even bulky disease.

INTENSITY-MODULATED RADIATION THERAPY. Intensity modulated radiation therapy delivers radiation from many small beams with nonuniform dose intensities, but the collective set of beams produces a more homogenous dose to the target volume. The multiple beams of variable intensity are achieved by the use of a multileaf collimator. **The end result is a high dose delivered to the target volume and acceptably low dose to the surrounding normal tissues.**

Brachytherapy

INTRACAVITARY RADIATION. Intracavitary therapy is used particularly in the treatment of cervical and vaginal cancer. **All applicators now in use should be *afterloaded*,** which means that they are placed in the patient and their position checked by radiography before the radioactive substance is loaded into the applicator. Traditionally, brachytherapy has been given at a low dose rate using radioactive substances such as cesium-137 (^{137}Cs). Applicators for the management of cervical cancer are placed under general anesthesia. For low–dose-rate therapy, the applicators are left in situ for 48 to 72 hours. Remote afterloading devices, such as the Selectron, allow the radioactive sources to be removed from the applicators when medical or nursing personnel enter the room, thereby significantly limiting staff exposure to radiation. **More recently, high–dose-rate brachytherapy has been given, using radioactive sources such as iridium** (^{192}Ir) (Figures 37-3 and 37-4). Treatment is given as an outpatient, which is much more acceptable for patients.

Radioactive colloids, such as chromic phosphate (^{32}P), may be instilled directly into the peritoneal cavity to treat minimal residual disease, particularly in patients with ovarian cancer. To be effective, these agents must achieve a uniform distribution throughout the cavity, which is difficult to achieve, so such agents are rarely used at present. ^{32}P is a pure β (electron) emitter.

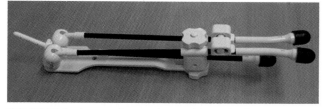

FIGURE 37-3   Intrauterine tandem and vaginal colpostats used for high–dose-rate intracavitary radiation in cervical cancer.

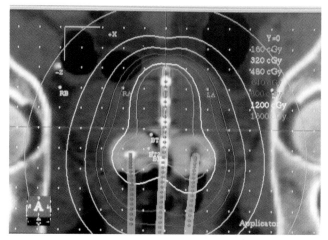

FIGURE 37-4   Posteroanterior view of brachytherapy applicator in situ, loaded with ^{192}Ir, for the treatment of cervical cancer. Note the isodose contours showing how the dose of radiation decreases with distance from the applicator.

INTERSTITIAL RADIATION. Interstitial therapy (in which the radioactive source is placed directly in the tumor) may be delivered by removable or permanent implants. **Permanent implants are used for inaccessible tumors. They use radioisotopes such as radon-222 (^{222}Rn) or iodine-125 (^{125}I) seeds** and are usually placed in an unresectable tumor nodule at the time of laparotomy.

Removable implants are placed in tumors that are accessible (e.g., cervical or vaginal tumors). Interstitial therapy has the theoretical advantage of better dose distribution within the tumor but the disadvantage that it is easier to overdose normal tissues, thereby increasing the complication rate. As with intracavitary devices, afterloading devices are now available for interstitial therapy. **The radioisotope of choice for afterloading interstitial implants is iridium-192 (^{192}Ir).**

COMPLICATIONS ASSOCIATED WITH RADIATION

The success of radiation therapy depends on an exploitable gradient of susceptibility to injury in favor of normal tissue. Unfortunately, most malignant tumors are only marginally more sensitive to radiation than are normal tissues, so the total dose that can be delivered, and therefore the radiocurability, is limited by the associated complications.

Acute Complications

Acute reactions to radiation occur in the first 3 to 4 months and include the following pathologic changes: rapid cessation of mitotic activity, cellular swelling, tissue edema, and tissue necrosis.

In the management of gynecologic tumors, these acute reactions may produce the following effects: **acute cystitis,** manifested by hematuria, urgency, and frequency; **proctosigmoiditis,** manifested by tenesmus, diarrhea, and passage of blood and mucus in the stool; **enteritis,** manifested by nausea, vomiting, diarrhea, and colicky abdominal pain; and **bone marrow suppression,** which is uncommon with pelvic radiation, but common with whole-abdominal or extended-field (pelvic and para-aortic) radiation, particularly if the patient has had previous cytotoxic chemotherapy.

Chronic Complications

Chronic complications occur 6 months or more after completion of radiation and are characterized pathologically by the following changes: internal thickening and obliteration of small blood vessels (endarteritis), fibrosis, and permanent reduction in the epithelial and parenchymal cell populations.

Significant chronic complications occur in 5% to 10% of patients receiving 50 cGy or more of radiation, and they may be slowly progressive over several years.

Common chronic complications of radiation follow.

Radiation Enteropathy

Previous surgery, with resultant loops of small bowel adherent in the pelvis, predisposes the patient to radiation enteritis, particularly when intracavitary or interstitial radiation is used in addition to teletherapy.

Large bowel injuries, which are best diagnosed by sigmoidoscopy or colonoscopy, may include **proctosigmoiditis,** manifested by pelvic pain, tenesmus, diarrhea, and rectal bleeding; **ulceration,** manifested by rectal bleeding and tenesmus; **rectal or sigmoid stenosis,** manifested by progressive large bowel obstruction; and **rectovaginal fistula,** manifested by passage of stool through the vagina. Figure 37-5 shows a radiation-induced stricture of the sigmoid colon.

Small bowel injuries usually present with cramping abdominal pain and vomiting, or with alternating diarrhea and constipation.

Vaginal Vault Necrosis

This is associated with severe pain and tenderness of the vaginal vault and a profuse vaginal discharge.

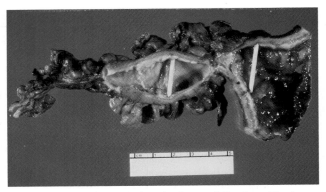

FIGURE 37-5   Radiation-induced stricture of the sigmoid colon. Note the tight fibrotic constriction, necessitating partial sigmoid colectomy for large bowel obstruction.

Urologic Injuries

The following are included in this category: **hemorrhagic cystitis,** which may necessitate frequent blood transfusions, and occasionally, urinary diversion; **ureteric stenosis,** which is manifested by progressive hydronephrosis; **vesicovaginal fistula,** manifested by the constant leakage of urine and demonstrable by cystoscopy; and **ureterovaginal fistula,** which is also manifested by constant leakage of urine and is demonstrable with an intravenous pyelogram.

Hormonal Therapy

The estrogen receptor (ER) status of primary and metastatic breast cancer has been shown to be of therapeutic and prognostic significance. The ER and progesterone receptor (PR) status of endometrial cancer also have prognostic and therapeutic significance.

MECHANISM OF ACTION OF HORMONAL RECEPTORS

Most steroid hormones influence their target tissues by the following series of steps: passive diffusion of the hormone through the cell membrane, specific binding in the cytoplasm with the hormone receptor, translocation of the receptor-hormone complex to the nucleus, binding of the receptor-hormone complex to an "acceptor" site on the chromatin, and transcription of DNA in a manner characteristic of the specific hormone–target cell interaction, eventually resulting in either an increase or a decrease in specific protein synthesis.

Tamoxifen binds with the ER and is translocated to the nucleus, where it binds to chromatin. It does not influence gene transcription, so functionally, tamoxifen acts as an antiestrogen.

Estrogen exposure increases the production of both ER and PR, whereas progesterone inhibits production of both ER and PR.

Aromatase inhibitors work by blocking aromatase, the enzyme that is responsible for the final step of estrogen synthesis. They prevent the production of estrogen, the substrate of the ER, in postmenopausal women.

Luteinizing hormone–releasing hormone agonists act by pituitary desensitization and receptor downregulation, suppressing gonadotropin release. They are as effective as surgical oophorectomy in premenopausal women with ER-positive advanced breast cancer.

CLINICAL APPLICATIONS

Because tumor growth in patients whose tumors contain ER and PR is likely to be stimulated by estrogen exposure, tumor regression should occur if endogenous estrogen production is abolished or if the patient is exposed to a progestin or antiestrogen. **In breast cancer, patients whose tumors contain ER and PR have an 80% response rate to hormonal manipulation,** whereas fewer than 10% of receptor-poor tumors respond.

An objective response to progestin therapy occurs in about one third of patients with recurrent or metastatic endometrial carcinoma. Progestin therapy is more likely to be effective in well-differentiated endometrial adenocarcinomas than in more poorly differentiated tumors because well-differentiated tumors are the ones that are most likely to contain ER and PR.

ER and PR have been demonstrated in some ovarian adenocarcinomas, particularly endometrioid carcinomas. **Tamoxifen is effective in up to 30% of women with recurrent ovarian cancer,** and early data suggest that aromatase inhibitors are also active agents.

Pain Management

More than 70% of patients with cancer develop significant pain at some point in their disease. Proper pain management requires an understanding of pain physiology, pain mechanisms, and the pharmacology of analgesics.

Pain in gynecologic cancer may be the result of soft tissue infiltration, bone involvement, neural involvement, muscle spasm (e.g., psoas spasm), infection within or near tumor masses, or bowel colic.

Therapeutic approaches vary according to the pain mechanism involved. Consideration must be given to the specific therapeutic measure that may be appropriate in the individual case, such as radiation therapy, chemotherapy, antibiotics, regional nerve block, or surgery.

Peripherally acting drugs such as acetaminophen (paracetamol) should rarely be omitted from analgesic regimes, and rectal suppositories are useful if oral intake is not appropriate. When pain is caused by bone metastases, nonsteroidal antiinflammatory drugs or bisphosphonates are helpful. Muscle spasm requires muscle relaxants such as diazepam, whereas bowel colic requires anticholinergics such as busulfan.

Opioid use will be necessary for severe pain, although nerve pain and muscle spasm are not well relieved by opioids. A variety of opioids are available, and in general, a low-potency opioid such as codeine or a high-potency opioid such as morphine is combined with a peripherally acting drug such as acetaminophen or aspirin.

Immediate-release morphine, which is best given orally or subcutaneously, should be given at regular 4-hour intervals. **Controlled-release morphine tablets are a significant advance in convenience of administration because they need to be given only every 12 to 24 hours,** once the total 24-hour requirement has been determined from the use of an immediate-release preparation. Constipation is a real problem with opioids, and prophylactic laxatives should be prescribed.

Alternative opioids (with equivalency to morphine 5 mg) include oxycodone (5 mg), hydromorphone (1 mg), pentazocine (45 mg), and meperidine (75 mg).

When pain is neurogenic in origin, an opioid and a peripherally acting drug should usually be supplemented by a tricyclic antidepressant, an anticonvulsant, or a corticosteroid.

◼ End-of-Life Issues

When it becomes clear that the patient is dying, the goals are to control symptoms, maintain dignity, and allow time and privacy for communication with loved ones.

Medications should usually be given subcutaneously or rectally, any unnecessary tubes or equipment should be removed to facilitate contact with loved ones, and nursing care should particularly focus on pressure areas, mouth care, and "grooming." Sedation, for example, with sublingual lorazepam, 0.5 to 2.5 mg every 4 to 6 hours, may be helpful if the patient is agitated.

Important issues from a patient's perspective are receiving adequate pain and symptom management, avoiding inappropriate prolongation of dying, achieving a sense of control, relieving the burden on caregivers, and strengthening relationships with loved ones.

SUGGESTED READING

Eifel PJ: Radiation therapy. *In* Berek JS, Hacker NF (eds): Practical Gynecologic Oncology, 4th ed. Philadelphia, Lippincott Williams & Wilkins, 2005, p 119-162.

Hortobagyi GN, Theriault RL, Lipton A, et al: Long-term prevention of skeletal complications of metastatic breast cancer with pamidronate. J Clin Oncol 16:2038-2044, 1998.

Lickiss JN, Philip JAM: Palliative care and pain management. *In* Berek JS, Hacker NF (eds): Practical Gynecologic Oncology, 4th ed. Philadelphia, Lippincott Williams & Wilkins, 2005, pp 835-862.

Markman M: Chemotherapy. *In* Berek JS, Hacker NF (eds): Practical Gynecologic Oncology, 4th ed. Philadelphia, Lippincott Williams & Wilkins, 2005, pp 89-118.

Singer PA, Martin DK, Kelner M: Quality end-of-life care: Patient's perspectives. JAMA 281:163-168, 1999.

Chapter 38

Cervical Dysplasia and Cancer

NEVILLE F. HACKER

Cervical cancer kills about 250,000 women a year worldwide and is the most common cause of death from cancer in women. About 80% of new cases reported each year occur in developing countries. **In developed countries, regular screening with Papanicolaou (Pap) smears has markedly decreased the incidence of the disease**, and most cases now occur in women who have not had regular Pap smears. In the United States, cervical cancer now ranks only 13th among cancers in women, with 11,150 new cases expected in 2007, and 3,670 deaths.

Studies have identified persistent infection with a high-risk human papillomavirus (HPV) as the cause of virtually all cervical cancers. Recent randomized clinical trials of prophylactic HPV vaccines have demonstrated dramatic efficiency in preventing HPV 16 and 18 infections as well as precancerous cervical lesions. Although it will take several decades to demonstrate a decreased incidence of invasive cervical cancer, **with widespread use, HPV vaccination has the potential to markedly decrease the incidence of cervical cancer in future generations.**

Etiology and Epidemiology

There are 15 high-risk HPV types, and types 16 and 18 are responsible for 70% of cervical cancers. Types 6 and 11 have been associated with cervical condylomas and low-grade cervical intraepithelial neoplasia (CIN).

The adolescent cervix is believed to be more susceptible to carcinogenic stimuli because of the active process of squamous metaplasia, which occurs within the transformation zone during periods of endocrine change. This squamous metaplasia is normally a physiologic process, but under the influence of the HPV, cellular alterations occur that result in an atypical transformation zone. These atypical changes initiate CIN, which is the preinvasive phase of cervical cancer.

Cervical cancer and its precursors have been associated with several epidemiologic variables (Box 38-1). These risk factors basically increase the likelihood of exposure to a high-risk HPV type.

The disease is relatively rare before 20 years of age, and the mean age is about 47 years.

Primary Prevention

Two prophylactic vaccines are presently available. The **quadrivalent vaccine Gardasil**, which is manufactured by Merck (Whitehouse Station, NJ) and protects against HPV types 6, 11, 16, and 18, was approved by the U.S. Food and Drug Administration in June 2006 for females aged 9 to 26 years. The **bivalent vaccine Cervarix**, which is manufactured by GlaxoSmithKline (Philadelphia, Pa) and protects against HPV types 16 and 18, was approved by the Australian Therapeutic Goods Administration in April 2007 for use in females aged 9 to 45 years.

HPV vaccination is most effective if performed before the onset of sexual activity. Vaccination is still recommended after commencement of sexual activity, and even after prior abnormal cytology or CIN, but it is likely to be less effective after HPV exposure. Australia was the first country in the world to introduce HPV vaccination into the National Immunization Program. In 2007, vaccination with Gardasil was introduced for all schoolgirls aged 12 years.

Screening of Asymptomatic Women

The American College of Obstetricians and Gynecologists has recommended that all women undergo an annual physical examination, including a Pap smear,

BOX 38-1   *Risk Factors for Cervical Cancer*

- Young age at first coitus (<20 yr)
- Multiple sexual partners
- Sexual partner with multiple sexual partners
- Young age at first pregnancy
- High parity
- Lower socioeconomic status
- Smoking

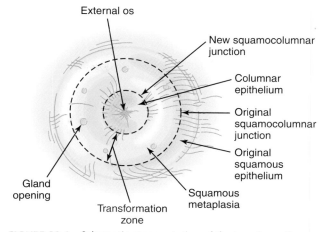

FIGURE 38-1   Schematic representation of the transformation zone.

within 3 years of sexual intercourse, or by age 21 years. Annual screening should occur until age 30 years. If there have been three consecutive negative tests, screening may occur every 2 or 3 years at the discretion of the treating physician. **Both the endocervical canal and the ectocervix should be sampled when taking the Pap smear.**

The false-negative rate for conventional Pap smears for high-grade intraepithelial lesions is generally reported to be about 20%, but it is higher for glandular lesions and for invasive cancers.

New technologies have been developed to decrease the false-negative rate. ThinPrep (Cytyc, Marlborough, Mass) and SurePath (BD Diagnostics–TriPath, Franklin Lakes, NJ) are automated liquid-based slide-preparation systems. With liquid-based cytology, the spatula or brush taking the smear is placed into a fixative solution, instead of smearing the cells directly onto a glass slide. Blood, mucus, and inflammatory cells are eliminated, and a monolayer smear is then automatically prepared by a machine. BD Focal Point (BD Diagnostics–TriPath) and ThinPrep Imager (Cytyc) are computerized image processors that select the most abnormal cells on a slide. They increase the sensitivity of slide reading, while decreasing the time needed by the cytotechnician to read each slide, thereby improving the cost-effectiveness of screening.

The cost-effectiveness of HPV DNA testing as a primary screening test, either alone or in combination with cervical cytology, in women aged 30 years or older, is currently under investigation. HPV DNA testing is much more sensitive than cervical cytology, but less specific.

Women should have regular cervical screening even if they have received the HPV vaccine because the vaccine does not protect against all high-risk HPV viral types.

Cervical Topography

During early embryonic development, the cervix and upper vagina are covered with columnar epithelium. During intrauterine development, the columnar epithelium of the vagina is progressively replaced by squamous epithelium. At birth, the vagina is usually covered with squamous epithelium, and the columnar

epithelium is limited to the endocervix and the central portion of the ectocervix. **In about 4% of normal female infants and about 30% of those exposed to diethylstilbestrol in utero, the columnar epithelium extends onto the vaginal fornices.** Macroscopically, the columnar epithelium has a red appearance because it is only a single cell layer thick, allowing blood vessels in the underlying stroma to show through it.

The embryologic squamous and columnar epithelia are designated the original and native squamous and columnar epithelia, respectively. The junction between them on the ectocervix is called the *original squamocolumnar junction.*

Throughout life, but particularly during adolescence and a woman's first pregnancy, metaplastic squamous epithelium covers the columnar epithelium so that a new squamocolumnar junction is formed more proximally. This junction moves progressively closer to the external os and then up the endocervical canal. **The transformation zone is the area of metaplastic squamous epithelium located between the original squamocolumnar junction and the new squamocolumnar junction** (Figure 38-1).

Classification of an Abnormal Papanicolaou Smear

In 1988, a consensus meeting was convened by the Division of Cancer Control of the National Cancer Institute to review existing terminology and to recommend effective methods of cytologic reporting. As a result of this meeting, **the Bethesda system** was devised and requires **(1) a statement regarding the adequacy of the specimen** for diagnosis, **(2) a diagnostic categorization** (normal or other), and **(3) a descriptive diagnosis.** A revised Bethesda system was developed in 2001 and is shown in Box 38-2.

BOX 38-2 *Bethesda Classification of Cytologic Abnormalities (2001, Abridged)*

Specimen Adequacy

Satisfactory for evaluation (note presence/absence of endocervical/transformation zone component)
Unsatisfactory for evaluation (specify reason)
Specimen rejected/not processed (specify reason)
Specimen processed and examined, but unsatisfactory for evaluation of epithelial abnormality (specify reason)

General Categorization (Optional)

Negative for intraepithelial lesion or malignancy
Epithelial cell abnormality
Other

Interpretation/Result

Negative for Intraepithelial Lesion or Malignancy

Organisms (e.g., *Trichomonas vaginalis*)
Reactive cellular changes associated with inflammation (includes typical repair), radiation, intrauterine contraceptive device
Atrophy

Epithelial Cell Abnormalities

Squamous Cell

Atypical squamous cells of undetermined significance (ASCUS) cannot exclude high-grade squamous intraepithelial lesion (HSIL) (ASC-H)
Low-grade squamous intraepithelial lesion (LSIL) encompassing: human papillomavirus/mild dysplasia/cervical intraepithelial neoplasia (CIN I)
HSIL encompassing: moderate and severe dysplasia, carcinoma in situ; CIN II and CIN III
Squamous cell carcinoma

Glandular Cell

Atypical glandular cells (AGC) (specify endocervical, endometrial, or not otherwise specified)
Atypical glandular cells, favor neoplastic (specify endocervical or not otherwise specified)
Endocervical adenocarcinoma in situ (AIS)
Adenocarcinoma

Other

For example, endometrial cells in a woman ≥40 years of age

CERVICAL INTRAEPITHELIAL NEOPLASIA

CIN represents a spectrum of disease, ranging from CIN I (mild dysplasia) to CIN III (severe dysplasia and carcinoma in situ). At least 35% of patients with CIN III develop invasive cancer within 10 years, whereas lower grades of CIN often spontaneously regress. With CIN, there is abnormal epithelial proliferation and maturation above the basement membrane. Involvement of the inner one third of the epithelium represents CIN I, involvement of the inner one half to two thirds represents CIN II, and full-thickness involvement represents CIN III (Figure 38-2). The disease is asymptomatic.

COLPOSCOPY

The colposcope is a stereoscopic binocular microscope of low magnification, usually 10× to 40×. Illumination is centered, and the focal length is between 12 and 15 cm.

To perform a colposcopic examination, an appropriately sized speculum is inserted to expose the cervix, which is cleansed with a cotton pledget soaked in 3% acetic acid to remove adherent mucus and cellular debris. A green filter can be employed to accentuate the vascular changes that frequently accompany pathologic alterations of the cervix.

At colposcopy, the original or native squamous epithelium appears gray and homogeneous. The columnar epithelium appears red and grape-like. **The transformation zone can be identified by the presence of gland openings that are not covered by the squamous metaplasia and by the paler color of the metaplastic epithelium compared with the original squamous epithelium. Nabothian follicles may also be seen in the transformation zone. Normal blood vessels branch like a tree.**

■ Evaluation of a Patient with an Abnormal Papanicolaou Smear

An algorithm for the evaluation of patients with abnormal Pap smears is presented in Figure 38-3.

Any patient with a grossly abnormal cervix should have a punch biopsy performed, regardless of the results of the Pap smear.

Patients with atypical squamous cells of undetermined significance (ASCUS) found on their smear may have a repeat test in 6 months. Alternatively, HPV testing, such as with the Hybrid Capture assay (Digene Diagnostics, Silver Spring, Md) may be used to triage such patients. About 6% to 10% of patients with an ASCUS smear will have high-grade CIN on colposcopy, and 90% of these can be detected by HPV testing for high-risk viral types.

The colposcopic hallmark of cervical intraepithelial neoplasia is an area of sharply delineated acetowhite epithelium, that is, epithelium that appears white after the application of acetic acid. It is thought that the acetic acid dehydrates the cells and that there is increased light reflex from areas of increased nuclear density. **Within the acetowhite areas, there may or may not be abnormal vascular patterns.**

There are two basic changes in the vascular architecture in patients with CIN: punctation and mosaicism. Punctation is caused by single-looped capillaries lying within the subepithelial papillae, seen end-on as a "dot" as they course toward the surface of the epithelium. Mosaicism is caused by a fine network of

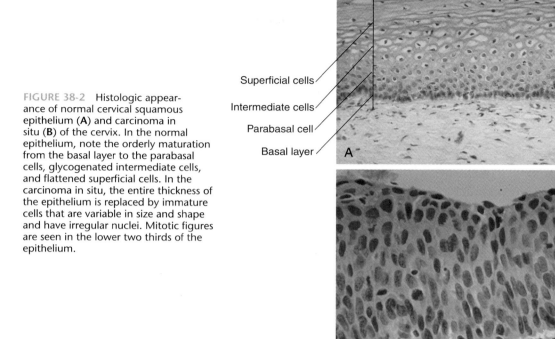

FIGURE 38-2   Histologic appearance of normal cervical squamous epithelium (**A**) and carcinoma in situ (**B**) of the cervix. In the normal epithelium, note the orderly maturation from the basal layer to the parabasal cells, glycogenated intermediate cells, and flattened superficial cells. In the carcinoma in situ, the entire thickness of the epithelium is replaced by immature cells that are variable in size and shape and have irregular nuclei. Mitotic figures are seen in the lower two thirds of the epithelium.

Superficial cells
Intermediate cells
Parabasal cell
Basal layer

capillaries disposed parallel to the surface in a mosaic pattern. Punctate and mosaic patterns may be seen together within the same area of the cervix. The more dilated and irregular the punctate and mosaic capillaries and the greater the intercapillary distance, the more atypical is the tissue on histologic examination. Similarly, the whiter the lesion, the more severe the dysplasia.

With microinvasive carcinoma, extremely irregular punctate and mosaic patterns are found, as are small atypical vessels. **The irregularity in size, shape, and arrangement of the terminal vessels becomes even more striking in frankly invasive carcinoma, with exaggerated distortions of the vascular architecture producing comma-shaped, corkscrew-shaped, and dilated, blind-ended vessels.**

BIOPSY AND ENDOCERVICAL CURETTAGE

If the colposcopic examination is satisfactory, which implies that the entire transformation zone has been visualized, a punch biopsy is taken from the worst area or areas, together with endocervical curettage. The endocervical curettage is not performed in patients who are pregnant.

A diagnostic cone biopsy of the cervix is indicated in the following circumstances:
1. **Pap smear shows a high-grade lesion, and the colposcopic examination is unsatisfactory.**
2. **Endocervical curettage shows a high-grade lesion.**
3. **Pap smear shows a high-grade lesion that is not confirmed on punch biopsy.**
4. **Pap smear shows adenocarcinoma in situ.**
5. **Microinvasion is present on the punch biopsy.**

▦ Treatment of Intraepithelial Neoplasia

It is reasonable to observe biopsy-proven CIN I without active treatment because many cases spontaneously regress. Active treatment is indicated for CIN II and III.

Superficial ablative techniques, such as large loop excision of the transformation zone (LLETZ), cryosurgery, and carbon dioxide laser, are appropriate if the entire transformation zone is visible.

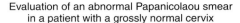

Evaluation of an abnormal Papanicolaou smear
in a patient with a grossly normal cervix

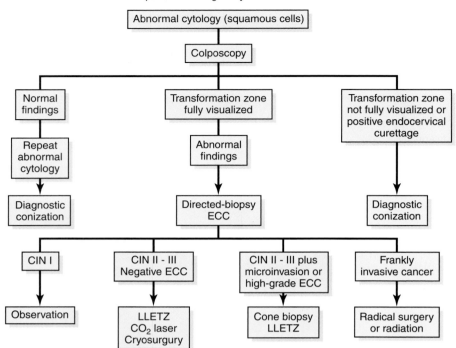

FIGURE 38-3 Algorithm for evaluation of patients with an abnormal Papanicolaou smear and a grossly normal-appearing cervix. CIN, cervical intraepithelial neoplasia; ECC, endocervical curettage; LLETZ, large loop excision of the transformation zone.

LARGE LOOP EXCISION OF THE TRANSFORMATION ZONE

LLETZ has gained popularity because **the equipment is relatively inexpensive, it can be performed on an outpatient basis under local anesthesia, and tissue is obtained for histologic evaluation.** Hence, occult invasive lesions should be more readily diagnosed. In unskilled hands, diathermy artifact may make histologic interpretation impossible.

LASER

Destruction of the transformation zone by carbon dioxide laser (*l*ight *a*mplification by *s*timulated *e*mission of *r*adiation) ablation can be performed as an outpatient procedure, under local anesthesia. Bleeding may sometimes occur, but scarring is minimal, and large lesions may be destroyed with low failure rates (5% to 10%). **The equipment is expensive, so laser has lost favor in most centers.**

CRYOSURGERY

The cryosurgery technique is a relatively painless outpatient procedure that can be performed without anesthesia. There is no bleeding, and the equipment is inexpensive. However, **there is a high failure rate for large lesions and for lesions extending down glandular crypts.** It is mainly useful for CIN I or II involving 1 or 2 quadrants. The major side effect is a rather copious vaginal discharge that persists for several weeks.

CERVICAL CONIZATION

Cervical conization is mainly a diagnostic technique, but it may be used for treatment. Provided that the margins of resection are clear, cure rates are as high as those with hysterectomy for intraepithelial lesions. **Bleeding, infection, cervical stenosis, and cervical incompetence are the major complications. Laser conization decreases the risk for cervical stenosis compared with cold-knife conization.**

HYSTERECTOMY

Hysterectomy is rarely necessary for the treatment of CIN. It may be applicable when there is concomitant uterine or adnexal disease.

Persistence and recurrence rates combined are about 2% to 3% after hysterectomy. This number should be significantly reduced by using colposcopy and Schiller's staining (Lugol's iodine) preoperatively to exclude intraepithelial neoplasia in the upper vagina.

■ *Invasive Cancer*

SYMPTOMS

Invasive cancer usually presents with postcoital, intermenstrual, or postmenopausal vaginal bleeding. In patients who are not sexually active, bleeding from cervical cancer usually does not occur until the disease is quite advanced (unlike patients with endometrial cancer, who almost always bleed early). **Persistent vaginal discharge, pelvic pain, leg swelling, and urinary frequency are usually seen with advanced disease.** In developing countries, it is not uncommon for patients to present with loss of urine or stool from the vagina, because of fistula formation.

PHYSICAL FINDINGS

Patients with cervical cancer usually have a normal general physical examination. Weight loss occurs late in the disease. With advanced disease, there may be enlarged inguinal or supraclavicular lymph nodes, edema of the legs, or hepatomegaly, but these are not commonly seen.

On pelvic examination, the cervix may be ulcerative or exophytic (Figure 38-4). It usually bleeds on palpation, and there is often an associated serous, purulent, or bloody discharge. The lesion may involve the adjacent vagina and extend toward the introitus.

A rectovaginal examination is essential to determine the extent of disease. **The diameter of the primary cancer and spread to the parametria are much more easily detected with a finger in the rectum, as is extension into the uterosacral ligaments.**

PATHOLOGIC FEATURES

Most uterine cervical cancers are squamous in origin. Adenocarcinomas and adenosquamous carcinomas are increasing in incidence and account for about 20% to 25% of cases. Melanomas and sarcomas occur rarely.

PATTERNS OF SPREAD

Invasive cervical cancer spreads by direct invasion of cervical stroma, corpus, vagina, and parametrium; lymphatic spread to pelvic and then para-aortic lymph nodes (Figure 38-5); and hematogenous spread, particularly to the lungs, liver, and bone.

PREOPERATIVE INVESTIGATIONS

The official International Federation of Gynecology and Obstetrics (FIGO) staging for cervical cancer is a clinical staging method based on physical examination and noninvasive testing (Table 38-1). **Studies allowed include biopsies, cystoscopy, sigmoidoscopy, chest and skeletal radiographs, intravenous pyelography, and liver function tests.** Lung metastases are seen in about 5% of patients with advanced disease and almost never in early disease.

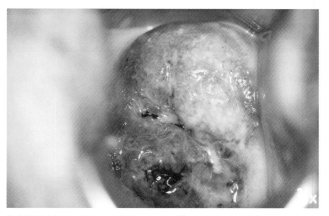

FIGURE 38-4   Invasive squamous cell carcinoma of the cervix. Note the irregular, ulcerated surface of the ectocervix. A biopsy of such a lesion is mandatory.

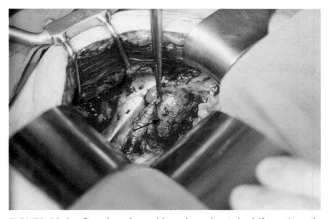

FIGURE 38-5   Grossly enlarged lymph node at the bifurcation of the common iliac artery in a patient with stage Ib2 carcinoma of the cervix. Large nodes such as this can cause ureteric obstruction.

Abdominal and pelvic computed tomography or magnetic resonance imaging (MRI) may be helpful in planning management, but the results do not influence the FIGO stage. MRI is particularly helpful in defining the extent of the primary lesion, including any extension into the parametrium, bladder, or rectum. Neither is particularly sensitive for detecting lymph node metastases, and **position-emission tomography is being increasingly used** for this purpose. **The incidence of para-aortic lymph node metastases is about 20% in stage II disease and 30% in stage III, and the status of the para-aortic nodes is the single most important prognostic factor.**

Laboratory studies may reveal abnormalities with advanced disease, the most common being anemia from bleeding, elevated blood urea nitrogen and creatinine levels if the ureters are obstructed, and abnormal liver function tests if there are liver metastases. **Ureteric obstruction occurs in about 30% of patients with**

TABLE 38-1

INTERNATIONAL FEDERATION OF GYNECOLOGY AND OBSTETRICS (FIGO) STAGING OF CERVICAL CARCINOMA

PREINVASIVE CARCINOMA

Stage 0	Carcinoma in situ, intraepithelial carcinoma (cases of stage 0 should not be included in any therapeutic statistics)

INVASIVE CARCINOMA

Stage I	The carcinoma is strictly confined to the cervix.
Stage Ia	Invasive cancer is identified only microscopically. All gross lesions even with superficial invasion are Ib cancers. Invasion is limited to a measured stromal invasion, with a maximal depth of 5 mm and a horizontal extension of not more than 7 mm.
Stage Ia1	Measured invasion of stroma not greater than 3 mm in depth and 7 mm in width
Stage Ia2	Measured invasion of stroma greater than 3 mm and not greater than 5 mm and width not greater than 7 mm
Stage Ib	Clinical lesions confined to the cervix or preclinical lesions greater than stage Ia
Stage Ib1	Clinical lesions not greater than 4 cm in size
Stage Ib2	Clinical lesions greater than 4 cm in size
Stage II	The carcinoma extends beyond the cervix but has not extended to the pelvic wall or to the lower third of the vagina.
Stage IIa	No obvious parametrial involvement
Stage IIb	Obvious parametrial involvement
Stage III	The carcinoma has extended to the pelvic wall. On rectal examination, there is no cancer-free space between the tumor and the pelvic wall. The tumor involves the lower third of the vagina. All cases with hydronephrosis or nonfunctioning kidney should be included, unless they are known to be due to another cause.
Stage IIIa	Tumor involves lower third of the vagina with no extension to the pelvic wall.
Stage IIIb	Extension onto the pelvic wall and/or hydronephrosis or nonfunctioning kidney
Stage IV	The carcinoma has extended beyond the true pelvis or has clinically involved the mucosa of the bladder or rectum. A bullous edema, as such, does not permit a case to be allotted to stage IV.
Stage IVa	Spread of the growth to adjacent organs
Stage IVb	Spread to distant organs

stage III disease and in 50% of patients with stage IV disease. Hypercalcemia may denote bone metastases.

TREATMENT

Stage Ia (Microinvasive Carcinoma)

A preoperative diagnosis of microinvasive carcinoma can be made only on the basis of a cone biopsy of the cervix, which allows multiple-step sections to be taken at 2-mm intervals. With a punch biopsy, the sampling of the cervix is too limited, and a more frankly invasive focus may be missed. The concept of microinvasive carcinoma has only been applied to squamous lesions in the past, but it is now accepted that it should also apply to glandular lesions, although an occasional adenocarcinoma will have a skip lesion higher in the endocervical canal.

When the depth of invasion on cone biopsy is 3 mm or less, the horizontal dimension is 7 mm or less (stage Ia1), and there is no lymphatic or vascular space involvement, an extrafascial abdominal or vaginal hysterectomy is appropriate treatment. Cervical conization alone may suffice if the patient desires to maintain her fertility, as long as the cone margins are free of disease and the endocervical curettings (taken after the conization) are negative. **For stage Ia2 disease, or if there is lymphatic or vascular space involvement, most gynecologic oncologists recommend modified radical hysterectomy and pelvic lymph node dissection.** If childbearing is desired, large-cone biopsy or radical trachelectomy combined with pelvic lymphadenectomy may be offered.

Stages Ib1 and Ib2

Stage Ib disease may be treated by either primary surgery (radical hysterectomy and bilateral pelvic lymphadenectomy) or primary chemoradiation therapy. The advantage of surgery is that the ovaries may be spared in younger women, surgical staging may be carried out, and chronic radiation complications may be avoided, particularly vaginal stenosis, radiation proctitis, and radiation cystitis. Primary surgery is regarded as the treatment of choice for stage Ib1 cervical cancer.

The results of treatment by either method are similar when both the surgeon and the radiotherapist are knowledgeable and skilled. Chemoradiation is often chosen for stage Ib2 lesions, but primary surgery followed by tailored external-beam therapy is a valid alternative approach. Patients with deep stromal penetration and extensive vascular space invasion but negative lymph nodes may receive a "small field" of pelvic radiation, whereas patients with positive common iliac or para-aortic nodes may receive extended-field radiation, often combined with cisplatin.

RADICAL HYSTERECTOMY. In this procedure, the uterus is removed along with adjacent portions of the vagina, cardinal ligaments, uterosacral ligaments, and bladder pillars.

The most common complication of radical hysterectomy is bladder dysfunction, which occurs as a result of interruption of the autonomic nerves traversing the cardinal and uterosacral ligaments. Normal bladder function is usually restored within 1 to 3 weeks, but 1% to 2% of patients have permanent dysfunction necessitating lifelong self-catheterization.

The most serious complication of radical hyster-ectomy is ureteric fistula or stricture, which occurs in 1% to 2% of cases. A less common but life-threat-ening complication is deep venous thrombosis, with or without pulmonary embolism. The incidence of ve-nous thromboembolism can be reduced with the use of external pneumatic calf compressors at the time of surgery, early ambulation, and prophylactic low-dose subcutaneous heparin or Clexane. Some degree of lymphedema occurs in 15% to 20% of patients having a pelvic lymphadenectomy.

RADICAL TRACHELECTOMY. For young women with early cancer (≤2 cm in diameter), radical vaginal or abdomi-nal trachelectomy and pelvic lymphadenectomy may allow fertility preservation, without significantly com-promising survival.

RADIATION THERAPY. For patients with stage Ib2 dis-ease, most centers use primary chemoradiation, using weekly cisplatin as the radiation sensitizer. Therapy usually begins with external radiation in an attempt to shrink the central tumor and improve the dosimetry of the subsequent intracavitary therapy.

External radiation may also be used postoperatively for patients with lymph node metastases or inadequate surgical margins. The addition of weekly cisplatin (40 mg/m^2, intravenously) during external-beam ther-apy has been shown to improve survival.

Stage IIa

In patients with minimal involvement of the vaginal fornix, radical surgery or chemoradiation therapy may be employed. With more extensive involvement of the upper vagina, chemoradiation therapy alone is the treatment of choice.

Stage IIb

Most patients with stage IIb lesions are treated with a combination of external-beam chemoradiation and intracavitary brachytherapy. If positive para-aortic or high common iliac lymph nodes are detected preop-eratively, extended-field radiation may be employed to treat all of the para-aortic lymph nodes up to the diaphragm.

Stages IIIa and IIIb

Patients with stage IIIa or IIIb disease are treated with chemoradiation therapy, usually external-beam followed by intracavitary brachytherapy. In patients with locally advanced disease, distortion of the cervix and vagina may make brachytherapy difficult to ap-ply. Therefore, a higher dose of external therapy, up to 7000 cGy, may be necessary. Alternatively, interstitial radiation may be given to get a better dose distribution than would be possible with intracavitary therapy.

Stage IVa

Pelvic chemoradiation therapy is used in most patients with stage IVa lesions. If radiation therapy results in only partial tumor regression, a "salvage" pelvic exen-teration may be performed. Primary pelvic exentera-tion is performed only rarely, usually when the patient presents with a rectovaginal or vesicovaginal fistula.

Stage IVb

Patients with stage IVb disease may receive some pelvic radiation therapy to palliate bleeding from the vagina, bladder, or rectum. Because distant metastases are present, however, chemotherapy is often employed but is only palliative.

Recurrent or Metastatic Disease

CHEMOTHERAPY. The effectiveness of chemotherapy is limited for metastatic cervical cancer.

Several drugs have been tested and found to be ac-tive in up to 35% of cases. Most responses are partial, and the patients usually progress within 12 months. The most active agents are cisplatin, bleomycin, mito-mycin C, methotrexate, and cyclophosphamide.

PELVIC EXENTERATION. Pelvic exenteration is gener-ally reserved for patients who have a central recur-rence following pelvic irradiation. Total exenteration involves removal of the pelvic viscera, including the uterus, tubes, vagina, ovaries, bladder, and rectum (Figure 38-6). Depending on the site and extent of the disease, the operation may be limited to an anterior exenteration, which spares the rectum, or a posterior exenteration, which spares the bladder.

Following the extirpative surgery, pelvic recon-struction is necessary. If the bladder is removed, the ureters must be implanted into a portion of the small or large bowel that has been isolated from the remainder of the gastrointestinal tract to form a conduit. A conti-nent conduit may be created, particularly in younger patients. When the disease is confined to the upper vagina and rectovaginal septum, the lower rectum and anal canal may be preserved and reanastomosed to the sigmoid colon. A temporary colostomy is often required to protect the reanastomosis because of the prior irradi-ation. Vaginal reconstruction can be performed using a split-thickness skin graft, bilateral gracilis myocuta-neous grafts, a rectus abdominis myocutaneous flap, or a segment of large intestine.

Relatively few patients with recurrent cancer of the cervix are suitable to undergo pelvic exenteration because of metastases outside the pelvis or fixation of the tumor to structures that cannot be removed, such as the pelvic side wall. If an extensive metastatic workup is negative for cancer, patients undergo explor-atory laparotomy with a view to pelvic exenteration. If the tumor is discovered to have spread to pelvic or

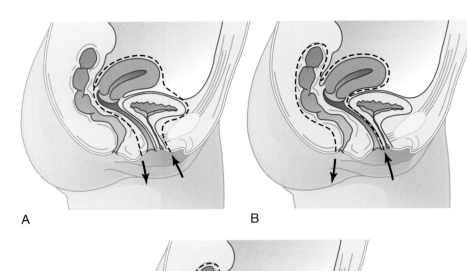

A

B

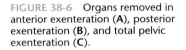

FIGURE 38-6 Organs removed in anterior exenteration (**A**), posterior exenteration (**B**), and total pelvic exenteration (**C**).

C

para-aortic lymph nodes or to intraabdominal viscera, the procedure is abandoned.

In selecting patients who may be suitable for pelvic exenteration, the triad of unilateral leg edema, sciatic pain, and ureteral obstruction is ominous and indicates unresectable disease in the pelvis.

Cervical Carcinoma in Pregnancy

Carcinoma of the cervix associated with pregnancy usually implies diagnosis during pregnancy or within 6 months postpartum. It is relatively uncommon; invasive carcinoma occurs in about 1 in 2200 pregnancies.

SYMPTOMS

The symptoms are similar to those in nonpregnant patients, with painless vaginal bleeding being the most common. During pregnancy, this symptom can readily be attributed to conditions such as threatened abortion or placenta previa, so there is often an unnecessary delay in diagnosis.

DIAGNOSIS

A prenatal Pap smear leads to the diagnosis in most cases. **Pregnancy tends to exaggerate the colposcopic features of CIN so that overdiagnosis is more likely than the reverse.** Endocervical curettage should not be performed during pregnancy because of the risk for rupturing the membranes. **Cone biopsy, if required, is best performed during the second trimester to avoid the possibility of induced abortion in the first trimester and severe hemorrhage and premature labor in the third trimester.** Unfortunately, about half of the patients are not diagnosed until the postpartum period. The later the diagnosis is made, the more likely the cancer is to be in an advanced stage.

MANAGEMENT

CIN III diagnosed during pregnancy should be managed conservatively, with the pregnancy allowed to proceed to term, vaginal delivery anticipated, and appropriate therapy carried out 6 to 8 weeks postpartum.

Microinvasive carcinoma of the cervix diagnosed by conization of the cervix during pregnancy may

also be managed conservatively, the pregnancy being allowed to continue to term. At term, either cesarean hysterectomy or vaginal delivery followed by postpartum extrafascial hysterectomy is appropriate, unless further childbearing is desired.

Frankly invasive cancer requires relatively urgent treatment. After 22 to 26 weeks, it is reasonable to continue the pregnancy until fetal viability (about 32 weeks) if the patient desires. The general principles of treatment are essentially the same as those in the nonpregnant patient. For early lesions, radical hysterectomy may be performed. Before 20 weeks' gestation, this is performed with the fetus in situ. After that time, hysterotomy through a high incision in the uterine fundus is performed to remove the fetus, followed by radical hysterectomy and bilateral pelvic lymphadenectomy.

For some patients with early disease and for all patients with advanced disease, the alternative to radical surgery is radiation therapy. For patients with disease diagnosed in the first trimester, external irradiation is initiated to shrink the tumor. Abortion usually occurs spontaneously during the course of external therapy; if it does not, uterine curettage should be performed before brachytherapy. After the first trimester, it is preferable to perform a hysterotomy through a high incision in the corpus before instituting radiotherapy.

If a decision is made to await fetal viability, it is important to be certain by ultrasonography that the fetus is apparently healthy and to obtain a mature lecithin-to-sphingomyelin ratio to ensure fetal lung maturity before delivery. Neoadjuvant chemotherapy using cisplatin and etoposide has been used to try to "contain" the disease. Because of the increased risk for hemorrhage and infection likely to be associated with delivery through a cervix containing gross cancer, classic cesarean delivery is the preferred method. For patients in whom inadvertent vaginal delivery has occurred, there is no evidence to indicate that the prognosis is altered.

▉ Prognosis for Cervical Cancer

Prognosis is related directly to clinical stage (Table 38-2). With more advanced stage of disease, the frequency of nodal metastasis escalates, and the 5-year survival rate

TABLE 38-2

CARCINOMA OF THE CERVIX: SURVIVAL BY FIGO STAGE

Stage	No. of Patients	Five-Year Survival (%)
Ia1	860	98.7
Ia2	227	95.9
Ib1	2530	88.0
Ib2	950	78.8
IIa	881	68.8
IIb	2375	64.7
IIIa	160	40.4
IIIb	1949	43.3
IVa	245	19.5
IVb	189	15.0

Data from the Annual Report on the Results of Treatment in Gynaecological Cancer. Patients treated 1996-1998. J Epidemiol Biostat 83:41-78, 2003.

diminishes. Adenocarcinomas and adenosquamous carcinomas have a somewhat lower 5-year survival rate than do squamous carcinomas, stage for stage.

Matched, controlled studies have demonstrated identical survival rates for pregnant and nonpregnant patients.

SUGGESTED READING

Goldie SJ, Kim JJ, Wright TC: Cost effectiveness of human papillomavirus DNA testing for cervical cancer screening in women aged 30 years or more. Obstet Gynecol 103:619-631, 2004.

Hacker NF: Cervical cancer. *In* Berek JS, Hacker NF (eds): Practical Gynecologic Oncology, 5th ed. Philadelphia, Lippincott Williams & Wilkins, 2009 (in press).

Koutsky LA: Quadrivalent vaccine against human papilloma virus to prevent high grade cervical lesions. The Future II Study Group. N Engl J Med 356:1915-1927, 2007.

Rocconi RP, Estes JM, Leath CA III, et al: Management strategies for stage IB2 cervical cancer: A cost-effective analysis. Gynecol Oncol 97:387-394, 2005.

Rose PG, Bundy B, Watkins EB, et al: Concurrent cisplatin-based radiotherapy and chemotherapy for locally advanced cervical cancer. N Engl J Med 340:1144-1153, 1999.

Shepherd JH, Spencer C, Herod J, Ind TEJ: Radical vaginal trachelectomy as a fertility-sparing procedure in women with early stage cervical cancer—cumulative pregnancy rate in a series of 123 women. Br J Obstet Gynaecol 113:719-724, 2006.

Chapter 39

Ovarian Cancer

JONATHAN S. BEREK

Ovarian cancer is the fifth most common cancer among females in the United States, accounting for one fourth of all gynecologic cancers. It is the leading cause of death from gynecologic cancer because it is difficult to detect before it disseminates. In 2007, 22,430 new cases and more than 15,280 deaths are expected from this disease. Most women with ovarian cancer are in the fifth or sixth decade of life.

■ Etiology and Epidemiology

The cause of ovarian cancer is unknown. The patient characteristics found to be associated with an increased risk for epithelial ovarian cancer include white race, late age at menopause, family history of cancer of the ovary, breast, or bowel, and prolonged intervals of ovulation uninterrupted by pregnancy. There is an increased prevalence of ovarian cancer in nulliparous women and those who have been infertile.

The incidence of ovarian cancer varies in different geographic locations. Western countries, including the United States, have rates that are 3 to 7 times greater than those in Japan. Second-generation Japanese immigrants to the United States have an incidence of ovarian cancer similar to that of American women. White Americans experience ovarian cancer about 1.5 times more frequently than do black Americans.

About 10% of epithelial ovarian cancers occur in women with a hereditary predisposition. In women with hereditary cancers, two or more first-degree relatives on either the paternal or maternal side typically have had breast or ovarian cancer. **The pattern of inheritance is autosomal dominant. Breast cancers generally occur in young premenopausal women,** whereas **ovarian cancers have a median age of about 50 years. The breast-ovarian cancer syndrome is due to germline mutations of *BRCA1*, which is located on chromosome 17, and *BRCA2*, which is located on chromosome 13. The Lynch II syndrome, nonpolyposis colorectal cancer syndrome, is associated with mutations in the mismatch repair genes.** Adenocarcinomas of the ovary, breast, colon, stomach, pancreas, and endometrium are seen in the families of these individuals.

The use of oral contraceptives has been found to protect against ovarian cancer, possibly because of suppression of ovulation. It has been postulated that **incessant ovulation may predispose to malignant transformation in the ovary.**

Patients with a known germline mutation (e.g., *BRCA1* and *BRCA2* mutations) may be offered prophylactic salpingo-oophorectomy once childbearing has been completed, and this operation is highly protective for ovarian and fallopian tube carcinomas. Indeed, the risk for subsequent breast cancer is also significantly reduced in these women. There is still a small risk for peritoneal carcinoma after prophylactic salpingo-oophorectomy.

Some case-control studies have suggested that the use of postmenopausal estrogen replacement therapy may increase the risk for ovarian cancer, but these data are controversial.

It has also been postulated that a causative agent could enter the peritoneal cavity through the lower genital tract. For example, the perineal use of asbestos-contaminated talc has been linked to the development of epithelial ovarian cancer. This possibility remains controversial, although **tubal ligation and hysterectomy are both associated with a decreased risk for the disease.**

Screening for Ovarian Cancer

Population screening for ovarian cancer is not feasible because ultrasonography and available tumor markers, for example, CA 125, lack specificity and sensitivity for early-stage disease. CA 125 is more useful in postmenopausal women because false-positive measurements occur commonly in premenopausal women in association with endometriosis, pelvic inflammatory disease, or uterine fibroids. Patients with a strong family history of epithelial ovarian cancer may benefit from surveillance with serial transvaginal ultrasonography and serum CA 125 titers.

Clinical Features

SYMPTOMS

Unfortunately, many patients in whom ovarian cancer develops have only nonspecific symptoms before dissemination takes place. In early-stage disease, vague abdominal pain or bloating is common, although symptoms of a mass compressing the bladder or rectum, such as urinary frequency or constipation, may bring the patient to a physician. Sometimes the patient complains of dyspareunia. Premenopausal women may experience menstrual irregularity. Only rarely does a patient present with acute symptoms, such as pain secondary to torsion, rupture, or intracystic hemorrhage.

In advanced-stage disease, patients most often present with abdominal pain or swelling. The latter may be from the tumor itself or from associated ascites. On careful questioning, there has usually been a history of vague abdominal symptoms, such as bloating, constipation, nausea, dyspepsia, anorexia, or early satiety. Premenopausal patients may complain of irregular menses or heavy vaginal bleeding. **Postmenopausal bleeding is occasionally a symptom of ovarian neoplasms, particularly functional stromal tumors.**

SIGNS

The disease is frequently misdiagnosed for several months because patients with nonspecific abdominal symptoms do not receive a vaginal and rectal examination. **A solid, irregular, fixed pelvic mass is suggestive of ovarian cancer, and if combined with an upper abdominal mass, ascites, or both, the diagnosis is almost certain.**

Preoperative Evaluation

The diagnosis of ovarian cancer requires a laparotomy or laparoscopy. Routine preoperative hematologic and biochemical studies should be obtained, as should a chest radiograph. A pelvic and abdominal computed tomography scan will exclude liver metastases, but it is not mandatory.

A Papanicolaou smear should be obtained to evaluate the cervix, but this test is of limited value in detecting ovarian cancer. **Endometrial biopsy and endocervical curettage are necessary in patients with abnormal vaginal bleeding because concurrent primary tumors occasionally occur in the ovary and endometrium.** In the presence of a pelvic mass, it is preferable not to perform abdominal paracentesis for cytologic evaluation of ascitic fluid, unless neoadjuvant chemotherapy is planned, because seeding of the abdominal wall may occur.

An abdominal radiograph may be useful in a younger patient to locate calcifications associated with a benign cystic teratoma (dermoid cyst), which is the most common neoplasm in patients younger than 25 years of age. **In patients with occult blood in the stool or significant intestinal symptoms, a barium enema or lower gastrointestinal endoscopy should be obtained** to rule out a primary colonic cancer with ovarian metastasis.

Similarly, **an upper gastrointestinal endoscopy is important if there are significant gastric symptoms.** Breast cancer may also metastasize to the ovaries, so **bilateral mammograms should be obtained if there are any suspicious breast masses.**

Pelvic ultrasonography, particularly transvaginal ultrasonography with or without color Doppler studies, **may be useful** for smaller (<8 cm) masses in premenopausal women. Masses that are predominantly solid or multilocular have a high probability of being neoplastic, whereas unilocular cystic masses are generally functional cysts. In postmenopausal women, ultrasonography may also be useful because small, unilocular cysts (<5 cm) that are stable are generally benign.

Several tumor markers have been investigated, but none has been consistently reliable. **The tumor-associated antigen CA 125 is elevated in only about 50% of women with stage I ovarian cancer.** When this assay is elevated, it is useful for monitoring the clinical course of the disease.

Differential Diagnosis

Ovarian malignancies must be differentiated from benign neoplasms and functional cysts of the ovaries. In addition, a variety of gynecologic conditions can simulate a neoplastic process, including tubo-ovarian abscess, endometriosis, and a pedunculated uterine leiomyoma. Nongynecologic causes of pelvic tumor must also be excluded, such as an inflammatory or neoplastic disease of the colon, or a pelvic kidney.

Mode of Spread

Ovarian cancer typically spreads by exfoliating cells that disseminate and implant throughout the peritoneal cavity. The distribution of intraperitoneal metastases

TABLE 39-1

INTERNATIONAL FEDERATION OF GYNECOLOGY AND OBSTETRICS (FIGO) STAGING FOR PRIMARY CARCINOMA OF THE OVARY

Stage I	Growth limited to the ovaries
Stage Ia	Growth limited to one ovary; no ascites. No tumor on the external surface; capsule intact
Stage Ib	Growth limited to both ovaries; no ascites. No tumor on the external surfaces; capsules intact
Stage Ic	Tumor either stage Ia or Ib but with tumor on the surface of one or both ovaries or with capsule ruptured or with ascites present containing malignant cells or with positive peritoneal washings
Stage II	Growth involving one or both ovaries with pelvic extension
Stage IIa	Extension or metastases, or both, to the uterus or tubes, or both
Stage IIb	Extension to other pelvic tissues
Stage IIc	Tumor either stage IIa or IIb but with tumor on the surface of one or both ovaries or with capsule or capsules ruptured or with ascites present containing malignant cells or with positive peritoneal washings
Stage III	Tumor involving one or both ovaries with peritoneal implants outside the pelvis or positive retroperitoneal or inguinal nodes, or both. Superficial liver metastasis equals stage III. Tumor is limited to the true pelvis, but with histologically proven malignant extension to small bowel or omentum
Stage IIIa	Tumor grossly limited to the true pelvis with negative nodes but with histologically confirmed microscopic seeding of abdominal peritoneal surfaces
Stage IIIb	Tumor of one or both ovaries with histologically confirmed implants of abdominal peritoneal surfaces, none exceeding 2 cm in diameter. Nodes negative for disease
Stage IIIc	Abdominal implants >2 cm in diameter or positive retroperitoneal or inguinal nodes, or both
Stage IV	Growth involving one or both ovaries with distant metastasis. If pleural effusion is present, there must be positive cytologic test results to allot a case to stage IV. Parenchymal liver metastasis equals stage IV.

BOX 39-1   *Requirements for Staging or Second-Look Operations**

Multiple Cytologic Assays
Free ascitic fluid, if present
Peritoneal "washings" (50 mL of normal saline)
Pelvic cul-de-sac
Both paracolic gutters
Both hemidiaphragms

Multiple Intraperitoneal Biopsies
Pelvis
Cul-de-sac peritoneum
Bladder peritoneum
Pedicles of infundibulopelvic ligaments
Any adhesions

Abdomen
Both paracolic gutters
Bowel serosa and mesenteries
Omentum
Any adhesions

Extraperitoneal Biopsies
Pelvic and para-aortic lymph nodes

*Procedures performed in patients with no visible evidence of metastatic disease.

not common, and parenchymal metastases to the liver and lungs are seen in only about 2% of patients at initial presentation.

Death from ovarian cancer usually results from progressive encasement of abdominal organs, leading to anorexia, vomiting, and inanition. The bowel obstruction caused by tumor growth is often incomplete and intermittent and may last for several months before the patient's demise.

▪ Staging

The standard staging system for ovarian cancer is presented in Table 39-1. **Ovarian cancer is surgically staged** according to the International Federation of Gynecology and Obstetrics (FIGO) staging system.

Even though all microscopic disease may appear to be confined to the ovaries at the time of laparotomy, microscopic spread may have already occurred; thus, patients must undergo a thorough surgical staging. Procedures necessary to stage ovarian cancer are shown in Box 39-1.

▪ Classification

The histologic classification of ovarian neoplasms is listed in Table 39-2. These lesions fall into four categories according to their tissue of origin. **Most ovarian neoplasms (80% to 85%) are derived from coelomic epithelium and are called *epithelial carcinomas*.** Less common tumors are derived from primitive germ cells,

tends to follow the circulatory path of peritoneal fluid, so **metastases are commonly seen on the posterior cul-de-sac, paracolic gutters, right hemidiaphragm, liver capsule, and omentum.** Implants are also common on the bowel serosa and its mesenteries. In general, they grow around the intestines, encasing them with tumor, without invading the bowel lumen. Widespread bowel metastases can lead to a functional obstruction known as *carcinomatous ileus*.

Lymphatic dissemination to the pelvic and para-aortic nodes is common, particularly with advanced disease. Extensive blockage of the diaphragmatic lymphatics is at least partially responsible for the development of ascites. Hematogenous metastases are

TABLE 39-2

HISTOGENETIC CLASSIFICATION OF PRIMARY OVARIAN NEOPLASMS

Derivation	Type of Tumor
Coelomic epithelial origin (80%-85%)	"Common" epithelial tumors; benign, borderline, malignant Serous tumor Mucinous tumor Endometrioid tumor Clear cell (mesonephroid) tumor Brenner tumor Undifferentiated carcinoma Carcinosarcoma or malignant mixed mesodermal tumors
Germ cell origin (10%-15%)	Teratoma Mature teratoma Solid adult teratoma Dermoid cyst Struma ovarii Malignant neoplasms secondarily arising from teratomatous tissues (squamous carcinoma, carcinoid tumor, sarcoma) Immature teratoma Dysgerminoma Endodermal sinus tumor Embryonal carcinoma Choriocarcinoma Gonadoblastoma* Mixed germ cell tumors
Specialized gonadal-stromal origin (3%-5%)	Granulosa-theca cell tumors Granulosa cell tumor Thecoma Sertoli-Leydig tumors Arrhenoblastoma Sertoli cell tumor Gynandroblastoma Lipid cell tumors
Nonspecific mesenchymal origin (fewer than 1%)	Fibroma, hemangioma, leiomyoma, lipoma Lymphoma Sarcoma

*Combined germ cell and specialized gonadal-stromal elements.
Data from Hart WR, Morrow CP: The ovaries. In Romney SL, Gray MJ, Little AO, et al (eds): Gynecology and Obstetrics: The Health Care of Women, 2nd ed. New York, McGraw-Hill, 1981.

specialized gonadal stroma, or nonspecific mesenchyme. In addition, the ovary can be the site of metastatic carcinomas, most often from the gastrointestinal tract or the breast.

▪ *Epithelial Ovarian Carcinomas*

PATHOLOGIC FEATURES

The main histologic subtypes of epithelial carcinomas are serous (about 55%), mucinous (about 20%), endometrioid (about 15%), and clear cell (about 5%). Malignant Brenner tumors and undifferentiated carcinomas are uncommon.

Serous tumors resemble fallopian tube epithelium histologically (Figure 39-1). About 30% of patients with stage I and stage IIa disease have bilateral involvement. On gross examination, serous carcinomas have an irregular and multilocular appearance (Figure 39-2).

Mucinous tumors histologically resemble endocervical epithelium and are often large, measuring 20 cm or more in diameter. They are bilateral in 10% to 20% of patients.

Endometrioid tumors closely resemble carcinomas of the endometrium and arise in association with primary endometrial cancer in about 20% of patients. In early-stage disease, they are bilateral in about 10% of cases. About 10% of endometrioid ovarian carcinomas are associated with endometriosis, although malignant transformation of endometriosis occurs in fewer than 1% of patients.

Clear cell carcinomas of the ovary are uncommon. **In about 25% of cases, they occur in association with endometriosis.**

The Brenner tumor represents only 2% to 3% of all ovarian neoplasms, and fewer than 2% of these tumors are malignant. **About 10% of Brenner tumors occur in conjunction with a mucinous cystadenoma or dermoid cyst in the same or opposite ovary.**

Tumors of low malignant potential or borderline histologic appearance exist for each histologic type. **About 5% to 10% of malignant serous tumors are borderline** (Figure 39-3), **whereas 20% of malignant mucinous tumors fall into this category.** The endometrioid, clear cell, and Brenner tumors are only rarely borderline.

MANAGEMENT OF EPITHELIAL OVARIAN CANCER

The initial approach to all patients with ovarian cancer is surgical exploration of the abdomen and pelvis.

Early-Stage Disease

Definitive diagnosis requires an intraoperative frozen section. In patients with no gross evidence of disease beyond the ovary, the standard operation is total abdominal hysterectomy, bilateral salpingo-oophorectomy, infracolic omentectomy, and thorough surgical staging, as shown in Box 39-1. Patients who wish to preserve fertility may have a unilateral salpingo-oophorectomy. **In patients with grade 1 or 2 tumors confined to one or both ovaries after surgical staging, no further treatment is necessary.** Patients with poorly differentiated (grade 3) tumors are subsequently treated with systemic chemotherapy.

Advanced-Stage Disease

In patients with advanced disease, cytoreductive surgery ("debulking") is required. The objectives are to remove the primary tumor and all of the metastases, if possible. If all macroscopic disease cannot be removed,

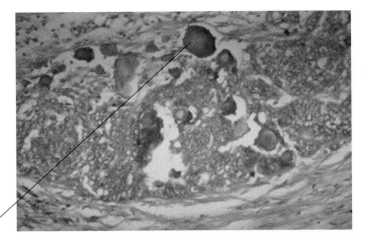

FIGURE 39-1 Papillary serous cystadenocarcinoma. This tumor frequently contains numerous psammoma bodies, which are shown here. Their origin is uncertain, but it has been suggested that they may reflect an immune reaction against the tumor or, more simply, represent alteration to the secretions from the malignant cells. There is no relationship between the presence of psammoma bodies and the malignancy of the tumor.

Psammoma bodies

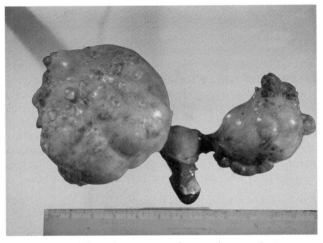

FIGURE 39-2 Bilateral serous cystadenocarcinomas. A uterus with both ovaries grossly enlarged by multilocular tumors with papillary excrescences on their serosal surfaces is shown.

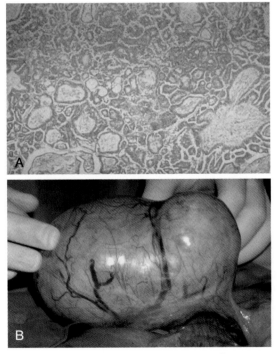

FIGURE 39-3 A: Serous tumor—borderline (papillary serous cystadenocarcinoma of low malignant potential). The papillary pattern filling the cyst lumen is very complex, and the epithelium is, in places, more than one cell thick. Mitotic figures are present, although not abundant. B: Large borderline tumor mobilized out of the pelvis. Note the smooth surface and large blood vessels coursing over the surface.

an attempt should be made to reduce individual tumor nodules to 1 cm or less in diameter. Patients in whom this goal is achieved are said to have had "optimal" cytoreduction, which can be achieved in about 70% of patients. In addition to a total or subtotal abdominal hysterectomy, bilateral salpingo-oophorectomy, omentectomy, and resection of peritoneal metastases, optimal cytoreduction may necessitate bowel resection; therefore, **all patients having surgery for suspected ovarian cancer should have a bowel preparation preoperatively.**

In retrospective studies, patients whose individual residual tumor nodules are 1 cm in diameter or less before the commencement of chemotherapy have been shown to have longer median survivals and more complete responses to therapy. The longest survival is seen in patients in whom all visible tumor has been removed before treatment.

In patients who are medically unfit or have a poor performance status, usually because of a large pleural effusion and massive ascites, it may be prudent to give two or three cycles of neoadjuvant chemotherapy

before undertaking radical surgery. If the disease does not respond to chemotherapy, as evidenced by the failure to resolve the malignant effusions, the patient should be offered palliative care only. **Usually, the effusions resolve completely, and an "interval" cytoreductive operation can be safely undertaken.**

Following primary cytoreductive surgery, combination chemotherapy is given, most commonly intravenous carboplatin and paclitaxel, or intraperitoneal cisplatin and paclitaxel. Intraperitoneal treatment is only useful for patients with minimal residual disease. Single-agent therapy with paclitaxel, or carboplatin, is occasionally used for frail or elderly patients. During chemotherapy, **the patient's response is monitored with serial CA 125 levels.** If the values rise or plateau within 6 months, it is advisable to change to second-line drugs, such as liposomal-encapsulated doxorubicin, topotecan, etoposide, gemcitabine, or experimental chemotherapeutic agents. If the progression-free interval has been longer than 6 to 12 months, the patient may respond to further paclitaxel or carboplatin chemotherapy. Response to second-line chemotherapy is in the range of 20% to 50%, but patients are not considered to be curable after their initial relapse. **Secondary cytoreduction may be appropriate if the disease-free interval is 24 months or longer.**

It is unclear whether patients with "metastatic" borderline tumors benefit from chemotherapy.

Second-Look Laparotomy

In patients who are clinically free of disease after completing a prescribed course of chemotherapy (usually about six cycles), **a second-look laparotomy** may be performed to determine whether the patient has had a complete response to chemotherapy. However, it is unclear whether the performance of a second-look laparotomy and the administration of further treatment ultimately prolong survival, so the surgery **should be confined to research settings.** If there is no macroscopic or microscopic evidence of disease at second-look laparotomy, essentially the same procedures as are carried out for surgical staging should be performed (see Box 39-1). If gross disease is present, an attempt should be made to resect persistent disease to facilitate a response to subsequent therapy.

PROGNOSIS

Patients with stage I disease have 5-year survival rates of 75% to 95%, depending on the histologic grade.

Almost all patients with carefully staged Ia grade 1 ovarian cancer are cured surgically, whereas the 5-year survival rate for patients with poorly differentiated bilateral lesions is as low as 75%. The 5-year survival rate for patients with stage II disease is about 65%. Despite aggressive primary surgery and combination chemotherapy, **the 5-year survival rate for patients with**

advanced-stage disease is about 20%, although the median survival is between 2 and 3 years. Patients with advanced-stage disease who have negative findings on second-look laparotomy have a 5-year survival rate of about 60%. Patients whose tumors are associated with *BRCA1* and *BRCA2* mutations may have a somewhat better prognosis, but this issue is unclear.

Patients who have borderline ovarian tumors can be expected to have a prolonged survival. If the disease is confined to the ovary, most tumors never recur. Five- and 10-year survival rates are 95% to 100%, but late recurrences may occur, and 20-year survival rates are about 85% to 90%. Patients who initially present with metastatic disease are more likely to exhibit subsequent clinical evidence of disease, although the rate of progression is slow; most live at least 5 years.

■ *Germ Cell Tumors*

Germ cell tumors of the ovary account for only about 2% to 3% of all ovarian malignancies. They occur predominantly in young patients and frequently produce either human chorionic gonadotropin (hCG) or alphafetoprotein (AFP), which serve as tumor markers. The most common germ cell tumors are the dysgerminoma and immature teratoma. Endodermal sinus tumors, embryonal tumors, and nongestational choriocarcinomas are less common. Mixed germ cell tumors are not uncommon.

DYSGERMINOMAS

Dysgerminomas occur predominantly in children and young women. About 10% are bilateral. **These tumors, of varying malignant virulence, are occasionally seen in patients with gonadal dysgenesis or the testicular feminization syndrome.** In such patients, the dysgerminoma may arise in a gonadoblastoma. In about two thirds of patients, the disease is confined to the ovaries at the time of diagnosis. About 10% of dysgerminomas are associated with other germ cell malignancies. **Pure dysgerminomas do not produce the tumor markers hCG and AFP but commonly produce lactate dehydrogenase.**

Treatment

In most patients, the contralateral ovary and the uterus can be preserved. **Surgical staging,** as outlined earlier in this chapter, **is important. Particular attention should be paid to the pelvic and para-aortic lymph nodes** because of the propensity of these tumors for lymphatic dissemination. If disease extends beyond one ovary, the treatment of choice is resection and chemotherapy. **The regimen employed for these patients is usually bleomycin, etoposide, and cisplatin.** Carboplatin and paclitaxel are also being tested in these patients. Dysgerminomas are uniquely radiosensitive, and radiotherapy was previously the treatment of choice. However, it is now best reserved for the management of recurrent, chemoresistant disease.

Prognosis

The 5-year survival rate for patients with stage Ia pure dysgerminoma treated with unilateral oophorectomy is about 95%, whereas it is 80% for stage II and 60% to 70% for stage III disease. Recurrences following conservative surgery have at least an 80% 5-year survival rate.

IMMATURE TERATOMAS

Immature teratomas are the second most common malignant ovarian germ cell tumor. About 75% of malignant teratomas are encountered during the first two decades of life. Bilateral lesions are rare, although the other ovary may contain a benign dermoid cyst in about 5% of cases. Like other germ cell tumors, immature teratomas grow fairly rapidly, cause pain early, and are found confined to the ovary in about two thirds of cases at the time of diagnosis. **Pure immature teratomas do not produce hCG or AFP.** Histologically, the tumors can be graded from 1 to 3 according to the degree of differentiation, with grade 3 tumors being the least differentiated. Neural elements are most frequently seen, but cartilage and epithelial tissues are also common.

Treatment

The primary tumor should be removed. **In young patients, the uterus and contralateral ovary should be preserved to maintain fertility.** All patients with other than stage Ia grade 1 immature teratomas should receive postoperative chemotherapy using bleomycin, etoposide, and cisplatin. Three cycles of chemotherapy should be given for stage I disease.

Prognosis

Survival correlates with grade and stage of disease. The 5-year survival rate for patients with grade 1 immature teratomas is about 95%, compared with 80% for grade 2 and 60% to 70% for grade 3 disease.

OTHER GERM CELL TUMORS

The endodermal sinus tumor is a rare malignancy. It is also referred to as a *yolk sac* tumor. **Endodermal sinus tumors produce AFP,** which can serve as a useful serum marker for this neoplasm. **Embryonal carcinomas produce both hCG and AFP, whereas choriocarcinomas produce hCG only.** All occur in children and young women, and all grow rapidly. **Bilateral tumors are rare.**

Therapy for these lesions includes surgical resection of the primary tumor followed by systemic combination chemotherapy with bleomycin, etoposide, and cisplatin. Before the advent of effective chemotherapy,

these tumors were usually fatal. The overall 5-year survival rate is now about 70% to 80%.

■ Specialized Gonadal-Stromal Tumors

A group of relatively uncommon tumors is derived from the specialized ovarian stroma. As such, they are often endocrinologically functional, many of them being capable of synthesizing gonadal or adrenal steroid hormones. Because the ovarian stroma has sexual bipotentiality, hormones that are secreted can be either female or male. **Estrogen and progesterone are typically associated with granulosa-theca cell tumors, whereas testosterone and other androgens may be secreted by many Sertoli-Leydig cell tumors. Rarely, lipid cell tumors**, which are usually virilizing, **produce adrenal corticoids** and a clinical cushingoid syndrome.

PATHOLOGIC FEATURES

Granulosa cell tumors are the most common stromal carcinomas. They have a distinct histologic pattern: **small groups of cells called Call-Exner bodies are the hallmark.** They may secrete large amounts of estrogen and can be associated with endometrial cancer in adults or sexual pseudoprecocity in children.

Thecomas, which are only one third as common as granulosa cell tumors, are rarely malignant. Mixtures of the two types of tumor exist.

Sertoli-Leydig cell tumors (arrhenoblastomas) contain both Sertoli-type and Leydig-type stromal cells and are classically associated with masculinization. **Only 3% to 5% of these tumors are malignant.**

Lipid cell tumors are often referred to as hilar cell tumors because they are located in the ovarian hilus. **Only a rare lipid tumor, usually larger than 8 cm in diameter, behaves in a malignant fashion.**

TREATMENT

Most stromal tumors occur in postmenopausal women and are best treated by a total abdominal hysterectomy and bilateral salpingo-oophorectomy. Conservation of the uterus and contralateral ovary is appropriate for carefully staged young patients with stage I disease provided that the possibility of an associated adenocarcinoma of the endometrium has been excluded by dilation and curettage. The tumors are not very chemosensitive.

PROGNOSIS

Granulosa cell tumors, which tend to grow slowly, are usually confined to one ovary at the time of diagnosis. **The 5-year survival rate is about 90% for stage I disease. Recurrences are usually detected late** and may result in death 15 to 20 years after removal of the primary lesion.

Metastatic Cancers

About 4% to 8% of ovarian malignancies are metastatic, most commonly from either the gastrointestinal tract or the breast. **The Krukenberg tumor is a specific type of metastatic tumor in which signet-ring cells are seen in the ovarian stroma histologically.** Most Krukenberg tumors are bilateral and metastatic from the stomach. Rarely, it has not been possible to locate a primary focus, and removal of the ovarian disease has produced apparent cures.

Fallopian Tube Carcinoma

Primary carcinoma of the fallopian tube accounts for only 0.1% to 0.5% of gynecologic cancers and is diagnostically confused with ovarian carcinoma. The incidence of fallopian tube carcinoma may be higher than previously suspected because some are misclassified as primary ovarian carcinomas. **Most are adenocarcinomas, but sarcomas and mixed tumors can occur.** There is no official staging system for fallopian tube carcinoma, but in general they are staged like ovarian cancer because the mode of dissemination is similar. Bilateral carcinomas are seen in 10% to 20% of patients.

CLINICAL FEATURES

Clinically, **patients can present with a vaginal discharge that is typically watery in nature,** as well as vaginal bleeding, pelvic pain, or some combination of symptoms. In postmenopausal patients, the vaginal discharge may be yellow, watery, and similar to that seen with a urinary fistula. Physical examination may reveal an adnexal mass but is often unremarkable. **A fallopian tube cancer should be suspected in a postmenopausal patient whose bleeding or abnormal cytologic findings are not explained by endometrial or endocervical curettage.** In most patients, the diagnosis is not made preoperatively.

TREATMENT

The treatment for fallopian tube carcinoma is total abdominal hysterectomy, bilateral salpingo-oophorectomy, and omentectomy. **Surgical staging should be performed in patients whose disease appears to be confined to the pelvis, and cytoreductive surgery is appropriate in patients with metastatic disease.** Postoperatively, combination chemotherapy, including carboplatin and paclitaxel, is usually used for patients with stages II or IV disease.

PROGNOSIS

The prognosis for fallopian tube carcinoma is similar to that for ovarian cancer.

SUGGESTED READING

Armstrong DK, Bundy B, Wenzel L, et al: Intraperitoneal cisplatin and paclitaxel in ovarian cancer. N Engl J Med 354:34-43, 2006.

Berek JS: Epithelial ovarian cancer. *In* Berek JS, Hacker NF (eds): Practical Gynecologic Oncology, 4th ed. Philadelphia, Lippincott Williams & Wilkins, 2004, pp 443-509.

Bristow RE, Tomacruz RS, Armstrong DK, et al: Survival effect of maximal cytoreductive surgery for advanced ovarian carcinoma during the platinum era: A meta-analysis. J Clin Oncol 20:1248-1259, 2002.

Haber D: Prophylactic oophorectomy to reduce the risk of ovarian and breast cancer in carriers of BRCA mutations. N Engl J Med 346:1660-1661, 2002.

Ozols RF, Bundy BN, Greer B, et al: Phase III trial of carboplatin and paclitaxel versus cisplatin and paclitaxel in patients with optimally resected stage III ovarian cancer: A Gynecologic Oncology Group study. J Clin Oncol 21:3194-3200, 2003.

Chapter 40

Vulvar and Vaginal Cancer

NEVILLE F. HACKER

■ *Vulvar Neoplasms*

Malignant tumors of the vulva are uncommon, representing about 4% of malignancies of the female genital tract. Most tumors are squamous cell carcinomas, with melanomas, adenocarcinomas, basal cell carcinomas, and sarcomas occurring much less frequently.

Squamous cell carcinoma of the vulva occurs mainly in postmenopausal women, and the mean age at diagnosis is 65 years. A history of chronic vulvar itching is common.

EPIDEMIOLOGY

Recent studies suggest two different etiologic types of vulvar cancer. **One type is seen mainly in younger patients, is related to human papillomavirus (HPV) infection and smoking, and is commonly associated with vulvar intraepithelial neoplasia (VIN) of the basaloid or warty type. The more common type is seen mainly in elderly women and is unrelated to smoking or HPV infection; concurrent VIN is uncommon, but long-standing lichen sclerosus is common. When VIN is present, it is of the differentiated type.** VIN III carries a significant risk for progression to invasive cancer if left untreated.

About 5% of patients have positive results on serologic testing for syphilis. In the latter group of patients, vulvar cancer occurs at an earlier age and carries a graver prognosis. Although rarely seen in the United States, **vulvar cancer also occurs in association with lymphogranuloma venereum and granuloma inguinale.**

■ *Intraepithelial Neoplasia*

The International Society for the Study of Vulvar Disease recognizes two varieties of intraepithelial neoplasia: squamous cell carcinoma in situ (Bowen's disease) or VIN III, and Paget's disease. With the introduction of the HPV vaccines, there should be a significant reduction in the incidence of VIN and invasive vulvar cancer, particularly in young patients, in the future.

SQUAMOUS CELL CARCINOMA IN SITU: VULVAR INTRAEPITHELIAL NEOPLASIA TYPE III

During the past 25 years, the incidence of VIN has increased markedly. Younger patients are being affected, and the mean age is about 45 years.

Clinical Features

Itching is the most common symptom, although some patients present with palpable or visible abnormalities of the vulva. About half of patients are asymptomatic. There is no absolutely diagnostic appearance. Most lesions are elevated, but the color may be white, red, pink, gray, or brown (Figure 40-1). **About 20% of the lesions have a "warty" appearance, and the lesions are multicentric in about two thirds of cases.**

Diagnosis

Careful inspection of the vulva in a bright light, with the aid of a magnifying glass if necessary, is the most useful technique for detecting abnormal areas. Colposcopic examination of the entire vulva after the application of 5% acetic acid will sometimes highlight additional acetowhite areas.

Management

The mainstay of treatment is local superficial surgical excision, with primary closure. The microscopic disease seldom extends significantly beyond the colposcopic lesion, so **margins of about 5 mm are usually adequate. For extensive lesions involving most of the vulva, a "skinning" vulvectomy,** in which the vulvar skin is removed and replaced by a split-thickness skin graft, **may be used.** Because the subcutaneous tissues

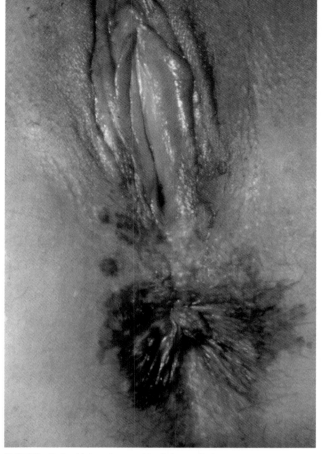

FIGURE 40-1   Vulvar intraepithelial neoplasia type III: carcinoma in situ of the vulva. Note the pigmented and multicentric nature of the lesions and the extensive perianal involvement in this patient.

are not excised, the cosmetic result is superior to that obtained with vulvectomy.

Laser therapy is also effective, particularly for multiple small lesions, or for lesions involving the clitoris, labia minora, or perianal area. No specimen is available for histologic study after laser ablation, so a liberal number of biopsies must be taken before treatment to exclude invasive cancer.

PAGET'S DISEASE

Paget's disease of the vulva predominantly affects postmenopausal white women. Paget's disease also occurs in the nipple areas of the breast.

Clinical Features

Itching and tenderness are common and may be long-standing. **The affected area is usually well demarcated and eczematoid in appearance,** with the presence of white plaquelike lesions. As growth progresses, extension beyond the vulva to the mons pubis, thighs, and buttocks may occur; rarely, it may extend to involve the mucosa of the rectum, vagina, or urinary tract. **In 10% to 20% of cases, Paget's disease is associated with an underlying adenocarcinoma.**

Histologic Features

The disease is an adenocarcinoma in situ and is characterized by large, pale, pathognomonic Paget's cells, which are seen within the epidermis and skin adnexa. **They are rich in mucopolysaccharide, a diastase-resistant substance that stains positive with periodic acid–Schiff stain.** The intracytoplasmic mucin may also be demonstrated by Mayer's mucicarmine stain. **The Paget's cells are typically located adjacent to the basal layer, both in the epidermis and in the adnexal structures.**

Management

The histologic extent of Paget's disease is frequently far beyond the visible lesion. Local superficial excision with 5- to 10-mm margins is required to clear the gross lesion, exclude underlying invasive cancer, and relieve symptoms. Recurrences are common and may be treated by further excision or laser therapy. **If an underlying invasive carcinoma is present, the treatment should be the same as for other invasive vulvar cancers.**

Invasive Vulvar Cancer

SQUAMOUS CELL CARCINOMA

Squamous cell carcinoma accounts for about 90% of vulvar cancers.

Clinical Features

Patients generally present with a vulvar lump, although long-standing pruritus is common. The lesions may be raised, ulcerated, pigmented, or warty in appearance, and **definitive diagnosis requires biopsy under local anesthesia.** Most lesions occur on the labia majora; the labia minora are the next most common sites. Less commonly, the clitoris or the perineum is involved (Figure 40-2). About 5% of cases are multifocal.

Methods of Spread

Vulvar cancer spreads by direct extension to adjacent structures, such as the vagina, urethra, and anus; **by lymphatic embolization to regional lymph nodes;** and **by hematogenous spread to distant sites,** including the lungs, liver, and bone. In most cases, the initial lymphatic metastases are to the inguinal lymph nodes, located between Camper's fascia and the fascia lata. From these superficial nodes, spread occurs to the

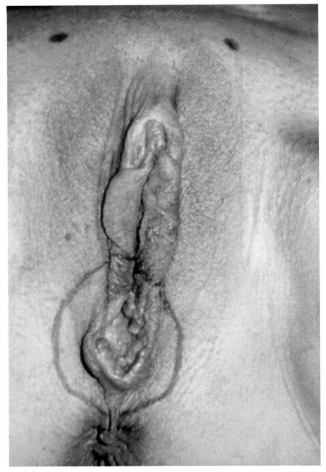

FIGURE 40-2   A small perineal carcinoma. Note that the remainder of the vulva is normal.

femoral nodes located medial to the femoral vein. Cloquet's node, which is situated beneath the inguinal ligament, is the most cephalad of the femoral node group. **From the inguinofemoral nodes, spread occurs to the pelvic nodes, particularly the external iliac group** (Figure 40-3).

The incidence of lymph node metastases in vulvar cancer is about 30%. It is related to the size of the lesion (Table 40-1). **About 5% of patients have metastases to pelvic lymph nodes. Such patients usually have three or more positive unilateral inguinofemoral lymph nodes.** Hematogenous spread usually occurs late in the disease and rarely occurs in the absence of lymphatic metastases.

Staging

In 1989, the International Federation of Gynecology and Obstetrics (FIGO) Cancer Committee introduced a surgical staging system for vulvar cancer. This system was revised in 1994, and the present FIGO staging system is shown in Table 40-2.

Management

In the past, en bloc radical vulvectomy and bilateral inguinofemoral lymphadenectomy, with or without pelvic lymphadenectomy, had been considered the standard treatment for invasive vulvar cancer. **During the past 30 years, a more conservative approach has been used for the primary lesion, and the groin dissection has frequently been performed through a separate groin incision.**

Using the separate incision technique, major wound breakdown is significantly reduced, so hospital stays are shorter. **Groin seromas and cellulitis are common acute complications,** whereas deep venous thrombosis and pulmonary embolism are uncommon. **Chronic complications include lower leg lymphedema, genital prolapse, and urinary stress incontinence.** Rarely, introital stenosis, pubic osteomyelitis, a femoral hernia, or a rectoperineal fistula may occur.

To decrease the morbidity associated with groin dissection, current research is focusing on identification of a sentinel node (or nodes). After the injection of a blue dye and a radiocolloid around the primary tumor, the sentinel nodes are identified and resected. They are subjected to thorough histopathologic analysis to detect any small micrometastases. Theoretically, patients with negative sentinel nodes should be at very low risk for disease in other nodes, so full groin dissection could be avoided. At the time of writing, this approach remains experimental.

EARLY VULVAR CANCER

During the past 30 years, much emphasis has been placed on vulvar conservation in an attempt to decrease psychological morbidity. With respect to the lymphadenectomy, **patients with stage Ia disease** (i.e., with T1 tumors and penetration depth of <1 mm from the overlying basement membrane) **do not need groin dissection. All other patients require at least an ipsilateral inguinal-femoral lymphadenectomy. For patients with midline lesions invading more than 1 mm, bilateral groin dissection is necessary.** For ipsilateral lesions, there is about a 1% risk for involvement of the contralateral nodes if the ipsilateral nodes are negative.

For patients with TI or T2 lesions (i.e., lesions confined to the vulva), a wide and deep local excision (radical local excision) is as effective as radical vulvectomy in preventing local recurrence provided that the remainder of the vulva is normal. For patients with stage I vulvar cancer, there is about a 10% risk for local recurrence, even with radical vulvectomy, and this incidence appears to be no higher with radical local excision. **Surgical margins should be at least 1 cm.**

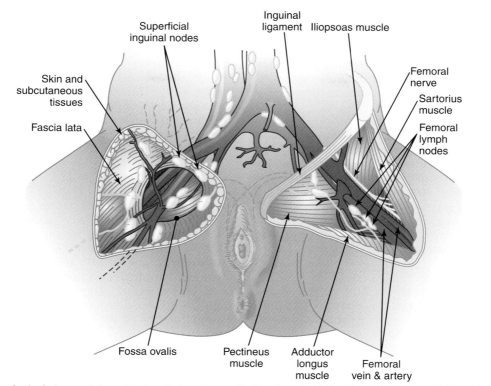

FIGURE 40-3 Lymphatic drainage of the vulva. Inguinal nodes are displayed on the right side of the groin, and femoral nodes are seen on the left side of the groin.

TABLE 40-1

INCIDENCE OF LYMPH NODE METASTASES IN RELATION TO LESION SIZE IN VULVAR CANCER

Lesion Size (cm)	Number	Positive Nodes	Percentage
0-1	43	3	7.0
1-2	63	14	22.2
2-4	52	14	26.9
>4	41	14	34.1

Data from Bosquet JG, Kinney WK, Russell AH, et al: Risk of occult inguinofemoral lymph node metastasis from squamous carcinoma of the vulva. Int J Rad Oncol Biol Phys 57:419, 2003.

ADVANCED VULVAR CANCER

If the cancer involves the proximal urethra, anus, or rectovaginal septum, radical surgery would necessitate a bowel or urinary stoma. For such patients, preoperative radiation or chemoradiation should be used to shrink the primary tumor, followed by more conservative surgical excision. Bilateral groin node dissection, or at least removal of any large, positive nodes, is usually performed before the radiation therapy. Most patients can be spared a stoma with this approach.

TABLE 40-2

INTERNATIONAL FEDERATION OF GYNECOLOGY AND OBSTETRICS (FIGO) STAGING OF VULVAR CARCINOMA (1994)

Stage 0	Carcinoma in situ, intraepithelial carcinoma
Stage I	Tumor confined to the vulva or perineum, or both, and 2 cm or less in greatest dimension; no nodal metastasis
Stage Ia	As above with stromal invasion ≤1 mm
Stage Ib	As above with stromal invasion >1 mm
Stage II	Tumor confined to the vulva or perineum, or both, and more than 2 cm in greatest dimension; no nodal metastasis
Stage III	Tumor of any size with: 1. Adjacent spread to the urethra and/or vagina and/or anus 2. Unilateral regional lymph node metastasis, or a combination
Stage IV	
Stage IVa	Tumor invades any of the following: upper urethra, bladder mucosa, rectal mucosa, pelvic bone or bilateral regional node metastasis, or a combination
Stage IVb	Any distant metastasis including pelvic lymph nodes

MANAGEMENT OF PATIENTS WITH POSITIVE NODES

Patients with more than one nodal micrometastasis (≤5 mm in diameter), one or more macrometastases, or evidence of extranodal spread should receive post-operative radiation to both groins and to the pelvis.

Prognosis

The overall survival rate for vulvar carcinoma is about 70%. Survival by FIGO stage is shown in Table 40-3. Survival also correlates significantly with lymph node status because **patients with positive nodes have a 5-year survival rate of about 50%, whereas those with negative nodes have a 5-year survival rate of about 90%.** Patients with one involved node have a good prognosis, regardless of stage, whereas those with three or more involved nodes do poorly, regardless of stage.

MALIGNANT MELANOMA

Malignant melanoma is the second most common type of vulvar cancer. Melanomas may arise de novo or from a preexisting junctional or compound nevus. They occur predominantly in postmenopausal white women and most commonly involve the labia minora or clitoris (Figure 40-4).

TABLE 40-3

SURVIVAL FOR VULVAR CANCER BY FIGO STAGE (EPIDERMOID INVASIVE CANCER ONLY)		
Stage	**No. of Patients**	**Five-Year Survival (%)**
I	160	76.9
II	202	54.8
III	125	30.8
IV	44	8.3

Data from the Annual Report on the Results of Treatment in Gynecological Cancer. Patients treated 1996-1998. J Epidemiol Biostat 83:7-26, 2003.

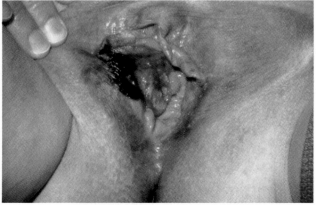

FIGURE 40-4 Malignant melanoma arising from the right labium minus.

Diagnosis and Staging

Any pigmented lesion on the vulva requires excisional biopsy for histologic diagnosis. The FIGO staging of vulvar cancer does not apply well to melanomas, which are usually smaller lesions and tend to metastasize early. **The prognosis correlates more closely with the depth of penetration into the dermis.** Those lesions that penetrate to a depth of 1 mm or less from the granular layer of the epidermis rarely metastasize. Clark's levels are not readily applicable to vulvar melanomas.

Management

For the superficial lesions referred to previously, radical local excision alone, with margins of at least 1 cm, is adequate therapy. For lesions with 1 mm or deeper invasion, **radical local excision of the primary tumor is usually combined with at least ipsilateral inguinal-femoral lymphadenectomy.** Adjuvant therapy with nonspecific immunostimulants or chemotherapeutic agents has been disappointing, although vaccines prepared from the patient's own tumor have shown some promise.

Prognosis

The overall 5-year survival rate for vulvar melanomas is about 30%, which is comparable to that for cutaneous melanomas of nongenital origin.

VERRUCOUS CARCINOMA

Verrucous carcinoma is a variant of squamous cell carcinoma and was originally described in the oral cavity. The lesions, which are cauliflower-like in nature, may occur in the cervix, vulva, or vagina. Invasion occurs with a broad "pushing" front, and unless the base of the lesion is submitted for histologic examination, these tumors may be difficult to differentiate from condyloma acuminatum or squamous papilloma. **Metastasis to regional lymph nodes is rare,** but the tumors are locally aggressive and prone to local recurrence unless wide surgical margins are obtained. **Radiation therapy may induce anaplastic transformation and is contraindicated.**

BARTHOLIN'S GLAND CARCINOMA

Adenocarcinomas, squamous cell carcinomas, and rarely, transitional cell carcinomas may arise from the Bartholin's gland and its duct. A history of preceding inflammation of Bartholin's gland is present in about 10% of patients, and malignancies may be mistaken for benign cysts or abscesses. Current management consists of hemivulvectomy and ipsilateral inguinofemoral lymphadenectomy. **Postoperative vulvar irradiation appears to decrease the local recurrence rate for patients with large lesions.**

BASAL CELL CARCINOMA

Basal cell carcinomas of the vulva are rare. They commonly present as a rolled-edged "rodent" ulcer, although nodules and macules may occur. They are locally aggressive but nonmetastasizing, so wide local excision is adequate treatment.

Vulvar Sarcoma

Vulvar sarcomas represent 1% to 2% of vulvar malignancies. Many histologic types have been reported, including leiomyosarcomas, fibrosarcomas, neurofibrosarcomas, liposarcomas, rhabdomyosarcomas, angiosarcomas, and epithelioid sarcomas. Leiomyosarcomas are the most common, and recurrences are most likely with lesions larger than 5 cm, with infiltrating margins, and with five or more mitotic figures per 10 high-power fields.

Vaginal Neoplasms

INTRAEPITHELIAL NEOPLASIA

Carcinoma in situ of the vagina, or vaginal intraepithelial neoplasia (VAIN), is much less common than its counterparts on the cervix or vulva. Most lesions occur in the upper third of the vagina, and the patients are usually asymptomatic.

Etiology

VAIN appears to be related to infection with the wart virus in many cases, and vaccination against HPV should decrease the incidence of VAIN and vaginal cancer in the future. Patients with a past history of in situ or invasive carcinoma of the cervix or vulva are at increased risk. Some lesions may occur after irradiation for cervical cancer.

Diagnosis

The diagnosis is usually considered because of an abnormal Papanicolaou smear in a woman who either has had a hysterectomy or has no demonstrable cervical abnormality. Definitive diagnosis requires vaginal biopsy, which should be directed by colposcopy or Lugol's iodine staining. Colposcopic findings are similar to those seen with cervical lesions, although thorough colposcopy of all vaginal walls is technically more difficult. **In postmenopausal patients, a 4-week course of topical estrogen before colposcopy is indicated to enhance the colposcopic features and eliminate those patients with Papanicolaou smear abnormalities because of inflammatory atypia.**

Management

When the lesion involves the vaginal vault, surgical excision is indicated to treat the VAIN and to exclude invasive cancer. For multifocal disease, laser therapy or topical 5-fluorouracil may be used. Extensive disease may require total vaginectomy and creation of a neovagina using a split-thickness skin graft.

SQUAMOUS CELL CARCINOMA OF THE VAGINA

Squamous cell carcinoma of the vagina is uncommon. The mean age of patients at presentation is about 60 years. **Up to 30% of patients with primary vaginal cancer have a history of in situ or invasive cervical cancer that was treated at least 5 years earlier.** Symptoms consist of abnormal vaginal bleeding, vaginal discharge, and urinary symptoms. On physical examination, ulcerative, exophytic, and infiltrative growth patterns may be seen. About half of the lesions are in the upper third of the vagina, particularly on the posterior wall. Punch biopsy is required to confirm the diagnosis.

Patterns of Spread

Vaginal cancer spreads by direct invasion as well as by lymphatic and hematogenous dissemination. **Direct tumor spread may result in involvement of the bladder, urethra, or rectum, or progressive lateral extension to the pelvic side wall.** The lymphatic drainage from the upper vagina is to the obturator, hypogastric, and external iliac nodes, whereas the lower third of the vagina drains primarily to the inguinofemoral nodes. Hematogenous spread is uncommon until the disease is advanced.

Staging

The FIGO staging for vaginal cancer is clinical, as shown in Table 40-4. In practice, all patients should have at least a chest radiograph and pelvic and abdominal computed tomography or magnetic resonance imaging to detect evidence of metastatic spread, including bulky pelvic or para-aortic lymph nodes. Positron emission tomography is increasingly used to look for metastatic disease.

Management

Radiotherapy or chemoradiation is the main method of treatment for primary vaginal cancer. Initial treatment usually consists of 4500 to 5000 cGy of external

TABLE 40-4	
INTERNATIONAL FEDERATION OF GYNECOLOGY AND OBSTETRICS (FIGO) STAGING OF VAGINAL CANCER	
Stage I	Carcinoma limited to the vaginal wall
Stage II	Carcinoma has involved the subvaginal tissue but has not extended onto the pelvic side wall
Stage III	Carcinoma has extended to the pelvic side wall
Stage IV	Carcinoma has extended beyond the true pelvis or has involved the mucosa of the bladder or rectum
Stage IVa	Spread to bladder or rectum
Stage IVb	Spread to distant organs

irradiation to the pelvis to shrink the primary tumor and treat the pelvic lymph nodes and paravaginal tissues. Brachytherapy is then given, either with intracavitary vaginal applicators or by interstitial techniques. **When the lower third of the vagina is involved, the groin nodes should either be included in the treatment field or surgically removed.**

Radical surgery has a limited role in the management of vaginal cancer. **Radical hysterectomy, partial vaginectomy, and pelvic lymphadenectomy may be performed for early lesions in the posterior fornix.** Surgery should otherwise be reserved for medically fit patients in whom a central recurrence develops after irradiation. Pelvic exenteration with creation of a neovagina may be appropriate in such patients provided there are no lymph node metastases at the time of exploratory laparotomy and adequate surgical margins can be attained.

Prognosis

The overall 5-year survival rate for vaginal cancer is about 50%. When corrected for death from intercurrent disease, 5-year survival rates should be about 85% to 90% for stage I lesions, 55% to 65% for stage II lesions, 30% to 35% for stage III lesions, and 5% to 10% for stage IV lesions.

RARE VAGINAL CANCERS

Adenocarcinoma

Most adenocarcinomas of the vagina are metastatic, usually from the cervix, endometrium, or ovary, but occasionally from more distant sites such as the kidney, breast, or colon. **Most primary vaginal adenocarcinomas are clear cell carcinomas in female offspring of women who ingested diethylstilbestrol (DES) during pregnancy** (see later in this chapter). Primary adenocarcinomas of the vagina not related to DES are rare but may arise in residual glands of müllerian (paramesonephric) origin, Gartner's duct (a remnant of the embryonic wolffian or mesonephric duct), or foci of endometriosis.

Malignant Melanoma

Vaginal melanomas account for fewer than 2% of vaginal malignancies. The mean age at diagnosis is 55 years. The carcinoma usually occurs on the distal anterior wall. **Radical surgery has been the traditional treatment, but comparable local control and overall survival maybe obtained with conservative tumor resection and postoperative radiation therapy.** The use of high-dose fractions (>400 cGy) may be beneficial. The prognosis is poor, with an overall 5-year survival rate of 5% to 10%.

Sarcoma

Vaginal sarcomas are rare. In adults, leiomyosarcomas are most common, whereas **in infants and children, sarcoma botryoides predominates.** The latter term comes from the Greek *botrys* (bunch of grapes), which these lesions usually grossly resemble. The mean age at diagnosis of sarcoma botryoides is 2 to 3 years, with a range of 6 months to 16 years. **Histologically the tumor is an embryonal rhabdomyosarcoma. Treatment consists of conservative surgical resection followed by adjuvant chemotherapy, with or without radiation therapy.**

▪ Diethylstilbestrol Exposure in Utero

In 1971, an association between in utero exposure to DES and the later development of clear cell adenocarcinoma of the vagina was reported. Since that time, numerous non-neoplastic uterine and vaginal anomalies have been reported in young women exposed in utero to DES. **Vaginal adenosis (vaginal columnar epithelium) is the most common anomaly and is present in about 30% of exposed females.** This tissue behaves similarly to the columnar epithelium of the cervix and is replaced initially by immature metaplastic squamous epithelium. With progressive squamous maturation, complete resolution of this anomaly usually occurs.

Structural changes of the cervix and vagina occur in about 25% of exposed females. Possible changes include a transverse vaginal septum, cervical collar, cockscomb (a raised ridge, usually on the anterior cervix), or cervical hypoplasia. Most of these changes tend to disappear as the individual matures. The risk is insignificant if the drug was given after the 22nd week of gestation.

In addition to these changes in the lower genital tract, upper genital tract anomalies occur in at least half of patients and may be associated with exposure later in pregnancy. **The most common abnormalities are a T-shaped uterus and a small uterine cavity** (<2.5 cm in length). Exposed individuals have an increased risk for miscarriage, premature delivery, or ectopic pregnancy, but most are able to deliver a viable infant successfully.

CLEAR CELL ADENOCARCINOMA

The risk for developing a clear cell adenocarcinoma following DES exposure in utero is somewhat less than 1 in 1000. The tumors are rare before age 14 years, and the mean age of patients at diagnosis is about 19 years. A few cases have been reported in women in their 40s and 50s. Not all patients with vaginal clear cell adenocarcinomas give a history of prior DES exposure in utero. **For early tumors, radical hysterectomy and vaginectomy (with creation of a neovagina) or radiation therapy is effective. Overall, the 5-year survival rate is about 80%,** which is considerably better than that for squamous cell cancer of the cervix or vagina.

SUGGESTED READING

Chan JK, Sugiyama V, Pham H, et al: Margin distance and other clinico-pathologic factors in vulvar carcinoma: A multivariate analysis. Gynecol Oncol 104:636-641, 2007.

Hacker NF: Vulvar cancer. *In* Berek JS, Hacker NF (eds): Practical Gynecologic Oncology, 5th ed. Philadelphia, Lippincott Williams & Wilkins, 2009 (in press).

Hakim AA, Terada KY: Sentinel node dissection in vulvar cancer: Current treatment options in oncology. 7:85–91, 2006.

Jones RW, Baranyai J, Stables S: Trends in squamous cell carcinoma of the vulva: The influence of vulvar intraepithelial neoplasia. Obstet Gynecol 90:448-452, 1997.

Landrum LM, Lanneau GS, Skaggs VJ, et al: Gynecologic Oncology Group risk groups for vulvar carcinoma: Improvement in survival in the modern era. Gynecol Oncol 106:521-525, 2007.

Tran PT, Su Z, Lee P, Lavori P, et al: Prognostic factors for outcome and complications for primary squamous cell carcinoma of the vagina treated with radiation. Gynecol Oncol 105:641-649, 2007.

Chapter 41

Uterine Corpus Cancer

NEVILLE F. HACKER

Cancer of the endometrium is the most common gynecologic malignancy in the United States. For 2007, it is estimated that there will be more than 39,000 new cases and 7400 deaths. It is the fourth most common malignancy found in American women after breast, colorectal, and lung cancer and is predominantly a disease of affluent, obese, postmenopausal women of low parity.

▣ *Epidemiology and Etiology*

The median age for endometrial cancer is about 58 years. The risk factors associated with the development of carcinoma of the endometrium are listed in Box 41-1. **Any factor that increases the exposure to unopposed estrogen increases the risk for endometrial cancer.** If the proliferative effects of estrogen are not counteracted by a progestin, endometrial hyperplasia and possibly adenocarcinoma can result.

Obesity results in an increased extraovarian aromatization of androstenedione to estrone. Androstenedione is secreted by the adrenal glands, whereas the increased peripheral conversion occurs predominantly in fat depots but also in the liver, kidneys, and skeletal muscles. **Granulosa-theca cell tumors of the ovary produce estrogen,** and up to 15% of patients with these tumors have an associated endometrial cancer.

Unopposed estrogenic stimulation from anovulatory cycles occurs in patients who have polycystic ovarian syndrome (Stein-Leventhal syndrome) **and in patients with a late menopause.** In postmenopausal women taking estrogen replacement without a progestin for menopausal symptoms, the risk for cancer developing appears to be both dose and duration dependent. This increased risk varies from 2-fold to 14-fold compared with nonusers. The addition of progestin in a cyclic fashion for 10 to 14 days of the month or in a continuous fashion daily throughout the month eliminates this increased risk. **Women taking tamoxifen for breast cancer have a twofold to threefold increased risk for endometrial cancer.** Young women who use oral contraceptives have been shown to have a lower incidence of subsequent endometrial cancer.

About 5% of endometrial cancers occur in women with the hereditary nonpolyposis colon cancer syndrome (HNPCC), which is caused by germ line mutations in the DNA repair genes. Women with the HNPCC syndrome have about a 40% risk for developing endometrial cancer, usually before the menopause.

▣ *Screening of Asymptomatic Women*

Population screening for endometrial cancer is not feasible because there is no simple method of cancer detection available. However, screening may be justified for high-risk women, including those with a family history of HNPCC syndrome, those with polycystic ovarian disease, and any woman with an intact uterus taking unopposed estrogen. **Only about 50% of women with endometrial cancer will have malignant cells on a Papanicolaou smear.**

Since the 1990s, transvaginal ultrasonography has been increasingly used for endometrial evaluation. Almost all women with endometrial hyperplasia or carcinoma will have an endometrial thickness of 5 mm or more. **Tamoxifen produces a confusing ultrasonic image, which leads to frequent false-positive reports.**

▣ *Symptoms*

The most common symptom of endometrial cancer is abnormal vaginal bleeding, which is present in 90% of patients. **Postmenopausal bleeding is**

- Obesity
- Nulliparity
- Late menopause
- Diabetes mellitus
- Hypertension
- Family history of breast, colon, or ovarian cancer (HNPCC syndrome)
- Chronic unopposed estrogen stimulation
- Chronic tamoxifen use

HNPCC—hereditary nonpolyposis colon cancer syndrome.

TABLE 41-1

ETIOLOGY OF POSTMENOPAUSAL BLEEDING

Factor	Approximate Percentage
Exogenous estrogens	30
Atrophic endometritis, vaginitis	30
Endometrial cancer	15
Endometrial or cervical polyps	10
Endometrial hyperplasia	5
Miscellaneous (e.g., cervical cancer, uterine sarcoma, urethral caruncle, trauma)	10

always abnormal and must be investigated. The most common conditions associated with postmenopausal bleeding are listed in Table 41-1. In the premenopausal patient, especially after age 35 years, menorrhagia or intermenstrual bleeding may signal an endometrial malignancy.

Signs

The general physical examination may reveal obesity, hypertension, and the stigmata of diabetes mellitus. Evidence of metastatic disease is unusual at initial presentation, but the chest should be examined for any effusion and the abdomen carefully palpated and percussed to exclude ascites, hepatomegaly, or evidence of upper abdominal masses.

On pelvic examination, the external genitalia are usually normal. The vagina and cervix are also usually normal but should be carefully inspected and palpated for evidence of involvement. **A patulous cervical os or a firm, expanded cervix may indicate extension of disease from the corpus to the cervix.** The uterus may be of normal size or enlarged, depending on the extent of the disease and the presence or absence of other uterine conditions, such as adenomyosis or fibroids. The adnexa should be carefully palpated for evidence of extrauterine metastases or an ovarian neoplasm. **A granulosa cell tumor or an endometrioid ovarian carcinoma may occasionally coexist with endometrial cancer.**

Diagnosis

Any woman who presents with postmenopausal bleeding should have a transvaginal ultrasound. If the endometrial thickness is greater than 5 mm, endometrial evaluation is necessary. Outpatient techniques for endometrial sampling include the use of the Kevorkian curette, Vabra aspirator, Gravlee jet washer, and Pipelle cannula. These techniques have a diagnostic accuracy of about 90%. If the endometrial biopsy reveals endometrial cancer, definitive treatment can be arranged. **If the endometrial biopsy is negative for cancer or reveals endometrial hyperplasia, a hysteroscopy and fractional dilation and curettage should be performed under general anesthesia.** Specimens from the endometrium and endocervix should be submitted separately for histologic evaluation to determine whether the tumor has extended to the endocervix.

In a premenopausal patient with high-risk factors and abnormal uterine bleeding, the endometrium must be sampled. Failure to respond to medical management or a suspicious transvaginal ultrasound is another indication for hysteroscopy and uterine curettage. A grossly obvious lesion of the cervix or vagina should be biopsied directly.

STAGING

The International Federation of Gynecology and Obstetrics (FIGO) changed from a clinical to a surgical staging system for endometrial cancer in 1988. The new surgical staging, based on pathologic confirmation of the extent of spread, is shown in Table 41-2.

Preoperative Investigations

In addition to a thorough physical examination, blood studies should include a complete blood count, determinations of hepatic enzymes, serum electrolytes, blood urea nitrogen, serum creatinine, and a coagulation profile. A routine urinalysis should be performed. The only radiologic study necessary is a chest x-ray. Additional radiographic procedures, including abdominopelvic computed tomography or magnetic resonance imaging, may be performed, particularly for poorly differentiated cancers, to look for metastatic disease.

Pathologic Features

About 75% of endometrial cancers are endometrioid adenocarcinomas. When squamous elements are present, the tumor is called an *adenocarcinoma with*

TABLE 41-2

INTERNATIONAL FEDERATION OF GYNECOLOGY AND OBSTETRICS (FIGO) STAGING OF ENDOMETRIAL CARCINOMA (1988)

Stage Ia	Tumor limited to endometrium
Stage Ib	Invasion through less than half of the myometrium
Stage Ic	Invasion equal to or more than half of the myometrium
Stage IIa	Endocervical glandular involvement only
Stage IIb	Cervical stroma invasion
Stage IIIa	Tumor invades serosa or adnexa or both, or positive peritoneal cytologic findings, or both
Stage IIIb	Vaginal metastases
Stage IIIc	Metastases to pelvic or para-aortic lymph nodes, or both
Stage IVa	Tumor invasion of bladder or bowel mucosa, or both
Stage IVb	Distant metastases including intraabdominal or inguinal lymph nodes, or both

Histologic grade does not change the stage
Grade 1	Well differentiated
Grade 2	Moderately differentiated
Grade 3	Poorly differentiated

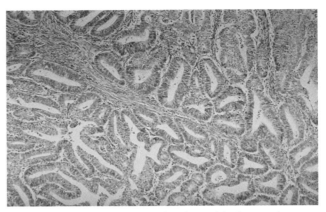

FIGURE 41-1   Well-differentiated endometrial adenocarcinoma (histologic study). Note the back-to-back glands with minimal intervening stroma and the gland-within-gland pattern.

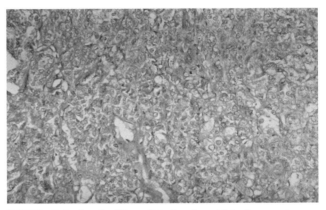

FIGURE 41-2   Poorly differentiated endometrial adenocarcinoma (histologic study). Note the predominantly solid nature of the tumor with minimal gland formation.

squamous differentiation. Such tumors are graded on the glandular component of the lesion. Less often, **clear cell, squamous, or serous carcinomas occur, and all carry a worse prognosis.**

Invasive adenocarcinoma of the endometrium demonstrates proliferative glandular formation with minimal or no intervening stroma. Tumor grade is determined by both the degree of abnormality of the glandular architecture and the degree of nuclear atypia. A lesion that is well differentiated (grade 1) forms a glandular pattern similar to normal endometrial glands (Figure 41-1). A moderately well-differentiated lesion (grade 2) has glandular structures admixed with papillary, and occasionally solid, areas of tumor. In a poorly differentiated lesion (grade 3), the glandular structures have become predominantly solid with a relative paucity of identifiable endometrial glands (Figure 41-2).

▨ *Pattern of Spread*

Endometrial cancer spreads by (1) direct extension, (2) exfoliation of cells that are shed through the fallopian tubes, (3) lymphatic dissemination, and (4) hematogenous dissemination.

The most common route of spread is direct extension of the tumor to adjacent structures. The tumor may invade through the myometrium and eventually penetrate the serosa. It may also grow downward and involve the cervix. Although uncommon, progressive growth may eventually involve the vagina, parametrium, rectum, or bladder.

Exfoliated cells may pass through the fallopian tubes and implant on the ovaries, the visceral or parietal peritoneum, or the omentum.

Lymphatic spread occurs most commonly in patients with deep myometrial penetration. **Spread mainly occurs to the pelvic lymph nodes and subsequently to the para-aortic lymph nodes, although simultaneous spread to both nodal groups may occur.** In stage I endometrial cancer, the overall incidence of pelvic lymph node metastases is about 12%, and para-aortic metastases occur in about 8% of cases. **In patients with deeply invasive, poorly differentiated stage I adenocarcinomas,** however, **pelvic lymph node metastases occur in up to 40%** of cases. Lymphatic spread is also responsible for vaginal vault recurrences.

Hematogenous dissemination is less common, but it results in parenchymal metastases, particularly in the lungs, liver, or both.

■ *Treatment*

STAGE I

Surgery

An exploratory laparotomy with total abdominal hysterectomy and bilateral salpingo-oophorectomy is performed on all patients, unless there are absolute

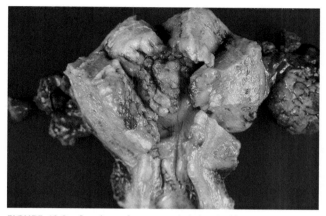

FIGURE 41-3   Specimen from a total abdominal hysterectomy and bilateral salpingo-oophorectomy. The uterus has been opened to reveal an exophytic carcinoma on the posterior wall of the corpus.

medical contraindications (Figure 41-3). On opening the abdomen, peritoneal washings are taken with normal saline for cytologic evaluation. **About 15% of patients with disease confined to the corpus have positive peritoneal cytology.** Retroperitoneal spaces should be opened and evaluated, and any enlarged pelvic or para-aortic lymph nodes should be resected. **Formal surgical staging, including at least pelvic lymphadenectomy, should be performed on high-risk patients, including those with serous, clear cell, or grade 3 histology; outer-half myometrial invasion; or cervical extension.** Laparoscopic surgery, including laparoscopic-assisted vaginal hysterectomy and bilateral salpingo-oophorectomy, with or without laparoscopic lymph node dissection, is being increasingly used, particularly for obese patients, and those with grade 1 or 2 cancers.

Radiation Therapy

With the advent of surgical staging, less reliance has been placed on adjuvant radiation therapy in the management of patients with endometrial cancer.

Recommendations are as follows (Figure 41-4).
1. Patients with grade 1 or 2 endometrioid carcinomas confined to the inner half of the myometrium may be followed **without adjuvant therapy** (i.e., **stage Ia or Ib, grade 1 or 2**).

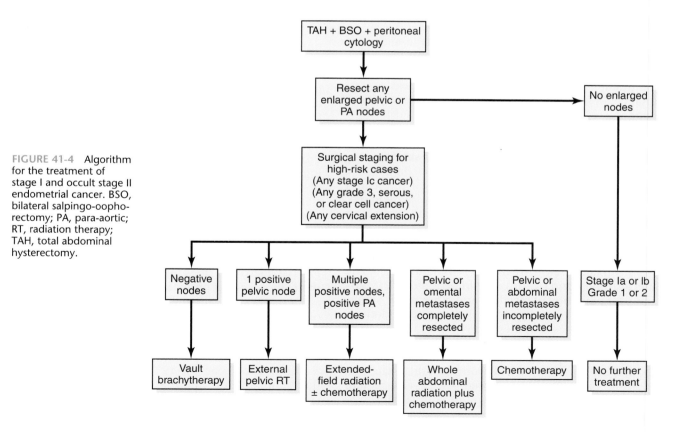

FIGURE 41-4   Algorithm for the treatment of stage I and occult stage II endometrial cancer. BSO, bilateral salpingo-oophorectomy; PA, para-aortic; RT, radiation therapy; TAH, total abdominal hysterectomy.

2. Patients with **high-risk carcinomas with negative pelvic nodes** (i.e., any stage Ic cancer; any grade 3, clear cell, or serous cancer; or any stage II cancer) may have **vault brachytherapy** (without external-beam pelvic radiation).
3. Patients with one positive pelvic node should receive **external pelvic radiation.**
4. Patients with multiple positive pelvic nodes or proven positive para-aortic nodes should receive **extended-field radiation** (i.e., pelvic and para-aortic).
5. For patients with adnexal or omental metastases, chemotherapy with carboplatin and paclitaxel (Taxol) should be given.

In patients medically unfit for surgery, radiation therapy alone may be employed. A combination of intracavitary plus external-beam radiation is used. The overall 5-year survival rate is about 20% lower than for patients treated with hysterectomy.

Hormonal Therapy

Endometrial cancer occasionally occurs **in women younger than 40 years**. These tumors are usually early-stage and low-grade, and there is frequently a desire to preserve fertility. **High-dose medroxyprogesterone acetate** (200 mg twice daily) **for 3 to 6 months will reverse the changes in about two thirds of patients**, but recurrences are common, so careful monitoring is essential.

STAGE II

If the cervix is grossly normal and involvement is detected only on the histologic evaluation of the endocervical curettage material (occult stage II disease), treatment may be the same as for stage I disease (i.e., total abdominal hysterectomy, bilateral salpingo-oophorectomy, surgical staging, and tailored postoperative radiotherapy).

Alternatively, regardless of the size of the cervix, primary radical hysterectomy, bilateral salpingo-oophorectomy, together with pelvic and para-aortic lymphadenectomy, may be performed. If the lymph nodes are negative, no brachytherapy is required. If positive, postoperative external-beam pelvic or extended-field radiation is required.

ADVANCED STAGES

For advanced disease, treatment is individualized. The uterus, tubes, and ovaries should be removed, if possible, for palliation of bleeding and other pelvic symptoms. If gross disease is present in the upper abdomen, tumor metastases that are readily removable, such as an omental "cake," should be extirpated in an attempt to improve the patient's quality of life by temporarily decreasing abdominal discomfort and ascites. In addition, patients with advanced disease also require chemotherapy, radiation therapy, or both, as shown in Figure 41-4.

Chemotherapy

There is increasing evidence for the use of chemotherapy in patients with advanced endometrial cancer. The combination of cisplatin and doxorubicin has been studied recently and may be used alone or in combination with radiation therapy, as shown in Figure 41-4.

RECURRENT DISEASE

Seventy-five percent of recurrences develop within 2 years of treatment. If recurrent disease is detected, the patient should undergo a complete physical examination and metastatic workup. Careful follow-up is particularly important for patients treated without adjuvant therapy. Most recurrences in these patients are at the vaginal vault, and 70% to 80% of isolated vault recurrences can be salvaged by radiation therapy.

Metastases in other sites, such as the upper abdomen, lungs, or liver, are treated initially with high-dose progestins or antiestrogens. About one third of recurrent endometrial carcinomas contain estrogen and progesterone receptors, with the more well-differentiated tumors more likely to contain such receptors. As with breast cancer, the likelihood of a patient responding to progestin treatment is increased in patients whose tumor contains estrogen and progesterone receptors. About 80% of such patients respond to progestin therapy, compared with fewer than 10% of patients whose tumor is receptor negative.

Medroxyprogesterone acetate (Provera, 50 mg 3 times daily; Depo-Provera, 400 mg intramuscularly weekly) or megestrol acetate (Megace), 80 mg twice daily, may be given. **If disease progresses while the patient is receiving progestins, chemotherapy may be offered.** The combination of carboplatin and paclitaxel (Taxol) gives a response rate of about 50%.

Prognosis

Prognosis is dependent on several variables, including uterine size, histologic type, grade of tumor, depth of myometrial penetration, status of lymph nodes, status of peritoneal cytologic features, and presence or absence of occult adnexal or upper abdominal metastases. **Serous and clear cell endometrial carcinomas have a particularly bad prognosis, and both of these histologic types are prone to early dissemination. Five-year survival rates for these tumor types are less than 50%, even for patients with stage I disease.**

Five-year survival rates for each stage of endometrioid endometrial cancer are presented in Table 41-3.

Follow-Up

Follow-up examinations should be performed every 3 months for 2 years, every 6 months for 3 years, and then annually. It is important to take a vault Papanicolaou smear on patients who have not had radiation therapy.

TABLE 41-3

SURVIVAL FOR ENDOMETRIAL CANCER BY FIGO STAGE (N = 5694)		
Stage	No. of Patients	Five-Year Survival (%)
Ia	1063	91.1
Ib	2735	89.7
Ic	1219	81.3
IIa	364	78.7
IIb	426	71.4
IIIa	484	60.4
IIIb	73	30.2
IIIc	293	52.1
IVa	47	14.6
IVb	160	17.0

Data from the Annual Report on the Results of Treatment in Gynecological Cancer. Patients treated 1996-1998. J Epidemiol Biostat 83:79-118, 2003.

TABLE 41-4

CLASSIFICATION OF UTERINE SARCOMAS		
Type	Homologous	Heterologous
Pure	Leiomyosarcoma Endometrial stromal sarcoma Endometrial sarcoma	Rhabdomyosarcoma Chondrosarcoma Osteosarcoma Liposarcoma
Mixed	Carcinosarcoma	Malignant mixed mesodermal tumor

◼ Uterine Sarcomas

Uterine sarcomas account for about 3% of uterine cancers. They arise from the stromal components of the uterus, either the endometrial stroma or the mesenchymal and myometrial tissues. As a group, sarcomas tend to be more advanced at the time of diagnosis, are more likely to disseminate hematogenously, and have much lower 2- and 5-year survival rates.

CLASSIFICATION

A classification system for uterine sarcomas is presented in Table 41-4.

Uterine sarcomas can be classified as either *pure,* **in which the only malignant tissue is of mesenchymal origin, or mixed, in which malignant mesenchymal and malignant epithelial tissues are present. They may also be classified as homologous,** implying that the tissue that is malignant is normally present in the uterus (e.g., endometrial stroma, smooth muscle), **or heterologous,** implying that the tissue that is malignant is not normally present in the uterus (e.g., bone or cartilage). Most pure uterine sarcomas are leiomyosarcomas and endometrial stromal sarcomas.

LEIOMYOSARCOMA

Leiomyosarcomas may be associated with a benign leiomyoma of the uterus, but the risk for malignant transformation in a benign fibroid is less than 1%. **The histologic criteria for distinguishing leiomyosarcomas from leiomyomas are the mitotic count (usually greater than 10 per 10 high-power fields), the presence or absence of coagulative necrosis, and the presence or absence of cellular atypia.**

Clinically, the mean age of patients with leiomyosarcoma is about 55 years. Patients with this disease may present with pelvic pain, abnormal uterine bleeding, or a pelvic or lower abdominal mass. A sensation of pressure on the bladder or rectum may also be noted.

Most cases are not diagnosed preoperatively but are discovered at the time of exploratory surgery for a probable fibroid. Curettings are usually normal. **If a known fibroid uterus appears to be rapidly enlarging, especially postmenopausally, malignancy should be suspected.**

The treatment of a uterine leiomyosarcoma consists of total abdominal hysterectomy and bilateral salpingo-oophorectomy. Adjuvant pelvic radiation appears to decrease local pelvic recurrence but does not prolong survival because most patients die with distant metastases.

Response rates to chemotherapy are very low.

ENDOMETRIAL STROMAL TUMORS

The three types of stromal tumors are (1) endometrial stromal nodule; (2) endometrial stromal sarcoma, previously known as endolymphatic stromal myosis; and (3) high-grade endometrial sarcoma. The first of these, **the stromal nodule, is a rare benign condition.** There are typically three or fewer mitoses per 10 high-power fields. A hysterectomy is curative.

Endometrial stromal sarcoma is a low-grade lesion. Histologically, there is minimal to no cellular atypia, with usually fewer than five mitoses per 10 high-power fields. There is always evidence of vascular channel invasion. These patients usually present with abnormal vaginal bleeding and often with pelvic pain.

Most patients are cured with total abdominal hysterectomy and bilateral salpingo-oophorectomy. Local and distant recurrences may occur even 10 to 20 years later and require reexploration and resection of disease. Prolonged survival is possible after resection of recurrent disease, and response to progestins is good. Pelvic disease may respond to radiation therapy.

High-grade endometrial sarcoma generally causes abnormal uterine bleeding, and more than half of patients are premenopausal. **The diagnosis can often be**

made by endometrial biopsy or uterine curettage. Histologically, there are 10 or more mitoses per 10 high-power fields, and the lesion is composed of very poorly differentiated cells. Aggressive myometrial invasion occurs, and hematogenous spread is common at the time of diagnosis.

The treatment of high-grade endometrial sarcoma is total abdominal hysterectomy and bilateral salpingo-oophorectomy. A thorough exploration of the peritoneal cavity and retroperitoneum should be made for evidence of metastases. **Postoperative pelvic irradiation improves local control but does not improve survival.** In patients with metastatic disease, progestogens or chemotherapy may be offered. The best chemotherapeutic agents are cisplatin, doxorubicin, and ifosfamide, but the prognosis is poor.

MALIGNANT MIXED MESODERMAL TUMORS

Malignant mixed mesodermal tumors or carcinosarcomas account for about 40% of uterine sarcomas. Most patients are postmenopausal and present with vaginal bleeding or discharge. About one third of patients have tumor growing through the cervix into the vagina as a polypoid mass. **Up to 50% of patients with this lesion have evidence of metastatic disease at the time of diagnosis if surgically staged.** The tumors aggressively invade the myometrium and disseminate through the lymphatics and the bloodstream.

The primary treatment of malignant mixed mesodermal tumors or carcinosarcomas is total abdominal hysterectomy, bilateral salpingo-oophorectomy, and surgical staging. Patients with negative nodes should receive vault brachytherapy, and patients with positive nodes should receive external-beam pelvic or extended-field radiation. Adjuvant chemotherapy may improve the prognosis.

Prognosis

The prognosis for uterine leiomyosarcomas and endometrial sarcomas is poor because of the propensity for hematogenous dissemination. The overall 5-year survival rate is about 35%. Patients with endometrial stromal sarcomas have a good prognosis, whereas patients with stage I or II carcinosarcomas have a 5-year survival of about 70% if treated with surgical staging and adjuvant radiation and chemotherapy.

SUGGESTED READING

Aalders JG, Thomas G: Endometrial cancer—revisiting the importance of pelvic and paraaortic lymph nodes. Gynecol Oncol 104:222-231, 2007.

Hacker NF: Endometrial cancer. In Berek JS, Hacker NF (eds): Practical Gynecologic Oncology, 5th ed. Philadelphia, Lippincott Williams & Wilkins, 2009 (in press).

Leath CA III, Huh WK, Hyde J, et al: A multi-institutional review of outcomes of endometrial stromal sarcoma. Gynecol Oncol 105:630-634, 2007.

Lee NK, Cheung MK, Shin JY, et al: Prognostic factors for uterine cancer in reproductive-aged women. Obstet Gynecol 109:655-662, 2007.

Parazzini F, La Vecchi C, Bocciolone L, Franceschi S: The epidemiology of endometrial cancer. Gynecol Oncol 41:1-16, 1991.

Prat J, Gallardo A, Cuatrecasas M, Catasus L: Endometrial carcinoma: Pathology and genetics. Pathology 39:1-7, 2007.

Secord AA, Havrilesky LJ, Bae-Jump V, et al: The role of multimodality adjuvant chemotherapy and radiation in women with advanced stage endometrial cancer. Gynecol Oncol 107:285-291, 2007.

Chapter 42

Gestational Trophoblastic Neoplasia

JONATHAN S. BEREK

Gestational trophoblastic neoplasia (GTN) represents a unique spectrum of diseases that includes benign hydatidiform mole; invasive mole (chorioadenoma destruens), which can metastasize; and the frankly malignant variety, choriocarcinoma. Most molar pregnancies are sporadic, but a familial syndrome of recurrent hydatidiform mole has been described. Future research should lead to identification of the genetic defect responsible for this uncommon syndrome.

Most patients (80% to 90%) with GTN follow a benign course, with their disease remitting spontaneously. Most patients with metastatic disease can be effectively cured with chemotherapy. This diverse group of diseases has a sensitive tumor marker, human chorionic gonadotropin (hCG), which is secreted by all these tumors and allows accurate follow-up and assessment of the disease.

▇ Epidemiology and Etiology

The incidence of molar pregnancy is about 1 in every 1500 to 2000 pregnancies among whites in the United States. There is a much higher incidence among Asian women in the United States (1 in 800) and an even higher incidence among women in Asia, for example, Taiwan (1 in every 125 to 200 pregnancies). **The risk for the development of a second molar pregnancy is 1% to 3%,** or as much as 40 times greater than the risk for developing the first molar pregnancy.

Although the cause of GTN is unknown, it is **known to occur more frequently in women younger than 20 years and in those older than 40 years.** It appears that GTN may result from defective fertilization, a process that is more common in both younger and older individuals. Diet may play a causative role. **The incidence of molar pregnancy has been noted to be** higher in geographic areas where people consume less β-carotene (a retinoid) and folic acid.

▇ Genetics of Gestational Trophoblastic Disease

The cytogenetic analysis of tissue obtained from molar pregnancies offers some clue to the genesis of these lesions. Figure 42-1 illustrates the genetic composition of molar pregnancies.

COMPLETE MOLE

Most hydatidiform moles are "complete" moles and have a 46 XX karyotype. Specialized studies indicate that both of the X chromosomes are paternally derived. This androgenic origin probably results from fertilization of an "empty egg" (i.e., an egg without chromosomes) by a haploid sperm (23 X), which then duplicates to restore the diploid chromosomal complement (46 XX). Only a small percentage of lesions are 46 XY. **Complete molar pregnancy is only rarely associated with a fetus, and this may represent a form of twinning.**

PARTIAL MOLE

In the "incomplete" or partial mole, the karyotype is usually a triploid, often 69 XXY (80%). Most of the remaining lesions are 69 XXX or 69 XYY. Occasionally mosaic patterns occur. **These lesions, unlike complete moles, often present with a coexistent fetus.** The fetus usually has a triploid karyotype and is defective.

CHORIOCARCINOMA

Genetic analysis of choriocarcinomas usually reveals aneuploidy or polyploidy, typical for anaplastic carcinomas.

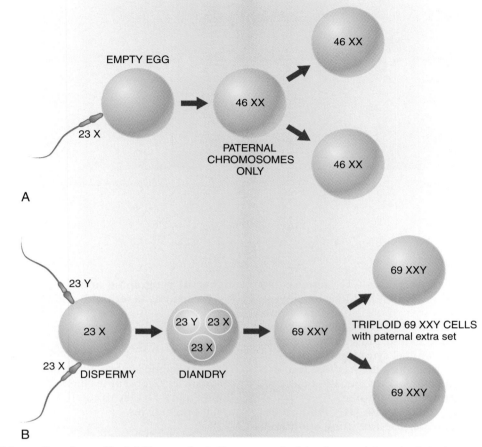

FIGURE 42-1 Cytogenetic makeup of hydatidiform mole. **A:** Chromosomal origin of a complete mole. A single sperm fertilizes an "empty egg." Reduplication of its 23 X set gives a completely homozygous diploid genome of 46 XX. A similar result follows fertilization of an empty egg by two sperms with two independently drawn sets of 23 X or 23 Y; note that both karyotypes, 46 XX and 46 XY, can ensue. **B:** Chromosomal origin of the triploid, partial mole. A normal egg with a 23 X haploid set is fertilized by two sperms that can carry either sex chromosome to give a total of 69 chromosomes with a sex chromosome configuration of XXY, XXX, or XYY. A similar result can be obtained by fertilization with a sperm carrying the unreduced paternal genome 46 XY (resulting sex complement, XXY only). *(Adapted from Szulman AE: Syndromes of hydatidiform moles: Partial vs. complete. J Reprod Med 29:789-790, 1984.)*

▓ *Classification*

The term *gestational trophoblastic neoplasia* is of clinical value because often the diagnosis is made and therapy instituted without definitive knowledge of the precise histologic pattern. GTN may be benign or malignant and nonmetastatic or metastatic (Box 42-1).

The benign form of GTN is called hydatidiform mole. Although this entity is usually confined to the uterine cavity, trophoblastic tissue can occasionally embolize to the lungs. **The malignant forms of GTN are invasive mole and choriocarcinoma. Invasive mole is usually a locally invasive lesion,** although it can be associated with metastases. This lesion accounts for most patients who have persistent hCG titers following molar evacuation. **Choriocarcinoma is the frankly malignant form of GTN.**

Metastatic GTN can be subdivided into good prognosis and poor prognosis groups, depending on the sites of metastases and other clinical variables (Box 42-2).

▓ *Pathologic Features*

Grossly, a hydatidiform mole appears as multiple vesicles that have been classically described as a "bunch of grapes" (Figure 42-2). **The characteristic histopathologic findings associated with a complete molar pregnancy are (1) hydropic villi, (2) absence of fetal blood vessels, and (3) hyperplasia of trophoblastic tissue** (Figure 42-3). Invasive mole differs from hydatidiform mole only in its propensity to invade locally and to metastasize.

BOX 42-1 *Classification of Gestational Trophoblastic Neoplasia*

Benign

Hydatidiform mole
* Complete mole
* Incomplete ("partial") mole

Malignant

Invasive mole ("chorioadenoma destruens")
Choriocarcinoma
Malignant gestational trophoblastic disease may be:
* Nonmetastatic
* Metastatic
  Good prognosis
  Poor prognosis

BOX 42-2 *Clinical Features of Metastatic Gestational Neoplasia with a Poor Prognosis*

* Urinary hCG level > 100,000 IU/24 hr, or serum hCG level > 40,000 IU
* Disease presents more than 4 mo from the antecedent pregnancy
* Metastasis to the brain or liver (regardless of hCG titer or duration of disease)
* Prior failure to respond to single-agent chemotherapy
* Choriocarcinoma after a full-term delivery

hCG, human chorionic gonadotropin.

A partial mole has some hydropic villi, whereas other villi are essentially normal. Fetal vessels are seen in a partial mole, and the trophoblastic tissue exhibits less striking hyperplasia.

Choriocarcinoma in the uterus appears grossly as a vascular-appearing, irregular, and "beefy" tumor, often growing through the uterine wall. Metastatic lesions appear hemorrhagic and have the consistency of currant jelly. **Histologically, choriocarcinoma consists of sheets of malignant cytotrophoblast and syncytiotrophoblast with no identifiable villi.**

▌ *Hydatidiform Mole*

SYMPTOMS

Most patients with hydatidiform mole present with irregular or heavy vaginal bleeding during the first or early second trimester of pregnancy (Box 42-3). The bleeding is usually painless, although it can be associated with uterine contractions. In addition, **the patient may expel molar "vesicles" from the vagina and occasionally may have excessive nausea, even hyperemesis gravidarum.** Irritability, dizziness, and photophobia may occur because **some patients experience preeclampsia. Patients may occasionally exhibit symptoms**

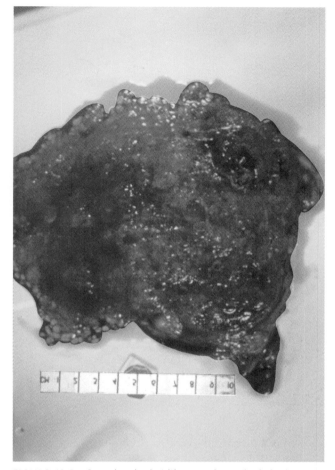

FIGURE 42-2 Complete hydatidiform mole. Multiple hydropic villi (vesicles), resembling a bunch of grapes, are admixed with areas of necrosis *(white areas)* and hemorrhage. Note the absence of a fetus.

relating to hyperthyroidism, such as nervousness, anorexia, and tremors.

SIGNS

The patient's vital signs may reveal tachycardia, tachypnea, and hypertension, reflecting the presence of preeclampsia or clinical hyperthyroidism. Funduscopic examination may show arteriolar spasm. In the rare case of trophoblastic emboli to the pulmonary system, wheezing and rhonchi may be noted on chest examination. Abdominal examination may reveal an enlarged uterus. **Auscultation of the uterus is typically remarkable for the absence of fetal heart sounds.**

On pelvic examination, the grape-like vesicles of the mole may be detected in the vagina. Blood clots may be present. **About half of patients with molar pregnancy present with a uterus that is bigger than expected based on their last menstrual period,** whereas about

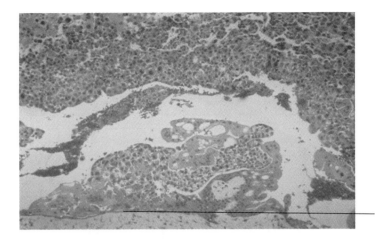

FIGURE 42-3 Histologic appearance of a complete hydatidiform mole. Note the marked trophoblastic proliferation.

— Edge of chorionic villus

BOX 42-3 *Diagnosis of Hydatidiform Mole*

Clinical Data
- Bleeding in the first half of pregnancy
- Lower abdominal pain
- Toxemia before 24 weeks' gestation
- Hyperemesis gravidarum
- Uterus "large for dates" (only 50% of cases)
- Absent fetal heart tones and fetal parts
- Expulsion of vesicles

Diagnostic Studies
- Ultrasonography
- Chest film
- Serum β-human chorionic gonadotropin higher than normal pregnancy values

one fourth have a size compatible with or smaller than gestational age. **Ovarian enlargement by theca-lutein cysts occurs in about one third of women with molar pregnancies.** This may be difficult to detect until the uterus has been evacuated.

DIAGNOSIS

The β-hCG titers can be high for early pregnancy. This should alert the physician that the patient might have GTN or a multiple gestation. The condition must also be distinguished from a threatened spontaneous abortion or an ectopic pregnancy.

Definitive diagnosis of hydatidiform mole can usually be made ultrasonographically. Ultrasonography is noninvasive and reveals a "snowstorm" pattern that is diagnostic.

CLINICAL INVESTIGATIONS

Patients who have the presumptive or definitive diagnosis of hydatidiform mole should have a complete blood count obtained to exclude anemia, which

might require a transfusion. They require an assessment of the platelet count, prothrombin time, partial thromboplastin time, and a fibrinogen level because an occasional patient may experience disseminated intravascular coagulation. Liver and renal function tests should be performed. Blood should be typed and crossmatched in the event that excessive bleeding is encountered at the time of evacuation of the mole. A chest film should be obtained, as should an electrocardiogram if tachycardia is present or if the patient is older than 40 years.

STAGING

The International Federation of Gynecology and Obstetrics (FIGO) staging system for gestational trophoblastic tumors is shown in Table 42-1.

Stage I: Patients with persistently elevated hCG levels and tumor confined to the uterine corpus

Stage II: Patients with metastases to the vagina, pelvis, or both

Stage III: Patients with pulmonary metastases with or without uterine, vaginal, or pelvic involvement. The diagnosis is based on a rising hCG level in the presence of pulmonary lesions on chest film.

Stage IV: Patients with advanced disease and involvement of the brain (Figure 42-4), **liver, kidneys, or gastrointestinal tract.** These patients are in the highest risk category because their disease is most likely to be resistant to chemotherapy. The histologic pattern of choriocarcinoma is usually present, and disease commonly follows a nonmolar pregnancy.

TREATMENT

Evacuation

The standard therapy for hydatidiform mole is suction evacuation followed by sharp curettage of the uterine cavity, regardless of the duration of pregnancy.

TABLE 42-1

INTERNATIONAL FEDERATION OF GYNECOLOGY AND OBSTETRICS (FIGO) STAGING OF GESTATIONAL TROPHOBLASTIC NEOPLASIA

Stage I	Disease confined to uterus
Stage Ia	Disease confined to uterus with no risk factors
Stage Ib	Disease confined to uterus with one risk factor
Stage Ic	Disease confined to uterus with two risk factors
Stage II	Gestational trophoblastic tumor extending outside uterus but limited to genital structures (adnexa, vagina, broad ligament)
Stage IIa	Gestational trophoblastic tumor involving genital structures without risk factors
Stage IIb	Gestational trophoblastic tumor extending outside uterus but limited to genital structures with one risk factor
Stage IIc	Gestational trophoblastic tumor extending outside uterus but limited to genital structures with two risk factors
Stage III	Gestational trophoblastic disease extending to lungs with or without known genital tract involvement
Stage IIIa	Gestational trophoblastic tumor extending to lungs with or without genital tract involvement and with no risk factors
Stage IIIb	Gestational trophoblastic tumor extending to lungs with or without genital tract involvement and with one risk factor
Stage IIIc	Gestational trophoblastic tumor extending to lungs with or without genital tract involvement and with two risk factors
Stage IV	All other metastatic sites
Stage IVa	All other metastatic sites without risk factors
Stage IVb	All other metastatic sites with one risk factor
Stage IVc	All other metastatic sites with two risk factors

Risk factors affecting staging include the following: (1) human chorionic gonadotropin greater than 100,000 IU/mL and (2) duration of disease longer than 6 months from termination of antecedent pregnancy. The following factors should be considered and noted in reporting: (1) prior chemotherapy has been given for known gestational trophoblastic tumor, (2) placental-site tumors should be reported separately, (3) histologic verification of disease is not required.

This should be performed in the operating room with general or regional anesthesia. **Intravenous oxytocin is given simultaneously to help stimulate uterine contractions and reduce blood loss.** This technique is associated with a low incidence of uterine perforation and trophoblastic embolization.

Most patients have an uncomplicated course in the immediate postoperative period. Some require transfusion, however, because of excessive blood loss. Abnormal clotting parameters should be treated with fresh frozen plasma and platelet transfusions, as indicated. Rarely, a patient can experience acute respiratory distress from trophoblastic embolization or fluid overload. Such patients may require respiratory support through a ventilator and careful cardiopulmonary monitoring.

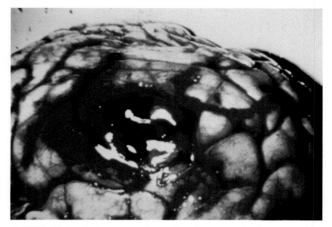

FIGURE 42-4 Autopsy specimen showing a cerebral metastasis from choriocarcinoma. Brain metastases carry a high mortality.

Monitoring Levels of the β Subunit of Human Chorionic Gonadotropin

After the evacuation of a hydatidiform mole, the patient must be monitored with weekly serum assays of β-hCG. Because the titers drop to a low level, a nonspecific pregnancy test cannot be used because of the possibility of cross-reactivity with luteinizing hormone. The radioimmunoassay, sensitive to levels of 1 to 5 mIU/mL, should be used. There are currently several reference standards used to measure hCG in serum, each with its own scale. It is very important, therefore, either to use the same standard each time for measurement or to accurately adjust for any differences between reference standards before making any comparisons between test results. Following the evacuation, the β-hCG levels should steadily decline to undetectable levels, usually within 12 to 16 weeks. A normal regression curve for β-hCG levels following evacuation of a molar pregnancy is shown in Figure 42-5.

Chemotherapy

Prophylactic chemotherapy is not indicated in patients with molar pregnancy because 90% of these individuals have spontaneous remissions. If the β-hCG levels plateau or rise at any time, chemotherapy should be initiated. This is discussed later in this chapter.

■ *Partial Mole*

The incomplete or partial mole is usually associated with a developing fetus. **Patients with a partial mole display most of the pathologic and clinical features of patients with a complete mole, although usually in a less severe form.** Partial moles are usually diagnosed later than are complete moles and generally present as a spontaneous or missed abortion.

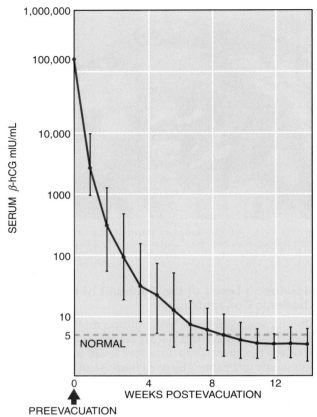

FIGURE 42-5 Normal regression curve of β-human chorionic gonadotropin after molar evacuation. *(Adapted from Morrow CP, Nakamura R, Schaerth J, et al: Clinical and laboratory correlates of molar pregnancy and trophoblastic disease. Am J Obstet Gynecol 128:428, 1977.)*

It is unusual for a partial mole to be detected before the spontaneous termination of a pregnancy. **Ultrasonography performed for other indications may indicate possible molar degeneration of the placenta associated with the developing fetus. Under these circumstances, an amniocentesis should be performed to determine whether the karyotype of the coexisting fetus is normal.**

Uterine enlargement is much less common; **most patients with partial moles are** actually "**small for dates.**" When preeclampsia occurs with a partial mole, it may be severe, but the condition usually occurs between 17 and 22 weeks, about 1 month later than with a complete mole. The most striking difference between partial and complete moles is related to the malignant potential of the two lesions. **Partial moles rarely metastasize, and only rarely is there the need for chemotherapy because of β-hCG levels that have plateaued or risen.**

Invasive Mole

Invasive mole is usually a locally invasive tumor. It constitutes about 5% to 10% of all molar pregnancies, representing most of those with persistent β-hCG levels after molar evacuation. The lesion may penetrate the entire myometrium, rupture through the uterus, and result in hemorrhage into the broad ligament or peritoneal cavity. **Rarely, invasive mole is associated with metastases, particularly to the vagina or lungs, although brain metastases have been documented.**

Histologic confirmation of invasive mole is almost always made at the time of hysterectomy. The latter is usually performed in patients with persistent β-hCG levels following evacuation of a molar pregnancy or in patients with persistent titers despite chemotherapy who have no evidence of metastatic disease. The hysterectomy is usually curative.

PLACENTAL-SITE TROPHOBLASTIC TUMOR

Placental-site trophoblastic tumor is an uncommon but important variant of GTN that consists predominantly of intermediate trophoblast and a few syncytial elements. These tumors produce small amounts of hCG and human placental lactogen relative to their mass, tend to remain confined to the uterus, and metastasize late in their course. In contrast to other trophoblastic tumors, placental-site tumors are relatively insensitive to chemotherapy, so surgical resection of disease is important.

Choriocarcinoma

The frankly malignant form of GTN is choriocarcinoma. **About one half of patients with gestational choriocarcinoma have had a preceding molar pregnancy. In the remaining patients, the disease is preceded by a spontaneous or induced abortion, ectopic pregnancy, or normal pregnancy.** Trophoblastic disease following a normal pregnancy is always choriocarcinoma. The tumor has a tendency to disseminate hematogenously, particularly to the lungs, vagina, brain, liver, kidneys, and gastrointestinal tract.

SYMPTOMS

Most patients with choriocarcinoma present with symptoms of metastatic disease. Vaginal bleeding is a common symptom of uterine choriocarcinoma or vaginal metastasis. Because of the gonadotropin excretion, amenorrhea may develop, simulating early pregnancy. **Hemoptysis, cough, or dyspnea** may occur as a result of lung metastasis. In the presence of central nervous system metastases, the patient may complain of **headaches, dizzy spells, "blacking out,"** or other symptoms referable to a space-occupying lesion in the brain.

Rectal bleeding or dark stools could represent disease that has metastasized to the gastrointestinal tract.

SIGNS

The signs, like the symptoms, are common to many pathologic entities.

Uterine enlargement may be present, with blood coming through the os, as seen on examination with a speculum. A tumor metastatic to the vagina may present with a firm, discolored mass. Occasionally, the patient presents with an **acute abdomen because of rupture of the uterus, liver, or theca-lutein cyst. Neurologic signs,** such as partial weakness or paralysis, dysphasia, aphasia, or unreactive pupils, indicate probable central nervous system involvement.

DIAGNOSIS

Choriocarcinoma is a great imitator of other diseases, so unless it follows a molar pregnancy, it may not be suspected. **In females of reproductive age, a β-hCG measurement to screen for choriocarcinoma should be performed when any unusual symptoms or signs develop.**

INVESTIGATIONS

If the β-hCG level is elevated, the workup of a patient with choriocarcinoma is the same as that for patients with hydatidiform mole, but it should also include computed tomography (CT) scans of the abdomen, pelvis, and head. In addition, a lumbar puncture should be performed if the CT scan of the brain is normal because simultaneous evaluation of the β-hCG level in the cerebrospinal fluid and serum may allow detection of early cerebral metastases. **Because the β subunit does not readily cross the blood-brain barrier, a ratio of serum to cerebrospinal fluid β-hCG levels of less than 40:1 suggests central nervous system involvement,** with secretion of the β-hCG directly into the cerebrospinal fluid.

Treatment of Gestational Trophoblastic Neoplasia

An approach to treatment of GTN with nonmetastatic disease (good prognosis) and metastatic disease (poor prognosis) follows.

NONMETASTATIC AND METASTATIC GESTATIONAL TROPHOBLASTIC NEOPLASIA WITH A GOOD PROGNOSIS

The chemotherapy most often employed is either methotrexate or actinomycin D (Box 42-4). Methotrexate is usually given as a daily dose for 5 consecutive days or every other day for 8 days, alternating with folinic acid (leucovorin). This folinic acid "rescue" regimen is associated with significantly less bone marrow,

---

BOX 42-4 *Single-Agent Chemotherapy for Molar Pregnancy*

Actinomycin D Treatment

Five-Day Actinomycin D

Actinomycin D, 12 μg/kg IV daily for 5 days
CBC, platelet count, SGOT determination daily
With response, re-treat at the same dose
Without response, add 2 μg/kg to the initial dose or switch to methotrexate protocol

Pulse Actinomycin D

Actinomycin D, 1.25 mg/m² every 2 wk

Methotrexate Treatment

5-Day Methotrexate

Methotrexate, 0.4 mg/kg IV or IM daily for 5 days
CBC, platelet count daily
With response, re-treat at the same dose
Without response, increase dose to 0.6 mg/kg or switch to actinomycin D protocol

Pulse Methotrexate

Methotrexate 40 mg/m² IM weekly

Protocol for Methotrexate with Folinic Acid "Rescue"

Methotrexate, 1 mg/kg/day IM or IV on days 1, 3, 5, 7 followed 24 hr later by 0.1 mg/kg/day of folinic acid "rescue" on days 2, 4, 6, and 8

CBC, complete blood count; IM, intramuscularly; IV, intravenously; SGOT, serum glutamic oxaloacetic transaminase.

---

gastrointestinal, and liver toxicity. Actinomycin D is given for 5 consecutive days intravenously or every other week as a single dose.

In appropriately selected patients, hysterectomy may be the primary therapy for hydatidiform mole. Women older than 40 years have an increased incidence of choriocarcinoma after molar pregnancy. These patients may decrease their risk for malignant sequelae by undergoing hysterectomy.

METASTATIC GESTATIONAL TROPHOBLASTIC NEOPLASIA WITH A POOR PROGNOSIS

For patients with disease having a poor prognosis, combination chemotherapy is always used. Regimens that have been successfully employed include **methotrexate, actinomycin D, and cyclophosphamide (MAC),** or the **modified Bagshawe regimen (EMA-CO),** which is a six-drug chemotherapy regimen. The drugs used include etoposide (VP-16), actinomycin D, vincristine, cyclophosphamide, methotrexate, and folinic acid. For patients whose disease fails to improve with these agents, combinations of cisplatin and etoposide or vinblastine, with or without bleomycin, have been used.

In patients with disease metastatic to the brain or liver, radiation is often employed to these areas in conjunction with chemotherapy. The whole brain tolerates an initial dose of 2000 to 3000 cGy, with fractions of about 200 cGy per day. Together with systemic chemotherapy, a 50% cure rate can be expected. Liver metastases are usually treated with about 2000 cGy.

Surgery plays a role in selected cases, especially hysterectomy and pulmonary resection for chemotherapy-resistant disease.

FOLLOW-UP STUDIES

Following three normal β-hCG levels, patients with a good prognosis should be followed with monthly levels for 1 year. Patients with a poor prognosis should have monthly titer determinations for 2 years or more. Thereafter, levels should be checked every 3 months until 5 years have elapsed. **Patients should be advised to not become pregnant again within the first 9 to 12 months after molar evacuation and should be given a reliable contraceptive.** If a patient's levels become normal and later are found to be rising, a second metastatic workup must be undertaken before the initiation of secondary therapy.

PROGNOSIS

About 95% to 100% of patients with GTN having a good prognosis are cured of their disease. Patients with poor prognostic features can be expected to be cured in only 50% to 70% of cases. **Most patients who die have brain or liver metastases.**

SUGGESTED READING

El-Helw LM, Hancock BW: Treatment of gestational trophoblastic neoplasia (Review). Lancet Oncol 8:715-724, 2007.

Garner EI, Goldstein DP, Feltmate CM, Berkowitz RS: Gestational trophoblastic disease. Clin Obstet Gynecol 50:112-122, 2007.

Lurian JR, Singh DK, Schink JC: Role of surgery in the management of high-risk gestational trophoblastic neoplasia. J Reprod Med 51:773-776, 2006.

Ngan S, Seckl MJ: Gestational trophoblastic neoplasia management: An update (Review). Curr Opin Oncol 19:486-491, 2007.

Soper JT, Spillman M, Sampson JH, et al: High-risk gestational neoplasia with brain metastases: Individualized multidisciplinary therapy in the management of four patients. Gynecol Oncol 104:691-694, 2007.

Index

A

Abdominal examination, 16, 16f
  in chronic pelvic pain, 260
Abdominal mass, palpation of, 16
Abdominal pain
  abruptio placentae with, 130
  ectopic pregnancy with, 291-292
  gynecologic causes of, 15
  uterine rupture with, 131
Abdominal pregnancy, 290, 291f, 297
Abdominal trauma, during pregnancy, 217
  Rh sensitization and, 196
Abdominal wall
  anatomy of, 31-32, 32f
  incisions in, 31-33, 33f
  myofascial trigger points in, 260-261,
    264, 264f
Abnormal uterine bleeding (AUB)
  hysteroscopic evaluation of, 337
  nondysfunctional causes of, 369, 369b
  patterns of, 368, 368b
ABO blood group incompatibility,
  maternal-fetal, 69
Abortion, induced, 312-314
  adjuvant chemotherapy and, 331
  complications of
    cervical incompetence as, 76
    duty to care for, 6-7
    preterm delivery subsequent to, 147
    Rh isoimmunization and, 184, 189
  by suction curettage, 314, 333
Abortion, spontaneous
  chromosomal abnormalities and, 75,
    76, 77, 79
  complete, 75
  definition of, 312-314
  etiologic factors in, 75-77
  human chorionic gonadotropin and,
    292-293
  hypothyroidism and, 75, 77, 196
  incidence of, 74-75
  incomplete, 75, 77
  inevitable, 75
  inflammatory bowel disease and, 202
  management of, 77
  missed, 75, 77

Abortion, spontaneous (Continued)
  partial mole as, 439, 440
  patient history of, 13
  preterm delivery subsequent to, 147
  recurrent, 75, 77
    chromosomal abnormalities and,
      77, 79
    immunologic factors in, 77
  Rh isoimmunization and, 77, 184,
    189
  systemic lupus erythematosus and,
    75, 77
  teratogens and, 82
  threatened, 75, 77
    vs. ectopic pregnancy, 292
  types of, 75
Abruptio placentae, 130-131
  abdominal trauma with, 217
  amniotic fluid embolus secondary to,
    132-133
  diagnosis of, 130
  fetal risks with, 131
  management of, 130-131
  maternal risks with, 131
  pathophysiology of, 130
  preeclampsia with, 130, 177
  risk factors for, 130, 130b
Abscess
  breast, 328
  fetal scalp, 126
  pelvic, puerperal, 136, 138
  tubo-ovarian, 274, 274-275f, 275
    rupture of, 259
Abuse. See Child abuse; Family violence;
  Intimate partner violence.
Acanthosis nigricans
  hyperandrogenic insulin resistance
    with, 365-366, 365f
  of vulva, 235
Acardiac twin, 163
Acceleration phase of labor, 139-140, 140f
ACE (angiotensin-converting enzyme)
  inhibitors, contraindicated in
  pregnancy, 181, 198
Acetaminophen, in cancer pain
  management, 400-401

Acetowhite epithelium
  of cervical intraepithelial neoplasia, 404
  of vulvar squamous cell carcinoma
    in situ, 420
Acetylcholinesterase, neural tube defect
  and, 81
Acid aspiration syndrome, in pregnancy,
  202
Acidosis
  at birth
    management of, 117
    in preterm infant, 150
  fetal
    blood sampling and, 117, 120,
      124-125
    cerebral dysfunction and, 125
    diabetic mother and, 191
    etiology of, 119-122
    heart rate monitoring and, 120, 122,
      124, 150
    management of, 124
    in preterm infant, 150
    respiratory distress syndrome and,
      157
Acne, premenstrual, 389
Acrosin, 42-43
Acrosome, 42-43, 43f
ACTH. See Adrenocorticotropic hormone
  (ACTH).
Actinomycin D, for gestational tropho-
  blastic neoplasia, 441-442, 441b
Active management of labor, 141-142
Active phase of labor, 98-99, 99t, 100f,
  139-140
  abnormalities of, 141-145
Acupressure, for nausea and vomiting, 201
Acupuncture
  for chronic pelvic pain, 264
  for labor pain, 112
Acute fatty liver of pregnancy, 203
Acute tubular necrosis, 200
Acyclovir, neonatal herpes infection and,
  211
Adaptive developmental plasticity, 4, 5, 10
Adaptive immune system, 67-68
  fetal, 68

Note: Page numbers followed by b indicate boxed material; those followed by f indicate figures; those followed by t indicate tables

Adenocarcinoma in situ, 421
Adenomyosis, 298-304, 304f
　chronic pain and, 261-262
　dysmenorrhea secondary to, 258
Adenosis, vaginal, 26, 236, 238f, 426
Adhesions
　chronic pelvic pain and, 263-264
　endometriosis with, 302
　intrauterine
　　in Asherman's syndrome, 247
　　hysteroscopic incision of, 337
　　pregnancy loss and, 76
　pelvic inflammatory disease and, 261,
　　274, 274f
　periadnexal, infertility and, 376
Adnexa
　bimanual examination of, 18, 18f, 19, 19f
　definition of, 248
　masses of, 19. See also Ovarian
　　masses.
　　diagnostic modalities for 250, 250t,
　　　335
　　in pregnancy, 217-218
　　tubal, 254
　torsion of, 255
　　acute pain secondary to, 258
　　in pregnancy, 217
Adolescent growth spurt, 349-350
Adolescent patient
　genital trauma in, 19-20
　life-course perspective and, 4-5
　special needs of, 19
Adolescent sexuality, 315
Adrenal glands
　androgen production by, 362
　androgen-secreting neoplasms of,
　　350-351
　fetal, 49, 50, 51, 54, 55
　hyperandrogenic disorders of, 363b,
　　363-364. See also Congenital
　　adrenal hyperplasia.
　　polycystic ovaries and, 364
　placental transfer of hormones and, 62t
　pregnancy-related changes and, 63
　prepubertal androgens and, 347
Adrenal hyperplasia
　congenital, 231, 351, 357f, 363-364
　　evaluation in, 366
　　treatment of, 367
　congenital lipoid, 354
　nonclassic, 351, 352, 363-364
Adrenal neoplasms, 364, 366
Adrenarche, 347, 349, 350f,
　premature, 352
α-Adrenergic stimulants, for stress
　urinary incontinence, 283
Adrenocorticotropic hormone (ACTH)
　fetal, 50
　pituitary production of, 34
　in pregnancy, 62t, 63
Adult respiratory distress syndrome
　(ARDS)
　acid aspiration and, 202
　pyelonephritis with, 212
Adverse drug event, 5
Adverse drug reaction, 5
AFI. See Amniotic fluid index (AFI).
AFP. See Alpha-fetoprotein (AFP).

African Americans
　leiomyomas in, 241
　ovarian cancer in, 412
　preterm deliveries in, 146
　puberty onset in, 349, 350t
　Rh D pseudogene in, 185
Age. See Gestational age; Maternal age.
Airway
　fetal, clearing of, 102, 115, 117
　maternal, anesthetic complications
　　and, 113, 113t
Albumin
　binding by
　　of calcium, 53
　　of steroids, 38-39, 362
　edema in pregnancy and, 58
Alcohol consumption in pregnancy, 13
　fetal effects of, 82, 83b
　spontaneous abortion and, 75
Alcoholism, pancreatitis in, 217
Aldosterone, in pregnancy, 53
Aldosterone antagonists
　fetal effects of, 197
　for hirsutism, 366-367
Algorithms, clinical, 8
Alkaloids, as chemotherapy agents,
　395-396t, 396
Alkalosis, respiratory
　hyperventilation in labor and, 112
　in pregnancy, 60, 61
Alkylating agents, 394, 395-396t
　as teratogens, 83
Allostasis, 4-5, 71
Allostatic overload, 4-5
Alpha-fetoprotein (AFP)
　in amniotic fluid, 221
　in maternal serum, 81, 82
　as tumor marker, 417, 418
Alveolar ventilation, in pregnancy, 60
Alveolar-arterial gradient, in pregnancy, 60
Ambiguous genitalia, 19, 231-232, 232f
　luteoma and, 249
　in testicular regression syndrome,
　　357
Amenorrhea, 355-367
　with breast development and normal
　　Müllerian structures, 355, 356t,
　　359-362
　in hyperandrogenism, 355, 362-363
　and normal estrogen, 362
　classification of, 355, 356t
　common causes of, 15
　lactational, 311
　primary, 355-358, 356t
　　with breast development and
　　　Müllerian anomalies, 356t, 358
　　mutations associated with, 354
　　with sexual infantilism, 355-358,
　　　356t
　secondary, 355
Aminopterin, as teratogen, 83
Amniocentesis, 220-221
　in cytomegalovirus infection, 209
　in premature rupture of membranes,
　　152
　procedure for, 220
　　in suspected hemolytic disease, 186
　respiratory distress syndrome and, 153

Amniocentesis (Continued)
　Rh isoimmunization and, 185,
　　186, 189
　risks associated with, 220
　therapeutic, 163, 221
Amnioinfusion
　meconium and, 124
　for variable decelerations, 123-124
Amniotic cavity, initial development of,
　43, 44f, 45f
Amniotic fluid
　bacteria in, 152
　bilirubin in, 186
　biophysical profile and, 220b
　functions of, 45
　testing for, in suspected PROM, 151, 221
Amniotic fluid embolus, 132-133, 135
Amniotic fluid index (AFI)
　definition of, 88-89, 151
　in intrauterine growth restriction, 156
　in oligohydramnios, 88-89
　in polyhydramnios, 88-89
　in postterm pregnancy, 157-158
　in premature rupture of membranes,
　　151
Amniotic fluid spectrophotometry, 186,
　187f, 188f
Amniotomy, 100, 141, 142
Anal incontinence, after episiotomy, 102
Anal lacerations, obstetric, 102, 104
Anal triangle, 22
Analgesia and anesthesia, obstetric,
　110-114. See also General
　anesthesia; Regional anesthesia.
　adverse effects of labor pain and, 112
　for cesarean delivery, 112-114
　for forceps delivery, 223-224
　goal of, 110 -111
　high-risk patients in, 114
　maternal mortality due to, 110-111,
　　113, 113t
　options for, 112
　pain pathways and, 111, 111f
　regional emphasis in, 110-111
　spinal vs. epidural for, 113, 113t
　unintended consequences of, 114
　uterine blood flow and, 111
Anastrazole, for breast cancer, 330
Anatomic conjugate (true conjugate),
　93, 94f
Anatomy
　of bony pelvis, 93-94, 94f, 94t, 95f
　of external genitalia, 22-24, 24f, 25f
　of fetal head, 91-93, 92f
　of internal genitalia, 26-28, 27f, 28f, 29
　reproductive, female, 22–33
Androgen insensitivity syndrome,
　231-232, 232f, 248, 358
Androgens. See also Hyperandrogenism;
　Steroids.
　fetal, 49, 51, 55
　normal metabolism of, 357f, 362-363
　ovarian cycle and, 35, 36f, 38, 39-40
　postmenopausal, 380
　in pregnancy, 49, 51
　in prepubertal period, 347
　from Sertoli-Leydig cell tumors, 418
　serum proteins and, 38-39, 362

Androgen-secreting tumors, 350-351, 365-366
Android pelvis, 95f, 96
Androstenedione, 35, 36f, 38, 38f, 362
  congenital adrenal hyperplasia and, 364
  obesity and, 428
  postmenopausal, 379-380
  puberty and, 347
Anemia
  fetal, Doppler assessment of, 185, 185f, 188-190, 220
  neonatal. *See also* Hemolytic disease of newborn.
    after blood loss, 117
  in pregnancy
    with cardiac disease, 197
    with multiple fetuses, 163
    physiologic, 56
  radiation therapy and, 397
Anencephaly, 80-81
  face presentation in, 170
  postterm pregnancy with, 157
Anesthesia. *See* Analgesia and anesthesia, obstetric; General anesthesia; Regional anesthesia.
Angiomas
  tubal, 254
  vulvar, 233
Angiotensin, in pregnancy, 53, 61
Angiotensin II receptor blockers, contraindicated in pregnancy, 181
Angiotensin sensitivity, in preeclampsia, 176
Angiotensin-converting enzyme (ACE) inhibitors, contraindicated in pregnancy, 181, 198
Anorexia nervosa
  amenorrhea in, 359
  delayed puberty in, 353-354
Anorgasmia, 320, 321
Antacids
  during labor, 202
  during pregnancy, 202
Antepartum care, 71-90. *See also* Prenatal care.
Antepartum hemorrhage
  causes of, 129b. *See also specific causes.*
  evaluation of, 128
Anterior fontanelle (bregma), 91, 92, 92f
Anteroposterior diameters, pelvic, 94, 94f, 94t, 95f, 96
Anthropoid pelvis, 95f, 96
Antianxiety agents, teratogenicity and, 83
Antibiotic agents
  breastfeeding and, 111t
  as chemotherapy agents, 395-396t, 396
  vaginal microflora and, 266, 288
Antibiotic prophylaxis
  of endocarditis, 198
  for HIV-infected pregnant women, 207
  intrapartum, of group B streptococcal infection, 212-213
  perioperative, with vaginal hysterectomy, 341
  in preterm labor, 147, 148, 150
    with PPROM, 152
  of urinary tract infection, 289

Antibiotic therapy
  for asymptomatic bacteriuria, 211-212
  for cervical infection, 375
  for chlamydial infection, 271
  for chorioamnionitis, 152
  for gonorrhea, 271
  for less common sexually transmitted infections, 275
  for mastitis, 110
  for pelvic inflammatory disease, 273-274, 273t
  for puerperal sepsis, 137-138
  for pyelonephritis, 212
  for syphilis, 214
  for toxoplasmosis, 214
  for tubo-ovarian abscess, 274, 275
  for urinary tract infection, 288-289, 289t
    recurrent, 289
Anticardiolipin, 199-200
Anticoagulants. *See also* Heparin.
  for deep venous thrombosis, 204
  mechanical valves and, 197
  prophylactic, in pregnancy, 204
  as teratogens, 83-84
Anticonvulsants
  breastfeeding and, 111t, 206
  contraceptive implants and, 306
  menstrual cycle and, 389
  oral contraceptive efficacy and, 389
  in pregnancy, 84, 84b, 205-206
Antihypertensive therapy
  for chronic hypertension, in pregnancy, 181
  in preeclampsia, 179-180, 180t
Antimetabolites, 394, 395t
Antineoplastic agents, 394-396, 395-396t
  as teratogens, 83
Antiphospholipid antibodies, 199-200
  intrauterine growth restriction and, 153-154, 156, 199-200
  lupus anticoagulant as, 199-200
    recurrent abortion and, 77
  neonatal lupus and, 199
Antiphospholipid antibody syndrome, 153-154, 199-200
Antiretroviral therapy, 207, 208
Antithyroid drugs, 195. *See also* Propylthiouracil.
Anxiety
  drugs for, teratogenicity and, 83
  premenstrual, 386, 388
Aortic compression, in pregnancy, 58
Apgar score, 115, 116t, 118
  asphyxia and, 125
  cerebral dysfunction and, 125
  fetal scalp pH and, 124-125
  magnesium sulfate and, 149
Aphthous ulcers, of labia, 235
Apneic newborn. *See* Asphyxiated infant.
Appendectomy, at time of hysterectomy, 339
Appendiceal mucocele, 251, 253
Appendicitis
  acute pain in, 259
  in pregnancy, 215-216
    anatomical changes and, 215, 215f
    differential diagnosis of, 215, 215b

Appendicitis *(Continued)*
    imaging studies in, 215-216, 216t
    laparoscopic surgery for, 216, 216t
    referred pain of, 259
ARDS. *See* Adult respiratory distress syndrome (ARDS).
Arias-Stella reaction, 292
Aromatase deficiency, 354
Aromatase inhibitors
  for breast cancer, 330
  mechanism of action of, 400
  for ovarian cancer, recurrent, 400
Aromatization, 38, 38f, 39-40
  extraovarian, 428
Arrest of descent, 141, 142f
  cephalopelvic disproportion with, 145
  transverse, 143
Arrest of dilation, 141, 142f
Arrhenoblastomas. *See* Sertoli-Leydig cell tumors.
Arrhythmias, cardiac, 197
Arterial blood gases. *See* Blood gases.
Arteriovenous malformation, uterine, 240
Arteriovenous oxygen difference, in pregnancy, 59, 60
Ascites
  abdominal examination and, 16
  fetal, dystocia secondary to, 144
  ovarian neoplasms and, 252, 253-254, 413, 414
    chemotherapy and, 416-417
ASCUS (atypical squamous cells of undetermined significance), 404, 404b
Asherman's syndrome, 247, 359
Asphyxiated infant. *See also* Acidosis; Fetal distress.
  with breech presentation, 169-170
  cerebral dysfunction in, 125, 126-127
  defined by acid-base status, 125
  intrauterine growth restriction and, 156, 157
  in multifetal gestation, 165
  postterm delivery and, 158
  resuscitation of, 115-118
    anticipating need for, 114
    drugs used for, 117, 118t
    flowchart for, 116f
    goals of, 114
    oxygen for, 115, 117
    personnel for, 115
    at term vs. preterm, 115
Aspirin, low-dose
  antiphospholipid antibody syndrome and, 199-200
  to prevent recurrent IUGR, 156
Assault, sexual, 322-325
Assisted reproductive technologies, 371-378, 377f. *See also* In vitro fertilization (IVF).
  ectopic pregnancy and, 290, 291f
  multifetal gestation secondary to, 166
Assisted vaginal delivery, 124. *See also* Operative vaginal delivery.
Asthma
  in pregnancy, 204-205
  premenstrual, 389
Asynclitism, 96, 97f

Atherosclerosis, developmental
  programming for, 4
Atosiban, 149
Atrial fibrillation, in pregnancy, 196,
  197
Atrophic vaginitis, 267, 269, 381
Atypical squamous cells of undetermined
  significance (ASCUS), 404, 404b
AUB. *See* Abnormal uterine bleeding
  (AUB).
Augmentation of labor. *See* Induction or
  augmentation of labor.
Autoimmune disease, in pregnancy,
  198-200, 198t
Autoimmune ovarian failure, 359
Autonomy, 6-8
Autosomal dominant disorders, 79-80
Autosomal recessive disorders, 80, 80t
Axillary hair, development of, 348-349
  premature, 352

B

B cells, 67-69
  fetal, 68
Back, examination of, 16
Back pain
  chronic pelvic pain and, 262
  epidural analgesia and, 114
  in parturients, 114
  in pregnancy, 86
Bacterial vaginosis, 267, 267t
  diagnosis of, 148, 266, 266f, 267
  intrauterine devices and, 274
  mucopurulent cervicitis associated
    with, 267
  preterm labor and, 147, 148
Bacteriuria
  asymptomatic, 286
    incidence of, 286
    in pregnancy, 84, 211-212
  definition of, 286
  group B streptococcal, in pregnancy,
    212-213
  persistent, 286, 288
  prolonged, 286
  sexual intercourse and, 286, 289
  significant, 286
  urinalysis and, 287
Bag-mask ventilation, for newborn, 117
Bagshawe regimen, 441
Balloon catheter, for postpartum
  hemorrhage, 134
Bardenheuer incision, 32-33, 33f
Barker hypothesis, 4, 5, 10
Bartholin's cyst, 237, 238f
Bartholin's glands
  anatomy of, 22, 24f, 25f
  carcinoma of, 424
  examination of, 16
  sexual response and, 316
  vaginal atrophy and, 239
Basal arteries, 40
Basal body temperature
  menstrual migraines and, 388
  ovulation and, 38, 374
Basal cell carcinoma, vulvar, 425
Basalis, endometrial, 40

Bearing down, 100-102
  epidural analgesia and, 114
Behçet's syndrome, 235
Beneficence, 6-7
β-blockers, in pregnancy, 181
β-carotene, gestational trophoblastic
  neoplasia and, 435
Bethesda system, 403-404, 404b
Bicarbonate, for severe acidosis,
  in newborn, 117, 118t
Bicornuate uterus, 240 241f
Bilirubin, amniotic fluid, 186
Bimanual pelvic examination, 17-19, 18f,
  19f
Bimanual rectovaginal examination, 19,
  20f
Biochemical pregnancy, 74-75
Biophysical profile, 88-89, 88f, 89t, 220
  definition of, 220b
  in intrauterine growth restriction, 156
  in multifetal gestation, 164
  in postterm pregnancy, 157-158
Biopsy
  breast, 327, 327b
  cervical, 334, 334f, 404, 405
    of microinvasive carcinoma, 408
  cutaneous, 235-236, 235f
  endometrial
    in dysfunctional uterine bleeding,
      369
    endometrial cancer and, 429
    infertility and, 374
    ovarian cancer and, 413
  vaginal, 425
Biparietal diameter, 92f, 93
Birth control. *See* Contraception.
Birth defects. *See* Chromosomal abnormalities; Congenital and hereditary
  disorders; Fetal abnormalities;
  Teratogenic agents.
Birth trauma
  to brachial plexus, 144, 169-170
  breech presentation and, 169-170
  in twins, 165
Bisexuality, 316
Bishop score, 107-108, 108t
Bisphosphonates
  in cancer pain management, 400-401
  for osteoporosis, 382, 384
Bispinous diameter, 93, 94
Bitemporal diameter, 92f, 93
Bituberous diameter, 93, 94, 95f
Bladder
  overactive, 282, 284-285, 284b
  post-hysterectomy dysfunction of, 408
Blastocyst, 43, 44
Bleeding. *See* Hemorrhage; Uterine
  bleeding; Vaginal bleeding.
Blood flow, in pregnancy
  regional, 58
  renal, 58, 60
  umbilical, 63-64, 64f
  uterine, 58
    regional analgesia/anesthesia and,
      111
Blood gases
  fetal and neonatal
    in acidosis, 117, 122, 125

Blood gases *(Continued)*
  blood sampling for, 115, 117, 125 126
  normal ranges of, 126t
  in pregnant woman, 60
Blood pressure. *See also* Hypertension,
  Hypotension.
  measurement of, 173
  in pregnancy, 56-58, 57t, 173
    elevated in preeclampsia, 177
    in supine position, 58, 124, 173
Blood products, characteristics of, 136t
  136b
Blood sampling. *See* Fetal blood
  sampling.
Blood transfusion
  fetal, intrauterine, 186-189
  maternal
    for amniotic fluid embolism, 135
    as massive replacement, 136
    for postpartum hemorrhage, 132, 133
  for neonatal blood loss, 117
  refused by patient, 7
Blood volume, in pregnancy, 56, 58-59
  with multiple fetuses, 163
Bloody show, 98
Body composition, puberty and, 347-348,
  350
Body mass index (BMI)
  leiomyomas and, 241
  obstetric complications and, 73
Bohr effect, 65, 122
Bone age
  precocious puberty and, 352
  puberty and, 350
Bone marrow suppression,
  radiation-induced, 399
Borderline tumor, serous, 416f
Bowel obstruction
  by endometriosis, 302
  in ovarian cancer, 414
  in pregnancy, 217
  radiation-induced, 399, 400f
Bowen's disease (squamous cell
  carcinoma in situ, vulvar),
  420-421, 421f
Brachial plexus injury
  breech presentation and, 169-170
  shoulder dystocia and, 144
Brachytherapy, 397-399, 398b, 399f
  for cervical cancer, 398, 399, 399f, 409
  for endometrial cancer, 432
  for uterine carcinosarcoma, 434
  for vaginal cancer, 425-426
Braxton Hicks contractions, 54-55, 97-98
BRCA1 and *BRCA2* mutations, 412, 417
Breast(s)
  benign disorders of, 327-328
  cyst(s) in, 327
    aspiration of, 327, 328f
    galactocele as, 328
  development of, 348f, 349, 350t
    premature, 352
  disease of, 326-331
  examination of, 16, 326
  pregnancy-related changes in, 58
  screening of, 326
  self-examination of, 326
Breast biopsy, 327, 327b

Breast cancer, 328
    clinical features of, 329, 329f
    epidemiology of, 328
    hormonal contraceptives and, 310, 311
    hormonal therapy for, 330, 400
    metastatic to ovaries, 413, 419
    ovarian cancer and, 412
    postmenopausal hormone therapy and, 382-384, 383f, 384t
    in pregnancy, 331
        inflammatory, 326-331
    prognosis of, 330
    raloxifene and, 384
    risk factors for, 328-329, 328t
    screening for, 326
    spread of, 329
    staging of, 329
    treatment of, 329-330
    types of, 329
Breast reconstruction, 330
Breastfeeding, 109-110
    antenatal recommendations, 87
    complications of, 110
    as contraceptive, 311
    diabetic mother's diet and, 194
    drug ingestion by mother and, 110, 111t
        anticonvulsants, 111t, 206
        fluoxetine, 83
    infection and
        herpes simplex, 211
        HIV, 207, 208
        rubella, 208-209
        tuberculosis, 213
    prenatal discussion of, 74, 86
    suppression of lactation and, 110
    vaginal atrophy secondary to, 239
Breathing initiation
    for asphyxiated infant, 116f, 117
    for normal newborn, 115
Breathing movements, fetal, 64
    in biophysical profile, 88-89, 220, 220b
    onset of labor and, 114-115
Breech presentation, 166-170
    cesarean delivery for, 167, 169
        preterm, 150, 169, 226
        rate of, 226
    in twins, 165
    classification of, 166, 167f
    complications with, 169-170
    diagnosis of, 166
    etiology of, 166
    external cephalic version and, 166-167, 226
    incidence of, 166
    labor management with, 167-169
    in multiple gestation, 165
    outcome with, 169-170
    pregnancy management with, 166-167
    preterm, 150
        cesarean delivery for, 150, 169, 226
    vaginal delivery with, 167-169, 167b, 168f
    forceps in, 167-169, 168f, 223, 224f
        Bregma (anterior fontanelle), 91, 92, 92f,

Brenner tumor, 251, 251f, 415
Broad ligaments
    anatomy of, 26-31, 27f, 28f
    neoplasms in, 254-255
Bromocriptine
    for cyclic mastalgia, 388
    for hyperprolactinemia, 361-362
        male infertility and, 373
        ovulatory infertility and, 374
Brow presentation, 171, 171f
Brucella infection, recurrent abortion and, 77
Burch procedure, 283
Buspirone, for premenstrual anxiety, 388
Busulfan, as teratogen, 83

C

CA 125
    adnexal masses and, 250, 250t, 253
    endometriosis and, 302
    ovarian cancer and, 413, 417
Cabergoline, for hyperprolactinemia, 361, 362
    ovulatory infertility and, 374
Calcium carbonate, for premenstrual syndromes, 388
Calcium channel blockers
    avoided in congestive heart failure, 198
    for hypertension, in pregnancy, 181
    male factor infertility and, 372
Calcium hydroxylapatite, for stress urinary incontinence, 283-284
Calcium metabolism, in pregnancy, 53-54
Call-Exner bodies, 418
Cancer. *See also* Chemotherapy; Hormonal therapy for cancer; Radiation therapy; and specific cancers.
    cellular biology of, 393
    end-of-life issues in, 401
    pain management in, 400-401
    therapy for, principles of, 391-401
Candida glabrata, 268
Candidiasis
    urinary tract, 288
    vulvovaginal, 267, 267t, 268
        discharge in, 266, 267f, 268, 268f
Caput, 100-101
Carbamazepine, 206
    as teratogen, 84
Carbon dioxide. *See also* Blood gases.
    arterial partial pressure of
        maternal-fetal gradient of, 63-64
        in pregnancy, 60, 61
        placental transfer of, 63-65, 64f
Carboplatin, 395t, 396
Carcinomatous ileus, 413-414
Carcinosarcoma, uterine, 434
Cardiac disease. *See* Heart disease.
Cardiac massage, in neonatal resuscitation, 117
Cardiac output, in pregnancy, 56-57, 57t, 58, 60
Cardinal (Mackenrodt's) ligaments, 26-28, 27f, 30-31

Cardiomyopathy, peripartum, 197
Cardiovascular system
    of fetus, 65-67, 67f, 67t
        changes after birth, 67
    of pregnant woman, 56-59, 57t
        postpartum changes in, 109
Caruncle, urethral, 232, 233f
Catamenial epilepsy, 388-389
Catheterization
    for epidural anesthesia, 114
    intrauterine, for cervical ripening, 106-107
    in postpartum hemorrhage treatment, 134
    for umbilical cord blood sampling, 117
    urinary tract infection and, 289, 289b
Caval compression, in pregnancy, 58
Cell cycle, 393, 394f
    chemotherapy agents and, 393, 394f
Cellulitis, pelvic, puerperal, 137
Cephalic curve, of forceps, 222-223, 223f
Cephalohematoma, vacuum extraction and, 225
Cephalopelvic disproportion, 145
Cerclage, cervical
    in multifetal gestation, 164
    to prevent recurrent abortion, 77
    procedure for, 222, 222f
    transabdominal, 222
Cerebral palsy
    etiology of, 125-127
    fetal monitoring and, 126-127
    low birth weight and, 118
    in twins, 165-166
Cervarix, 402
Cervical cancer, 402-411
    brachytherapy for, 398, 399, 399f, 409
    HPV infection and, 402
    HPV vaccination and, 9-10, 270, 402, 403
    hysterectomy for
        diagnosis in pregnancy and, 410-411
        in microinvasive disease, 408
        radical, 339, 408-409
    microinvasive
        biopsy of, 405
        in pregnancy, 410-411
        treatment of, 408
        vascular architecture of, 405
    pathologic features of, 407, 411
    physical findings in, 407, 407f
    in pregnancy, 410-411
    preoperative studies in, 407-408
    prevalence of, 402
    prognosis for, 411, 411t
    rectovaginal examination in, 19, 407
    recurrent or metastatic, 409-410, 410f
    risk factors for, 402, 403b
    screening of asymptomatic women, 402-403
    spread of, 407, 407f
    staging of, 407-408, 408t
    symptoms of, 407
    treatment of, 408-410
Cervical cap, 311
Cervical carcinoma in situ, 404, 405, 405f
Cervical collar deformity, 240, 242f

Cervical conization, 334, 334f
    See also Cone biopsy of cervix.
    for cervical intraepithelial neoplasia, 406
    for microinvasive carcinoma, 408
    in pregnancy, 410-411
Cervical dilation, 98-99
    active-phase abnormalities and,
        141-145, 141f, 142f
    arrest of, 141, 142f
    Bishop score and, 107-108, 108t
    phases of labor and, 98, 100f, 139-140,
        140f
    in preterm labor, 148
    rate of, during active phase, 99t
    vaginal examination and, 100
Cervical dysplasia, 402-411, 404b
Cervical effacement, 98, 99, 99f,
    See also Cervical ripening.
    Bishop score and, 107-108, 108t
    phases of labor and, 139-140
    in preterm labor, 148
    vaginal examination and, 100
Cervical factor infertility, 375
Cervical incompetence, 247. *See also*
    Cerclage, cervical.
    management of, 77
    in multifetal gestation, 164
    pregnancy loss caused by, 76, 77
Cervical intraepithelial neoplasia (CIN),
    404, 404b, 405f
    human papillomavirus and, 402, 404
    in pregnancy, 410
    treatment of, 405-406, 406f
    vascular architecture of, 404-405
Cervical polyps, 246
Cervical pregnancy, 291f, 297
Cervical procedures, 334
Cervical ripening. *See also* Cervical
    effacement.
    induction of labor and, 105-107
Cervical stenosis, noncongenital, 247
Cervicitis
    chlamydial, 270, 272
    infertility secondary to, 375
    mucopurulent, 267, 270-272, 272f
Cervidil, 106
Cervix
    anatomy of, 26, 27f
    benign conditions of, 240–247
    bimanual examination of, 17
    cone biopsy of, 405, 408. *See also*
        Conization, cervical.
    in pregnancy, 410
    congenital abnormalities of, 240-247
        241f, 242f
    agenesis as, 358
    atresia as, 241f
    diethylstilbestrol-induced changes in, 426
    ectropion of, 245, 246
    embryology of, 24-26, 240
    labor-related changes in, 139
    laceration of, in delivery, 132, 133
        inspection for, 103
        repair of, 103, 134, 134f
    length of, preterm labor and, 147, 164,
        219
    lymphatic drainage of, 30-31
    Nabothian cysts of, 246, 246f

Cervix *(Continued)*
    normal, 245, 245f
    pain sensitivity of, 259-260
    pregnancy-related changes in, 14
    speculum examination of, 16-17, 17f
    topography of, 403, 403f
    trauma to, 246
Cesarean delivery, 225-227
    active management of labor and,
        141-142
    anesthesia for, 112-114
    benefits of, 225
    for breech presentation, 167, 169
        preterm, 150, 169, 226
        rate of, 226
        in twins, 165
    for brow presentation, 171
    in cardiac patient, 197-198
    for cephalopelvic disproportion, 141
    for chorioamnionitis, 152
    classic, 226
    court-ordered, 7
    epidural analgesia and, 145
    for face presentation, 170
    for failure to progress, 141
    for fetal developmental abnormalities,
        144-145
    fetal heart decelerations and, 124
    hemorrhage secondary to, 132
    herpes simplex infection and, 211
    for HIV-infected women, 207-208
    hospital facilities required for, 225
    incisions in, types of, 226, 226f
    indications for, 226
    intrauterine growth restriction and, 157
    macrosomia and, 143
    with diabetic mother, 194
    maternal morbidity with, 226, 227
    maternal mortality with, 225-226
    perinatal morbidity and mortality
        with, 225, 227
    for placenta previa, 129-130, 226
    in preeclampsia, 178
        antihypertensive therapy and, 179
    in premature rupture of membranes,
        152
    prevention of, 226-227
    rate of, 222, 225
    repeat, 226, 227
    for shoulder presentation, 144, 171-172
    for transverse arrest of descent, 143
    of twins
        with breech presentation, 165
        monoamniotic, 164
    of very-low-birth-weight baby, 150
Chadwick's sign, 14
Chancroid, 275
Chemoradiation, 397
    for advanced vulvar cancer, 423
    for cervical cancer, 408-409
    for vaginal cancer, 425-426
Chemotherapy
    agents for, 394-396, 395-396t
        as teratogens, 83
    for breast cancer, adjuvant, 330, 331
    cell cycle and, 393
    for cervical cancer, metastatic, 409
    for endometrial cancer, 432

Chemotherapy *(Continued)*
    for fallopian tube carcinoma, 419
    for gestational trophoblastic neoplasia,
        439-442
    for ovarian cancer
        epithelial, 415-417
        germ cell, 417-418
        principles of, 393, 393-394
    for uterine sarcomas, 433, 434
    Cherney incision, 31-32, 33f
Chickenpox. *See* Varicella-zoster virus
    infection.
Child. *See* Adolescent patient; Pediatric
    patient.
Child abuse, 322
    healthcare provider's responsibilities
        with, 20
    telephone resources for, 325b
Childbirth preparation classes, 90, 112,
    142
Chlamydia infection, 265, 270-271
    lymphogranuloma venereum and,
        275
    mucopurulent cervicitis in, 267
    pelvic inflammatory disease and,
        270-274
    salpingitis in, ectopic pregnancy and,
        290
Chloasma, 14
Chlorambucil, as teratogen, 83
Chlordiazepoxide, as teratogen, 83
Cholecystitis
    acute, in pregnancy, 216-217
    pancreatitis with, 217
Cholelithiasis
    hormonal contraceptives and, 310
    pancreatitis with, 217
    in pregnancy, 216-217
Cholestasis, intrahepatic, of pregnancy,
    202-203
Cholesterol screening, recommendations
    for, 10t
Chorioamnionitis
    amniotic fluid analysis for, 221
    fetal demise with, 158
    management of, 152
    PROM management and, 151-152
    signs and symptoms of, 151-152
    subclinical
        delaying diagnosis of, 151-152
        preterm labor and, 150
Choriocarcinoma, 436, 439f, 440-441
    diagnosis of, 441
    genetics of, 435
    investigations of, 441
    ovarian, 418
    pathologic features of, 437
    signs of, 441
    staging of, 438
    symptoms of, 440-441
    treatment of, 441-442
Chorion, 44, 45f
Chorion frondosum, 44, 45f
Chorion laeve, 44, 45f
Chorionic villus sampling (CVS), 221
    fetal Rh status and, 185
Chorioretinitis, in congenital
    toxoplasmosis, 214

Chromic phosphate, 398
Chromosomal abnormalities, 78-80.
   See also Down syndrome (trisomy
   21); Fetal abnormalities.
   diagnosis of
      amniocentesis for, 220
      chorionic villus sampling for, 221
   ectopic pregnancy and, 290
   first-trimester screening for, 77, 81, 219
   gonada1 dysgenesis and, 357
   gonadal development and, 248
   hypergonadotropic hypogonadism
      and, 353-354
   maternal age and, 78, 79t
   nuchal translucency and, 81
   spontaneous abortion and, 75, 76, 77, 79
Chronic fatigue syndrome, 262
Chronic hypertension, 174-175
   management of, 181
   with superimposed preeclampsia, 175,
      181
Chvostek's sign, in preeclampsia, 178-179
CIN. *See* Cervical intraepithelial
   neoplasia (CIN).
Cisplatin, 395-396t, 396
   for cervical cancer
      metastatic, 409
      radiation with, 408, 409
      radiation with, 397
Clear cell adenocarcinoma, vaginal, 84, 426
Clear cell carcinoma
   endometrial, 429-432
   ovarian, 415
   Cleavage, 43
   timing of, in twinning, 160, 160t
Climacteric, 379-385. *See also* Menopause;
   Postmenopausal women.
   alternative treatments for, 385
   clinical manifestations of, 381
   definition of, 379
   hormonal changes in, 379-380
   lifestyle changes for, 384-385
   osteoporosis and, 381-382
   ovarian hormone therapy and,
      382-384, 383f
   ovarian senescence in, 380-381
   selective estrogen receptor modulators
      and, 384
Clinical guidelines, 8-9
Clinical pathways, 8, 9
Clinical pelvimetry, 13, 74, 96-97, 98f
Clinical trials, 8
Clitoral vacuum device, 320
Clitoris
   agenesis of, 231
   anatomy of, 22, 23, 24f, 25f, 27f
   bifid, 231
   embryology of, 22, 23f
   female genital mutilation and, 234b
   sexual sensitivity of, 316
Clitoromegaly, 231, 233, 362, 365-366
Cloaca, 231
Clomiphene citrate, 374-375, 377, 384
   catamenial epilepsy and, 388-389
Clonazepam, 206
Clue cells, 266, 266f
CMV. *See* Cytomegalovirus (CMV)
   infection.

Coagulopathy. *See also* Disseminated
      intravascular coagulopathy (DIC).
   acute fatty liver of pregnancy with, 203
   amniotic fluid embolism with, 135
   fetal demise and, 159
   missed abortion and, 75
   postpartum hemorrhage secondary to,
      132-133
      management of, 135-136
   preeclampsia with, 174, 176, 177
   rapid subjective test for, 128
Cocaine, as teratogen, 85
Coccyx, 93
Coitus interruptus, 311
Colitis, ulcerative, pregnant patient with,
      202
Collagen injections, for stress urinary
      incontinence, 283-284
Colles' fascia, 27f
Colostrum, 110
Colpocleisis, 279
Colpopexy, 279
Colporrhaphy
   anterior, 279
   posterior, 279
Colposcopy, 404-406
   in pregnancy, 410
   of vaginal intraepithelial neoplasia,
      425
   vulvar squamous cell carcinoma in situ
      and, 420
Complete abortion, 75
Compound presentation, 171-172
Computed tomography (CT)
   of adnexal mass, 250t
   of cervical cancer, 407
   in pregnancy, 215-216, 216t
Conception, 42, 371
Condoms
   female, 311
   male, 311
Conduit, urinary, after pelvic
      exenteration, 409
Condylomata acuminata, 270
   cervical, 402
   cryoablation of, 334
   vaginal, 239
Cone biopsy of cervix, 405, 408.
   See also Conization, cervical.
   in pregnancy, 410
Confidentiality, 7-8
Congenital adrenal hyperplasia, 351,
      357f, 363-364
   evaluation in, 366
   treatment of, 367
Congenital and hereditary disorders,
      78-81 See also Chromosomal
      abnormalities; Fetal abnormalities;
      "Genetic" entries.
   intrauterine growth restriction
      secondary to,154
   prenatal screening for, 81-82
Congenital anomalies
   of cervix, 240, 241f, 242f
      agenesis as, 358
      atresia as, 241f
   of fallopian tubes, 248
   of ovaries, 248

Congenital anomalies *(Continued)*
   of urinary tract, 358
   of uterus, 240, 241f, 358
      pregnancy loss due to, 76,
         77
      septum as, 337
   of vagina, 236, 237f, 238f, 358
   of vulva, 231-232, 232f
Congenital heart disease, 196-197
Congenital lipoid adrenal hyperplasia,
      354
Congestive heart failure, in pregnancy
   atrial fibrillation and, 196
   postpartum, 198
Conization, cervical, 334, 334f. *See also*
      Cone biopsy of cervix.
   for cervical intraepithelial
      neoplasia, 406
   for microinvasive carcinoma, 408
   in pregnancy, 410-411
Conjoined twins, 162
   dystocia secondary to, 145
Conjunctivitis, neonatal, 271
Consent, informed, 7, 7t
   for gynecologic procedures, 333
Constipation, in pregnancy, 87
Contact dermatitis, of vulva, 235-236
Contraception. *See also* Oral
      contraceptives.
   barrier methods of, 311
   behavioral methods of, 311
   combined hormonal methods of,
      307-309t, 310-311
   after ectopic pregnancy, 295,
      296
   efficacy of, 305, 306t
   emergency, 310, 311-312
      after sexual assault, 324
   failure rates of, 305, 306t
   implant methods of, 306-309, 307-309t
   incorrect use of, 305
   intrauterine, 309-310, 307t, 310f
   mechanism of action of, 305-306
   Medical Eligibility Criteria of WHO,
      306, 307t
   progestin-only injections and pills for,
      307t, 310-311
   public health significance of, 305
   sexually transmitted infections and,
      305, 311
Contraceptive history, 13, 15
Contraction stress test, 90
   in multifetal gestation, 164
Contractions. *See* Uterine contractions.
Cordocentesis (percutaneous umbilical
      blood sampling), 125, 186, 221-222
Corona radiata, 39, 40, 43
Corona-dispersing enzyme, 42-43
Coronal suture, 91, 92f
Corpus albicans, 40, 41f
Corpus luteum, 35-36, 38, 39, 40,
      41f, 368
   in excised ovary, during pregnancy,
      217
   regression of, 41-42
Corpus luteum cysts, 217-218, 249
   in ectopic pregnancy, 292
Corticosteroid-binding globulin, 63

Corticosteroids (glucocorticoids).
See also Cortisol; Dexamethasone; Prednisone.
for adrenal hyperandrogenism, 367
for asthma, in pregnancy, 205
for contact dermatitis, 235-236
endogenous
from lipid cell tumors, 418
PPROM and, 152
in pregnancy, 51
for fetal pulmonary maturation, 107, 150
for immune (idiopathic) thrombocytopenia, 199
for lichen sclerosis, 234
for preterm premature rupture of membranes, 152
for systemic lupus erythematosus, 199
Corticotropin-releasing factor (CRF).
See Corticotropin-releasing hormone (CRH).
Corticotropin-releasing hormone (CRH)
hypothalamic secretion of, 36
parturition and, 55
in pregnancy, 50
preterm birth and, 147-148
Cortisol, in pregnancy, 51, 63
fetal adrenal and, 51
fetal thyroid and, 114
labor and, 51, 54
placental transfer of, 62t
preterm birth and, 147-148
Cotton swab test, 281, 281f
Coumadin. *See* Warfarin (Coumadin).
COX. *See* Cyclooxygenase (COX).
Crab lice, 275
Craniopagus twins, 162
Craniopharyngioma, 360-361
Creatinine clearance
in preeclampsia, 177
in pregnancy, 60
Cretinism, 196
CRF (corticotropin-releasing factor).
See Corticotropin-releasing hormone (CRH).
CRH. *See* Corticotropin-releasing hormone (CRH).
Critical paths, 9
Crohn disease
pregnant patient with, 202
vulvar ulcers in, 235
Crowning, 102
Crown-rump length, 78
Cryoablation, of condylomas, 334
Cryomyolysis, 244-245
Cryoprecipitate, 135, 136t, 136b
Cryosurgery, for cervical intraepithelial neoplasia, 406
CT. *See* Computed tomography (CT).
Cul-de-sac. *See* Pouch of Douglas (cul-de-sac).
Cumulus oophorus, 39, 40, 40f
Curettage
dilation and (D&C), 333-334
endocervical, 405, 408
ovarian cancer and, 413
suction, for pregnancy termination, 314, 333

Cushing's disease, 364
Cushing's syndrome, 364, 366
lipid cell tumors and, 418
CVS (chorionic villus sampling), 221
fetal Rh status and, 185
Cyanotic newborn. *See* Asphyxiated infant.
Cyclooxygenase (COX), 53
primary dysmenorrhea and, 256
Cyclooxygenase inhibitors, 53
Cyclophosphamide, as teratogen, 83
Cyclosporine, in pregnancy, 201
Cyst(s)
Bartholin's, 237-239, 238f
breast, 327
aspiration of, 327, 328f
galactocele as, 328
corpus luteum, 217-218, 249
in ectopic pregnancy, 292
dermoid, 250, 252-254, 252f, 413
Brenner tumor with, 415
Gartner's duct, 26, 26f, 236
inclusion
tubal, 254
vaginal, 237
vulvar, 232
Nabothian, 246, 246f
ovarian. *See* Ovarian cysts.
parovarian, 254-255
tubal, 254, 258
vaginal, 237, 238f, 239
vulvar, 232
Cystadenocarcinoma, serous, ovarian, 251
Cystadenofibroma, ovarian, 252-253
Cystadenoma, ovarian
mucinous, 250-251, 251f, 253
serous, 250-251, 251f
Cystic fibrosis
genetics of, 80, 80t, 205
pregnant patient with, 205
Cystic teratoma, benign, 250, 252, 252f, 254, 413
Cystitis
acute, 211-212
antimicrobial therapy for, 288-289, 289t
pain in, 259
definition of, 286
honeymoon, 287, 286
interstitial, chronic pain in, 262
radiation-induced
acute, 399
hemorrhagic, 400
Cystocele, 239, 276
Cystometrogram, 282, 282f
Cytokines, 67-68
Cytomegalovirus (CMV) infection, 209
amniotic fluid analysis for, 221
congenital, 209, 209b
recurrent abortion and, 77
Cytotec, 106

D

D&C (dilation and curettage), 333-334
D&E (dilation and evacuation), for fetal demise, 158, 314

Da Vinci surgical system, 342, 342f
Danazol
for endometriosis pain, 302-303
for tubal occlusion, 376
Danocrine, for cyclic mastalgia, 388
Darifenacin, 284
Deceleration phase of labor, 139-140, 140f
Decelerations. *See* Fetal heart rate decelerations.
Decidua basalis, 43-44, 44f, 45f
Decidua capsularis, 43-44, 44f, 45f
Decidua vera (parietalis), 43-44, 44f, 45f
Decubitus ulcers, of vulva, 235
Deep venous thrombosis, 203-204
combined hormonal contraceptives and, 310
after radical hysterectomy, 409
Dehydroepiandrosterone (DHEA), 38, 51f, 52f, 362
puberty and, 347
Dehydroepiandrosterone sulfate (DHEA-S), 38, 50-51, 51f, 52f, 362
hyperandrogenism and, 366
puberty and, 347
Delivery, 102-103
in cardiac patient, 197-198
of fetal head, 102, 103f
genital trauma during, 132.
See also Lacerations, obstetric; Uterine rupture.
management of, 134
maternal position for, 102
normal, 91–118
of shoulders, 103, 104f
Dendritic cells, 67-68
Depression
chronic pelvic pain and, 263
postmenopausal, 381
postpartum, 109
in pregnancy, fluoxetine for, 83
premenstrual dysphoric disorder and, 386-387
Dermatitis, contact, of vulva, 235-236
Dermoid cyst, 250, 252-254, 252f, 254, 413
Brenner tumor with, 415
DES. *See* Diethylstilbestrol (DES).
Descent, fetal
arrest of, 141, 142f
cephalopelvic disproportion with, 145
transverse, 143
mechanism of, 101
molding or caput and, 100-101
monitoring of, 100-101
plotting normal rate of, 139-140, 140f
protraction disorder of, 141, 141f
Desquamative vaginitis, 267
Detrusor areflexia, 282f, 285
Detrusor hyperreflexia, 282, 282f
Developmental plasticity, adaptive, 4, 5, 10
Developmental programming, 4-5
Dexamethasone
for ovulatory infertility, 374
for thyroid storm, 196
Dexamethasone suppression test, 366

DHEA. *See* Dehydroepiandrosterone (DHEA).
DHEA-S. *See* Dehydroepiandrosterone sulfate (DHEA-S).
DHT (dihydrotestosterone), 51, 362-363
Diabetes mellitus. *See also* Gestational diabetes mellitus.
  contraceptives and, 307t, 310
  developmental programming for, 4
  developmental vulnerability to, 154
  diet and
    postpartum, 194
    in pregnancy, 192
  exercise and, in pregnancy, 192
  overflow incontinence in, 285
  polycystic ovary syndrome and, 365, 366, 367
  postpartum management with, 194
  in pregnancy, 191-194
    antepartum management with, 192-194
    classification of, 191, 192t
    complications of, 191, 193t
    diagnosis of, 191-192, 194t
    incidence of, 191
    intrapartum management with, 194
    macrosomia and, 143, 191, 192-194, 193t
    management of, 192, 194b
    shoulder dystocia and, 144
  premenstrual effects in, 389
  spontaneous abortion and, 75, 77
Diagonal conjugate, 94f, 96-97, 98f
Diameters, pelvic, 93-94, 94, 94t, 94f, 95f
Diamniotic twins, 160t, 161-162, 161f
Diaphragmatic hernia, in newborn, 117-118
Diaphragms, 311
Diarrhea, in pregnancy, with inflammatory bowel disease, 202
Diazepam
  for eclamptic seizures, 180
  for status epilepticus, 206
DIC. *See* Disseminated intravascular coagulopathy (DIC).
Dichorionic twins, 160, 161-162, 160t, 161f
Diet. *See also* Nutrition.
  for cardiac patient, in pregnancy, 197
  for diabetic patient
    postpartum, 194
    in pregnancy, 192
  for inflammatory bowel disease, in pregnancy, 202
Diethylstilbestrol (DES)
  anomalies caused by, 240, 242f, 426
    cervical incompetence and, 247
    in columnar epithelium, 403
    of fallopian tubes, 248
    vaginal adenosis as, 26, 236, 238f, 426
  as teratogen, 84
  vaginal clear cell adenocarcinoma and, 84, 426
Dihydrotestosterone (DHT), 51, 362-363
Dilantin. *See* Phenytoin (diphenylhydantoin).
Dilation. *See* Cervical dilation.
Dilation and curettage (D&C), 333-334

Dilation and evacuation (D&E), for fetal demise, 158, 314
Dinoprostone, to expel dead fetus, 158-159
Diphenylhydantoin. *See* Phenytoin (diphenylhydantoin).
Disabled women, 21
  abuse of, 324, 325b
Discriminatory zone, of human chorionic gonadotropin, 293-294, 294f
Disseminated intravascular coagulopathy (DIC)
  acute fatty liver of pregnancy with, 203
  fetal demise with, 158, 159
  placenta previa with, 130
  placental abruption with, 131
  preeclampsia and, 176, 177
  rapid subjective test for, 128
  retained dead fetus syndrome with, 163
Diuretics
  for acute tubular necrosis, 200
  for premenstrual syndrome, 388
Dizygotic twins, 160-162, 162f
DMPA. *See* Medroxyprogesterone acetate, depot (DMPA).
Docetaxel, 395t, 396
Domestic violence. *See* Child abuse; Family violence; Intimate partner violence.
Doppler sonography
  of adnexal masses, 250t
  in deep venous thrombosis, 203-204
  intrauterine growth restriction and, 154, 157
  middle cerebral artery, fetal anemia and, 185, 185f, 186, 188-190, 220
  umbilical artery, 89-90, 90f, 125, 220
    IUGR and, 154, 157
  uterine artery, IUGR and, 154
Double-ring sign, of ectopic pregnancy, 292
Douching, vaginal microflora and, 266
Down syndrome (trisomy 21), 78, 79
  karyotype in, 78, 78f
  maternal age and, 78, 79t
  screening for, 80, 81
Drospirenone, premenstrual syndromes and, 388
Drugs
  adverse reactions to, 4
  in breast milk, 110, 111t
    anticonvulsants, 111t, 206
    fluoxetine, 83
  hyperprolactinemia caused by, 360b, 361
  male factor infertility and, 372
  in pregnancy. *See* Teratogenic agents.
  sexual dysfunction associated with, 319, 319b
DUB. *See* Dysfunctional uterine bleeding (DUB).
Duchenne muscular dystrophy, prenatal diagnosis of, 80
Ductus arteriosus, 65, 66f, 67, 67t
Ductus venosus, 65, 66f, 67, 67t
Due date. *See* Estimated date of confinement (EDC).

Duffy antigen, 189-190
Dyschezia, endometriosis with, 300
Dysfunctional uterine bleeding (DUB)
  definition of, 368
  diagnosis of, 369, 369b
  management of, 369-370, 370b
  overview of, 368
Dysgerminoma, 357, 417-418
Dysmaturity syndrome, 157
Dysmenorrhea, 256-258
  definition of, 256
  patient history of, 15
  prevalence of, 256
  primary, 256-258
    clinical features of, 256, 257b
    pathophysiology of, 256, 257f
    treatment of, 256-258, 257b
  secondary, 256, 258
    adenomyosis with, 304
    clinical features of, 258, 258b
    endometriosis with, 300, 302, 303
    leiomyomas with, 243-244
    pathophysiology of, 258
    treatment of, 258
Dyspareunia, 320
  adenomyosis with, 304
  endometriosis with, 300, 302
  lichen planus with, 234-235
  lichen sclerosis with, 234
  in residual ovary syndrome, 255
  urethral diverticula with, 236-237
  uterine retroversion with, 262
  vaginal atrophy with, 239
  vulvar vestibulitis with, 232, 236
  vulvodynia with, 236
Dyspnea of pregnancy, 60
Dystocia, 139-145
  active management of labor and, 141-142
  active phase, 141-145, 141f, 142f
  causes of, 139
  cesarean delivery secondary to, 226
  definition of, 139
  latent phase, 140-141
  recognition of, 140
Dysuria, analgesics for, 288

E

E3. *See* Estriol (E3).
Eclampsia, 174
  clinical and laboratory manifestations of, 176
  etiology of, 175-176
  management of, 177, 180-181
  pathology of, 176
  pathophysiology of, 176
  prodromal signs and symptoms of, 178-179
  seizures in, 174, 177, 180-181
ECMO (extracorporeal membrane oxygenation), 117-118
Ectopic pregnancy, 290-297
  acutely ruptured, 291-292
    pain secondary to, 259
  clinical diagnosis of, 291-292
  clinical presentations of, 291-292
  contraception after, 295, 296

Ectopic pregnancy (Continued)
definition of, 290
diagnostic algorithm for, 293f
diagnostic tests for, 292-294, 294f
differential diagnosis of, 292, 292b
epidemiology of, 290
etiology of, 290
fertility subsequent to, 295, 297
high index of suspicion for, 290
locations of, 290, 291f
management of, 294-296
expectant, 296
laparoscopic, 294-296, 295f, 296f, 335
with methotrexate, 295-297, 297b
with salpingocentesis, 295-296
surgical, 294-295, 295f, 296f
for uncommon types, 297
possible, 292
probable, 292
repeated, 297
Rh isoimmunization and, 184, 189, 296
risk factors for, 290, 291b
spontaneous resolution of, 296
symptoms of, 291-292
after tuboplasty, 376
uncommon types of, 290, 291f, 297
untreated, natural history of, 290-291
Ectropion, cervical, 245, 246
Eczema, vulvar, 235
EDC (estimated date of confinement), 13, 77-78
Edema
lymphedema after groin dissection, 422
in pregnancy
in cardiac patient, 197
lower extremity, 58
preeclampsia and, 174, 177
Effacement. See Cervical effacement.
Egg donation, 378
Eisenmenger's syndrome, 73, 196-197
Elder abuse, 322, 324, 325b
Elective abortion. See Abortion, induced.
Electromagnetic radiation, 396
Electron beam therapy, 396
Electronic fetal monitoring. See Fetal heart rate monitoring.
Embryo transfer, 377-378, 377f
Embryology
of external genitalia, 22, 23f
of internal genitalia, 24-29, 25f, 26f, 240
reproductive, female, 22-33
structural homologues in males and females, 29, 30t
Embryonal carcinoma, 418
Empty sella syndrome, 360-361
Endocarditis, infectious, delivery and risk of, 198
Endocervical curettage, 405, 408
ovarian cancer and, 413
Endocervix, 403
Endocrine disorders, in pregnancy, 191-196
Endodermal sinus tumor, 418
Endoglin, preeclampsia and, 175
Endometrial ablation, 247, 337-338
for adenomyosis, 304
for dysfunctional uterine bleeding, 370

Endometrial ablation (Continued)
hyperplasia as contraindication to, 247
for leiomyomas, 244, 245t
Endometrial biopsy
in dysfunctional uterine bleeding, 369
endometrial cancer and, 429
infertility and, 374
ovarian cancer and, 413
Endometrial cancer
clear cell, 429-432
diagnosis of, 429
endometrioid, 429-430
follow-up of, 432
granulosa cell tumors and, 418
hormonal therapy for, 400, 432
hyperplasia progressing to, 246
ovarian cancer concurrent with, 413, 415, 418
pathologic features of, 429-430, 430f
pelvic lymphadenectomy for, 431, 432
perimenopausal, 380-381
polycystic ovary syndrome and, 367
postmenopausal hormone therapy and, 384
preoperative investigations in, 429
prevalence of, 428
prognosis of, 432, 433t
radiation therapy for, 431-432, 431f
brachytherapy, 432
extended-field, 432
recurrent, 432
risk factors for, 428, 429b
screening for, 428
serous, 429-432
signs of, 429
spread pattern of, 430
squamous cell, 429-430
staging of, 429, 430t, 431, 431f
symptoms of, 428-429, 429t
tamoxifen for, 428
treatment of, 431-432, 431f
Endometrial hyperplasia, 246-247, 247f
anovulatory cycles and, 368-369
granulosa-theca cell tumors and, 246, 252
perimenopausal, 380-381
polycystic ovary syndrome and, 367
postmenopausal hormone therapy and, 384
Endometrial polyps, 245
infertility secondary to, 375, 375f
removal of, 333, 337
Endometrial sampling procedures, 333-334, 333f, 429
Endometrial sarcomas, 434, 433-434
Endometrial stromal tumors, 433-434
Endometrioid adenocarcinoma, endometrial, 429-430
Endometrioid ovarian tumors, 415
endometrial cancer coexisting with, 429
Endometriomas, of ovary, 299
Endometriosis, 298-304
adenomyosis associated with, 303
chronic pelvic pain and, 261
congenital abnormalities associated with, 303

Endometriosis (Continued)
diagnosis of, 302
differential diagnosis of, 301
dysmenorrhea secondary to, 258
importance of, 298
infertility secondary to, 298, 301, 302, 376-377
management of, 302-303, 303b
ovarian tumors associated with
clear cell, 415
endometrioid, 415
pathogenesis of, 298-299
pathology of, 299, 300f
patient characteristics with, 298
prevalence of, 298
prevention of, 303
signs of, 301
sites of, 299, 299f
vaginal, 239
staging of, 299-300, 301f
symptoms of, 300-301
Endometritis
acute pain secondary to, 259
puerperal, 136, 137
Endometrium
anatomy of, 26
histophysiology of, 40-42
implantation and, 43-44
involution of, 41-42
lymphatic drainage of, 30-31
Endomyometritis, postpartum, group B streptococcal, 212
Endomyoparametritis, 137
Endopelvic fascia, 276, 279, 280
Endoscopy, gynecologic, 334. See also Hysteroscopy; Laparoscopic surgery; Laparoscopy, diagnostic.
Endotracheal intubation. See Intubation, endotracheal.
Energy substrates, maternal homeostasis of, 61
Engagement, 96
Enteritis, radiation-induced, 399
Enterocele, 239, 276
rectovaginal examination and, 19, 20f, 278
repair of, 279
uterosacral ligaments and, 26-28
Epidermal inclusion cyst. See Inclusion cyst.
Epidural analgesia, for labor pain, 112, 114
dystocia secondary to, 145
shoulder dystocia and, 144
unintended consequences of, 114, 124
Epidural anesthesia
compared to spinal block, 113, 113t
headache secondary to, 114
in preeclampsia, 178
preemptive catheter placement for, 114
unintended consequences of, 114
Epigenetics, 3-4
Epilepsy
catamenial, 388-389
pregnant patients with, 205-206
Epinephrine, for asphyxiated newborn, 117, 118t

Epipodophyllotoxins, 396

Episiotomy
anal lacerations secondary to, 102
analgesia for, 112
concealed hemorrhage secondary to, 133
mechanism of labor and, 102
for occipitoposterior position, 143
for preterm infant, 150
repair of, 105, 106f
analgesia for, 112
scarring secondary to, 233
technique of, 105f

Epithelial neoplasms, benign
ovarian, 250-251, 251f, 253
tubal, 254

Epithelial ovarian cancer. *See* Ovarian cancer, epithelial.

Epophoron, 26, 26f

Erb's palsy
breech presentation and, 169-170
shoulder dystocia and, 144

Ergonovine maleate, for uterine atony, 133-134

Ergot compounds, for hyperprolactinemia, 361

Error, medical, 5-6

Esophagitis, reflux, during pregnancy, 201-202

Estimated date of confinement (EDC), 13, 77-78

Estradiol (E2)
biosynthesis of, 38f, 51f
fetal, 345-346
menstrual cycle and, 35-40, 36f
postmenopausal decline in, 380
in pregnancy, 50-51
seizure threshold and, 388-389
serum, in amenorrheic patient, 359, 361

Estriol (E3), in pregnancy, 50-51, 52f
unconjugated (UE3), 82

Estrogen(s). *See also* Estradiol; Estriol (E3); Estrone; Steroids.
endometrial hyperplasia and, 246
from granulosa-theca cell tumors, 418
menstrual cycle and, 368-369
migraine headaches and, 388
ovarian cycle and, 38
parturition and, 55
postmenopausal decline in, 380, 381, 381t
in pregnancy, 49, 50-51
serum proteins and, 38-39
unopposed, endometrial cancer risk and, 428

Estrogen deficiency
adolescent presenting with, 354
amenorrhea and oligomenorrhea with, 359-360
cervical stenosis secondary to, 247
postmenopausal, genital atrophy and, 233-234, 239
sexual arousal disorder in, 320

Estrogen receptors, 384
cancer therapy and, 400, 432

Estrogen therapy
for dysfunctional uterine bleeding, 369-370

Estrogen therapy *(Continued)*
ovarian cancer and, 412
for permanent hypoestrogenism, 354
postmenopausal, 382-384
breast cancer risk and, 328, 328t
endometrial cancer risk and, 428
for sexual dysfunction, 320
for sexual infantilism, 357-358
for stress urinary incontinence, 283
topical, for urethral syndrome, 286

Estrogenic phase. *See* Proliferative phase.

Estrogen-progestin combinations. *See* Oral contraceptives.

Estrone (E1)
biosynthesis of, 38, 38f, 51f
after menopause, 379-380
obesity and, 428
ovarian cycle and, 38
in pregnancy, 50-51

Ethambutol, for tuberculosis, in pregnancy, 213

Ethical practice, 3, 5, 6-8, 11

Etonogestrel, 306-309

Etoposide, 395-396t, 396

Etretinate, as teratogen, 85

Evidence-based practice, 8-9, 11

Examination. *See* Physical examination.

Exercise
excessive, amenorrhea and, 359
in pregnancy
of cardiac patient, 197
cardiovascular response to, 56
of diabetic patient, 192
recommendations for, 86
puberty onset and, 345

Expulsion of child, 102

Extended-field radiation, for endometrial cancer, 432

Extension of fetal head, 102

External cephalic version, 166-167, 226
Rh sensitization and, 189

External rotation of fetal head, 102

External-beam radiation therapy, 398, 398b

Extracorporeal membrane oxygenation (ECMO), 117-118

Extraembryonic celom, 44, 44f, 45f

Extremities, examination of, 16

F

Face presentation, 170, 170f, 171f

Fallopian tubes. *See also* "Tubal" entries.
adenoma of, 254
anatomy of, 28, 29
benign conditions of, 248-255
bimanual examination of, 17, 18f, 19, 19f
carcinoma of, 412, 419
congenital anomalies of, 248-255
cysts of, 254, 258
embryology of, 24-26
fertilized ovum in, 43
implantation in. *See* Ectopic pregnancy.
infectious or inflammatory masses of, 254, 254f
infertility associated with, 375-376, 376f

Fallopian tubes *(Continued)*
rupture of
with cystic tube, 258
in ectopic pregnancy, 291
torsion of, 255, 258

False labor (prelabor), 97-98, 140

False pelvis, 93

Family planning, 305-314. *See also* Abortion, induced; Contraception; Sterilization.

Family violence, 322-325. *See also* Child abuse.
healthcare provider's responsibilities with, 323, 324b
telephone resources for, 325b

Fatigue, in pregnancy, 86

Fatty liver of pregnancy, acute, 203

Female circumcision. *See* Female genital mutilation.

Female genital mutilation, 233, 234b

Female pseudohermaphroditism, 231

Female sexual dysfunction. *See* Sexual dysfunction, female.

Femoral thrombophlebitis, 138

Fentanyl, for labor pain, 112

Fertility. *See* Infertility.

Fertility awareness methods of contraception, 311

Fertilization, 42-43
sperm defect and, 377

Fetal abdomen
circumference of, 154-155, 155f, 156f
enlarged, dystocia and, 144

Fetal abnormalities. *See also* Chromosomal abnormalities; Congenital and hereditary disorders; Congenital anomalies; Teratogenic agents.
amniotic fluid leakage and, 45
commonly detected with ultrasound, 219, 220b
diabetic mother and, 192-194, 193t
dystocia secondary to, 144-145
fetal demise secondary to, 159
multifactorial, 80-81, 82
oligohydramnios resulting in, 151
pregnancy termination and, 314
screening for, 81-82, 219
with amniocentesis, 220-221
spontaneous abortion and, 75, 76
in twins, 162, 163, 165

Fetal alcohol syndrome, 83, 83b

Fetal anemia, 185
due to Rh sensitization, 185
middle cerebral artery assessment, 185

Fetal bladder, enlarged, dystocia secondary to, 144

Fetal blood sampling, 124-125
scalp, 124-125, 125f, 126t
complications of, 126
in suspected diabetes, 191-192
umbilical cord. *See* Umbilical cord blood sampling.

Fetal breathing movements, 64
in biophysical profile, 88-89, 220, 220b
onset of labor and, 114-115

Fetal circulation, 65-67, 66f, 67t

Fetal demise, intrauterine, 158-159.
   See also Missed abortion.
   abortion for, 314
   coagulopathy caused by, 75, 159
   diagnosis of, 74, 75, 158
   etiology of, 158
      intrahepatic cholestasis
         of pregnancy and, 202
      maternal diabetes and, 191
      maternal epilepsy and, 206
   follow-up of, 159
   management of, 158-159
Fetal distress. *See also* Asphyxiated infant;
      Fetal blood sampling; Fetal heart
      rate monitoring.
   abruptio placentae with, 130
   cesarean delivery secondary to, 226
   conditions associated with, 120, 121f
   late decelerations and, 123f
   meconium and, 124
   respiratory distress syndrome and, 157
   uterine rupture with, 131
Fetal fibronectin, 147
Fetal growth. *See also* Intrauterine growth
      restriction (IUGR).
   abdominal circumference and, 154-
      155, 155f, 156f
   ultrasound measurements of, 154,
      219-220
Fetal head. *See also* Station.
   anatomy of, 91-93, 92f
   circumference of, 154-155, 155f, 156f
   compression of, early decelerations
      and, 121
   delivery of, 102, 103f
   mechanism of labor and, 101-102
   molding of, 91, 100-101
Fetal heart
   detection of heartbeat, 14
   ultrasonography of, 14, 74
Fetal heart rate. *See also* Nonstress test
      (NST).
   baseline assessment of, 120-121, 121t
   in hypoxic conditions, 120
      decelerations and, 122
   nonreactive, 124
   opioids and, 112
   patterns of, 120-122, 121t, 122f, 123f,
      123t
   tachycardia, 124
Fetal heart rate decelerations
   beat-to-beat variability and, 120-121,
      122
   classification of, 121
   definition of, 121
   early, 121, 122f
   intervention and, 123-124
   late, 121, 122, 123f, 123t
   mixed, 121, 122
   normal, 102, 121
   in postterm pregnancy, 157-158
   variable, 121, 122, 123t
Fetal heart rate monitoring
   algorithm for management with, 125,
      126f
   complications of, 126
   controversies about, 126-127
   in first stage of labor, 100

Fetal heart rate monitoring *(Continued)*
   intervention and, 122-124
   methods of, 100, 119, 120f
   patterns observed in, 120-122, 121t,
      122f, 123f, 123t
   in postterm pregnancy, 158
   of preterm fetus, 150
   in second stage of labor, 102
   of twins, 165
Fetal hydantoin syndrome, 84
Fetal immunity, 68
Fetal interventions, maternal risk
      associated with, 8
Fetal monitoring. *See* Fetal heart rate
      monitoring.
Fetal movement. *See also* Fetal breathing
      movements; Nonstress test (NST).
   in biophysical profile, 220, 220b
   maternal assessment of, 87, 156, 158
      hypertension and, 181
   maternal recognition of, 14
   prenatal discussion of, 87
   ultrasound assessment of, 88-89
Fetal oxygenation, 63-64, 64f, 65f
   biophysical profile and, 220
Fetal position
   abnormal, dystocia caused by, 142-143
   prenatal identification of, 87
Fetal presentation. *See also*
      Malpresentation, fetal.
   in multifetal gestation, 165
   prenatal identification of, 87
Fetal pulmonary maturity. *See* Pulmonary
      maturity, fetal.
Fetal surveillance, 119-127. *See also* Fetal
      blood sampling; Fetal heart rate
      monitoring.
   in multifetal gestation, 164
   in suspected IUGR, 156, 157
Fetal tone, in biophysical profile, 220b
Fetal weight
   estimation of, 143, 219-220
   viability limit of, 150
Fetal well-being, assessment of, 87-90,
      88f. *See also specific tests*.
Fetomaternal (transplacental)
      hemorrhage, 183, 184
   detection of, 184
   fetal demise caused by, 159
   procedure-related, 186
   Rh immune globulin and, 189
Fetoplacental unit, 49
   hormones produced by, 49-53
Fetus
   adrenal glands of, 49, 50, 51, 54, 55
   developmental programming of, 4-5
   energy substrates of, 62
   hemoglobin dissociation curve of,
      64-65, 65f
   hypothalamic-pituitary-gonadal axis
      in, 345-346, 346f, 347f
   labor-related changes in, 114-115
   lungs of. *See* Pulmonary maturity, fetal.
   radiation dose to, diagnostic, 215-216,
      216t
   Rh status of, determining, 185
   thyroid of
      normal physiology of, 194

Fetus *(Continued)*
   physiology at term, 114
   thyrotoxicosis and, 196
Fetus papyraceus, 163
Fibrin split products, 136b
Fibrinogen
   fetal demise and, 159
   fresh frozen plasma and, 136, 136t,
      136b
Fibroadenoma, of breast, 328
Fibrocystadenoma, ovarian, 252-253
Fibrocystic changes, of breast, 327
Fibroids. *See* Leiomyomas, uterine
      (fibroids).
Fibroma
   ovarian, 251-252, 252f, 253-254
   vulvar, 233
Fibromyalgia, 262
Fibronectin, fetal, 147
Fibrothecoma, ovarian, 252
FIGO (International Federation
      of Gynecology and Obstetrics)
      staging
   of cervical cancer, 407, 408t
   of endometrial cancer, 429, 430t
   of gestational trophoblastic neoplasia,
      438, 439t
   of ovarian cancer, 414, 414t
   of vulvar cancer, 422, 423t
Fine-needle aspiration biopsy, 327
First trimester screening, 81-82
FISH (fluorescent in situ hybridization),
      chromosomal abnormalities and,
      79, 220
Fistulas
   rectovaginal, 239
      cervical cancer with, 407
      radiation-induced, 399
   urinary, 239, 285
      cervical cancer with, 407
      after hysterectomy, 409
      radiation-induced, 285, 400
Flexion of fetal head, 101, 101f, 102
Flow cytometry, fetal Rh status and, 185
Fluid administration
   in acute renal failure, 200
   for hyperemesis gravidarum, 201
   in labor, 99
   before regional anesthesia, 112-113
Fluid balance
   in preeclampsia, 180
   in pregnancy, 61
Fluid resuscitation
   for neonatal blood loss, 117, 118t
   for postpartum hemorrhage, 133
   for shock
      in amniotic fluid embolism, 135
      in uterine inversion, 134-135
Fluid volumes, in pregnancy, 61
Fluorescent in situ hybridization (FISH),
      chromosomal abnormalities and,
      79, 220
Fluoxetine
   during pregnancy, 83
   for premenstrual dysphoric disorder,
      388
FOCUS-PDCA (Plan, Do, Check, Act)
      cycle, 8, 9f

Folic acid
  with antiepileptic drugs, 206
  gestational trophoblastic neoplasia
    and, 435
  neural tube defects and, 80-81
  preconception recommendation for, 73
Follicles. *See* Ovarian follicles.
Follicle-stimulating hormone (FSH)
  in amenorrheic patient, 359
  in fetal life through puberty, 345-348,
    346f
  follicular development and, 35-36, 36f,
    39-40
  gene mutations affecting, 354
  hypogonadism and, 355
  infertility and
    male, 373
    ovulatory, 374-375
  menstrual cycle and, 35-36, 36f
  pituitary synthesis of, 34, 36-37
  postmenopausal, 381
  in vitro fertilization and, 377
Follicular cysts, 249-250
  in polycystic ovary syndrome, 364, 364f
Follicular phase, 35, 36f, 37f, 39
Fontanelles, 91, 92, 92f
Footling, 166, 167f
Foramen ovale, 65-67, 67t
Forceps delivery
  for breech extraction, 167-169, 168f,
    223, 224f
  in cardiac patient, 197-198
  failed, 224, 225
  indications for, 223
  instruments for, 222-223, 223f
  for persistent occipitoposterior
    position, 143
  prerequisites for, 223-224
  of preterm infant, 150
  technique of, 224
  for transverse arrest of descent, 143
  trauma caused by, 132, 225
  types of, 223-224
  vs. vacuum extraction, 225
Foreign body, vaginal, 239, 266, 267, 269
  atrophic vaginitis and, 269
Fornix (fornices), vaginal, 26, 27f
Fourchette, 23-24, 25f
Fox-Fordyce disease, 232
Fragile X syndrome, 80
Frank method of vaginal dilation, 358
Fraternal twins. *See* Dizygotic twins.
Fresh frozen plasma, 136, 136t, 136b
Frontal suture, 91, 92f
FSH. *See* Follicle-stimulating hormone
  (FSH).
Functionalis, endometrial, 40
Furosemide, for acute tubular necrosis,
  200

G

Galactocele
  of breast, 328
  of vulva, 232
Galactorrhea
  hyperprolactinemia with, 360-362
  precocious puberty with, 352

Gallstones, in pregnancy, 216-217
Gamete intrafallopian transfer (GIFT),
  377-378
Gamma rays, 396
Ganaxolone, as seizure prophylactic, 389
Gap junctions, of myometrium, 139
Gardasil, 270, 402
Gartner's duct cyst, 26, 26f, 236
Gastrointestinal disorders
  chronic pelvic pain in, 262
  during pregnancy, 201-202
Gastroschisis, alpha-fetoprotein and, 81, 221
GBS. *See* Group B streptococci (GBS).
Gender identity disorder, 315
General anesthesia
  for cesarean delivery, 113-114
  risks of, 333
Genetic counseling
  indications for, 78-80, 78b
  screening programs and, 82
Genetic diagnosis, 82-83
  amniocentesis for, 220-221
  chorionic villus sampling for, 221
  pregnancy termination and, 314
Genetic disorders. *See* Congenital
  and hereditary disorders.
Genetic screening
  for autosomal recessive disorders, 80
  vs. diagnostic testing, 82
Genetics, disease risk and, 3-4, 5
Genital ambiguity. *See* Ambiguous
  genitalia.
Genital folds, 22, 30t
Genital mutilation, female, 233, 234b
Genital ridge, 29, 29f
Genital tubercle, 22, 23f
Genitalia
  external. *See also* Vulva.
    anatomy of, 22-24, 24f, 25f
    development of, 22, 23f, 30t
    masculinization of, by progestins, 84
  internal
    anatomy of. *See also specific structures.*
    embryology of, 24-29, 25f, 26f
Genitofemoral nerve, 23-24
Genitourinary dysfunction, 276-289
Geriatric patient, 21
Germ cell tumors, 250, 252, 252f, 415t,
  417-418
Germ cells, primordial, 29, 29f
German measles. *See* Rubella.
Gestation, multifetal, 160-172
Gestational age
  factors in determining, 154b
  initial estimate of, 13, 77-78
  postterm pregnancy and, 157, 158
  teratogenic susceptibility and, 82-83
  viability limit of, 150
Gestational diabetes mellitus
  classification of, 191, 192t
  definition of, 191
  diagnosis of, 191-192, 194t
  incidence of, 191
  management of, 192, 194b
  postpartum management with, 194
  predisposition to, 191
  protease inhibitors and, 207
  screening for, 87

Gestational hypertension, 175
  chronic hypertension subsequent to,
    181-182
  in multifetal gestation, 163
Gestational length, hormonal control of,
  54-55
Gestational sac, ultrasonography of,
  14, 74
  with empty sac, 76
Gestational thrombocytopenia, 198-199
Gestational trophoblastic neoplasia,
  435-442
  chemotherapy for, 439-442
    combination, 441
    single-agent, 441, 441b
  as choriocarcinoma, 436, 439f, 440-441
    diagnosis of, 441
    genetics of, 435
    investigations of, 441
    pathologic features of, 437
    signs of, 441
    staging of, 438
    symptoms of, 440-441
    treatment of, 441-442
  classification of, 436, 437b
  epidemiology of, 435
  etiology of, 435
  follow-up studies with, 442
  genetics of, 435, 436f
  as hydatidiform mole, 435-439
    chemotherapy for, 439
    clinical investigations of, 438
    complete, 437f, 438f
    diagnosis of, 438, 438b
    genetics of, 435, 436f
    monitoring of β-hCG and, 439, 440f
    pathologic features of, 436-437,
      437f
    signs of, 437-438
    staging of, 438, 439t
    symptoms of, 437
    treatment of, 438-439, 441
  as invasive mole, 435, 436, 440
  metastatic, 439f
    follow-up of, 442
    with good prognosis, 441, 442
    with poor prognosis, 441-442
  as partial mole, 189, 435, 436f, 437,
    439-440
  pathologic features of, 436-437, 437f,
    438f
  as placental-site trophoblastic tumor,
    435
  prognosis of, 435, 442
  prognostic groups in, 437b, 436
  Rh sensitization and, 189
  staging of, 438, 439t
  treatment of, 441-442, 441b
GFR. *See* Glomerular filtration rate
  (GFR).
GIFT (gamete intrafallopian transfer),
  377-378
Glabella, 92, 92f
Glomerular capillary endotheliosis,
  in preeclampsia, 176
Glomerular filtration rate (GFR),
  in pregnancy, 60
  with preeclampsia, 176

Glucocorticoids. *See* Corticosteroids (glucocorticoids).
Glucose
for asphyxiated newborn, 117
hyperosmolar, for ectopic pregnancy, 295-296
Glucose challenge test, 191-192
Glucose metabolism, in pregnancy, 61
placental transfer and, 62, 62t, 191
Glucose tolerance test
antepartum, 192, 194t
postpartum, 194
GnRH. *See* Gonadotropin-releasing hormone (GnRH).
GnRH stimulation test, 351-352
Goiter
fetal
antithyroid drugs in utero and, 195
maternal Graves' disease and, 196
neonatal, 196
in pregnant woman, 194
Gonadal agenesis, 357
Gonadal dysgenesis, 355, 356-358
Gonadal-stromal tumors, specialized, 415t, 418
Gonadoblastoma, 253, 254, 357, 417
Gonadostat, 346-347, 347f, 347-348
Gonadotrophs, 34, 36-37
Gonadotropin-releasing hormone (GnRH), 35, 36-37, 37f
hypogonadotropic hypogonadism and, 355-356, 357-358
for ovulatory infertility, 374
postmenopausal, 381
precocious puberty and, 351, 352
receptor for, mutations of, 354
Gonadotropin-releasing hormone (GnRH) agonists
for catamenial epilepsy, 389
for chronic pelvic pain, 263
for endometriosis, 302-303
for leiomyomas, 244
mechanism of action of, 37
for precocious puberty, 352, 353f
for premenstrual syndromes, 388
in vitro fertilization and, 377
Gonadotropins, 35-36, 36f. *See also* Follicle-stimulating hormone (FSH); Luteinizing hormone (LH).
in fetal life through puberty, 345-348, 346f, 347f
for infertility, 374
postmenopausal, 381
Gonorrhea, 265, 271
mucopurulent cervicitis in, 267
pelvic inflammatory disease in, 271-274
Graafian follicle, 39, 41f
Granular cell myoblastoma, vulvar, 233
Granuloma inguinale, 275
vulvar cancer and, 420
Granulosa cell tumors, 251-252, 418
endometrial cancer with, 429
Granulosa cells, 29, 35, 36f, 38, 39-40
fertilization and, 43
Granulosa-theca cell tumors, 251-252, 418
endometrial cancer with, 428
endometrial hyperplasia and, 246, 252

Graves' disease, in pregnancy, 198t
fetal goiter and, 196
Graves speculum, 17f
Gray (Gy), 397
Groin dissection, 422, 424
bilateral, 422, 423
with separate incision, 422
Group B streptococci (GBS), 212-213
prenatal screening for, 87, 212-213
preterm labor and, 148, 212-213
vaginitis caused by, 267
Growth hormone, 34
Growth restriction. *See* Intrauterine growth restriction (IUGR).
Growth spurt, adolescent, 349-350
Guaiac test, 19
Guidelines, clinical, 8-9
Gunshot wounds, abdominal, in pregnancy, 217
Gynandroblastoma, 251
Gynecoid pelvis, 94-96, 95f
Gynecologic history, 14-15
Gynecologic physical examination, 15-19
Gynecologic procedures, 332-342. *See also* Cervical procedures; Endometrial sampling procedures; Hysterectomy; Hysteroscopy; Laparoscopic surgery; Laparoscopy, diagnostic.
appropriateness of, 332, 332b
credentialing and privileging for, 332-333
informed consent for, 333
risks associated with, 333
robotic, 342, 342f
training for, 332-333

H

H$_2$ (histamine-2) receptor blockers
in pregnancy, 202
preoperative, 215
HAIR-AN (hyperandrogenic insulin resistance and acanthosis nigricans) syndrome, 365, 365f, 365-366, 366
HBsAg (hepatitis B surface antigen), 74, 210, 211b
hCG. *See* Human chorionic gonadotropin (hCG).
Head, fetal. *See* Fetal head.
Head and neck, physical examination of, 16
Headache
menstrual migraine, 388
postdural puncture, 114
in preeclampsia, 178-179
Health care, women's, life-course perspective for, 3-11
Heart, examination of, 16. *See also* Fetal heart.
Heart disease
congenital, 196-197
in pregnancy, 196-198
categories of, 196
functional classification of, 197, 197t
management of, 197-198
Heart failure. *See* Congestive heart failure.

Heart rate
fetal. *See* Fetal heart rate.
in pregnancy, 56, 57t
Heartburn, in pregnancy, 85, 201, 202
Hegar's sign, 14
HELLP syndrome, 174, 176, 177
hepatic rupture in, 177
hypertension in, 179
Hematocrit
fetal
amniotic fluid spectrophotometry and, 186
cordocentesis and, 222
Doppler sonography and, 220
packed red cell transfusion and, 135-136
in pregnancy
fluctuations in, 56, 59
screening measurements of, 87
Hematoma
of neonatal head, vacuum extraction and, 225
postpartum, 133
management of, 134
vaginal, 239
vulvar, 233
Hematometra, 247
Hemoglobin
cord blood, 186
percutaneous sampling and, 186
normal fetal values of, 186
packed red cell transfusion and, 135-136
in pregnancy, 59
screening measurement of, 87
Hemoglobin A$_{1C}$, in diabetes control, 191, 192t
Hemoglobin dissociation curves
fetal, 64-65, 65f
maternal, 64-65, 65f
hyperventilation during labor and, 112
Hemolysis, in HELLP syndrome, 174, 177
Hemolytic disease of newborn, 69
non-Rh antigens and, 69, 189-190
Rh antigen and. *See* Rhesus (Rh) isoimmunization.
Hemorrhage. *See also* Uterine bleeding; Vaginal bleeding.
acute renal failure secondary to, 200
antepartum
causes of, 129b. *See also specific causes.*
evaluation of, 128
fetomaternal (transplacental), 183, 184
detection of, 184
fetal demise caused by, 159
procedure-related, 186
Rh immune globulin and, 189
intraventricular, in preterm infants, 150
postpartum. *See* Postpartum hemorrhage.
retinal
in preeclampsia/eclampsia, 176
vacuum extraction and, 225
Hemorrhagic cyst, ovarian, 249, 250
Hemorrhagic cystitis, radiation-induced, 400
Hemorrhoids, 85

Heparin
  for pelvic thrombophlebitis, postpartum, 138
  during pregnancy
    antiphospholipid antibody syndrome and, 199-200
    for DVT prophylaxis, 204
    for DVT treatment, 204
    mechanical valves and, 197
    to reduce risk of IUGR, 156
    risks of, 83-84
Hepatic disorders of pregnancy, 202-203
Hepatic tumors, benign, hormonal contraceptives and, 310
Hepatitis A vaccine, 10
Hepatitis B surface antigen (HBsAg), 74, 210, 211b
Hepatitis B vaccine, 10, 74, 210
  after sexual assault, 324
Hepatitis B virus, 210-211
Hepatitis C virus, 210-211
Herceptin. See Trastuzumab (Herceptin).
Hereditary disorders. See Congenital and hereditary disorders.
Hereditary nonpolyposis colon cancer (HNPCC) syndrome, endometrial cancer risk and, 428
Hermaphroditism, 232
Hernial sac, as vulvar mass, 231
Herpes simplex virus (HSV) infection
  of fetal scalp, 126
  genital, 265, 269-270
    vaginitis as, 267
  in pregnancy, 211
    ruptured membranes and, 152
  in vaginal vault, 239
Herpes zoster, 209, 210
Heterosexual precocious puberty, 350-351, 351b
Heterosexuality, 315-316
Heterotopic implantation, with assisted reproductive technologies, 290, 291f
Hidradenoma, vulvar, 233
High-risk pregnancy
  antepartum assessment of, 87-90, 88f
  incidence of, 119
  monitoring of contractions during labor, 100
  preterm delivery in, 146
  transfer to tertiary care center, 115
Hilar cell tumors. See Lipid cell tumors.
HIPAA (Health Insurance Portability and Accountability Act), 7-8
Hippocratic Oath, 3, 6-7
Hirsutism, 362, 362-363, 363f. See also Hyperandrogenism.
  idiopathic, 365
  laboratory tests in, 366
  physical examination and, 365-366
  in polycystic ovary syndrome, 364, 366-377
  treatment of, 366
Histamine-2 (H₂) receptor blockers
  in pregnancy, 202
  preoperative, 215
History, patient
  in amenorrhea, 359
  approach for, 12, 12b
  in chronic pelvic pain, 260, 260b

History, patient (Continued)
  contraceptive, 13, 15
  gynecologic, 14-15
  in hyperandrogenic disorders, 365-366
  medical, 13, 15
  menstrual, 13, 15
  obstetric, 12-13, 15
  in prenatal visit, 73
  of previous pregnancies, 12-13
  sexual, 15, 318-319
  social, 13, 323
  surgical, 15, 13
HIV. See Human immunodeficiency virus (HIV) infection.
hMG. See Human menopausal gonadotropin (hMG).
HNPCC (hereditary nonpolyposis colon cancer) syndrome, endometrial cancer risk and, 428
Homans' sign, 203
Homosexuality, 315-316, 318-319
Honeymoon cystitis, 286, 287
Hormonal therapy for cancer, 400
  breast, 330, 400
  endometrial, 400, 432
  ovarian, 400
Hormone replacement therapy, menopausal, 382-384
  breast cancer risk and, 328, 328t
  endometrial cancer risk and, 428
Hot flashes, 379-385
HPA (hypothalamic-pituitary-adrenal) axis, 4
hPL (human placental lactogen), 50
  insulin and, 61
HPV. See Human papillomavirus (HPV) infection.
HSG. See Hysterosalpingography (HSG).
HSV. See Herpes simplex virus (HSV) infection.
Human chorionic gonadotropin (hCG), 49-50
  assays for, 293
  dynamics of, 292-293
  in ectopic pregnancy
    diagnosis and, 292-294, 294f
    with expectant management, 296
    with methotrexate treatment, 295
    from residual trophoblast, 295
  implantation and, 44, 292-293
  for infertility, 374-375, 377
  pregnancy tests based on, 14, 50, 74
  in screening for fetal abnormalities, 81, 82
  spontaneous pregnancy loss and, 292-293
  thyroid function and, 62
  as tumor marker, 49-50, 417, 418. See also Gestational trophoblastic neoplasia.
  in vitro fertilization and, 377
Human immunodeficiency virus (HIV) infection, 206-208
  contraceptive methods and, 305, 311
  disease course of, 207
  hepatitis C coinfection with, 210-211
  infections amplifying susceptibility to, 275
  in pregnancy, 207-208

Human immunodeficiency virus (HIV) infection (Continued)
  screening for, 208
  tuberculosis testing and, 213
  sexual assault and, 324, 325
  testing for
    intrapartum, 208
    methods of, 206-207
    prenatal, 74, 208
  treatment and management of, 207-208
  vertical transmission of, 206-208
  viral characteristics in, 206
Human menopausal gonadotropin (hMG)
  for male factor infertility, 373
  for ovulatory factor infertility, 374-375
  in vitro fertilization and, 377
Human papillomavirus (HPV) infection, 265, 270
  cervical cancer and, 402
  condylomata acuminata and
    cervical, 402
    vaginal, 239
  DNA testing for, 403, 404
  vaccination against, 9-10, 10, 270, 402, 403
  vaginal neoplasia and, 425
  vulvar cancer and, 420
Human placental lactogen (hPL), 50
  insulin and, 61
Hydatid of Morgagni, 26f
Hydatidiform mole, 435, 436, 437-439
  chemotherapy for, 439
  clinical investigations of, 438
  complete, 437f, 438f
  diagnosis of, 438, 438b
  genetics of, 435, 436f
  monitoring of β-hCG and, 439, 440f
  partial, 435, 436f, 437, 439-440
  pathologic features of, 436-437, 437f, 438f
  signs of, 437-438
  staging of, 438, 439t
  symptoms of, 437
  treatment of, 441, 438-439
Hydralazine, for severe hypertension, in pregnancy, 179, 180t
Hydrocephalus
  in congenital toxoplasmosis, 214
  dystocia secondary to, 144
Hydronephrosis, physiologic, of pregnancy, 200
Hydrops fetalis
  dystocia secondary to, 144
  Rh isoimmunization and, 183-184, 185
    intrauterine transfusion and, 187
  ultrasound diagnosis of, 185
Hydrosalpinx, 254, 254f
  hysterosalpingography of, 376f
  in vitro fertilization and, 376
17-Hydroxylase deficiency, 354, 357, 358
21-Hydroxylase deficiency, 19, 351, 363-364, 366
Hymen
  anatomy of, 23, 27f
  embryology of, 22
  imperforate, 236, 237f
Hyperandrogenic insulin resistance and acanthosis nigricans (HAIR-AN) syndrome, 365-366, 365f, 366

Hyperandrogenism, 356t, 362-363
  disorders associated with, 362, 363b,
    363-365
  evaluation in, 365-367
  treatment of, 366-367
Hyperemesis gravidarum, 85, 201
Hypergonadotropic hypogonadism,
  353-358
Hyperinsulinism
  acanthosis nigricans with, 365
  in polycystic ovary syndrome, 365
Hyperosmolar glucose, by salpingocentesis,
  for ectopic pregnancy, 295-296
Hyperprolactinemia
  amenorrhea secondary to, 359,
    360-362, 360b
  hypothyroidism with, 37, 360, 361
  infertility and
    male, 373
    ovulatory, 374
Hyperstimulation syndrome, 374-375
Hypertension
  developmental programming for, 4
  diagnosis of, 173
  hormonal contraceptives and, 310
  screening for, 10t
Hypertensive disorders of pregnancy,
  173-182. *See also* Eclampsia;
  Preeclampsia.
  abruptio placentae and, 130
  aldosterone and, 53
  chronic hypertension as, 174-175
    management of, 181
    with preeclampsia, 175, 181
    sequelae of, 182
  classification and definitions of,
    173-175, 174b
  complications of, 173
  gestational hypertension as, 175
    chronic hypertension subsequent
      to, 181-182
    in multifetal gestation, 163
  incidence of, 173
  intrauterine growth restriction and, 154
  sequelae and outcome of, 181-182
Hyperthyroidism
  hydatidiform mole with, 437
  maternal, 195
  normal neonatal state of, 114
Hyperventilation
  during contractions, 112
  of pregnancy, 60, 61
Hypervolemia, physiologic, in pregnancy,
  61
Hypoestrogenism, amenorrhea and
  oligomenorrhea in, 359
Hypoglycemia
  in asphyxiated newborn, 117
  diabetes in pregnancy and, 191
  intrauterine growth restriction and, 157
Hypoglycemic agents, oral, in pregnancy,
  192
Hypogonadotropic hypogonadism, 353-358
Hypotension in pregnancy
  acute renal failure secondary to, 200
  regional analgesia/anesthesia and, 111
    late decelerations and, 124
  in supine position, 58, 124, 173

Hypotensive syndrome, supine, 58, 124
Hypothalamic amenorrhea, 359
Hypothalamic-pituitary axis, 34-37
Hypothalamic-pituitary dysfunction
  amenorrhea and oligomenorrhea with,
    359
  male infertility and, 373,
Hypothalamic-pituitary-adrenal (HPA)
  axis, 4
Hypothalamic-pituitary-gonadal axis,
  developmental changes in, 345-348,
  346f, 347f
Hypothalamic-pituitary-ovarian axis,
  dysfunctional uterine bleeding and,
  369
Hypothalamus, 34-37
  hypogonadotropic hypogonadism
    and, 355-356
  ovulatory infertility and, 374
  postmenopausal hot flashes and, 381
  tumors of, hyperprolactinemia and,
    360-361
Hypothermia, in newborn, 117
Hypothyroidism
  congenital, 196
  hyperprolactinemia with, 37, 360, 361
  maternal, 196
    spontaneous abortion and, 75, 77,
      196
  neonatal, 196
  precocious puberty caused by, 352
Hypotonic bladder, 282, 282f, 285
Hypoventilation, between contractions,
  112
Hypovolemic shock, placental abruption
  and, 131
Hypoxia, fetal, during labor, 119-122
  acid-base status and, 120, 125
  decelerations and, 122
  heart rate and, 120
  resuscitation of newborn and, 114
Hysterectomy, 338-342
  abdominal, 338-340. *See also* Total
    abdominal hysterectomy and
    bilateral salpingo-oophorectomy
    (TAH-BSO).
  for cervical cancer
    diagnosed in pregnancy, 410-411
    in microinvasive disease, 408
    radical, 339, 408-409
  for cervical intraepithelial neoplasia,
    406
  complications of, 341-342, 408, 409
  for endometrial cancer, 431, 431f, 432
  for endometrial hyperplasia, complex,
    247
  for gestational trophoblastic neoplasia,
    442, 441
  indications for, 338t
    abdominal, 339
    vaginal, 340
  laparoscopic, 335-336
    for endometrial cancer, 431
    for leiomyomas, 244
  for leiomyomas, 244, 245t
  oophorectomy at time of, 339
  for postpartum hemorrhage, intractable,
    134

Hysterectomy *(Continued)*
  types of, 338, 339f
  vaginal, 340-341
    for dysfunctional uterine bleeding,
      370
Hysterosalpingography (HSG)
  of hydrosalpinges, 376f
  infertility and, 372, 375
  normal, 376f
  procedure for, 375
Hysteroscopy, 334, 336-338, 337f

I

ICSI (intracytoplasmic sperm injection),
  373, 377
Identical twins. *See* Monozygotic twins.
Idiopathic (immune) thrombocytopenia
  (ITP), 132-133, 198-199, 198t
Ileus, carcinomatous, 413-414
Ilioinguinal nerve, 23-24
Ilium, 93
Imipramine, for urinary incontinence,
  284-285
Immature teratoma, 418
Immune hydrops, 144
Immune system
  breastfeeding and, 109-110
  fetal, 68
  hemolytic disease of newborn and,
    69
  maternal-fetal interaction and, 67-69
    preterm birth and, 147
  overview of, 67-68
  of pregnant woman, 69
  spontaneous abortion and, 77
Immune (idiopathic) thrombocytopenia
  (ITP), 132-133, 198-199, 198t
Immunization
  against human papillomavirus, 9-10,
    270, 402, 403
  recommended, 9-10
  for travel during pregnancy, 86
Immunoglobulins
  B-cell production of, 68
  in breast milk, 109-110
  in colostrum, 110
  fetal production of, 68
  intravenous, for immune
    thrombocytopenia, 199
  maternal-fetal transfer of, 62t, 68
Imperforate hymen, 236, 237f, 358
Implanon, 306
Implantation, 43-44, 44f
  immune system and, 69
  relaxin and, 52
In vitro fertilization (IVF), 377-378,
  377f
  ectopic pregnancy and, 290, 291f
  heterotopic implantation with, 290
  vs. laparoscopic surgery, 376-377
  in male factor infertility, 373, 377
  relaxin excess and, 52
Incisions
  abdominal wall, 31-33, 33f
    for hysterectomy, 339
  uterine, for cesarean delivery, 226,
    226f

Inclusion cyst
  tubal, 254
  vaginal, 237
  vulvar, 232
Incomplete abortion, 75, 77
Incontinence. *See* Anal incontinence;
    Urinary incontinence.
Indomethacin, for tocolysis, 149
Induction or augmentation of labor,
    105-109. *See also* Oxytocin.
  in active management protocols, 142
  with artificial rupture of membranes,
      106-107, 108, 141
  Bishop score and, 107-108, 108t
  complications of, 108-109
  epidural analgesia and need for, 145
  to expel dead fetus, with misoprostol,
      159
  genetic thrombophilias and, 146
  in HIV-infected women, 207-208
  indications and contraindications for,
      107, 108t
  infusion method for, 108, 109t
  macrosomia and, 143
  monitoring of contractions with, 100
  in multifetal gestation, 165
  in postterm pregnancy, 157-158
  in preeclampsia, 178
  for premature rupture of membranes,
      151
  for prolonged latent phase, 140-141
  for protraction and arrest disorders,
      141
  shoulder dystocia and, 144
  for transverse arrest of descent, 143
Inevitable abortion, 75
Infant. *See* Neonate.
Infant mortality. *See also* Perinatal mortality.
  prematurity and, 146
  United States ranking in, 3
Infection. *See also* Sexually transmitted
    infections (STIs); Urinary tract
    infection (UTI); Vulvovaginitis.
  mastitis, 110
    galactocele with, 328
  in pregnancy. *See also* Chorioamnionitis;
      Sepsis.
    abortion for, 314
    amniotic fluid analysis and, 221
    bacterial, 211-214
    chlamydial, 271
    fetal effects of, 82, 85
    intrauterine growth restriction
        secondary to, 154
    parasitic, 214
    preterm labor and, 53, 147-148, 150
    PROM management and, 151-152
    recurrent abortion and, 75, 77
    viral, 206-211
Infectious endocarditis, delivery and, 198
Infertility, 371-378
  age and, 371
  definition of, 371
  after ectopic pregnancy, 295, 297
  endometriosis and, 298, 301, 302,
      376-377
  etiologic factors in, 372-377, 373t
    cervical, 375

Infertility *(Continued)*
    male, 372-373, 373t, 377
    ovulatory, 373-375
    peritoneal, 376-377
  evaluation of, 371-372, 372t.
      See also specific etiologic factors.
    laparoscopic, 335, 372
    hyperprolactinemia with, 361
    in hypogonadotropic hypogonadism,
        358
    hysteroscopic procedures for,
        337, 372
    leiomyomas and, 243
    in polycystic ovary syndrome, 364
    prevalence of, 371
    primary vs. secondary, 371
    treatment options for, 372b
      success of, 378
    unexplained, 372, 377
Inflammatory bowel disease, pregnancy
    and, 202
Inflammatory breast cancer, 329
Influenza vaccine, 10
Informed consent, 7, 7t
  for gynecologic procedures, 333
Infundibulopelvic ligament, 28, 28f,
    29-31
Inguinofemoral lymphadenectomy
  for vaginal cancer, 425-426
  for vulvar cancer, 422, 423, 424
Inhibin A, 81
Injury. *See* Trauma.
Innate immune system, 67-68
  fetal, 68
Innominate bones, 93
Inositol triphosphate, 54, 54f
  oxytocin receptor antagonists and, 149
Insulin
  in metabolism during pregnancy, 61
  use in pregnancy, 192, 194b
    fetal testing and, 194
    intrapartum, 194
    postpartum, 194
Insulin resistance
  acanthosis nigricans and, 235, 365,
      365f
  developmental programming for, 4
  in polycystic ovary syndrome,
      365, 367
    infertility and, 374
  in pregnancy, 61, 191
Insurance companies, ethical practice
    and, 8
Integrins, implantation and, 43-44
Intensity-modulated radiation therapy,
    398
Interconception care, 110
Intermenstrual bleeding
  definition of, 368b
  patient history of, 15
Internal rotation, 101-102
International Federation of Gynecology
    and Obstetrics. *See* FIGO (Interna-
    tional Federation of Gynecology and
    Obstetrics) staging.
Interstitial brachytherapy, 397, 398b, 399
  for cervical cancer, 409
  for vaginal cancer, 425-426

Intimate partner violence, 322-325
  clinical manifestations of, 322, 323b
  cycle of, 323, 323f
  healthcare provider's responsibilities
      with, 323, 324b
  prenatal screening for, 73
  telephone resources for, 325b
Intracavitary brachytherapy, 397, 398,
    398b, 399f
  for cervical cancer, 409
  for endometrial cancer, 432
  for vaginal cancer, 425-426
Intracytoplasmic sperm injection (ICSI),
    373, 377
Intraductal papilloma, 328
Intrahepatic cholestasis of pregnancy,
    202-203
Intrapartum fetal asphyxia, 126
Intraperitoneal transfusion, fetal, 187-188
Intrauterine devices (IUDs), 307t, 309-310,
    310f
  levonorgestrel-releasing, 309, 310
    for adenomyosis, 304
    endometriosis and, 302, 303
    for leiomyomas, 243-244
  retained in pregnancy, 13
Intrauterine fetal demise. *See* Fetal
    demise, intrauterine.
Intrauterine growth restriction (IUGR),
    153-157
  cerebral palsy and, 118
  in twins, 165-166
  chronic hypertension and, 181
  clinical manifestations of, 154
  definition of, 153, 154
  diagnosis of, 154-155
  disorders associated with, 153
  etiology of, 153-154
  genetic thrombophilias and, 146
  labor and delivery with, 157
  management of, 156-157
  postterm pregnancy with, 157
  prognosis with, 157
Intrauterine insemination (IUI), 373, 375,
    377
Intrauterine transfusion, 186-188,
    188-189, 188
Intravenous immunoglobulin (IVIG), for
    immune thrombocytopenia, 199
Intraventricular hemorrhage, in preterm
    infants, 150
Intubation, endotracheal
  difficult, 112, 113, 113b, 113t
  for general anesthesia, in cesarean
      delivery, 113-114
  of newborn, 115, 117
Invasive mole, 435, 436, 440
Inverse square law, 397
Iodine supplementation, in pregnancy, 194
Iron, requirement in pregnancy, 59
Ischial tuberosities, 22, 24f
Ischiopagus twins, 162
Ischium, 93
Isoimmunization, rhesus, 183-190
Isoniazid, 213
Isosexual precocious puberty, 351-352, 351b
  incomplete, 351b, 352
Isotretinoin, as teratogen, 84-85

Isthmus
    fallopian tube, 29
    uterine, 26, 27f
ITP. *See* Immune (idiopathic)
    thrombocytopenia (ITP).
IUDs. *See* Intrauterine devices (IUDs).
IUGR. *See* Intrauterine growth restriction
    (IUGR).
IUI (intrauterine insemination), 373, 375,
    377
IVF. *See* In vitro fertilization (IVF).
IVIG (intravenous immunoglobulin), for
    immune thrombocytopenia, 199

J

Jadella 2 implant system, 309
Justice, 6, 7

K

Kallmann syndrome, 354
Karyotype, in Down syndrome, 78, 78f
Karyotyping, fetal
    cordocentesis for, 222
    in recurrent abortion, 77
Kegel exercises, 109, 283, 284
Kell antigen, 69, 189-190
Kernicterus, neonatal, Rhesus
    isoimmunization and, 183
Ketoacidosis, in pregnancy, 61
Ketosis, in hyperemesis gravidarum, 201
Kick count, fetal, 87, 156, 158
    in hypertensive patient, 181
Kidd antigen, 189-190
Kielland forceps, 223f
Kleihauer-Betke test, 159, 184, 189
Klinefelter's syndrome (47 XXY), 248
Klumpke's palsy, 144
KOH test, 266
Korotkoff sound, 173
Krukenberg tumor, 419

L

Labetalol, for hypertension in pregnancy
    chronic, 181
    severe, 179, 180t
Labia. *See also* Vulva.
    agglutination of, 232
    anatomy of, 23, 23-24, 25f
    aphthous ulcers of, 235
    benign growths on, 233
    contact dermatitis of, 235-236
    embryology of, 22, 23f
    examination of, 16
    galactocele in, 232
    injuries to, 19-20
    postmenopausal atrophy of, 233-234
Labioscrotal folds, fusion of, 231
Labor. *See also* Uterine contractions.
    acid aspiration syndrome in, 202
    active management of, 141-142
    active phase of, 98-99, 99t, 100f, 139-140
        abnormalities of, 141-145
    adequate, 141
    of cardiac patient, 197-198
    definition of, 54, 91

Labor *(Continued)*
    diagnosis of, 139
    dysfunctional
        active management and, 141-142
        active phase, 141-145, 141f, 142f
        causes of, 139
        cesarean delivery secondary to, 226
        definition of, 139
        latent phase, 140-141
        recognition of, 140
    false, 97-98, 140
    fetal changes associated with, 114-115
    fetal surveillance during, 119-127
    first stage of, 98-100, 99t
    fourth stage of, 98, 105
    hormonal control of, 54-55
    initiation of, 54-55
    latent phase of, 98-99, 100f, 139-140, 140f
        abnormalities of, 140-141
    maternal position in
        first stage, 99
        second stage, 102
        mechanism of, 101-102, 101f
    muscle contraction in, 54
    normal, 91-118, 139-140
    obstetrician's role in, 91
    phases of, 98, 139-140, 140f
    physiologic changes of, 139
    physiologic preparations for, 97-98
    second stage of, 98, 99t, 100-103,
        See also Delivery.
    stages of, 98-105
    symptoms of, instructing patient
        about, 87
    third stage of, 98, 99t, 103-105
Labor curve, 140
Labor induction. *See* Induction or
    augmentation of labor.
Labor pain. *See also* Analgesia
    and anesthesia, obstetric.
    adverse effects of, 112
    neural pathways of, 111, 111f
Laboratory tests
    in acute renal failure, 200
    in cervical cancer, 407-408
    in chronic pelvic pain, 261
    in delayed puberty, 353b
    for gynecologic patient, 19
    in labor, first stage, 99
    normal values in pregnancy, 56, 57t
    in precocious puberty, 351b
    in preeclampsia, 178, 178b
    for pregnancy diagnosis, 14, 50, 74
    in premature rupture of membranes,
        151
    prenatal, 74
    in preterm labor, 148
    in virilization or hirsutism, 366
Lacerations
    obstetric, 233
        classification of, 104
        hemorrhage secondary to, 132, 133
        inspection for, 103
        repair of, 103, 105, 134, 134f
    uterine, abdominal trauma with, 217
    vaginal, 239
    vulvar, 233
Lactation, 110

Lactation suppression, 110
Lactational amenorrhea, 311
Lactotrophs, 34-35, 37
Lambda (posterior fontanelle), 91, 92, 92f
Lambdoid suture, 91, 92f
Lamellar bodies, amniotic fluid, 221
Lamellar body number density, 153
Laminaria, for pregnancy termination,
    314, 314f
Laparoscopic surgery, 334-336, 335f
    for bladder neck suspension, 283
    for ectopic pregnancy, 294-296, 295f,
        296f, 335
    for endometrial cancer, 431
    for endometriosis, 302, 335, 376
    for leiomyomas, 244, 335
    for "ovarian drilling," 374
    for periadnexal adhesions, 376
    in pregnancy, 216, 216t
    for sterilization, 312, 312t, 335
    for tubal occlusion, 375-376
Laparoscopically assisted vaginal
    hysterectomy, 340, 341
Laparoscopy, diagnostic, 334-336
    in chronic pelvic pain, 261, 335
    in endometriosis, 261, 300f, 302, 335
    in infertility, 335, 372, 376
    with ovarian masses, 253, 335
    in pelvic inflammatory disease, 272,
        274, 335
Large for gestational age, 143
Laser technology, 334
    in cervical procedures, 406
    in hysteroscopic procedures, 337-338
    in laparoscopic procedures, 335
    in Paget's disease, 421
    in squamous cell carcinoma in situ, 421
Last menstrual period (LMP), 13, 15
Latent phase of labor, 98-99, 100f,
    139-140, 140f
    abnormalities of, 140-141
Latex allergy, condom use and, 311
Latzko's operation, 285
Lecithin/sphingomyelin (L/S) ratio, 153,
    221
LeFort colpocleisis, 279
Leg cramps, 85
Legal issues
    child abuse and, 322
    physician liability and, 6, 8
    for Erb's palsy, 144
Leiomyomas, uterine (fibroids), 241-245
    characteristics of, 242, 242f
    chronic pain secondary to, 261-262
    differential diagnosis of, 243, 243f, 244f
        vs. leiomyosarcoma, 433
    dysmenorrhea secondary to, 258
    hormonal contraceptives and, 310
    infertility secondary to, 375
    management of, 243, 245t
        hysteroscopic, 337
        laparoscopic, 244, 335
    parasitic, 242, 242f
    pathogenesis of, 241-242
    in pregnancy, 241-242, 261-262
    pregnancy loss secondary to, 76
    risk factors for, 241
    significance for women's health, 241

Leiomyomas, uterine (fibroids) *(Continued)*
  signs of, 243
  symptoms of, 243
  tubal, 254
Leiomyosarcoma
  uterine, 433, 434
  vaginal, 426
  vulvar, 425
Lentigo, labial, 233
Leopold maneuvers, 87, 166
Leptin, 345, 347-348, 354
Leukotrienes, 53, 53f
Leuprolide, 352. *See also* Gonadotropin-
  releasing hormone (GnRH) agonists.
Levator ani muscles, 22, 24f, 27f, 276
  continence and, 280
  prolapse repair and, 279
Levator hiatus, 276
Levonorgestrel. *See also* Intrauterine
  devices (IUDs).
  as emergency contraception, 311-312
  in Mirena intrauterine system, 370
  in Norplant-6, 309
Leydig cell agenesis, 357
Leydig cells, 29
LH. *See* Luteinizing hormone (LH).
LH-RH (luteinizing hormone-releasing
  hormone), 36-37
Lichen planus
  of vagina, 239, 267
  of vulva, 234-235
Lichen sclerosis
  of vulva, 234, 235f
  vulvar cancer and, 420
Lichen simplex chronicus, of vulva, 234, 234f
Lie, prenatal identification of, 87
Life-course perspective, 1-11, 10b
Ligaments
  broad
    anatomy of, 26-31, 27f, 28f
    neoplasms in, 254-255
  cardinal (Mackenrodt's), 26-28, 27f,
    30-31
  infundibulopelvic, 28, 28f, 29-31
  ovarian, 28, 28f, 29-30
  of pelvic support system, 276
  round, 26-29, 27f, 28f
  sacrospinous, 97
  uterosacral, 26-28, 28f
    endometriosis and, 299, 299f, 300-302
Lightening, 97
Liley chart, 186, 187f
Linea nigra, 14
Linear accelerator, 397, 398f
Lipid cell tumors, 418
Lipid metabolism, in pregnancy, 61
Lipoid adrenal hyperplasia, congenital, 354
Lipoma, vulvar, 233
Listeria infection, recurrent abortion and,
  75, 77
Liver disorders of pregnancy, 202-203
Liver function, in preeclampsia, 177
LLETZ (large loop excision of transforma-
  tion zone), 405, 406, 406f
LMP (last menstrual period), 13, 15
Lochia, 109, 137
Lochia alba, 109
Lochia rubra, 109

Lochia serosa, 109
Loop excision
  electrosurgical, 334, 334f
  of transformation zone, 405, 406, 406f
Low birth weight. *See also* Intrauterine
  growth restriction (IUGR).
  adult health and, 4
  cerebral palsy and, 118
  in twins, 165-166
  small for gestational age (SGA), 153
  very low, cesarean delivery and, 150
Low forceps, 223
Low transverse cesarean delivery,
  226-227, 226f
Low vertical cesarean delivery, 226, 226f
Lower uterine segment, 139
L/S (lecithin/sphingomyelin) ratio, 153, 221
Lung disease, obstructive, in pregnancy,
  204-205
Lung profile, 153
Lung volumes and capacities,
  in pregnancy, 59, 59t
Lungs
  examination of, 16
  fetal. *See* Pulmonary hypoplasia;
    Pulmonary maturity, fetal.
Lupus, neonatal, 199
Lupus anticoagulant, 199-200
  recurrent abortion and, 77
Lupus erythematosus. *See* Systemic lupus
  erythematosus (SLE).
Luteal cysts, dysmenorrhea secondary
  to, 258
Luteal phase, 35-36, 37f, 38, 39
  infertility and, 374, 374-375
Lutein cysts, 249-250
Luteinization, 40
Luteinizing hormone (LH)
  in fetal life through puberty, 345-347,
    346f, 347f
  follicular development and, 35, 36f,
    39-40
  hypogonadism and, 355
  hypothalamus and, 36-37
  infertility and, 374, 374-375
  menstrual cycle and, 35-36, 36f, 368
  ovulation and, 35, 36f, 40, 374
  pituitary production of, 34, 36-37
  polycystic ovary syndrome and, 364
  postmenopausal, 381
Luteinizing hormone-releasing hormone
  (LH-RH), 36-37
Luteinizing hormone-releasing hormone
  (LH-RH) agonists, for breast cancer,
  400
Luteoma of pregnancy, 249, 249f
Lymph node metastases
  in breast cancer, 330, 331
  in endometrial cancer, 430, 431, 431f, 432
Lymphadenectomy
  inguinofemoral
    for vaginal cancer, 425-426
    for vulvar cancer, 422, 423, 424
    para-aortic, for endometrial cancer,
    432
  pelvic
    for cervical cancer, 408-409
    for endometrial cancer, 431, 432

Lymphatic drainage, of genital organs,
  30-31, 31f, 423f
Lymphatic spread theory
  of endometriosis, 298
Lymphedema, after groin dissection, 422
Lymphogranuloma venereum, 275
  vulvar cancer and, 420

M

Mackenrodt's (cardinal) ligaments,
  26-28, 27f, 30-31
Macrophages, 67-68
  fetal
Macrosomia, 143
  maternal diabetes and, 143, 191,
    192-194, 193t, 194
  postterm pregnancy with, 157
  shoulder dystocia with, 144
Magnesium sulfate
  for eclampsia, 180
  for preeclampsia, 179, 179t
  for tocolytic therapy, 148-149, 149b
Magnesium toxicity, 179
Magnetic resonance imaging (MRI)
  of adnexal mass, 250t
  of breast, 327
  of cervical cancer, 407
  of pelvic thrombosis, 203-204
  for pelvimetry, 97
  in pregnancy, 215-216
  of tubo-ovarian abscess, 274, 275f
  in urinary incontinence, 283
Male factor infertility, 372-373, 373t, 377
Male pseudohermaphroditism, 232
Male sexual response cycle, 316, 318f,
  317-318
Males, structural homologues in females
  and, 29, 30t
Malignant melanoma
  vaginal, 426
  vulvar, 424, 424f
Malignant mixed mesodermal tumors, 434
Malpresentation, fetal, 160-172
  breech. *See* Breech presentation.
  brow, 171, 171f
  compound, 171-172
  definition of, 166
  dystocia caused by, 142
  face, 170, 170f, 171f
  placenta previa with, 130
  shoulder, 171-172, 171f
Mammography, screening, 326
  recommendations for, 10t, 326
Maneuvers of Leopold, 87, 166
Marshall-Marchetti-Krantz procedure,
  283
Mask of pregnancy, 14
Mastectomy, 330
Mastitis, 110
  galactocele with, 328
Maternal age
  chromosomal abnormalities and,
    78, 79t
  placenta previa and, 129
  preterm delivery and, 146
  in screening for fetal abnormalities, 81
  spontaneous abortion and, 75, 76t

Maternal mortality
  anesthesia-related, 110-111,
    113, 113t
  cesarean delivery and, 225-226
  in ectopic pregnancy, 290
  legal abortion and, 313-314
  in placenta previa, 130
  in uterine rupture, 131
  worldwide, 305
Mauriceau-Smellie-Veit maneuver, 168f
Mayer-Rokitansky-Küster-Hauser
    syndrome. *See* Rokitansky-Küster-
    Hauser syndrome.
Maylard incision, 32-33, 33f
MCA. *See* Middle cerebral artery (MCA),
    fetal, Doppler studies of.
McBurney incision, 33f
McCune-Albright syndrome, 352
McDonald's cerclage, 222, 222f
McIndoe vaginoplasty, 358
McRoberts' maneuver, 144
Mechanical ventilation, for newborn,
    117
Meconium, 124
  aspiration of, 117-118
  clearing airway and, 115, 117
  intrahepatic cholestasis of pregnancy
    and, 202
Medical error, 5-6
Medical history, 13, 15
Medication errors, 4
Medroxyprogesterone acetate
  depot (DMPA)
    for adenomyosis, 304
    for contraception, 307-309t, 311
    leiomyomas and, 241
    to prevent recurrent endometriosis,
      302
  for endometrial cancer, 432
  for endometriosis, 302-303
  in postmenopausal hormone therapy,
    382-383, 384
  for primary dysmenorrhea, 257
Megavoltage radiation therapy, 397, 398b
Meigs' syndrome, 252, 253-254
Meiotic division, 40
Melanoma, malignant
  vaginal, 426
  vulvar, 424, 424f
Melasma, hormonal contraceptives and,
    311
Menarche, 348-350, 350f
  historical decrease in age of, 345, 346f
  race and, 350t
  weight and, 345
Mendelson's syndrome, in pregnancy,
    202
Meningitis, neonatal, group B
    streptococcal, 212
Meningocele, 80-81, 144-145
Meningococcal vaccine, 10
Meningomyelocele, 144-145
Menometrorrhagia
  definition of, 368, 368b
  management of, 370b
Menopause, 379. *See also* Climacteric;
    Postmenopausal women.
  premature 379, 383-384

Menorrhagia
  adenomyosis and, 304
  definition of, 368b
  endometrial ablation for, 337-338
  leiomyomas and, 243-244
  in pelvic congestion syndrome, 262
Menstrual cramps, 15
Menstrual cycle, 34, 38-40. *See also*
    Corpus luteum; Ovarian follicles;
    Ovulation.
  estrogens in, 38
  gonadotropin secretion and, 35-36,
    36f, 37, 37f
  postpartum, 109
  progestins in, 38
  summary of events in, 368-369
Menstrual cycle-influenced disorders,
    386-389
  acne, 389
  asthma, 389
  diabetes mellitus, 389
  epilepsy, 388-389
  migraine headache, 388
  premenstrual dysphoric disorder,
    386-387, 387f, 387t
  premenstrual syndrome, 386-388, 387f,
    387t
  epilepsy and, 388
Menstrual history
  expected date of confinement and, 13,
    77-78
  in gynecologic patient, 15
Menstrual phase, endometrial, 40
Mentum, fetal, 170
Meprobamate, as teratogen, 83
Mesonephric ducts, 24-26, 25f, 29f, 30t, 240
  remnants of, 26, 26f,
Mesosalpinx, 28, 29
Metabolic syndrome, 191, 365
Metformin, for ovulatory infertility, 374
Methergine, avoided in cardiac patient, 198
Methimazole, for maternal
    hyperthyroidism, 195
Methotrexate
  for ectopic pregnancy, 295, 296, 297
    elimination from body, 296
    patient selection for, 297b
    by salpingocentesis, 295-296
    after surgery, 295
    of uncommon types, 297
  for gestational trophoblastic neoplasia,
    441-442, 441b
  to induce abortion, 314
  mechanism of action of, 394
  as teratogen, 83
Methyldopa, for hypertension, in
    pregnancy, 181
Methylergonovine, for uterine atony,
    133-134
Metronidazole, for trichomoniasis,
    268-269
Metrorrhagia, 15, 368b
Mexican Americans, puberty onset in,
    349, 350t
Mid forceps, 223
Middle cerebral artery (MCA), fetal,
    Doppler studies of, 185, 185f, 186
    188-190, 220

Midpelvis, cephalopelvic disproportion
    at, 145
Mifepristone (RU 486)
  to induce abortion, 314
  for leiomyomas, uterine, 244
Migraine headache, menstrual, 388
Minute ventilation, in pregnancy, 60
Mirena intrauterine system, 370
Miscarriage, 312. *See also* Abortion,
    spontaneous.
Misoprostol
  to expel dead fetus, 158-159, 314
  for induced abortion, 314
  Missed abortion, 75, 77
Mitosis, 393
Mitral stenosis, 196, 197
Mittelschmerz, 15
Mixed mesodermal tumors, malignant, 434
MMR (measles, mumps, and rubella)
    vaccine, 10
Molar pregnancy. *See* Gestational
    trophoblastic neoplasia.
Molding of fetal head, 91, 100-101
Molluscum contagiosum, 275
Monoamniotic twins, 160, 160t, 161f
  delivery of, 164
Monochorionic twins, 160, 160t, 161f
  ultrasonography of, 161-162, 162f
  umbilical cord abnormalities of, 163
  vascular anastomoses of, 162
Monozygotic twins, 160-162, 161f,
  twin-twin transfusion syndrome in,
    162-163, 163f
Mons veneris, 23, 25f
Montevideo units, 141
Morgagni, hydatid of, 26f
Morphine, for cancer pain, 401
Mortality. *See* Fetal demise, intrauterine;
    Infant mortality; Maternal mortality;
    Perinatal mortality.
Morula, 43
Mosaicism, cervical pattern of, 404-405
Mosaicism, genetic, 357, 359
MRI. *See* Magnetic resonance imaging
    (MRI).
MSAFP (maternal serum
    alpha-fetoprotein), 82
Mucinous carcinoma, ovarian, 415
Mucinous cystadenoma, ovarian,
    250-251, 251f, 253
  Brenner tumor with, 415
Mucopurulent cervicitis, 267, 270, 271,
    272, 272f
Müllerian agenesis, 236, 240, 358, 358
Müllerian ducts. *See* Paramesonephric
    ducts.
Müllerian dysgenesis, 358
Müllerian inhibiting substance, 240
Müllerian metaplasia theory
    of endometriosis, 298
Müllerian tubercle, 24-26, 25f
Multip trap, 145
Multiple gestation, 160-172
  abnormalities of twinning process in,
    162-163
  antepartum management of, 163-164
  breech presentations in, 165
  cerebral palsy and, 165-166

Multiple gestation (*Continued*)
complications of, 164b
conjoined twins in, 162
dystocia secondary to, 145
diagnosis of, 163
etiology and classification of, 160, 160t, 161f
fetal abnormalities in, 162, 163, 165
incidence and epidemiology of, 160-161
intrahepatic cholestasis of pregnancy and, 202
intrapartum management of, 164-166, 165b
maternal physiologic adaptation in, 163
with more than two fetuses, 166
ovulation induction and, 166, 374-375
perinatal outcome in, 165-166, 165b
placenta previa and, 129
preterm labor in, 148, 164
reproductive technologies and, 160-161
retained dead fetus syndrome in, 163
timing of cleavage, 160f
twin-twin transfusion syndrome in, 162-163, 163f
amniocentesis for, 163, 221
ultrasonography in
diagnostic, 163
for monitoring, 164
for zygosity determination, 161-162, 162f
umbilical cord in
abnormalities of, 163
blood sampling from, 165
clamping and cutting of, 165
vertex-vertex presentations in, 165
zygosity determination in, 161-162, 162f, 165
Muscular dystrophy, prenatal diagnosis of, 80
Myasthenia gravis, in pregnancy, 198t
Mycoplasma infection
mucopurulent cervicitis in, 267
pelvic inflammatory disease in, 271-272, 273
puerperal endometritis in, 137
recurrent abortion and, 75, 77
Myelocele, 80, 144-145
Myoblastoma, granular cell, of vulva, 233
Myofascial trigger points
abdominal wall, 260-261, 264, 264f
pelvic floor, 262
Myomas. *See* Leiomyomas, uterine (fibroids).

N

Nabothian cysts, 246, 246f
Nabothian follicles, 17, 17f, 404
Nägele's rule, 13
Nalbuphine, for labor pain, 112
Naloxone, for respiratory depression, in newborn, 117, 118t
Narcotics. *See* Opioids (narcotics).
Nasion, 92, 92f
Natural killer (NK) cells, 67-68
fetal, 68
in uterus, 69
Nausea, in pregnancy, 201

Neonatal lupus, 199
Neonate. *See also* Apgar score; Asphyxiated infant.
airway clearing for, 102, 115, 117
cerebral dysfunction in, asphyxia-related, 125, 126-127
chlamydial infection in, 271
diaphragmatic hernia in, 117-118
drying of, 115
facilitating adaptation of, 115
gonococcal infection in, 271
herpes simplex infection in, 211
hypothalamic-pituitary-gonadal axis in, 345-346, 346f, 347f
normal, steps to follow after delivery, 115, 116f
thyroid in
changes at birth, 114
hypothyroidism of, 196
thyrotoxicosis of, 196
umbilical cord clamping and cutting, 102, 103, 115, 125
with twins, 165
Neosalpingostomy, for fimbrial occlusion, 376
Neovagina, creation of, 358
Nerve blocks, for chronic pelvic pain, 264
Neural tube defects, 80-81. *See also* Anencephaly.
alpha-fetoprotein and, 81, 221
Neurofibroma, vulvar, 233
Nevi, on labia, 233
Nifedipine
avoided in congestive heart failure, 198
for primary dysmenorrhea, 257
for severe hypertension, in pregnancy, 179-180
for tocolytic therapy, 149, 149b
Nipples, cracked, 110
Nitabuch's layer, 44
absent in placenta accreta, 130
Nitrazine test, 151
Nitrofurantoin, for urinary tract infection, 288, 289, 289t
Nitrogen mustard, as teratogen, 83
Nitroglycerin, for delivery of second twin, 165, 165f
for uterine inversion, 134-135
Nitroprusside, for severe hypertension, in preeclampsia, 179-180
NK cells. *See* Natural killer (NK) cells.
Noncompliance, patient, 5
Nonmaleficence, 6
Nonreactive fetal heart tracing, 124
Nonsteroidal anti-inflammatory drugs (NSAIDs)
for adenomyosis, 304
in cancer pain management, 400-401
for chronic pelvic pain, 263
for endometriosis pain, 302-303
for menstrual migraines, 388
for primary dysmenorrhea, 256-257
Nonstress test (NST), 87-88, 87f, 88f
β-blockers and, 181
in multifetal gestation, 164
in postterm pregnancy, 157-158
in preeclampsia, 178
in suspected IUGR, 156

Norgestrel, as emergency contraception, 311-312
Norplant-6, 309
NSAIDs. *See* Nonsteroidal anti-inflammatory drugs (NSAIDs).
NST. *See* Nonstress test (NST).
Nuchal translucency, 81, 81f, 219
Nurses, in decision-making process, 8
Nutrition. *See also* Diet.
fetal, adult consequences of, 4, 4f
gestational trophoblastic neoplasia and, 435
intrauterine growth restriction and, 156
multifetal gestation and, 164
preconception, 73
prenatal advice on, 86
preterm birth and, 147-148
puberty onset and, 345

O

Obesity
developmental vulnerability to, 4, 154
disease risk and, 3-4
endometrial cancer risk and, 428
endometrial hyperplasia and, 246
obstetric complications and, 73
polycystic ovary syndrome with, 364
postmenopausal estrogens and, 379-380
puberty onset and, 345
shoulder dystocia and, 144
Oblique diameter, 93-94, 94f
Observational studies
biases in, 382, 382t
of postmenopausal hormone therapy, 382, 384
Obstetric complications, 146-159
Obstetric conjugate, 93, 94f, 96-97
Obstetric history, 12-13, 15
Obstetric physical examination, 13
Obstetric procedures, 219-227
Obstetric shock, 133
amniotic fluid embolus with, 132-133, 135
causes of, 133
coagulopathy with, 135-136, 136b, 136t
definition of, 133
genital tract trauma with, 134, 134f
management of, 133-136
retained products of conception with, 134, 135f
uterine atony with, 133-134
uterine inversion with, 133, 134-135
Occipitofrontal diameter, 92, 92f, 101
Occiput, of fetal skull, 92, 92f
Occiputoanterior position, 101-102, 101f
Occiputoposterior position, 101-102
persistent, 143
Occiputotransverse position, persistent, 142-143
Oligohydramnios, 355-367
intrauterine growth restriction and, 156
in postterm pregnancy, 157-158
premature rupture of membranes and, 151, 152
prenatal detection of, 87-89, 87f
pulmonary hypoplasia and, 45, 151
ultrasonic definition of, 88-89, 151

Oligomenorrhea, 355-367
  with breast development and normal
      Müllerian structures, 359-362, 356t
    and hyperandrogenism, 362-363
    and normal estrogen, 362
  definition of, 359
  infertility associated with, 374
Omega-3 fatty acids
  in breast milk, 110
  in preconception diet, 73
Omphalocele, alpha-fetoprotein and, 81
Oocytes, 29, 39, 41f
  climacteric and, 379
  fertilization and, 42-43,
Oophorectomy. See
      Salpingo-oophorectomy.
Operative vaginal delivery. See also
      Assisted vaginal delivery; Forceps
      delivery; Vacuum extraction.
  indications for, 223
  rate of, 222
    epidural analgesia and, 145
Ophthalmia neonatorum, 271
Opioids (narcotics)
  for cancer pain, 401
  after cesarean delivery, 113-114
  for labor pain, 112
  respiratory depression caused by,
      in newborn, 117
Oral contraceptives, 307-309t, 310-311
  for adenomyosis, 304
  for amenorrheic patient, 361
  catamenial epilepsy and, 389
  child's ingestion of, 20
  in endometriosis treatment, 302-303
  intrahepatic cholestasis of pregnancy
      and, 202
  leiomyomas and, 241, 243-244
  for migraine prophylaxis, 388
  ovarian cancer and, 412
  premenstrual syndromes and, 388
  for primary dysmenorrhea, 256-257
  skin changes and, 14
  as teratogenic agents, 13, 84
Orgasmic disorder, 320, 321
Orgasmic phase, 316-317
Orthovoltage radiation therapy,
      397-398
Osmotic dilators
  for cervical ripening, 106-107
  for pregnancy termination, 314f
Oseoporosis, 381-383, 384
  in amenorrheic patient, 361
  statin drugs and, 384-385
Outcomes. See Quality improvement.
Outlet forceps, 223, 223-224
Ovarian arteries, 30, 31f
Ovarian cancer. See also Ovarian masses;
      Ovarian tumors.
  epithelial, 415-417
    classification of, 414-415, 415t
    clinical features of, 413
    differential diagnosis of, 413
    epidemiology of, 412
    etiology of, 412
    hormonal therapy for, 400
    management of, 415-417
    metastatic, 419

Ovarian cancer (Continued)
    pathologic features of, 415, 416f,
    preoperative evaluation of, 413
    prognosis of, 417
    radioactive colloids for, 398
    screening for, 413
    signs of, 413
    spreading mode of, 413-414
    staging of, 414, 414t, 414b
    symptoms of, 413
  germ cell, 415t, 417-418
  second-look laparotomy in, 414b
  specialized gonadal-stromal, 415t, 418
  staging laparotomy in, 414, 414b
Ovarian cycle, 38-40. See also Corpus
      luteum; Menstrual cycle; Ovarian
      follicles; Ovulation.
Ovarian cysts
  choriocarcinoma with, 441
  chronic pain secondary to, 261
  diagnosis of, 253
  dysmenorrhea secondary to, 258
  endometriomas as, 299, 302
  functional, 249-250, 249f, 249t, 335.
      See also Corpus luteum cysts,
      Follicular cysts.
    precocious puberty and, 20
    rupture of, 258
  management of, 253-254
    laparoscopic, 335
  molar pregnancy with, 437-438
  precocious puberty and, 20, 352
  rupture of, 253, 258
  torsion of, 258, 259f
Ovarian ectopic pregnancy, 291f, 297
Ovarian failure, premature, 359-360, 379
Ovarian fibroma, 252
Ovarian follicles
  development of, 39-40, 41f
  primordial, 29, 39, 41f
  secondary, 39
  visibility of, 29-30
Ovarian fossa, 29-30
Ovarian ligament, 28, 28f, 29-30
Ovarian masses. See also Ovarian cysts;
      Ovarian tumors.
  classification of, 248, 249t
  diagnostic modalities for, 250, 250t, 335
  risk of malignancy with, 250, 250t
Ovarian remnant syndrome, 255
  chronic pain in, 261
Ovarian senescence, 380-381
Ovarian tumors. See also Ovarian cancer;
      Ovarian masses.
  androgen-secreting, 350-351, 365, 366
  benign neoplastic, 248, 249t, 250-253
  classification of, 250
    diagnosis of, 253
    epithelial, 250-251, 251f, 253
    germ cell, 250, 252, 252f
    management of, 253-254
    mixed, 252-253
    sex cord-stromal, 251-252, 252f, 253-254
    torsion of, 255
    functional, 248-254, 249f
  functioning, 252
  histologic classification of, 414-415, 415t
  laparoscopic evaluation of, 335

Ovarian tumors (Continued)
  in pregnancy, 217-218
    ischemic, 217
  pseudoprecocious puberty caused by,
      20, 352
Ovaries
  anatomy of, 29-30
  androgen production by, 362
  benign conditions of, 248-255
  bimanual examination of, 18f, 19, 19f
  blood supply to, 30, 31f
  cancer of, 412-419
  congenital anomalies of, 248-255
  embryology of, 29-33, 29f, 30t
  endometriosis with involvement of,
      253, 299, 299f, 300
  hyperandrogenic disorders of, 363b,
      364-365, 364f
  infarcted, during pregnancy, 217
  injury to, hypergonadotropic
      hypogonadism and, 353-354
  lymphatic drainage of, 30-31
  pain sensitivity of, 259-260
  torsion of, 255, 258
  venous drainage of, 60
Overactive bladder, 282, 284-285, 284b
Overflow incontinence, 285
Ovulation, 40
  in chronic pelvic pain management,
      263
  confirmation of, 374
  hormonal patterns and, 35, 36f, 37, 37f
  infertility and, 373-375
  postpartum, 109
  signs and symptoms of, 14-15
Ovulation induction, 374-375
  multifetal gestation secondary to, 166,
      374-375
Ovum, 40
Oxazolidinedione anticonvulsants,
      as teratogens, 84
Oxybutinin chloride, 284
Oxygen. See also Blood gases.
  arterial partial pressure of
      maternal-fetal gradient of, 63-64, 65
    in pregnancy, 60
  placental transfer of, 63-65, 64f
Oxygen consumption, in pregnancy, 56,
      59-60
Oxygen supplementation
  during cesarean delivery, 112-114
  during labor, 112
    with late decelerations, 124
    with variable decelerations, 123
  for neonatal resuscitation, 115, 117
Oxygenation, fetal, 63-64, 64f, 65f
  biophysical profile and, 220
Oxytocin. See also Induction or
      augmentation of labor.
  in evacuation of hydatidiform mole,
      438-439
  to expel dead fetus, with misoprostol,
      159
  to induce or augment labor
    in active management protocols, 142
    adverse effects of, 108-109
    with artificial rupture of
        membranes, 106-107, 108, 141

Oxytocin (*Continued*)
  assessment and plan for, 107-108
  epidural analgesia and need for, 145
  in HIV-infected women, 207-208
  indications and contraindications
    for, 107, 108t
  infusion method for, 108-109, 109t
  monitoring of contractions with, 100
  in multifetal gestation, 165
  principles for use of, 108-109
  for prolonged latent phase, 140-141
  for protraction and arrest disorders,
    141
  synthetic preparation of, 107
  for transverse arrest of descent, 143
  as natural hormone, 34, 49, 51-52
  in final phase of labor, 55
  suckling and, 109-110
  for postpartum hemorrhage, with
    uterine atony, 133-134
  routine administration of, after
    delivery, 103-104
  in uterine inversion, after
    replacement, 134-135
Oxytocin challenge test, 88f, 90, 156
Oxytocin receptor antagonists, 149

P

Packed red blood cells, 135-136, 136t
  intrauterine transfusion of, 186-188
  for neonatal blood loss, 117, 118t
Paclitaxel, 395-396t, 396
Paget's disease
  of breast, 329
  of vulva, 420, 421
Pain. *See also* Abdominal pain;
    Dyspareunia; Labor pain; Pelvic pain.
  cancer, management of, 400-401
  endometriosis and, 300-302
  in urinary tract infection, 288
  vulvar with no obvious pathology, 236
Pancreatitis, acute, in pregnancy, 217
Papanicolaou (Pap) smear
  abnormal
    classification of, 403-404, 404b
    evaluation of patient with, 404-405,
      406f
    in atrophic vaginitis, 269
  endometrial cancer and, 428
  false negative rate with, 403
  new technologies for, 403
  ovarian cancer and, 413
  prenatal, 74, 410
  procedure for, 17
  recommendations for, 10t
  as screening test, 402-403
  vaginal intraepithelial neoplasia and,
    425
Papilloma, intraductal, 328
Papillomatosis, vestibular, 236
PAPP-A (pregnancy-associated plasma
    protein-A), 81, 82
Para-aortic lymphadenectomy, for
    endometrial cancer, 432
Paramesonephric ducts, 24-26, 25f, 26f,
    30t, 240
  anomalies and, 240

Paramethadione, as teratogen, 84
Parametritis, 137
Parasitic infections, in pregnancy, 214
Parathyroid function, maternal-fetal
    transfer and, 62t
Paroöphoron, 26, 26f
Parovarian masses, 254-255
Partial mole, 435, 436f, 437, 439-440
  Rh sensitization and, 189
Particulate radiation, 396
Parturition. *See also* Labor.
  definition of, 54
  endocrinology of, 49-55
  initiation of, 54-55
  muscle contraction in, 54
Parvovirus B19 infection, amniotic fluid
    analysis for, 221
Pathologic retraction ring of Bandl, 139
Patient, clinical approach to, 12-21, 12b
Patient education, for decreasing preterm
    birth, 147
Patient safety, 3, 5-6, 11
Peau d'orange, 329, 329f
Pederson speculum, 17f
Pediatric patient, 19. *See also* Child abuse.
  genital ambiguity in. *See* Ambiguous
    genitalia.
  genital trauma in, 19-20
  vaginal bleeding in, 20
Pediatric speculum, 17f
Pediculosis pubis, 275
Pelvic congestion syndrome, 262
Pelvic curve, of forceps, 222-223, 223f
Pelvic diameters, 93-94, 94f, 94t, 95f
Pelvic examination, 16-19. *See also*
    Vaginal examination.
  in abnormal uterine bleeding, 369
  approach to patient in, 16
  bimanual, 17-19, 18f, 19f
  in cervical cancer, 407, 407f
  in endometrial cancer, 429
  prenatal, 13
  speculum in, 16-17, 17f
  in stress urinary incontinence, 281
  third-trimester hemorrhage and, 128
  of vulva, 16
Pelvic exenteration
  for cervical cancer, 409-410, 410f
  for vaginal cancer, 426
Pelvic floor
  electrical stimulation of, 285
  Kegel exercises for, 283, 284
  myofascial trigger points in, 262
Pelvic inflammatory disease (PID),
    265-275
  acute pain secondary to, 259
  chronic pain secondary to, 261
  complications of, 272
    adhesions as, 261, 274, 274f
    tubo-ovarian abscess as, 259,
      274-275, 274f, 275f
  diagnosis of, 272, 335
  epidemiology of, 271-272
  intrauterine devices and, 274
  pathogenesis of, 271-272
  prevention of, 273-274
  symptoms of, 272
  treatment of, 272-273, 273b, 273t

Pelvic inlet, 93-94, 94f, 94t
  assessment of, 96
  cephalopelvic disproportion at, 145
Pelvic lymphadenectomy
  for cervical cancer, 408-409
  for endometrial cancer, 431, 432
Pelvic organ prolapse, 276-279
  definition of, 276
  diagnosis of, 278
  etiology of, 278
  management of, 278-279, 279f
  quantification and staging of, 278,
    278f, 278t
  types of, 276, 277, 277f
Pelvic Organ Prolapse Quantification
    (POP-Q), 278
Pelvic outlet, 93, 94, 94t, 95f
  assessment of, 97
  cephalopelvic disproportion at, 145
Pelvic pain, 256-264. *See also*
    Dysmenorrhea.
  acute
    adnexal torsion and 258, 259f
    causes of, 258-259, 258b
    laparoscopic evaluation in, 335
  anatomy and physiology of, 259-260,
    260t
  chronic, 259
    definition of, 259
    diagnostic studies in, 261
    differential diagnosis of, 261-263,
      261b
    laparoscopic evaluation in, 335
    management of, 263-264
    myofascial trigger points and,
      260-261, 262, 264, 264f
    patient history in, 260, 260b
    physical examination in, 260-261
    psychological evaluation in, 261
    psychological factors in, 262-263
  classification of, 256
Pelvic planes, 93, 94t
Pelvic thrombophlebitis, 136, 137, 138
Pelvimetry, clinical, 13, 74, 96-97, 98f
Pelvis
  anatomical supports of, 276
  bony anatomy of, 93-94, 94f, 95f, 95t
  shapes of, 94-96, 95f
Pemphigus, 235
Peptic ulcer, during pregnancy, 202
Percutaneous umbilical blood sampling
    (cordocentesis), 125, 186, 221-222
Perinatal mortality. *See also* Infant
    mortality.
  with breech presentation, 169-170
  cesarean delivery and, 225
  in multifetal gestation, 166
  placental abruption and, 130, 131
  postterm pregnancy and, 157
  uterine rupture and, 131
  vasa previa and, 131
Perineal body, 22, 23-24, 276, 279
Perineorrhaphy, 279
Perineum
  anatomy of, 22, 23, 24f, 25f
  lacerations of, 103, 104-105, 107f
Peritoneal cavity, tubal abortion into, 291
Peritoneal factor infertility, 376-377

Peritoneal folds, 28
Peritonitis, pelvic, puerperal, 137
Pessaries
  for pelvic organ prolapse, 279, 279f
  for stress urinary incontinence, 283
Peutz-Jeghers syndrome, 352
Pfannenstiel incision, 31-33, 33f
Phenazopyridine, 288
Phenobarbital, in pregnancy
  neonatal effects of, 84
  for Rh isoimmunization, 188
  for seizure disorders, 206
  teratogenicity of, 84
Phenotype, 4
Phenytoin (diphenylhydantoin)
  fetal syndrome caused by, 84
  use in pregnancy, 206
  Phospholipase A_2, 52-53, 53f
Phospholipids, amniotic fluid, 221. *See
  also* Antiphospholipid antibodies.
Physical examination. *See also* Pelvic
    examination.
  approach to patient for, 12, 12b
  appropriate boundaries in, 319
  chaperone during, 319, 324
  in chronic pelvic pain, 260-261
  general, 15-16
  gynecologic, 15-19
  in hyperandrogenic disorders, 366
  obstetric, 13
  prenatal, 74
  rectal, 13, 19
  rectovaginal, 13, 19, 20f
  of sexual assault victim, 324
Physiologic adaptation to pregnancy.
    See Pregnancy, physiologic
    adaptation to.
Phytoestrogens, 385
PID. *See* Pelvic inflammatory disease
    (PID).
Piercings, genital, 233
PIF (prolactin release-inhibiting factor),
    36, 37
Piper forceps, 223f
  for breech extraction, 167-169, 168f, 224f
Piskacek's sign, 14
Pitocin, 107. *See also* Oxytocin.
Pituitary gland, 34-35
  adenomas of
    Cushing's disease and, 364
    with hyperprolactinemia, 360-361, 362
  anatomy of, 35f
  hormonal deficiencies of, 356, 359, 362
    anovulation secondary to, 374
  hypogonadotropic hypogonadism
    and, 355-356
  portal system of, 35f
  postpartum necrosis of, 131
Placenta
  chorionic villus sampling of, 221
    fetal Rh status and, 185
  delivery of, 103-104
  development of, 44, 45f
  fetal distress and, 120, 121f
  hemorrhages across, 183, 184
  detection of, 184
    Rh immune globulin and, 189
  hormones produced by, 49-53, 55

Placenta *(Continued)*
  immunobiology of, 69, 147
  infarction of, in preeclampsia, 176, 177
  intrauterine growth restriction and,
    154
  ischemia of, preeclampsia and,
    175, 176
  low implantation of, 129f
    postpartum hemorrhage secondary
    to, 132
  low-lying, 129f, 130
  manual removal of, 134, 135f
  oxygen consumption by, 63
  postterm pregnancy and, 157
  preeclampsia/eclampsia and, 176,
    176, 177
  preterm birth and, 147-148
  prostaglandins produced by, 52-53
  retained tissue from, 132, 133,
    134, 135f
  separation of, 55, 103
  transfer of substances across, 61-62,
    62t
    oxygen and carbon dioxide, 64f,
      63-65
    thyroid hormone, 194-195
  of twins, 160, 161-162, 161f
    problems with, 162-163
  ultrasonic imaging of, transvaginal,
    129, 130, 219
Placenta accreta, 130
Placenta increta, 130
Placenta percreta, 130
Placenta previa, 128-130, 129f
  cesarean delivery for, 129-130, 226
  placental abruption with, 130
  ultrasonic imaging of, 129, 130, 219
Placental abruption. *See* Abruptio
    placentae.
Placental growth factor (PlGF),
    preeclampsia and, 175
Placental-site trophoblastic tumor, 440
Placental transfer, 62
  of immunoglobulins, 64
  of nutrients, 61
  of oxygen and carbon dioxide, 64
Planes, pelvic, 93, 94t
Plant alkaloids, as chemotherapy agents,
    396, 395-396t
Plasma, fresh frozen, 136, 136b, 136t
Plasmapheresis, maternal, for Rh
    isoimmunization, 188
Plasticity, developmental, 4, 5, 10
Platelet concentrate, 135, 136, 136t, 136b
  for immune (idiopathic)
    thrombocytopenia, 199
Platypelloid pelvis, 95f, 96
PlGF (placental growth factor),
    preeclampsia and, 175
PMDD. *See* Premenstrual dysphoric
    disorder (PMDD).
PMS. *See* Premenstrual syndrome (PMS).
Pneumococcal vaccine, 10
Pneumonia
  Pneumocystis carinii, 207
  varicella, 209-210
Pneumothorax, in newborn, 117
Polar bodies, 40

Polycystic ovary syndrome, 249, 249f,
    364-365
  endometrial cancer risk and, 428
  endometrial hyperplasia in, 246
  infertility in, 374
  laboratory evaluation in, 366
  premature pubarche and, 347, 351
  premature thelarche or adrenarche
    and, 352
  subclinical, 362
  treatment of, 366, 367
Polyhydramnios
  amniocentesis for, 221
  definition of, 87-89, 221
  prenatal detection of, 88-89
  preterm birth and, 148
Polymenorrhea, definition of, 368b
Polyps
  cervical, 246
  endometrial, 245
    infertility secondary to, 375, 375f
    removal of, 333, 337
  tubal, 254
Pomeroy method of tubal ligation, 312, 313f
POP-Q (Pelvic Organ Prolapse
    Quantification), 278
Posiero effect, 58, 124
Position of fetus
  abnormal, dystocia caused by, 142-143
  prenatal identification of, 87
Postcoital test, 375
Posterior fontanelle (lambda), 91, 92, 92f
Posterior sagittal diameter, 94, 94t, 94f, 95f
Postmaturity syndrome, 157
Postmenopausal women. *See also*
    Climacteric; Menopause.
  estrogen deficiency in
    genital atrophy and, 233-234
    sexuality and, 315
    vaginal infections and, 266
  vaginal bleeding in, 428-429, 429t
Postpartum depression, 109
Postpartum hemorrhage, 131-133
  causes of, 132, 132b. *See also specific
    causes.*
  coagulopathy and, 132-133
    management of, 135-136
  concealed, 133
  differential diagnosis of, 133
  macrosomia and, 143
  management of, 133-136
  observation of patient for, 105
  prophylactic measures for, 103-104, 133
  retained placental tissue and, 132, 133,
    134, 135f
  uterine atony and, 132
  differential diagnosis in, 133
    management of, 133-134
    uterine inversion and, 133
  uterine inversion and, 133
    management of, 134-135
  uterine rupture and, 131, 132
    management of, 134
Postpartum period. *See also* Puerperium.
  acute renal failure in, 200
  in cardiac patient, 198
  care during, 91-118
  thromboembolic disorders in, 203-204

Postterm pregnancy, 157-158
shoulder dystocia and, 144
Posttraumatic stress disorder, in rape
victims, 325
Potassium balance, in pregnancy, 61
Potassium hydroxide test, 266
Pouch of Douglas (cul-de-sac), 18, 26, 28
herniation of, 276
masses in, 19
PPROM. *See* Preterm premature rupture
of membranes (PPROM).
Practice management, 3-5
Precocious puberty. *See* Puberty,
precocious.
Preconception care, 71-73, 78f
genetic counseling in, 78
life-course perspective and, 4-5
Prednisone, for immune (idiopathic)
thrombocytopenia, 199
Preeclampsia, 173-174
acute fatty liver coexisting with, 203
angiotensin sensitivity in, 176
blood pressure elevation in, 177
cardiomyopathy and history of, 197
central nervous system effects in, 177
chronic hypertension prior to, 181, 175
chronic renal disease and, 201
clinical and laboratory manifestations
of, 176
coagulopathy and, 174, 176, 177
diagnosis of, 173-174
eclampsia with, 174
edema in, 174, 177
etiology of, 175-176
evaluation in, 177-181, 178b
vs. gestational hypertension, 175
hydatidiform mole with, 437, 440
liver function in, 177
lupus and, 199
management of, 177-181
antihypertensive therapy in,
179-180, 180t
assessment for, 177-181, 178b
fluid balance in, 180
goal of, 177
intrapartum, 178
seizure prophylaxis in, 178-179, 179t
in multifetal gestation, 163, 164
pathology of, 176
pathophysiology of, 176
placenta and, 130, 175, 176, 177
prophylaxis of, 181, 182
proteinuria in, 173-174, 177
hypertension and, 181, 175
pathophysiology of, 176
severe, 174
renal function in, 177
sequelae and outcome of, 181-182
severe
criteria for, 174, 174b
HELLP syndrome in, 174, 177
hypertensive emergency in, 179
management of, 178, 179
seizures in, 174
sequelae of, 181-182
thrombophilias and, 146, 176
warning symptoms of, 87
weight gain in, 177

Pregnancy. *See also* High-risk pregnancy;
Prenatal care.
amenorrhea secondary to, 358-359
autoimmune disease in, 198-200, 198t
back pain in, 86
blood flow in
regional, 58
renal, 58, 60
umbilical, 63-64, 64f
uterine, 58, 111
blood gases in, 60
blood pressure in, 56, 57t, 58, 173
elevation of, 177
in supine position, 58, 124, 173
breast cancer in, 331
inflammatory, 329
cervical cancer in, 410-411
constipation in
cystic fibrosis in, 205
diabetes in. *See* Diabetes mellitus,
in pregnancy.
diagnosis of, 14, 74-77
dyspnea of, 60
ectopic. *See* Ectopic pregnancy.
endocrine disorders in, 191-196
endocrinology of, 49-55
fluid volumes in, 61
glucose metabolism in, 61
placental transfer and, 62, 62t, 191
heart disease in, 196-198
heartburn in, 85
hemoglobin dissociation curve in,
64-65, 65f
hyperventilation in labor and, 112
hemorrhoids in, 58, 85
hepatic disorders of, 202-203
hypertension in. *See* Hypertensive
disorders of pregnancy.
immunology of, 67-69
infection in. *See* Infection, in
pregnancy.
leg cramps in, 85
leiomyomas during, 241-242, 243,
261-262
medical/surgical conditions
complicating, 191-218
nausea in, 85, 201
normal laboratory values in, 56, 57t
obstructive lung disease in, 204-205
physiologic adaptation to, 56-70
adrenal, 63
cardiovascular, 56-59, 57t
energy substrates and, 61
hormonal, 49-53
metabolic, 49, 53-54
with multifetal gestation, 163
placental transfer of oxygen and
carbon dioxide in, 63-65, 64f
placental transfer of substances in,
61-62, 62t
in puerperium, 109
renal, 60-61
respiratory, 59-60, 59t
thyroid, 62-63, 194-195
pituitary adenoma during, 362
previous, history of, 12-13
renal disorders in, 200-201
seizures in. *See* Seizures.

Pregnancy *(Continued)*
surgical conditions in, 214-218
symptoms of, 14
alleviating, 85
thromboembolic disorders in, 203-204
thyroid diseases in, 194-196
unintended, 305
urinary tract changes in, 60
viability determination of, 74
weight gain in. *See* Weight gain,
in pregnancy.
Pregnancy loss. *See* Abortion,
spontaneous.
Pregnancy tests, 14, 50, 74
Pregnancy-associated plasma protein-A
(PAPP-A), 81, 82
Prelabor (false labor), 97-98, 140
Premature adrenarche, 352
Premature labor. *See* Preterm labor and
delivery.
Premature pubarche, 352
Premature rupture of membranes
(PROM), 150-152
chorioamnionitis and, 151-152
definition of, 150
diagnosis of, 151
with indigo dye, 221
etiology and risk factors for, 150
incidence of, 150
labor and delivery with, 152
management of, 151-152
outpatient management of, 152
preterm (PPROM)
definition of, 150
management of, 151-152
as proportion of preterm births,
146-147, 147t
Premature thelarche, 352
Premenstrual dysphoric disorder
(PMDD), 386-388, 387f, 387t
Premenstrual syndrome (PMS), 386-388,
387f, 387t
epilepsy and, 388-389
Prenatal care, 73-74. *See also*
Ultrasonography, prenatal.
advice to patient in, 85-87
on breastfeeding, 86
on lifestyle, 85-86
on nutrition, 86
on preventive health care, 90
on symptom management, 85-86
on weight gain, 86, 86t
of cardiac patients, 197
confirming pregnancy in, 74-77
estimated date of confinement and,
13, 77-78
fetal abnormalities and
diagnosis of, 82
screening for, 81-82
fetal assessment in, 87-90
algorithm for, 88f
first visit in, 73-74
follow-up visits in, 86-87
genetic counseling in, 78-80, 78b
gestational age estimation in, 13, 77-78
patient history in, 12-13
physical examination in, 13
viability determination in, 74-77

Present illness, in gynecologic history, 14-15
Presentation, fetal. *See also*
    Malpresentation, fetal.
    in multifetal gestation, 165
    prenatal identification of, 87
Preterm infant
    cerebral palsy and, 118
    intraventricular hemorrhage in, 150
    respiratory distress syndrome in
        antenatal corticosteroids and, 150,
            152
        surfactant therapy and, 153
Preterm labor and delivery, 146-150
    bacterial vaginosis and, 147, 148
    with breech presentation, 150, 169, 226
    definition of, 146
    delivery recommendations for, 150
    diagnosis of, 148
    etiology and risk factors for, 146-147, 147t
        fetal fibronectin in, 147
    glucocorticoids for pulmonary
        maturation in, 107, 150
    incidence of, 146
    infection and, 53, 147, 148, 150
    management of, 148
    in multiple gestation, 148, 164, 166
    occupational stress and, 85-86
    pathways leading to, 147-148
    phospholipase A$_2$ and, 53
    prenatal nutrition and, 86
    prevention of, 147-148
        in multifetal gestation, 164
    spontaneous, 146, 147t
    tocolytic therapy in, 148
        agents for, 148-150, 149b
        contraindications to, 150
        efficacy of, 150
        in multifetal gestation, 164
        with premature rupture of
            membranes, 152
    warning symptoms of, 87
Preterm premature rupture of
    membranes (PPROM)
    definition of, 150
    management of, 151-152
    as proportion of preterm births, 146, 147t
Preventive health care, 3, 4-5, 9-10
    life-course perspective on, 10b
    prenatal advice on, 90
    recommended screening for women,
        10, 10t
PRF (prolactin-releasing factors), 37
Primordial follicles, 29, 39, 41f
Primum non nocere, 6
Procedures. *See* Gynecologic procedures;
    Obstetric procedures.
Procidentia, uterine, 277, 277f
Proctosigmoiditis, radiation-induced, 399
Progesterone
    anticonvulsant effect of, 389
    from granulosa-theca cell tumors, 418
    menstrual cycle and, 35-36, 36f, 38,
        39, 368
    ovulation and, 374
    postmenopausal, 380-381
    in pregnancy, 49, 50
        ectopic, 294
        quiescence and, 54-55

Progesterone *(Continued)*
    as respiratory stimulant, 60
    ureteral dilation and, 60
    premenstrual syndromes and, 388
Progesterone receptors, cancer therapy
    and, 400, 432
Progesterone withdrawal, 55
Progestin challenge test, 359
Progestins. *See also*
    Medroxyprogesterone acetate.
    in chronic pelvic pain management, 263
    in contraceptives
        as implants, 306-309, 307t
        as injections and pills, 307t, 310-311
        as IUDs, 309-310, 307t
    for dysfunctional uterine bleeding,
        370, 370b
    for endometrial cancer, 432
    for endometrial carcinoma, 400
    for endometrial hyperplasia, 247
    for endometriosis pain, 302-303
    for leiomyoma symptoms, 243-244
    ovarian cycle and, 38
    in postmenopausal hormone therapy,
        384
    premenstrual syndromes and, 388
    for primary dysmenorrhea, 257
    use in pregnancy, 84
    for uterine sarcomas, 433, 434
Prolactin, 34-35, 37. *See also*
    Hyperprolactinemia.
    big, 360
    menstrual cycle and, 39
    precocious puberty and, 352
    in pregnancy, 49, 50
    suckling and, 110
Prolactin release-inhibiting factor (PIF),
    36, 37
Prolactinomas, 360
Prolactin-releasing factors (PRF), 37
Prolapse. *See* Pelvic organ prolapse.
Proliferative phase, endometrial, 41, 41f,
    368
Prolonged gestation. *See* Postterm
    pregnancy.
PROM. *See* Premature rupture of
    membranes (PROM).
Promontory, sacral, 93
Propranolol, for thyroid storm, 196
Propylthiouracil
    breastfeeding and, 111t
    for maternal hyperthyroidism, 195
    for thyroid storm, 196
Prostaglandin analogues, 52
    to expel dead fetus, 158-159
    for uterine atony, 134
Prostaglandin synthetase inhibitors, 53
    for tocolytic therapy, 149, 149b
Prostaglandins, 52-53
    biosynthesis of, 52-53, 53f
    for cervical ripening, 53, 106
    dysmenorrhea and, 256-257, 257f, 258
    for ectopic pregnancy,
        by salpingocentesis, 295-296
    endometrial cycle and, 368-369
    to expel dead fetus, 158-159
    parturition and, 54, 55
    preeclampsia and, 175-176

Proteinuria
    diagnosis of, 173-174
    in preeclampsia/eclampsia, 173-174, 177
        hypertension and, 175, 181
        pathophysiology of, 176
        severe, 174
Protocols, disease management, 8, 9
Proton pump blockers, in pregnancy, 202
Protraction disorder, 141, 141f
Pruritus
    intrahepatic cholestasis of pregnancy
        with, 202-203
    vulvar, 232, 233b
        intraepithelial neoplasia and, 420
        squamous cell carcinoma and, 420,
            421
Psammoma bodies, in serous ovarian
    tumors, 251, 416f
Pseudohermaphroditism
    female, 231
    male, 232
Pseudoisosexual precocious puberty, 20,
    351-352, 351b
Pseudomyxoma peritonei, 251
Psoriasis, vulvar, 232, 235
Pubarche, 347, 349
    premature, 352
Puberty, 343-354
    age of, historical decrease in, 345, 346f
    definition of, 345
    delayed, 352-354, 356-357
        diagnostic tests in, 353b
    endocrinologic changes of, 345-349,
        346f, 347f
    factors determining onset of, 345
    precocious, 20, 350-352
        classification of, 351b, 350
        GnRH agonist therapy for, 352, 353f
        laboratory tests in, 351b
        pseudoisosexual, 20, 351b, 352, 418
    sexuality during, 315
    somatic changes of, 349-350
        body composition in, 350
        bone age in, 350
        breast stages in, 349, 348f
        growth spurt in, 349-350
        pubic hair stages in, 347, 349f, 348-349
        race and, 349, 350t
        stages of, 349, 350f
Pubic hair, development of, 347, 349, 349f
    premature, 352
    race and, 350t
Pubis, 93
Pubocervical ligaments, 26-28
Pudendal nerve, 23-24
    electrical stimulation of, for
        incontinence, 285
    urethral sphincter and, 280
Pudendal nerve block, 23-24
    for labor pain, 112
Puerperal sepsis, 128-138
    group B streptococcal, 212
    macrosomia and, 143
    predisposing factors for, 137, 137b
Puerperium, 109. *See also* Postpartum
    period.
Pulmonary aspiration, in anesthetized
    patient, 215

Pulmonary embolism
 combined hormonal contraceptives
  and, 310
 in pregnancy, 204
Pulmonary hypertension, pregnancy
 and, 196-197
Pulmonary hypoplasia, oligohydramnios
 leading to, 45, 151
Pulmonary maturity, fetal. *See also*
 Respiratory distress syndrome
 (RDS); Surfactant.
 amniotic fluid analysis and, 221
 glucocorticoids and, 107, 150
 induction of labor and, 107
 intrauterine growth restriction and, 156
 tests of, 152-153
Punch biopsy, cutaneous, 235f
Punctation, cervical pattern of, 404-405
Pyelonephritis, 286, 287
 antibiotics for, 288
 in pregnancy, 211-212
Pygopagus twins, 162
Pyosalpinx, 254, 254f
Pyridoxine
 for nausea and vomiting, in pregnancy,
  201
 for premenstrual syndromes, 388
Pyuria, 287, 288

Q

Q-tip test, 281, 281f
Quadruple screen, 81
Quality improvement, 3, 5, 8-9f, 9, 11
 medical error reporting and, 5-6
Queenan curve, 186, 188f

R

Race. *See also* African Americans.
 pubertal changes and, 345, 349, 350t
Radiation
 definition of, 396
 types of, 396
 units for measurement of, 397
Radiation therapy 396-400 *See also*
 Brachytherapy; Chemoradiation.
 for Bartholin's gland carcinoma, 424
 biologic considerations in, 397
 for breast cancer, 330
 cell cycle and, 393
 for cervical cancer, 408-409
  in pregnancy, 411
 complications of, 399-400, 400f
  urinary fistulas, 285, 400
 for endometrial cancer, 431-432, 431f
 factors influencing outcome of, 397, 397b
 fractionated, 397
 for gestational trophoblastic neoplasia,
  441-442
 intensity-modulated, 398
 modalities of, 397-399, 398b
 physics of, 396, 397
 in pregnancy, fetal effects of, 85
 unit of radiation in, 397
 for uterine sarcomas, 433, 434
 for vaginal cancer, 425-426
 for vulvar cancer, 423, 424

Radical hysterectomy, 339, 408-409
Radical mastectomy, 330
Radical trachelectomy, 408, 409
Radical vulvectomy, 422
Radiofrequency ablation,
 for leiomyomas, 244-245
Radiologic studies
 in chronic pelvic pain, 261
 in delayed puberty, 353b
 in precocious puberty, 351b
 in pregnancy
  fetal dose from, 215-216, 216t
  fetal effects of, 85
 in urinary tract infection, 288
Raloxifene, 382, 384
Randomized controlled trials, 8
Rape. *See also* Sexual Assault.
 community resources for, 325, 325b
Rationing of health-care resources, 7, 7f
RDS. *See* Respiratory distress syndrome
 (RDS).
Records, health-care, confidentiality of, 7-8
Rectal examination, 13, 19
Rectal injury
 in episiotomy repair, 105
 obstetric laceration as, 104, 107f
 radiation-induced, 399
 in young girl, 20
Rectocele, 239, 276
 rectovaginal examination and, 19, 278
Rectouterine fold, 28
Rectovaginal examination, 13, 19, 20f
 in cervical cancer, 19, 407
Rectovaginal fistula, 239
 cervical cancer with, 407
 radiation-induced, 399
Rectus sheath, anatomy of, 31-32, 32f
Recurrent abortion, 75, 77
 chromosomal abnormalities and, 76, 79
 immunologic factors in, 77
Red blood cells. *See* Packed red blood cells.
Referred pain, 259
Reflux esophagitis, during pregnancy,
 201-202
Regional anesthesia
 for cesarean delivery, 112, 113, 114
 contraindications to, 112, 112b, 113
 for forceps delivery, 223-224
 risks of, 333
 for surgery in pregnancy, 215
 unintended consequences of, 114
Regional enteritis, pregnant patient with,
 202
Relaxin, 52, 60
Renal blood flow, in pregnancy, 58, 60
 with preeclampsia, 176
Renal changes, in pregnancy, 60-61
Renal failure, acute
 hyperprolactinemia in, 361
 in pregnancy or postpartum, 200
  preeclampsia and, 177
Renal failure, chronic
 hyperprolactinemia in, 361
 pregnancy with, 201
 IUGR and, 154
Renal function, preeclampsia and, 177
Renal function tests, in urinary tract
 infection, 288

Renal lesions, in preeclampsia, 176
Renal transplantation, pregnancy
 following, 201
Renal tuberculosis, 287
Renin-angiotensin system, in pregnancy,
 61
Reproductive life plan, 71-73
Resectoscopic endometrial ablation,
 337-338
Residual ovary syndrome, 255
Respiratory alkalosis
 hyperventilation in labor and, 112
 in pregnancy, 60, 61
Respiratory changes, in pregnancy, 59-60,
 59t
Respiratory depression, narcotic-
 induced, in newborn, 117
Respiratory distress syndrome, adult
 (ARDS)
 acid aspiration and, 202
 pyelonephritis with, 212
Respiratory distress syndrome (RDS).
 See also Pulmonary maturity, fetaI;
 Surfactant.
 amniotic fluid testing and, 153, 221
 intrauterine growth restriction
  and, 157
 in preterm infants
  antenatal corticosteroids and, 150,
   152
  surfactant therapy and, 153
 surfactant deficiency and, 115
Respiratory onset. *See also* Breathing
 movements, fetal.
 in asphyxiated infant, 116f, 117
 in normal newborn, 115
Resuscitation. *See also* Asphyxiated
 infant, resuscitation of; Fluid
 resuscitation.
 of normal newborn, 115, 116f
Retained dead fetus syndrome, 163
Rete ovarii, 29
Retinal hemorrhage
 in preeclampsia/eclampsia, 176
 vacuum extraction and, 225
Retinoids, as teratogens, 84-85
Retrograde menstruation theory of
 endometriosis, 298-299
Retropubic urethropexy, 283
Review of systems, 15
Rh complex, 183
 immune thrombocytopenia and, 199
Rh immune globulin (Rh$_0$GAM), 189-190
 indications for, 74, 184, 189-190
  amniocentesis as, 220
  chorionic villus sampling as, 221
  ectopic pregnancy as, 296
  spontaneous abortion as, 77, 184, 189
Rhesus (Rh) isoimmunization, 183-190
 definition of, 183
 detecting hemorrhage related to, 184
 detecting risk of, 184-188
  amniotic fluid for, 185, 186 187f, 188f,
  fetal Rh status for, 185
  maternal antibody titer for, 184-185,
   189
  ultrasound for, 185, 185f
  umbilical blood for, 186

Rhesus (Rh) isoimmunization *(Continued)*
  ectopic pregnancy and, 184, 189, 296
  ethnicity and, 183
  fetal distress in, 120
  incidence of, 184
  intrauterine transfusion for, 186-189
  maternal plasmapheresis for, 188
  pathophysiology of, 69, 183-184
  phenobarbital for, 188
  prevention of, 189-190. *See also* Rh
    immune globulin (Rh$_o$GAM).
  timing of delivery in, 188-189
Rheumatic heart disease, 196
Rheumatoid arthritis, in pregnancy, 198t
Rifampin, in pregnancy, 213
Risk for malignancy index, for ovarian
  mass, 250, 250t, 253
Ritgen maneuver, 102, 103f
Robotic surgery, 342, 342f
Rokitansky-Küster-Hauser syndrome,
  236, 358
Round ligaments, anatomy of, 26-28, 27f,
  28f, 29
RU 486. *See* Mifepristone (RU 486).
Rubella, 82
  congenital syndrome caused by,
    208-209, 208b
  diagnosis of, 208
  vaccination for, 74, 208
Rupture of membranes
  artificial, 106-107, 108, 141
  premature. *See* Premature rupture
    of membranes (PROM).

S
Sacrococcygeal joint, 93
Sacrococcygeal teratoma, dystocia
  secondary to, 145
Sacroiliac joints, 93
Sacrospinous ligament, 97
Sacrospinous notch, 95f, 97
Sacrum, 93
  curve and length of, 93, 97
Safety, patient, 3, 5-6, 11
Sagittal suture, 91, 92f
Salpingectomy
  for ectopic pregnancy, 294, 295, 296f
  for tubal neoplasm, 254
Salpingitis
  ectopic pregnancy and, 290
  infertility secondary to, 375
Salpingocentesis, for ectopic pregnancy,
  295-296
Salpingo-oophorectomy
  for benign ovarian neoplasm, 253-254
  hysterectomy with, 339, 341
  laparoscopic, 335
  prophylactic, 412
Salpingostomy, for ectopic pregnancy,
  294, 295, 296f
Salpingotomy, for ectopic pregnancy,
  294, 295
Sarcoma botryoides, 20, 426
Sarcomas
  uterine, 433-434, 433t
  vaginal, 426
  vulvar, 425

Scabies, 275
Scalp, fetal
  abscess or injury of, 126
  blood sampling from, 124-125, 125f, 126t
    complications of, 126
    in suspected diabetes, 191-192
Screening, recommended procedures for
  women, 10, 10t
Sebaceous cysts, vulvar, 232
Second trimester screening, 81-82
Secretory phase, endometrial, 41-42, 42f
Secundines, 137
Seizures
  in eclampsia, 174, 177, 180-181
  in neonate, asphyxia-related, 125
  pregnancy with history of, 205-206
  prophylaxis of, in preeclampsia,
    178-179, 179t
Selective estrogen receptor modulators
  (SERMs), 382, 384
Selective serotonin re-uptake inhibitors
  (SSRIs), 388, 389
Semen analysis, 372-373, 373t
Sentinel nodes, 422
Sepsis
  incomplete abortion and, 77
  missed abortion and, 77
  neonatal
    bacteria in amniotic fluid and, 152
    group B streptococcal, 212
  puerperal, 128-138
    group B streptococcal, 212
    macrosomia and, 143
    predisposing factors for, 137, 137b
Septate uterus, 240
Septic abortion, 314
Septic shock, 136
  pyelonephritis with, 212
SERMs (selective estrogen receptor
  modulators), 382, 384
Serous borderline tumor, 415, 416f
Serous carcinoma, endometrial, 429-430,
  431, 432
Serous cystadenocarcinoma, ovarian,
  251, 415, 416f
Serous cystadenoma, ovarian, 250-251, 251f
Sertoli-Leydig cell tumors, 251-252, 418
Sertraline, for premenstrual dysphoric
  disorder, 388
Serum triple screen, 81, 154
Sex chromosomal abnormalities, 78
Sex cords, primary, 29
Sex cord-stromal tumors, 251-252, 252f,
  253-254
Sex flush, 316, 317, 320
Sex hormone-binding globulin, 362, 365
Sex-linked disorders, 80
Sexual abuse, of pediatric or adolescent
  patient, 20
  vaginal discharge and, 269
Sexual activity, in pregnancy, 86
Sexual arousal disorder, 320
Sexual assault, 322-325
  community resources for, 325, 325b
  in pediatric or adolescent patient, 19-20
  vaginal trauma in, 239
Sexual aversion disorder, 319-320
Sexual desire disorders, 319-320, 321

Sexual development, 315
Sexual dysfunction, female, 315-321
  classification of, 319-320, 319b
  drugs and, 319, 319b
  etiology of, 319
  history and physical examination in,
    318-319
  management of, 320
  prevalence of, 318
  treatment outcomes with, 321
Sexual expression, variation in, 315-316,
  316b
Sexual history, 15, 318-319
Sexual infantilism, 355-358, 356t
Sexual intercourse, vaginal microflora
  and, 266
Sexual pain disorders, 320. *See also*
  Dyspareunia.
Sexual response cycle
  female, 316-317, 317f
  male, 316-318, 318f
Sexuality, 315-321
Sexually transmitted diseases (STDs). *See*
  Sexually transmitted infections (STIs).
Sexually transmitted infections (STIs),
  265-275. *See also* Pelvic inflammatory
  disease (PID).
  candidiasis as, 268
  contraceptive methods and, 305,
    311
  definition of, 265
  HIV risk and, 275
  intrauterine devices and, 274
  less common, 275
  most common, 265, 269-271
  prenatal testing for, 74, 87
  sexual assault and, 324, 325
  trichomoniasis as, 268
  vaginal microflora and, 265, 266
SGA (small for gestational age), 153, 155
Sheehan's syndrome, 131
Shingles. *See* Herpes zoster.
Shirodkar's cerclage, 222
Shock
  obstetric. *See* Obstetric shock.
  septic, 136
    pyelonephritis with, 212
Shoulder dystocia, 143-144
Shoulder presentation, 171-172, 171f
Sickle cell disease, genetics of, 80, 80t
Sildenafil (Viagra), 320
Simpson forceps, 222-223, 223f
Sims-Huhner test, 375
Sinciput, 92, 92f
Single gene disorders, 79
  prenatal diagnosis of, 221
Skene's glands, examination of, 16
Skin, in pregnancy, 14
Skinning vulvectomy, 420-421
SLE. *See* Systemic lupus erythematosus (SLE).
Sling procedures, for stress urinary
  incontinence, 283-284
Small for gestational age (SGA), 153, 155
Smoking
  in pregnancy
    history-taking and, 13
    intrauterine growth restriction and, 156
    spontaneous abortion and, 75

Smoking *(Continued)*
  teratogenicity of, 85
  vulvar cancer and, 420
Social history, 13, 323
Sodium balance, in pregnancy, 61
Sodium bicarbonate, for severe acidosis, in newborn, 117, 118t
Sodium iodide, for thyroid storm, 196
Solifenacin, 284
Somatostatin, 36
Somatotropin release-inhibiting factor, 36
Special needs patients, 19-20
Speculum, 16-17, 17f
Speculum examination, 16-17
Sperm, antibodies against, 377
Sperm capacitation, 42-43
Sperm head, 42-43, 43f
Spermatogenesis, 42
Spermicides, 311
Spina bifida, 80-81
Spinal anesthesia, 113, 113t
  headache secondary to, 114
Spinnbarkeit, 375
Spiral arteries, 40, 41-42
  preeclampsia and, 176
Spiramycin, for toxoplasmosis, 214
Spironolactone
  for hirsutism, 366-367
  for premenstrual syndromes, 388
Spontaneous abortion. *See* Abortion, spontaneous.
Squamocolumnar junction, 26, 245, 245f, 403, 403f
Squamous cell carcinoma
  Bartholin's gland, 424
  endometrial, 429-430
  vaginal, 425-426
  vulvar, 420
Squamous cell carcinoma in situ, vulvar, 420-421, 421f
Squamous cell hyperplasia, vulvar, 234, 234f
Squamous metaplasia, cervical, 402-404
SSRIs (selective serotonin re-uptake inhibitors), 387-388, 389
St. John's Wort, contraceptive implants and, 306
Statin drugs, for postmenopausal women, 384-385
Station, 96, 100, 100f
  active-phase abnormalities and, 141, 141f, 142f
  Bishop score and, 107-108, 108t
  at crowning, 102
  plotting versus time, 140f
Status epilepticus, 206
Stein-Leventhal syndrome, 428
Sterility, 371
Sterilization, 312, 312t, 313f
  laparoscopic, 312, 312t, 335
  reversal of, 312, 375-376
Steroids. *See also* Androgens; Estrogen(s).
  binding of, by serum proteins, 38-39, 362
  biosynthesis of, 38f, 39-40, 50, 51f, 380f
    enzyme defects in, 357, 357f
  receptors for, 384, 400

Stillbirth
  placental abruption and, 131
  in twins, 165
STIs. *See* Sexually transmitted infections (STIs).
Straddle injuries, 19-20, 239
Streak gonads, 357
Streptococci group B (GBS), 212-213
  prenatal screening for, 87, 212-213
  preterm labor and, 148, 212-213
  vaginitis caused by, 267
Streptomycin, contraindicated in pregnancy, 213
Stress response, 4-5
  preconception care and, 71
  preterm birth and, 147-148
Stress test, for urinary incontinence, 281
Stress urinary incontinence, 280-284
  definition of, 280
  diagnostic tests in, 281-283, 281f, 282f
  etiology of, 280-281
  pelvic examination in, 281
  treatment of, 283
    electrical stimulation for, 285
Stroke, developmental programming and, 4
Stroke volume, in pregnancy, 56, 57t, 58-59
Subgaleal hematoma, vacuum extraction and, 225
Submentobregmatic diameter, 92, 92f
Subocciputobregmatic diameter, 92, 92f, 101
Subpubic angle, 93
Substance abuse, in pregnancy, 13
Suction, of fetal airway, 102, 115, 117
Suction curettage, for pregnancy termination, 314, 333
Sufentanil, epidural, for labor pain, 112
Superficial thrombophlebitis, 203
Superinfection, 286
Supine hypotensive syndrome, 58, 124
Supraoccipitomental diameter, 92, 92f
Supraventricular tachycardia, 197
Surfactant. *See also* Pulmonary maturity, fetal; Respiratory distress syndrome (RDS).
  acidosis and, 157
  chemistry and physiology of, 153
  cortisol and, 51
  initiation of labor and, 55
  laboratory assessment of, 153
  therapy with, 115, 153
Surgical conditions in pregnancy, 214-218
Surgical history, 13, 15
Sutures, cranial, 91, 92f
Swyer syndrome, 357
Symphysis pubis, 93
Synclitism, 96, 97f
Synechiae. *See* Adhesions.
Syphilis, 275
  congenital, 213
  in pregnancy, 213-214
  vaginitis in, 267
  vulvar cancer and, 420
Syphilis testing
  prenatal, 74, 213
  after treatment, 214

Syringoma, vulvar, 233
Systemic lupus erythematosus (SLE)
  diagnostic criteria for, 199, 199t
  in pregnancy, 199, 198t
  spontaneous abortion and, 75, 77
Systemic review, 15

T

T cells, 67, 68, 69
  fetal, 68
  in pregnant women, 207
Tachycardia
  fetal, 124
  supraventricular, 197
TAH-BSO. *See* Total abdominal hysterectomy and bilateral salpingo-oophorectomy (TAH-BSO).
Tamoxifen
  as antiestrogen, 400
  for breast cancer, 330
  endometrial cancer and, 428
  endometrial hyperplasia and, 246
  for ovarian cancer, recurrent, 400
  as selective estrogen receptor modulator, 384
Tattoos, genital, 233
Tay-Sachs disease, 80, 80t
Teletherapy, 398
Teratogenic agents, 82-85
  alcohol as, 83, 83b
  antianxiety agents as, 82-83
  anticoagulants as, 83
  anticonvulsants as, 84, 205, 206
  antineoplastic agents as, 83
    in breast cancer, 331
  cocaine as, 84
  definition of, 82
  diethylstilbestrol as. *See* Diethylstilbestrol (DES).
  estrogen-progestin combinations as, 84
  fetal susceptibility to, 82
  frequency of exposure to, 82
  historical recognition of, 82
  hormones as, 76, 84
  hyperglycemia as, 191
  infectious, 82, 85
  metronidazole and, 268-269
  occupation or lifestyle and, 13
  oral contraceptives as, 13, 84
  oral hypoglycemic agents as, 192
  radiation as, 84-85
  retinoids as, 84-85
  tobacco smoking as, 85
Teratology, principles of, 82
Teratoma
  benign cystic, 250, 252, 252f, 413
  immature
    sacrococcygeal, dystocia secondary to, 145
Terbutaline, variable decelerations and, 123
Testicular feminization. *See* Androgen insensitivity syndrome.
Testicular regression syndrome, 357
Testosterone
  conversion to estrogen, 35, 36f, 38, 38f
  for female sexual dysfunction, 320

Testosterone (Continued)
  hormone-binding proteins and, 38-39, 362
  in hyperandrogenism
    with congenital adrenal hyperplasia, 364
    laboratory evaluation of, 366
    with polycystic ovary syndrome, 365
  normal metabolism of, 357f, 362-363
  postmenopausal, 380
  secretion of, 38
    fetal, 51
  from Sertoli-Leydig cell tumors, 418
Tetanus-diphtheria-pertussis vaccine, 10
Thalassemia, 80, 80t
Thalidomide, 82
Theca cell tumors, 251-252
Theca cells, 29, 35, 36f, 39-40
Theca externa, 39
Theca interna, 39-40
Theca-lutein cysts, 249
  choriocarcinoma with, 441
  molar pregnancy with, 437-438
Thecoma, 418
Thelarche, 349, 350f
  absent, aromatase deficiency and, 354
  delayed, 352-353
  premature, 352
Therapeutic abortion. See Abortion, induced.
Thoracopagus twins, 162
Threatened abortion, 75, 77
  acute pain secondary to, 259
  vs. ectopic pregnancy, 292
Thrombocytopenia
  gestational, 198-199
  immune (ITP), 132-133, 198-199, 198t
  neonatal, maternal ITP and, 199
  platelet concentrate for, 135, 136, 136t, 136b
    in ITP, 199
  preeclampsia with, 174, 175, 177
  thrombotic, in pregnancy, 132-133
Thromboembolic disorders, in pregnancy, 203-204
Thromboembolism
  combined hormonal contraceptives and, 310
  pelvic, 138
  venous, after radical hysterectomy, 409
Thrombophilias, hereditary
  fetal demise and, 159
  induction of labor secondary to, 146
  intrauterine growth restriction and, 153-154, 156
  preeclampsia and, 146, 176
  pulmonary embolism and, 204
Thrombophlebitis
  femoral, 138
  pelvic, 136, 137, 138
  superficial, 203
Thrombosis
  deep venous, 203-204
    combined hormonal contraceptives and, 310
    after radical hysterectomy, 409
  in pregnancy

Thrombosis (Continued)
  in antiphospholipid antibody syndrome, 199-200
  predisposition to, 58
Thrombotic thrombocytopenia, in pregnancy, 132-133
Thyroid
  fetal
    normal physiology of, 194
    physiology at term, 114
    thyrotoxicosis and, 196
  neonatal
    changes at birth, 114
    hypothyroidism and, 196
    thyrotoxicosis and, 196
  in pregnancy
    hyperthyroidism and, 195
    hypothyroidism and, 196
    normal physiology of, 62-63, 194-195
    placental transfer and, 62-63, 62t, 194-195
    thyroid storm and, 195-196
Thyroid drugs, breastfeeding and, 111t
Thyroid function tests
  on cord blood, 195t
  in nonpregnant women, 195t
  in pregnancy, 194, 195t
Thyroid storm, 195-196
Thyroid-stimulating hormone (TSH), 34
  fetal, 194
  in newborn, 114
  in pregnancy, 62
    with hyperthyroidism, 195
    with hypothyroidism, 196
    placental transfer and, 194-195
Thyrotoxicosis
  fetal, 196
  maternal, 195-196
  neonatal, 196
Thyrotrophs, 34
Thyrotropin-releasing hormone (TRH), 36, 37, 39
  placental barrier and, 195
Tinidazole, for trichomoniasis, 269
Tobacco. See Smoking.
Tocolytic therapy
  agents for, 148-150, 149b
  for late decelerations, 124
  for preterm labor, 148
    contraindications to, 150
    efficacy of, 150
    in multifetal gestation, 164
    with premature rupture of membranes, 152
  for primary dysmenorrhea, 257
  for variable decelerations, 123
Tolterodine, 284
TORCH (toxoplasmosis, other, rubella, cytomegalovirus, herpes), 159
Total abdominal hysterectomy and bilateral salpingo-oophorectomy (TAH-BSO)
  for endometrial cancer, 431, 431f, 432
  for endometriosis, 302
  for fallopian tube carcinoma, 419
  for ovarian cancer, 415-416, 418
  for ovarian neoplasms, 253
  for uterine sarcomas, 433, 434

Toxemia of pregnancy, 173
Toxoplasmosis
  amniotic fluid analysis for, 221
  cats in patient history and, 13
  congenital, 214, 214b
  in pregnancy, 214
  recurrent abortion and, 75, 77
Trachelectomy, radical, 408, 409
Transcortin, 63
Transformation zone, 402, 403, 403f, 404, 405
  excision or ablation of, 405, 406
Transfusion. See Blood products; Blood transfusion.
Transgender individuals, 315, 316
Transplacental hemorrhage. See Fetomaternal (transplacental) hemorrhage.
Transsexuals
Transvaginal ultrasonography
  in ectopic pregnancy, 292, 293-294
  for endometrial evaluation, 428, 429
  in polycystic ovary syndrome, 364f
  prenatal, 219
    of low-lying placenta, 130
    of placenta previa, 129, 130
    for viability determination, 74
Transverse arrest, 143
Transverse diameter, 93-94, 94f, 94t, 95f
Trastuzumab (Herceptin), 330
Trauma. See also Abdominal trauma; Birth trauma.
  cervical incompetence secondary to, 76
  to cervix, 247, 246
  obstetric, 132, 246. See also Lacerations, obstetric; Uterine rupture.
    fistulas secondary to, 285
    management of, 134
  to uterus, 246
  to vagina, 239
  to vulva, 233
  in young girl, 19-20
Travel, in pregnancy, 86
Treponema infection, recurrent abortion and, 77
TRH. See Thyrotropin-releasing hormone (TRH).
Trichomoniasis, 267, 267t, 268-269, 268f
  testing for, 266, 266f, 267, 268
Trigger points, myofascial
  in abdominal wall, 260-261, 264, 264f
  in pelvic floor, 262
Triglycerides, in pregnancy, 61
Trimethadione, 206
  as teratogen, 84
Triple screen, 81, 154
Triptans, for menstrual migraines, 388
Trisomy 18, screening for, 81
Trisomy 21. See Down syndrome (trisomy 21).
Trophoblast, 43, 44. See also Gestational trophoblastic neoplasia.
  hCG secreted by, 49-50
  immune response and, 69
  residual, after tubal surgery, 295
Trospium chloride, 284
True conjugate (anatomic conjugate), 93, 94f
True pelvis, 93

TSH. *See* Thyroid-stimulating hormone (TSH).
Tubal factor infertility, 375-376, 376f
Tubal ligation, 312, 312t, 313f
  adnexal torsion secondary to, 255
  ectopic pregnancy after, 290
  reversal of, 312, 375-376
Tubal occlusion, infertility secondary to, 375, 376, 377
Tubal pregnancy. *See* Ectopic pregnancy.
Tubal reconstruction, ectopic pregnancy after, 290
Tuberculosis, 213
  congenital, 213
  prenatal testing for, 74, 213
  urinary tract, 287
Tubo-ovarian abscess, 274-275, 274f, 275f
  rupture of, acute pain with, 259
Turner syndrome (45 XO), 248, 357
Turtle sign, 144
Twins. *See* Multiple gestation.
Twin-twin transfusion syndrome, 162-163, 163f
  amniocentesis for, 163, 221
Two-gonadotropin, two-cell theory, 35, 36f

U

UE3 (unconjugated estriol), 81, 82
Ulcer diseases, genital. *See* Herpes simplex virus (HSV) infection; Syphilis.
Ulcerative colitis, pregnant patient with, 202
Ulcers
  peptic, during pregnancy, 202
  vulvar
    aphthous, 235
    in Behçet's syndrome, 235
    in Crohn disease, 235
    decubitus, 235
Ultrasonography. *See also* Doppler sonography; Transvaginal ultrasonography.
  of adnexal masses, 250, 250t, 261
  in appendicitis, 215-216
  breast, 326-327
  in dysfunctional uterine bleeding, 369
  in ectopic pregnancy, 292-294
  of endometrial thickness, 333
  in endometriosis, 302
  focused, in leiomyoma treatment, 244-245
  for guidance, in obstetric procedures, 220
  of hydatidiform mole, 437
  of leiomyomas, 243, 243f
  of ovarian tumors, 250, 250t, 253, 413
  prenatal, 219-220
    adnexal masses identified in, 217-218
    in cytomegalovirus infection, 209
    to diagnose pregnancy, 14
    fetal abnormalities detected with, 219, 220b
    fetal demise and, 158
    in fetal hydrops, 185
    for gestational age determination, 78
    in high-risk pregnancy, 88-89
    in hypertensive patient, 181

Ultrasonography (*Continued*)
    intrauterine growth restriction and, 154-156, 155f, 156f
    in multifetal gestation, 161-162, 162f, 163, 164
    overview of, 219-220
    of placenta previa, 129, 130
    of placental abruption, 130
    Rh sensitization and, 185, 185f
    routine, 87
    in screening for abnormalities, 81-82
    third-trimester hemorrhage and, 128
    transabdominal, 219-220
    transvaginal, 74, 129, 130
  in stress urinary incontinence, 283
  transvaginal
    in ectopic pregnancy, 292-294
    for endometrial evaluation, 428, 429
    in polycystic ovary syndrome, 364f
    prenatal, 74, 129, 130, 219
Umbilical artery, Doppler assessment of, 89-90, 90f, 125, 220. *See also* Umbilical vessels.
  IUGR and, 154, 157
Umbilical cord
  clamping and cutting of, 102, 103, 115, 125
    with twins, 165
  compression of, decelerations and, 122-124
  encircling neck during delivery, 102
  of twins
    abnormalities of, 163
    clamping and cutting of, 165
  velamentous, 131
Umbilical cord blood sampling, 115, 125, 126t
  with arterial catheter, 117
  in hemolytic disease, 186
  percutaneous (cordocentesis), 125, 186, 221-222
  thyroid function tests with, 195t
  with twins, 165
Umbilical vessels. *See also* Umbilical artery, Doppler assessment of.
  blood flow in, 63-64, 64f
  fetal circulation and, 65, 66f, 67, 67t
  obliteration of, after birth, 67
  rupture of, 131
Unconjugated estriol (UE3), 81, 82
Unicornuate uterus, 240, 241f
Upper uterine segment, 139
Ureteral stone, pain secondary to, 259
Ureteric fistula, after hysterectomy, 409
Ureterovaginal fistula, 239, 285
  radiation-induced, 400
Ureters
  anatomy of, 27f, 28, 28f, 30
  injury to, 28
    in hysterectomy, 340-342, 409
  obstruction of
    in cervical cancer, 407-410
    by endometriosis, 302
  ovaries adherent to, 29-30
  pregnancy-related changes in, 60
  stenosis of, radiation-induced, 400

Urethra
  anatomy of, 22, 24f, 280
  examination of, 16
  tears in region of, anesthesia for repair of, 23-24
Urethral caruncle, 232, 233f
Urethral closing pressure profile, 282
Urethral diverticula, 236-237
Urethral pressure measurements, 282
Urethral sphincter, 280
  intrinsic deficiency of, 280, 282, 283-284
Urethral syndrome, 259, 285-286
Urethritis
  acute
    chlamydial, 270
    gonococcal, 271
  atrophic, 286
  nongonococcal, 271-272
Urethrocystoscopy, 281
Urethropexy
  abdominal retropubic, 283
  laparoscopic, 335
Urethrovaginal fistula, 285
Urge urinary incontinence, 284-285
  electrical stimulation for, 285
Urinalysis, 287
Urinary conduit, after pelvic exenteration, 409
Urinary fistulas. *See* Fistulas, urinary.
Urinary incontinence, 280
  anatomical and physiological basis of, 280
  definition of, 280
  fistulas and, 285
  overflow, 285
  pelvic examination and, 16-17
  postmenopausal, 381
  prevalence of, 280
  stress. *See* Stress urinary incontinence.
  in urethral syndrome, 285-286
  urge, 284-285
Urinary retention, 285
Urinary tract
  chronic pelvic pain associated with, 262
  congenital abnormalities of, 358
  injury to, in young girl, 20
  lower, anatomy and physiology of, 280
  pregnancy-related changes in, 60
Urinary tract infection (UTI), 286-289
  clinical classification of, 287
  complicated, 287
  endoscopic studies in, 288
  hospital-acquired, prevention of, 289, 289b
  host defense mechanisms in, 286-289
  incidence and prevalence of, 286
  management of, 288-289, 289t
    for recurrent infection, 289
  pathogenesis of, 286-287
  perpetuating factors in, 287
  in pregnancy, 211-212
  radiologic studies in, 288
  recurrent, 286, 289
  renal function tests in, 288
  risk factors for, 286, 287b
  terminology of, 286
  urethral diverticula and, 236-237
  urinalysis in, 287
  urine culture and microbiology in, 288

Urinary tract obstruction
in cervical cancer, 407-410
by endometriosis, 302
infection and, 287
Urine collection, 288
Urine culture, 288
Uroflowmetry, 282
Urogenital diaphragm, 22, 24f, 276
Urogenital folds, 22, 23f, 30t
Urogenital ridges, 24-26, 29
Urogenital septum, 24-26, 240
Urogenital sinus, 24-26, 25f, 30t
Urogenital triangle, 22
Ursodeoxycholic acid, for intrahepatic
cholestasis, 203
Uterine artery(ies), 30
embolization of, for leiomyomas, 244, 245t
intraoperative laceration of, 134
ligation of, for postpartum
hemorrhage, 134
Uterine atony
obstetric shock and, 133
postpartum hemorrhage secondary
to, 132
differential diagnosis in, 133
management of, 133-134
uterine inversion and, 133
risk factors for, 132b
oxytocin infusion as, 108-109
Uterine bleeding. *See also* Postpartum
hemorrhage; Vaginal bleeding.
abnormal (AUB)
hysteroscopic evaluation of, 337
nondysfunctional causes of, 369,
369b
patterns of, 368, 368b
dysfunctional (DUB), 368-370
definition of, 368
diagnosis of, 369, 369b
management of, 369-370, 370b
overview of, 368
after placental delivery, 103-104
Uterine blood flow, in pregnancy, 58
regional analgesia/anesthesia and,
111
Uterine cancer, 428-434. *See also*
Endometrial cancer; Sarcomas,
uterine.
Uterine contractions, 139-145
biochemical basis of, 54
contraction stress test, 90
in multifetal gestation, 164
fetal heart rate and, 119, 120f, 121,
122f, 123f,
monitoring of, 100, 119, 120f, 122f,
123f
indications for, 127
physiology of, 139
after placental delivery, 103-104
preterm labor and, 148
prostaglandins and, 52, 53
Uterine corpus, anatomy of, 26, 28f
benign conditions of, 240-247
congenital anomalies of, 240-247
Uterine factor infertility, 375-376, 375f
Uterine inversion, 133
management of, 134-135
Uterine leiomyomas. *See* Leiomyomas,
uterine (fibroids).

Uterine prolapse, 277, 277f
Uterine rupture, 131, 132
cesarean incision and, 226, 227
management of, 134
oxytocin-related, 108-109
pathologic retraction ring and, 139
Uteroplacental insufficiency, 122, 124
Uterosacral ligaments, 26-28, 28f
endometriosis and, 299-300, 299f
Uterus
adenomyosis of, 303-304, 304f
chronic pain and, 261-262
dysmenorrhea secondary to, 258
adhesions in
in Asherman's syndrome, 247
hysteroscopic incision of, 337
pregnancy loss secondary to, 76
anatomy of, 26-28, 27f, 28f
bimanual examination of, 17-18, 18f
chronic pain associated with, 261-262
congenital abnormalities of, 241f,
240-247, 358
pregnancy loss due to, 76, 77
septum as, 337
development of
embryological, 24-26, 25f, 240
from infancy to adulthood, 27f
diethylstilbestrol-induced changes
in, 426
gravid, mechanical effects of
circulatory, 58
respiratory, 59
involution of, 109-110
lower segment of, 26
pain sensitivity of, 259-260
pregnancy loss due to abnormalities
of, 76, 77
pregnancy-related changes in, 14
blood flow as, 58
renin produced by, 61
retroversion of, chronic pain and,
262
segments of, during labor, 139
size of, gestational age and, 154, 154b
stretch of, preterm birth and, 148
trauma to, 246
upper segment of, 139
Uterus didelphys, 240, 241f
UTI. *See* Urinary tract infection (UTI).

V

Vaccination. *See* Immunization.
Vacuum curettage, for pregnancy
termination, 314, 333
Vacuum extraction, 224-225, 225f
in cardiac patient, 197-198
contraindications to, 224-225
vs. forceps delivery, 225
for persistent occipitoposterior
position, 143
trauma caused by, 132
Vagina
agenesis of, 236
anatomy of, 23-24, 26, 27f
atresia of, 236
atrophy of, estrogen deficiency and,
239, 320
benign conditions of, 231-239, 238f

Vagina *(Continued)*
congenital abnormalities of, 231-239,
237f, 238f, 358
cysts of, 237, 238f, 239
dermatologic conditions of, 239
development of, 24-27
diethylstilbestrol-induced changes
in, 426
foreign body in, 239, 266, 267, 269
atrophic vaginitis and, 269
inclusion cysts of, 237
laceration of, during delivery, 132, 133
classification of, 104
inspection for, 103
repair of, 103, 107f, 134
lichen planus of, 239
lymphatic drainage of, 30-31
microecology of, 265-266
in pregnancy, 136
urinary tract infection and, 289
normal physiology of, 265-266
pain sensitivity of, 259-260
postmenopausal changes in, 233-234, 239
postpartum recovery of, 109
speculum examination of, 16-17
trauma to, 239. *See also* Lacerations.
in young girl, 19-20
Vaginal adenosis, 26, 236, 238f, 426
Vaginal birth after cesarean (VBAC), 107,
226-227
Vaginal bleeding, 300. *See also* Uterine
bleeding.
abnormal, history of, 14-15
in cervical cancer, 407, 410
in ectopic pregnancy, 290-292, 297
endometrial cancer and, 428-429
endometriosis and, 300, 302
intermenstrual, history of, 15
in ovarian cancer, 413
postmenopausal, 428-429, 429t
in pregnancy
early, 74, 75
hydatidiform mole with, 437
Rh isoimmunization and, 189
spontaneous abortion and, 75
third-trimester causes of, 128, 129b.
See also specific causes.
in prepubertal child, 20
Vaginal cancers, 420-427
adenocarcinoma, 426
clear cell, 84, 426
malignant melanoma, 426
management of, 425-426
in prepubertal child, 20
prognosis for, 426
sarcoma, 426
spread patterns of, 425
squamous cell carcinoma, 425-426
staging of, 425, 425t
Vaginal carcinoma in situ, 425
Vaginal dilation, Frank method of, 358
Vaginal discharge, 266-269
Vaginal examination. *See also* Pelvic
examination.
during labor, 100, 102
Vaginal fluids, 266
testing of, 266
Vaginal fornix (fornices), 26, 27f
Vaginal plate, 25f, 26

Vaginal prolapse. *See* Pelvic organ prolapse.
Vaginal septum
    longitudinal, 236
    transverse, 236, 237f, 358
Vaginal tumors, in prepubertal child, 20
Vaginal vault necrosis, radiation-
    induced, 399
Vaginal vault suspension, 279
Vaginismus, 239, 320
Vaginitis. *See also* Vulvovaginitis.
    atrophic, 267, 269, 381
    desquamative, 267
    foreign-body, 267, 269
Vaginoplasty, McIndoe, 358
Vaginosis, bacterial. *See* Bacterial
    vaginosis.
VAIN (vaginal intraepithelial neoplasia),
    425
Valproic acid, 206
    as teratogen, 84, 205
Varicella vaccine, 10, 210
Varicella-zoster immune globulin (VZIG),
    210
Varicella-zoster virus infection, 209-210
    in pregnancy, 209-210
        amniotic fluid analysis for, 221
Varicose veins
    pelvic, chronic pain secondary to, 262
    in pregnancy, 58
    vulvar, 232
Vasa previa, 131
Vascular anastomoses, interplacental,
    162-163
    cord cutting and, 165
Vascular endothelial growth factor
    (VEGF), preeclampsia and, 175
Vasectomy, 312
Vasovagal shock, uterine inversion with, 133
Vault brachytherapy, for endometrial
    cancer, 432
VBAC (vaginal birth after cesarean), 107,
    226-227
Velamentous umbilical cord, 131
Velocimetry. *See* Doppler sonography.
Ventilation. *See also* Mechanical ventilation.
    in pregnancy, 60
Ventral wall defects, alpha fetoprotein
    and, 81
Verrucous carcinoma, 424
Version, external cephalic, 166-167, 226
    Rh sensitization and, 189
Vertex, of fetal skull, 92, 92f
Vertex-vertex presentations, in multiple
    gestation, 165
Vesicoureteral reflux, 287
Vesicouterine fold, 28
Vesicovaginal fistula, 239, 285
    radiation-induced, 400
Vestibular adenitis, 232
Vestibular bulbs, 22, 23, 24f, 27f
Vestibular papillomatosis, 236
Vestibule, vaginal, 23-24, 27f
Vestibulitis, vulvar, 232, 236
Viability of pregnancy, 74
Viagra. *See* Sildenafil (Viagra).
Video urodynamics, 283
VIN (vulvar intraepithelial neoplasia),
    420-421, 421f
Vinca alkaloids, 395t, 396

Violence. *See* Child abuse; Family
    violence; Intimate partner violence;
    Sexual assault.
Virilization
    androgen-secreting tumors and, 366, 418
    aromatase deficiency and, 354
    congenital adrenal hyperplasia and, 351
    definition of, 362
    laboratory tests in, 366
    maternal, luteoma and, 249
    onset of, 365-366
    Sertoli-Leydig cell tumors and, 252
Visceral pain, 259
Viscerosomatic convergence, 259
Visual disturbances, in preeclampsia, 177
Vital signs, in physical examination, 15
Vitamin B$_6$
    with isoniazid, in pregnancy, 213
    for nausea and vomiting, in pregnancy,
        201
    for premenstrual syndromes, 388
Vitamin D, with antiepileptic drugs, 206
Vitamin K, with antiepileptic drugs, 206
Voiding cystourethrogram, 282-283
Vomiting, in pregnancy, 85
Von Willebrand's disease, 132-133, 135
Vulva. *See also* Labia.
    anatomy of, 23-24, 25f
    benign conditions of, 231-239
    congenital anomalies of, 231-239, 232f
    cysts of, 232
    epithelial conditions of, 233-236
        234f, 235f,
    examination of, 16
    functional discomfort of, 236
    hematoma of, postpartum, 133
    lymphatic drainage of, 30-31, 423f
    pruritus of, 232, 233b
    traumatic lesions of, 233
Vulvar cancer, 420-427
    Bartholin's gland carcinoma, 424
    basal cell carcinoma, 425
    epidemiology of, 420
    etiology of, 420
    groin dissection in, 422, 424
        bilateral, 422, 423
        with separate incision, 422
    histologic types of, 420
    lymph node metastases from, 421-422,
        423t, 424
    malignant melanoma, 424, 424f
    radical local excision for, 422
    sarcomas, 425
    squamous cell carcinoma, 421-422, 422f
    staging of, 422, 423t
    survival rates of, 424, 424t
    verrucous carcinoma, 424
    vulvectomy for, 422
        radical, 422
        skinning, 420-421
Vulvar intraepithelial neoplasia (VIN),
    420-421, 421f
Vulvar vestibulitis, 232, 236
Vulvar-vaginal-gingival syndrome, 234-
    235
Vulvectomy
    for invasive vulvar cancer, 422
    radical, 422
    skinning, 420-421

Vulvectomy *(Continued)*
    for squamous cell carcinoma in situ,
        420-421
Vulvodynia, 236, 262
Vulvovaginal glands. *See* Bartholin's
    glands.
Vulvovaginitis, 265-275. *See also* Vaginitis.
    causes of, 265-269, 267t
    diagnostic methods in, 266, 267
    in prepubertal child, 20
VZIG (varicella-zoster immune globulin),
    210

W

Warfarin (Coumadin)
    for deep venous thrombosis, 204
    teratogenicity of, 83
Warts, genital. *See* Condylomata
    acuminata.
Water brash, 201
Weight
    birth. *See* Low birth weight.
    fetal
        estimation of, 143, 219-220
        viability limit of, 150
        puberty onset and, 345
Weight gain, in pregnancy
    average value of, 63
    of cardiac patient, 197
    components of, 63, 63t
    with multifetal gestation, 164
    preeclampsia and, 177
    recommended, 86, 86t
Weight loss, hyperemesis gravidarum
    with, 201
Whiff test, 266, 267
White's classification of diabetes in
    pregnancy, 191, 192t
Withdrawal method of contraception, 311
Wolffian ducts. *See* Mesonephric ducts.
Woods maneuver, 144

X

X-linked disorders, 80
X-rays, 396

Y

Y chromosome
    embryologic development and, 29
    gonadoblastoma and, 357
    hypergonadotropic hypogonadism
        and, 353-354
    mosaicism with, 359
Yeast infection. *See* Candidiasis,
    vulvovaginal.
Yolk sac, 29, 45f
    fetal immunity and, 68
Yolk sac tumor, 418

Z

Zavanelli maneuver, 144
Zidovudine, 207, 208
Zona pellucida, 39, 42-43
Zygosity determination, in multiple
    gestation, 161-162, 162f, 165